Cytokine Knockouts

Contemporary Immunology

Cytokine Knockouts, Second Edition
Edited by Giamila Fantuzzi, 2003

Therapeutic Interventions in the Complement System
Edited by John D. Lambris and V. Michael Holers, 2000

Chemokines in Disease: *Biology and Clinical Research*
Edited by Caroline A. Hébert, 1999

Lupus: *Molecular and Cellular Pathogenesis*
Edited by Gary M. Kammer and George C. Tsokos, 1999

Autoimmune Reactions
Edited by Sudhir Paul, 1999

Molecular Biology of B-Cell and T-Cell Development
Edited by John G. Monroe and Ellen V. Rothenberg, 1998

Cytokine Knockouts
Edited by Scott K. Durum and Kathrin Muegge, 1998

Immunosuppression and Human Malignancy
Edited by David Naor, 1990

The Lymphokines
Edited by John W. Haddon, 1990

Clinical Cellular Immunology
Edited by Howard H. Weetall, 1990

Cytokine Knockouts

Second Edition

Edited by

Giamila Fantuzzi, PhD

University of Colorado Health Sciences Center, Denver, CO

Foreword by

Scott K. Durum

National Cancer Institute, Frederick, MD

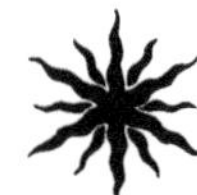

SPRINGER SCIENCE+BUSINESS MEDIA, LLC

Originally published by Humana Press Inc. in 2003
MyCopy version of the original edition 2003

All authored papers, comments, opinions, conclusions, or recommendations are those of the author(s), and do not necessarily reflect the views of the publisher.

This publication is printed on acid-free paper. ∞
ANSI Z39.48-1984 (American National Standards Institute) Permanence of Paper for Printed Library Materials.

Production Editor: Tracy Catanese

Cover illustration: Fig. 2 from Chapter 7, "IL-1 Receptor Antagonist-Deficient Mice" by Martin J. H. Nicklin and Joanna Shepherd.

Cover design by Patricia F. Cleary.

10 9 8 7 6 5 4 3 2 1
Library of Congress Cataloging in Publication Data

Cytokine Knockouts / edited by Giamila Fantuzzi ; foreword by Scott K. Durum.--2nd ed.
p. cm. -- (Contemporary immunology)
Includes bibliographical references and index.

DOI 10.1007/978-1-59259-405-4
1. Cytokines. 2. Gene targeting. I. Fantuzzi, Giamila. II. Series.

QR185.8.C95C9814 2002
616.07'9--dc21 2002191938
www.springer.com/mycopy

Foreword

This is the second edition of *Cytokine Knockouts*, an entirely new volume edited by Giamila Fantuzzi. The first edition, edited by Kathrin Muegge and me, was inspired by what we felt were the most important experiments in cytokinology. But at that time, their bold messages had not yet sunk in. For example, there were papers still being published and grants being funded studying effects of Interleukin (IL)-1 or IL-2 in the development of thymocytes, when in fact, the knockouts of IL-1 or IL-2 had shown no effect on the thymus (although now it looks like IL-2 does have a thymic effect—*see* Chapter 9). So we thought it was useful to compile the studies on cytokine knockout mice in a single volume.

Times have changed since the first edition of *Cytokine Knockouts*. These mice have become de rigueur for immunology studies; there were a dozen papers in a recent issue of the *Journal of Immunology* using knockout mice, and one paper actually used 10 different knockout lines. The second edition of *Cytokine Knockouts* therefore represents far more extensive studies than the first edition with many new knockouts, emergent phenotypic patterns, and a more precise understanding of the impact of each cytokine knockout. Many other fields in experimental biology have been redirected by the several thousand strains of knockout mice that have been created. How many knockouts will there be? Possibly more than the number of genes, because multiple regions of each gene are often deleted or replaced.

Molecular targets have been identified or eliminated based on knockout phenotypes and most of the cytokines were shown to be benign targets. For example, tumor necrosis factor (TNF) was hoped to be a desirable target for anti-inflammatory drugs. The knockout of TNF or its receptors clearly predicted there should be no dire effects from blocking TNF pharmacologically because mice completely lacking TNF from conception showed relatively subtle abnormalities. This prediction has been vindicated in the 250,000 or so patients being treated with TNF antagonists for rheumatoid arthritis and Crohn's disease; although it is now thought that TNF blockade awakens latent tuberculosis infections, that is still a modest risk, and was accurately predicted by the phenotype of knockout mice.

The technology bar has been raised. The major embryonic stem cell lines are still from the (weird) 129 mouse strain and the basic DNA reaction has not been improved over the extremely rare homologous recombination event. But there are new methods for creating the targeting construct without relying on restriction sites. The practice of simply replacing a critical gene segment with a *neo* cassette is now supplanted by methods for subsequently removing the troublesome *neo* cassette. The Cre-loxP and FLP-FRT recombinase systems are commonly used to perform this deletion, and these systems are also used to delete very large gene segments.

The original targeting strategy for creating knockouts deleted the gene in all tissues. Clever variations have allowed study of gene function in specific cell lineages and stages. Perhaps the first variation, Rag complementation, was used to study effects in the lymphocyte lineage; this was done by placing knockout ES cells into a Rag knockout blastocyst. For studying other hematopoietic cells, knockout fetal liver cells are used as hematopoietic stem cells in radiation chimeras. Combining knockouts and transgenes has allowed many strategies. For example, mice that lack a certain enzyme have a block in thymocyte development; the enzyme is reintroduced as a transgene restricted in expression to the thymocyte. T cells then leave the thymus, shut off the transgene, and the effect of the enzyme is examined on subsequent T cell survival. "Conditional knockout" has used the Cre-loxP and FLP-FRT systems to somatically delete genes in several specific lineages, such as T cells, B cells, and macrophages. Acute somatic deletion in specific lineages combines Cre-loxP with IFN or tetracycline regulation—this, for example, established that antigen receptors are required for long-term survival of lymphocytes, not just their generation.

It is disappointing that homologous recombination has not been improved to a higher efficiency, which among other applications could make it therapeutically useful in somatic cells in patients. For example, γc-deficient patients have been successfully treated by retroviral gene therapy, introducing a good γc gene under a viral promoter. But most virally introduced transgenes only function in patients for a few weeks and are then shut off. Moreover, the risk of retroviral insertion activating oncogenes proved to be far greater than imagined and several γc patients have developed lymphoma. A better alternative would be to fix a bad gene (for γc, IL-7 receptor, hemoglobin, etc.) by repairing the bad copy in a patient's hematopoietic stem cells ex vivo, then transferring them back to the patient. The major problem to overcome is the rare frequency of homologous recombination. An even greater problem would be to repair a nonhematopoietic gene, for example a bad collagen gene that affects tissues throughout the patient, or restoring tumor suppressor genes that have been deleted or mutated in cancer cells. Maybe the field needs new methods, perhaps a DNA repair enzyme, delivered with the gene of interest that would excise the old and insert the new.

Improving the frequency of homologous recombination would also be tremendously useful for experimental work, for example, in creating cell lines that have a specific gene deleted or altered. Imagine a variation on Cre-lox or FLP-FRT, like the Rag proteins which are extremely specific in cutting immune receptor genes and creating rearrangements, errors virtually never occur and efficiency is extremely high.

Knockout mice have created an expensive maintenance, storage and distribution problem for what could become 20–100,000 different mouse strains. Jackson Labs currently handles 300 knockout strains and Taconic distributes 40. The National Cancer Institute is cryopreserving and distributing knockout mouse strains that are relevant to cancer research. The American Type Culture Collection, which has preserved and distributed cell lines, is now considering taking on cryopreservation and distribution of a wide variety of mouse embryos. There is a real need for preserving these valuable strains and, sadly, many of the less popular strains may already have been lost. Ethical concerns have also developed, in that new knockouts and new genetic combinations can clearly create pain and suffering in mice. It is gratifying that at least here at NIH the PI is held responsible for anticipating and observing these problems.

When stem cell ceases to be a four letter word, future editions of this book will likely cover knockouts in lots of other species in addition to mice. Boneless fish and chickens. Fat-free beef. Shedless, clawless, unfinicky cats. Dogs with an aversion to garbage cans.

Diurnal hamsters. Deer that eat poison ivy and avoid roadways. Thrilling revelations await in pursuing the unnatural and undoing hundreds of millions of years of evolution.

But seriously, the second edition of *Cytokine Knockouts* brings together outstanding world authorities on these unique mice. It is a rich resource for researchers interested in the roles cytokines play in physiological and pathological processes and in selection of drug targets.

Scott K. Durum
National Cancer Institute

Preface

As mentioned in the preface to the first edition of *Cytokine Knockouts* (1998) by the editors S. K. Durum and K. Muegge, "The technique of gene targeting or 'knockout' has swept through biomedical research of the 1990s as if it were the Occam's razor of biology. The technique provides an acid test of the function of a gene." In the years since the first edition of *Cytokine Knockouts* was published, several factors have contributed to expand the use of gene-deficient mice in research. Advances in molecular biology techniques have facilitated gene cloning and the building of DNA constructs. Furthermore, the possibility of generating conditional or tissue-specific knockouts, as well as knock-in mice, has opened new avenues for more sophisticated use of gene-modified animals in research. At the same time, many universities and research centers have organized core laboratories for the generation of knockout and transgenic mice, therefore making this technique available even to nonexperts. These two factors have contributed to the incredibly rapid increase in the number of new knockout mice created every year and have led to a marked reduction in the time between the cloning of a new gene and generating the corresponding deficient mouse, thus speeding up the appreciation of the in vivo role of any given new gene. The commercial availability of several strains of gene-deficient mice has been the third factor greatly contributing to widening the use of knockout mice. After an initial characterization, a large number of investigators decided to make their mice available through commercial providers. This choice has allowed laboratories without expertise in molecular biology, but oftentimes with a great deal of knowledge in the characterization of in vivo processes, to have easy access to gene-deficient mice. In this way, a sort of long-distance collaboration has narrowed the gap between molecular biology and in vivo studies, a much appreciated result given the ever increasing technical specialization of many laboratories. Approximately 10% of the more than 300 different types of knockout mice that are currently commercially available is represented by cytokine- or cytokine receptor-deficient mice.

Research in the closely intertwined fields of immunology, infection, and inflammation is proceeding at a pace faster than ever before. Among the many types of mediators involved in the regulation of phenomena as varied as resistance to infectious pathogens, fever, pain, wound healing, autoimmune reactions, hematopoiesis, angiogenesis, and tumor surveillance—to cite only a few—the family of cytokines can, without any doubt, be considered one of the most prominent. Paraphrasing an Italian saying, "Cytokines are like parsley," you can find them everywhere. In fact, as attested by the reviews collected in this volume, the variety of physiological and pathological conditions in which cytokines have been implicated is staggering. Thanks to the factors mentioned above, the use of cytokine knockouts in research has literally exploded in the past 5 to 10 years. A PubMed search with the terms "cytokine" and "knockout mice" provides a list of approximately 4000 scientific reports, more than 3000 of which were published since 1998, the year of the first edition of *Cytokine Knockouts*.

As the reader will appreciate, several new types of cytokine knockout mice have been generated since the first edition was published. Thus, to cite only a few examples, osteoprotegerin (or RANK) ligand, a major player in bone metabolism and one of the most promising cytokines in terms of therapeutic developments, had just been cloned when the first edition of *Cytokine Knockouts* appeared; the generation of RANK and RANK- ligand-deficient mice soon followed (*see* Chapter 23). Despite the long history of Interleukin (IL)-1, reports describing the generation of IL-1α and double IL-1α/IL-1β knockouts were only published in 1998, the same year of the first report on IL-18-deficient mice (*see* Chapters 6 and 18). Moreover, novel important data have been published by investigators studying new phenomena in "old" knockouts. To cite only a few examples, the critical role for IL-1Ra in maintaining control of inflammatory responses had been reported by two separate groups in 2000 (*see* Chapter 7), a more detailed characterization of the pathogenesis of colitis development in IL-2- and IL-10-deficient mice appeared over the course of the past 5 years (*see* Chapter 14), the role of tumor necrosis factor-α and lymphotoxin in the development of germinal centers has been further clarified (*see* Chapter 25), and so have the roles of IL-2, IL-7 and the common γ chain of their receptor in lymphopoiesis (Chapters 8 and 9). From these and the many more examples that might have been listed, it is clear that the time is right for a new edition of *Cytokine Knockouts*.

Structure of the Volume

Cytokine Knockouts is comprised of two sections, *Cytokine Knockouts in Models of Human Disease*, and *Cytokine Knockout Mice*. Although both sections are addressed to researchers interested in the field of cytokines, Part I could also serve as an introduction to the use knockout mice for scientists who are not familiar with cytokine research.

Part I contains chapters dedicated to the use of cytokine knockout mice in different fields of research. Rather than providing a comprehensive overview of results obtained using each available knockout mouse, the intent of this first set of reviews is to present a constructive discussion of ways in which cytokine knockout mice have been employed in various fields, with clarification of the relative advantages and disadvantages of their use.

Several important points are raised by the authors of these chapters. Thus, the reader is reminded of how the use of different experimental models is subject to the "fashion" of the moment, so that novel cytokines or novel cytokine-deficient mice are rarely tested for "old" parameters of pro-inflammatory activities, such as induction of fever. At the same time, it is critical to use caution when trying to interpret data derived from different studies, given the variability of results obtained using apparently similar experimental models. We also need to use caution when trying to directly infer results for clinical practice, and avoid creating misleading interpretations. When dealing with knockout mice, researchers should always take into account the possible effects of redundancy and of unspecific perturbations of the immune (and other) systems when a single gene is deleted. The importance of crossing gene-deficient animals into different background strains appropriate for the study of various conditions is also touched upon in Part I. I am sure this section will be a helpful tool to stimulate reflection and discussion about research methodology and data interpretation.

Part II includes chapters dealing with individual cytokines. To avoid excessive repetition, some cytokines are grouped and presented in families. Similarly, to provide the reader with a "concentrated" source of information, mice knockouts for a given cytokine are generally discussed together with mice knockouts for that cytokine's receptor(s). Rather than presenting a brief summary of each of the chapters contained in Part II, I will point out how many unexpected discoveries were made possible by the use of cytokine knockout mice, and of gene-deficient models in general. Given the extreme pleiotropy and functional redundancy of many cytokines, it was only after the generation of mice deficient for each cytokine and each cytokine receptor that the specific in vivo role of a given molecule could be determined. As detailed in the various chapters, almost without exception there were big surprises awaiting investigators studying cytokine knockout mice. New phenotypes are being continually discovered, and some of them do not apparently have a relationship with immune responses, such as the recently described spontaneous obesity of IL-6 knockout mice (*see* Chapter 13). When working with cytokine-deficient mice, thus, one has to keep an open mind, be a careful observer and be ready to share results and materials with researchers in other disciplines. When these measures are carried out, cytokine knockout mice laboratories flourish and important results can quickly reach an eager audience.

***Giamila Fantuzzi,* PhD**

Contents

Contributors

LUCIANO ADORINI • *Chief Scientific Officer, BioXell, Milano, Italy*

SHIZUO AKIRA • *Institute for Microbial Diseases, Osaka University, Suita, Japan*

MASAHIDE ASANO • *Graduate School of Medical Science, Kanazawa University, Kanazawa, Japan*

JEFFREY S. BERMAN • *Pulmonary Center, Boston University School of Medicine, Boston, MA*

ALFONS BILLIAU • *Rega Institute, Leuven, Belgium*

HERVÉ BOUTIN • *School of Biological Sciences, University of Manchester, Manchester, UK*

SANDRA N. BROWN • *Department of Autoimmunity and Inflammation, Amgen Corp., Seattle, WA*

RICHARD BUCALA • *Section of Rheumatology, Department of Internal Medicine, Yale University School of Medicine, New Haven, CT*

ERIC A. BUTZ • *Department of Autoimmunity and Inflammation, Amgen Corp., Seattle, WA*

DYANA DALTON • *Trudeau Institute, Saranac Lake, NY*

CHARLES A. DINARELLO • *Department of Medicine, University of Colorado, Denver, CO*

GLENN DRANOFF • *Department of Adult Oncology, Dana-Farber Cancer Institute, and Department of Medicine, Brigham and Women's Hospital and Harvard Medical School, Boston, MA*

SCOTT K. DURUM • *Laboratory of Molecular Regulation, Center for Cancer Research, National Cancer Institute, National Institutes of Health, Frederick, MD*

THOMAS ENZLER • *Department of Adult Oncology, Dana-Farber Cancer Institute, and Department of Medicine, Brigham and Women's Hospital and Harvard Medical School, Boston, MA*

GUNTER FINGERLE-ROWSON • *Hematology and Oncology, Medical Clinic III, Klinikum Grosshadern, Ludwig-Maximilians University, Munich, Germany*

PAUL S. FOSTER • *Division of Molecular Biosciences, John Curtin School of Medical Research, Australian National University, Canberra, Australia*

PIETRO GHEZZI • *Laboratory of Neuroimmunology, Istituto Mario Negri, Milano, Italy*

ANANDA W. GOLDRATH • *Joslin Diabetes Center, Harvard Medical School, Boston, MA*

SERGEI I. GRIVENNIKOV • *Engelhardt Institute of Molecular Biology and Belozersky Institute of Physico-Chemical Biology, Moscow, Russia*

HUBERTINE HEREMANS • *Rega Institute, Leuven, Belgium*

DUNCAN R. HEWETT • *Medical Research Council, Cambridge, UK*

REIKO HORAI • *Center for Experimental Medicine, Institute of Medical Science, University of Tokyo, Tokyo, Japan*

CORY M. HOGABOAM • *Department of Pathology, University of Michigan, Ann Arbor, MI*

SIMON P. HOGAN • *Division of Molecular Biosciences, John Curtin School of Medical Research, Australian National University, Canberra, Australia*

THOMAS HÜNIG • *University of Wurzburg, Wurzburg, Germany*

YOICHIRO IWAKURA • *Center for Experimental Medicine, Institute of Medical Science, University of Tokyo, Tokyo, Japan*

HUMBERTO JIJON • *University of Alberta, Edmonton, Alberta, Canada*

MARY K. KENNEDY • *Department of Autoimmunity and Inflammation, Amgen Corp., Seattle, WA*

YOUNG-YUN KONG • *Division of Molecular and Life Sciences, Pohang University of Science and Technology, Pohang, Kyungbuk, South Korea*

YUTAKA KOMIYAMA • *Center for Experimental Medicine, Institute of Medical Science, University of Tokyo, Tokyo, Japan*

PASCALE KROPF • *Faculty of Medicine, Department of Immunology, Imperial College of Science, Technology and Medicine, London, UK*

STEVEN L. KUNKEL • *Department of Pathology, University of Michigan, Ann Arbor, MI*

DMITRY V. KUPRASH • *Engelhardt Institute of Molecular Biology and Belozersky Institute of Physico-Chemical Biology, Moscow, Russia*

JOHN J. LETTERIO • *Laboratory of Cell Regulation and Carcinogenesis, National Cancer Institute, Bethesda, MD*

GIAMAL N. LUHESHI • *Douglas Hospital Research Center, McGill University, Montreal, Quebec, Canada*

KAREN L. MADSEN • *University of Alberta, Edmonton, Alberta, Canada*

THOMAS R. MALEK • *University of Miami, Miami, FL*

MIZUKO MAMURA • *Laboratory of Cell Regulation and Carcinogenesis, National Cancer Institute, Bethesda, MD*

DIEGO MARITANO • *Department of Genetics, Biology, and Biochemistry, University of Torino, Torino, Italy*

PATRICK MATTHYS • *Rega Institute, Leuven, Belgium*

ANDREW N. J. MCKENZIE • *Medical Research Council, Cambridge, UK*

INGRID MÜLLER • *Faculty of Medicine, Department of Immunology, Imperial College of Science, Technology, and Medicine, London UK*

WILLIAM J. MURPHY • *University of Nevada, Reno, NV*

SUSUMU NAKAE • *Center for Experimental Medicine, Institute of Medical Science, University of Tokyo, Tokyo, Japan*

AKIO NAKANE • *School of Medicine, Hirosaki University, Hirosaki, Japan*

KENJI NAKANISHI • *Department of Immunology and Medical Zoology, Hyogo College of Medicine, Hyogo, Japan*

AYA NAMBU • *Center for Experimental Medicine, Institute of Medical Science, University of Tokyo, Tokyo, Japan*

SERGEI A. NEDOSPASOV • *National Caner Institute, Frederick, MD*

MARTIN J. H. NICKLIN • *Division of Genomic Medicine, Royal Hallamshire Hospital, University of Sheffield, Sheffield, UK*

ANTHONY W. O'REGAN • *Pulmonary Center, Boston University School of Medicine, Boston, MA*

HARUKI OKAMURA • *Institute for Advanced Medical Sciences, Hyogo College of Medicine, Hyogo, Japan*

FERENC OLOSZ • *University of Miami, Miami, FL*

JOSEF M. PENNINGER • *Institute of Molecular Biotechnology of the Austrian Academy of Science, Vienna, Austria*

EMMANUEL PINTEAUX • *School of Biological Sciences, University of Manchester, Manchester, UK*

VALERIA POLI • *Department of Genetics, Biology, and Biochemistry, University of Torino, Torino, Italy*

SUSAN R. RITTLING • *Department of Genetics, Rutgers University, Piscataway, NJ*

ANITA ROBERTS • *Laboratory of Cell Regulation and Carcinogenesis, National Cancer Institute, Bethesda, MD*

ABHAY R. SATOSKAR • *Yale University, New Haven, CT*

ANNELIESE SCHIMPL • *University of Wurzburg, Wurzburg, Germany*

JANE M. SCHUH • *Department of Pathology, University of Michigan, Ann Arbor, MI*

JOANNA SHEPHERD • *Division of Genomic Medicine, Royal Hallamshire Hospital, University of Sheffield, Sheffield, UK*

PALLAVUR V. SIVAKUMAR • *Immunology Department, Zymogenetics Inc., Seattle, WA*

HIROKO TSUTSUI • *Department of Immunology and Medical Zoology, Hyogo College of Medicine, Hyogo, Japan*

ANN RENEE VAN DER VUURST DE VRIES • *Department of Autoimmunity and Inflammation, Amgen Corp., Seattle, WA*

JOANNE L. VINEY • *Department of Autoimmunity and Inflammation, Amgen Corp., Seattle, WA*

JON M. WIGGINTON • *National Cancer Institute, Frederick, MD*

ROBERT H. WILTROUT • *Laboratory of Experimental Immunology, National Cancer Institute, Frederick, MD*

LAWRENCE WOLFRAIM • *Laboratory of Cell Regulation and Carcinogenesis, National Cancer Institute, Bethesda, MD*

TOMOHIRO YOSHIMOTO • *Department of Immunology and Medical Zoology, Hyogo College of Medicine, Hyogo, Japan*

I

Cytokine Knockouts in Models of Human Disease

1

Cytokine Knockouts in Inflammation

Pietro Ghezzi

Summary

The discovery of the role of cytokines as inflammatory mediators, particularly interleukin-1 (IL-1) and tumor necrosis factor (TNF), and later chemokines, has led to an evolution of the concept of inflammation. Although IL-1 receptor antagonist and TNF inhibitors are approved for the therapy of rheumatoid arthritis, the role of IL-1 and TNF in inflammation was discovered by studying their effect in models of endotoxin [lipopolysaccharide (LPS)] systemic toxicity. This model is still the first priority for studies with knockout mice. We review here the models of inflammation used to characterize the pathogenic role of cytokines using knockout mice, in an attempt to relate the results obtained with models of LPS jitoxicity and those using other models of autoimmune- or chemically induced inflammation.

1. Inflammation and Inflammatory Cytokines

As defined by Janeway and colleagues *(1)*, Inflammat ion is traditionally defined by the four Latin words calor, dolor, rubor, and tumor, meaning heat, pain, redness and swelling, all of which reflect the effect of cytokines on the local blood vessels."

Although we know that cytokines are not the only primary mediators of inflammation, the inflammatory role of cytokines has largely surpassed, in terms of popularity, that of cytokines in cancer and even that of cytokines in immunity. With the approval of use of anti-tumor necrosis factor (TNF) molecules (antibodies and soluble receptors) for the therapy of rheumatoid arthritis, cytokines have completed their rite of passage and become established pharmacologic targets for inflammatory diseases.

The two cytokines considered prototypic inflammatory mediators are interleukin-1 (IL-1) and TNF, as one can see from the abstracts presented at a meeting on "The Physiologic, Metabolic and Immunological Actions of Interleukin-1" held in Ann Arbor in 1985 *(2)* and the report by Anthony Cerami's group that TNF is identical to the inflammatory mediator cachectin, also published in 1985 *(3)*.

Since then, the number of known cytokines has increased enormously, the nomenclature has changed, and the different cytokines have been classified in many ways [e.g., glycoprotein (gp)130-user cytokines, IL-6 family, TNF superfamily, T-helper (Th)1 and Th2 cytokines]. However, classification into the categories of proinflammatory and antiinflammatory still holds, or at least is widely used, particularly in applied (pharmacologic and clinical) research. In the absence of standardized, established criteria for defining a cytokine as inflammatory, we should stick to the old-times definition of inflammation. Hence,

From: *Contemporary Immunology: Cytokine Knockouts, 2nd Edition*
Edited by: Giamila Fantuzzi © Humana Press Inc., Totowa, NJ

a cytokine should be defined as inflammatory when it induces fever, hyperalgesia, leukocyte infiltration, and increased vascular permeability. Very few cytokines, possibly only IL-1 and TNF, have all these effects. Furthermore, IL-1 and TNF do not induce all these effects directly: for instance, IL-1 is not chemotactic and induces leukocyte recruitment through the induction of "secondary" inflammatory cytokines, namely, chemokines.

The availability of pure, lipopolysaccharide (LPS)-free recombinant cytokines allowed easy testing of the effect of each of them on the activities just noted. Although the nomenclature has been to some extent standardized, the performance of certain some biologic assays is not necessary to assign an interleukin number.

Although the ability of a cytokine to induce one of the hallmarks of inflammation is certainly sufficient for us to define it as inflammatory, this is biologically relevant only if endogenous production of that cytokine mediates some of the effects of inflammation. This implies defining the animal or in vitro models in which the role of a cytokine in inflammation can be tested. As mentioned above, earlier studies relied on the use of antibodies, and the availability of good neutralizing antibodies against TNF has been very important in identifying it as an important pharmacologic target.

It should also be noted that the concept of "hallmark of inflammation" is time-sensitive, and scientists are also subject to attitudes that may well be defined as fashion. As adhesion molecules, and then chemokines, became the most fashionable molecules implicated in inflammation, leukocyte infiltration became the most studied inflammatory mechanism, so now the term inflammation is often invoked for diseases in which the old criteria are not really met. In particular, local infiltration or activation of leukocytes is often sufficient to speak of inflammatory components, as in the case of many inflammatory diseases of the central nervous system (multiple sclerosis, brain trauma, and ischemia), as well as in the ischemia-reperfusion injury to most organs.

On the other hand, fever, which was one of the first in vivo activities identified for IL-1, has not been much studied, and very few recently discovered cytokines were tested for pyrogenicity (at least this is the impression we obtain from the literature); as pointed out in a recent review, only IL-1, IL-6, TNF, and IL-10 knockouts were tested in models of LPS fever *(4)*. The same holds true for other in vivo activities such as hyperalgesia or induction of acute-phase protein synthesis.

2. Cytokine Knockouts and Their Problems

Antibodies are certainly a good choice for studying the role of cytokines in acute models of inflammation, but their use becomes problematic in chronic models, for which knockout mice represent a valuable tool. The downside of knockout mice is that, unless conditioned knockouts are developed, other cytokines may be overexpressed to act vicariously for the deleted one, and many other adaptive changes may take place.

However, the general difficulty of working with transgenic mice, in terms of number of mice available for the different experiments, requires a more careful identification of priority experiments. We have reviewed the literature on cytokine knockouts to identify the animal models most used for investigation of the role of cytokines in inflammation.

3. Animal Models of Inflammation

Inflammation is induced by various means, and inflammation is a reaction to diseases described at length in other chapters. In fact, the use of LPS as a tool (see below), at least in the cytokine field, has provided a wider definition of inflammation, which includes effects not covered by the Latin definition, such as induction of hepatic acute-phase proteins, hypoferremia, or cachexia. For this reason, we deal first with LPS-induced systemic or local inflammation.

Another way of inducing inflammation is to use live bacteria or other models of infection, such as that induced by cecal ligation and puncture. Since these are true models of infection, they are described in Chapter 2, and we discuss them here only in relation to the inflammatory response associated with infection.

A second group of inflammation models is composed of those induced by autoimmunity that target different tissues and systems (e.g., rheumatoid arthritis, experimental autoimmune encephalomyelitis, inflammatory bowel disease). In another group of models, inflammation is induced, particularly in the airways but also in the skin, by immunization (allergic inflammation).

A last group relies on the induction of inflammation by a chemical irritant.

3.1. LPS Toxicity and Septic Shock as a Model of Inflammation

For historical reasons, the concept of inflammatory cytokine does not stem from studies on chronic inflammatory diseases such as arthritis but rather from the model of LPS-induced systemic inflammation, also termed endotoxic shock or endotoxicosis. Treatment of mice with IL-1 or TNF reproduces most of the symptoms of LPS toxicity, including lethality. In fact, IL-1 was first characterized as the endogenous pyrogen that mediates fever associated with infection or LPS administration and as a "leukocyte endogenous mediator" that is responsible for the induction of hepatic acute-phase protein synthesis also observed after infection or LPS administration *(5)*. On the other hand, according to earlier studies, TNF was clearly implicated in the multiple organ failure (MOF) and acute respiratory distress syndrome (ARDS) observed after administration of LPS *(6)*.

The enthusiasm associated with the growing evidence of a role for TNF and IL-1 in the various aspects of septic shock triggered a discussion on the meaning of the terms septic or endotoxic shock in relation to MOF and ARDS that led to the introduction of a new term, the systemic inflammatory response syndrome (SIRS) *(7)*. It should be mentioned, however, that the new term did not resolve the ambiguity and complexity of the role of the cytokines whose administration, in some cases, induces only some of the changes associated with inflammation (e.g., IL-6 that does not make mice sick, at least within a reasonable dose range, but only induces elevated levels of acute-phase proteins). As a result, most papers dealing with animal models of ARDS and MOF still use the term septic shock. On the other hand, the term "systemic inflammation" better explains how anti-TNF antibodies, originally found to protect against septic and endotoxic shock, were then tested in models of arthritis, for which the use of anti-TNF was then approved.

The easiest model of LPS toxicity is induced in mice by a single injection of LPS. This model is easy, inexpensive, and induces the production of a large number of cytokines; it was the first model in which neutralization of endogenous TNF by an anti-TNF antibody was protective *(8)*. Depending on the dose of LPS injected, one can observe induction of cytokine levels in blood and tissues, elevation of plasma acute-phase proteins, damage to specific organs (such as pulmonary edema), hypothermia, and lethality. It should be noted that mice are extremely resistant to LPS, hence the high doses required, ranging from a few micrograms/per kilogram of body weight for the induction of cytokines up to 30 mg/kg to induce lethality. This model is probably the most widely used and the first choice for any knockout mice.

In a second model of LPS toxicity that is also used, and that allows observation of lethality at lower LPS doses (in the microgram/kg range), mice are sensitized to the lethal effect of LPS with the toxicants galactosamine or actinomycin D (see, for instance ref. *9*). However, the use of these toxins with LPS results in fulminant hepatitis that is not observed with a lethal dose of LPS alone. Thus, one should be aware that the sensitizing toxin changes the pattern of organ toxicity of LPS. Another means of increasing susceptibility of LPS is achieved by adrenalectomy, which removes the protective mechanism represented by endogenous glucocorticoids.

Table 1 summarizes the results obtained with various knockout mice tested in these models of LPS-induced lethality.

A third model that was widely used in the past for studying the role of interferon-γ (IFN-γ) in LPS toxicity was the so-called Shwartzman reaction, a local skin reactivity resulting in hemorrhagic necrosis observed when a first (preparative) intradermal injection of LPS is followed by a systemic, intravenous, injection (provoking) of the same agent. It was shown that cytokines can participate in the Shwartzman reaction, including IL-1 *(30)*, IL-1 receptor antagonist (Ra), TNF, IL-8 , IL-10, IL-12, IL-15, and IFN-γ *(31)*. However, we found that only IL-10 knockouts were tested by this model *(16)*.

3.2. Autoimmune Models of Inflammation

The various models in which autoimmunity results in an inflammatory reaction will be better described in specific chapters [*see* Chap. 3 for experimental autoimmune encephalomyelitis (EAE) and arthritis]. However, whereas in the case of EAE inflammation is only one component (and for inflammatory responses in the central nervous system those induced by autoimmunity are not the only ones, as inflammation can also be induced by meningitis or ischemic or traumatic injury), in the case of arthritis inflammation is the main result of autoimmunity.

The most valuable models of arthritis in mice or rats are autoimmune models: rats are immunized with Freund's adjuvant (adjuvant arthritis), and mice are immunized with collagen in adjuvant [collagen-induced arthritis (CIA)]. The CIA model has been used to test the role of various cytokines using knockout mice and is discussed in Chapter 3.

Among the variables to keep in mind in testing knockout mice in these experimental models is that cytokines, as shown for IFN-γ, may have opposite roles in the disease depending on the adjuvants used *(32)*.

Furthermore, the use of autoimmune models of inflammation should take into consideration that cytokines, in addition to their proinflammatory activity, might have immunosuppressive roles, as in the case of TNF *(33,34)*. The need for a critical evaluation of the results obtained in cytokine knockout mice have been pointed out by Steinman *(35)* for EAE, and this may well apply to arthritis.

3.3. Physical and Chemical Irritants

Many agents have been reported to induce inflammation and have been used to test the susceptibility of cytokine knockouts to inflammation. The most used models of inflammation of this kind are those induced by local (intradermal, intrapleural, or intraperitoneal)

Table 1
Susceptibility of Various Knockout Mice to the Lethal Effects of LPS[a]

Knockout	Model	Mortality	Ref.
CCR4	LPS	Decreased	*10*
CCR5	LPS	Decreased	*11*
GM-CSF	LPS	Decreased	*12*
ICE	LPS	Decreased	*13*
ICE/ IL-1RI[b]	LPS	Decreased	*14*
IFN-γR	LPS	Decreased	*15*
IL-1b	LPS	No change	*13*
IL-10	LPS	Increased	*16*
IL-12	*Propionibacterium acnes*/LPS	Decreased	*17*
IL-18	*P. acnes*/LPS	Increased	*17*
IL-18	Galactosamine/LPS	No change	*18*
IL-1RI	Galactosamine/LPS; LPS	No change	*14*
MIF	LPS	Decreased	*19*
TNF	Galactosamine/LPS	Decreased	*20,21*
TNF	LPS	No change	*20*
TNF/LT*	*Salmonella typhimurium* LPS	No change	*22*
TNF/LT*	LPS, BCG-sensitized	Decreased	*23*
TNF/LT*	LPS	No protection, slower lethality	*24*
TNF/LT*	*Escherichia coli* or *Klebsiella pneumoniae* LPS	Decreased	*22*
TNFRI	Adrenalactomy/LPS	Decreased	*25*
TNFRI	Galactosamine/LPS	Decreased	*26–28*
TNFRI	LPS	No change	*26,27*
TNFRI	LPS	Decreased	*29*
TNFRII	Galactosamine/LPS	Increased	*28*

[a]In some experiments increased/decreased toxicity is shown by noting the lethal dose (dose required to induce lethality; not always the LD_{50} or LD_{100}) changes (e.g., ref. *16*) and in others by a survival curve and one LPS dose (e.g., ref. *17*).

[b]Double knockout.

Abbreviations: BCG, bacille Calmette-Guérin; GM-CSF, granulocyte/macrophage colony-stimulating factor; ICE, IL-1-converting enzyme; IL, interleukin; IL-1RI, IL-1 receptor type I; LPS, lipopolysaccharide; LT, lymphotoxin; MIF, macrophage inhibitory factor; TNF, tumor necrosis factor.

administration of carrageenan or turpentine, as well as croton oil, the source of the tumor-promoting phorbol esters. Local inflammation induced by turpentine has been used to study inflammatory responses, including fever, in cytokine knockout mice *(36–38)*.

One particular route of administration of carrageenan is injection into an air pouch, previously induced in the back of mice by injection of air. This model has been used to study leukocyte infiltration, for instance in IL-6 knockout mice *(39)*.

For models of chemically induced inflammatory bowel diseases, acetic acid and 2,4,6-trinitrobenzene sulfonic acid are widely used.

For the sake of completeness, it should also be noted that anoxia/reoxygenation (models of ischemia) also induce an extensive inflammatory response in which the trigger is oxygen deprivation or reperfusion, with subsequent oxidative stress, and various knockout mice have been studied in animal models of ischemia in various organs.

4. From the Mouse Cage to the Bedside

The study of the role of cytokines in inflammation is normally targeted at curing inflammatory diseases, based on the assumption that inflammation is bad. Certainly, even when inflammation is not life-threatening (as it is in septic shock), its symptoms are undesirable (fever, for instance). However, we have to keep in mind that inflammation is part of the innate immune response to infections. It comprises activities such as leukocyte infiltration, fever, and hypoferremia that are part of the antibacterial defense. Serious infections are now controlled by antibiotic therapy, and we can afford to block fever without risking a worsening of the infection. Nevertheless, we must be aware that tampering with inflammation might actually increase the risk of infection.

Although this reasoning is quite obvious, since immunosuppressors such as glucocorticoids and methotrexate are among the approved drugs for rheumatoid arthritis, it is often overlooked. For instance, the warning that anti-TNF therapy for rheumatoid arthritis might worsen the underlying infection was not included in the label of Enbrel® until this safety issue arose in patients *(40)*. It should be mentioned that this issue might have been anticipated by animal studies showing that neutralization of TNF might actually worsen survival in sublethal models of sepsis induced by cecal ligation and puncture *(41)*.

Another consideration is that some of the changes observed in inflammation are actually protective, antiinflammatory mechanisms. For instance, activation of the hypothalamus-pituitary-adrenal axis (HPAA) is part of a protective response that is induced in many inflammatory conditions, particularly SIRS. Activation of the HPAA is mediated by various cytokines and is impaired in IL-6 knockout, leukemia inhibiting factor knockout, and TNF receptorII knockout mice *(42–44)*. Current evidence suggests that glucocorticoids may be beneficial in patients with catecholamine-dependent septic shock, indicating the importance of these endogenous mediators *(45)*.

In addition to glucocorticoids, inflammatory cytokines are responsible for the increased synthesis of hepatic acute-phase proteins. Although some of these, such as fibrinogen, might actually be important in the coagulation components of septic shock *(46)*, others, such as C-reactive protein, are protective *(47)*. Thus, not all the biochemical hallmarks of inflammation have negative effects.

References

1. Janeway, C. A., Travers, P., Walport, M., and Capra, J. D. (1999) *Immunobiology. The Immune System in Health and Disease, 4th ed.* Elsevier Science and Garland Publishing, London.
2. Kluger, M. J., Oppenheim, J. J., and Powanda, M. C. (1985) The physiologic, metabolic and immunological actions of interleukin-1. *J. Leukoc. Biol.* **37,** 671–755.
3. Beutler, B., Greenwald, D., Hulmes, J. D., et al. (1985) Identity of tumour necrosis factor and the macrophage-secreted factor cachectin. *Nature* **316,** 552–554.
4. Leon, L. R. (2002) Invited review: cytokine regulation of fever: studies using gene knockout mice. *J. Appl. Physiol.* **92,** 2648–2655.

5. Dinarello, C. A. (1984) Interleukin-1. *Rev. Infect. Dis.* **6,** 51–95.
6. Tracey, K. J., Lowry, S. F., and Cerami, A. (1988) Cachetin/TNF-alpha in septic shock and septic adult respiratory distress syndrome. *Am. Rev. Respir. Dis.* **138,** 1377–1379.
7. American College of Chest Physicians/Society of Critical Care Medicine Consensus Conference (1992) Definitions for sepsis and organ failure and guidelines for the use of innovative therapies in sepsis. *Crit. Care Med.* **20,** 864–874.
8. Beutler, B., Milsark, I. W., and Cerami, A. C. (1985) Passive immunization against cachectin/ tumor necrosis factor protects against lethal effect of endotoxin. *Science* **229,** 869–871.
9. Gadina, M., Bertini, R., Mengozzi, M., Zandalasini, M., Mantovani, A., and Ghezzi, P. (1991) Protective effect of chlorpromazine on endotoxin toxicity and TNF production in glucocorticoid-sensitive and glucocorticoid-resistant models of endotoxic shock. *J. Exp. Med.* **173,** 1305–1310.
10. Chvatchko, Y., Hoogewerf, A. J., Meyer, A., et al. (2000) A key role for CC chemokine receptor 4 in lipopolysaccharide-induced endotoxic shock. *J. Exp. Med.* **191,** 1755–1764.
11. Zhou, Y., Kurihara, T., Ryseck, R. P., et al. (1998) Impaired macrophage function and enhanced T cell-dependent immune response in mice lacking CCR5, the mouse homologue of the major HIV-1 coreceptor. *J. Immunol.* **160,** 4018–4025.
12. Basu, S., Dunn, A. R., Marino, M. W., et al. (1997) Increased tolerance to endotoxin by granulocyte-macrophage colony-stimulating factor-deficient mice. *J. Immunol.* **159,** 1412–1417.
13. Netea, M. G., Fantuzzi, G., Kullberg, B. J., et al. (2000) Neutralization of IL-18 reduces neutrophil tissue accumulation and protects mice against lethal *Escherichia coli* and *Salmonella typhimurium* endotoxemia. *J. Immunol.* **164,** 2644–2649.
14. Glaccum, M. B., Stocking, K. L., Charrier, K., et al. (1997) Phenotypic and functional characterization of mice that lack the type I receptor for IL-1. *J. Immunol.* **159,** 3364–3371.
15. Heremans, H., Dillen, C., Groenen, M., Matthys, P., and Billiau, A. (2000) Role of interferon-gamma and nitric oxide in pulmonary edema and death induced by lipopolysaccharide. *Am. J. Respir. Crit. Care Med.* **161,** 110–117.
16. Berg, D. J., Kuhn, R., Rajewsky, K., et al. (1995) Interleukin-10 is a central regulator of the response to LPS in murine models of endotoxic shock and the Shwartzman reaction but not endotoxin tolerance. *J. Clin. Invest.* **96,** 2339–2347.
17. Sakao, Y., Takeda, K., Tsutsui, H., et al. (1999) IL-18-deficient mice are resistant to endotoxin-induced liver injury but highly susceptible to endotoxin shock. *Int. Immunol.* **11,** 471–480.
18. Hochholzer, P., Lipford, G. B., Wagner, H., Pfeffer, K., and Heeg, K. (2000) Role of interleukin-18 (IL-18) during lethal shock: decreased lipopolysaccharide sensitivity but normal superantigen reaction in IL- 18-deficient mice. *Infect. Immun.* **68,** 3502–3508.
19. Bozza, M., Satoskar, A. R., Lin, G., et al. (1999) Targeted disruption of migration inhibitory factor gene reveals its critical role in sepsis. *J. Exp. Med.* **189,** 341–346.
20. Pasparakis, M., Alexopoulou, L., Episkopou, V., and Kollias, G. (1996) Immune and inflammatory responses in TNF alpha-deficient mice: a critical requirement for TNF alpha in the formation of primary B cell follicles, follicular dendritic cell networks and germinal centers, and in the maturation of the humoral immune response. *J. Exp. Med.* **184,** 1397–1411.
21. Marino, M. W., Dunn, A., Grail, D., et al. (1997) Characterization of tumor necrosis factor-deficient mice. *Proc. Natl. Acad. Sci. USA* **94,** 8093–8098.
22. Netea, M. G., Kullberg, B. J., Joosten, L. A., et al. (2001) Lethal Escherichia coli and Salmonella typhimurium endotoxemia is mediated through different pathways. *Eur. J. Immunol.* **31,** 2529–2538.
23. Jacobs, M., Brown, N., Allie, N., and Ryffel, B. (2000) Fatal *mycobacterium bovis* BCG infection in TNF-LT-alpha-deficient mice. *Clin. Immunol.* **94,** 192–199.
24. Amiot, F., Fitting, C., Tracey, K. J., Cavaillon, J. M., and Dautry, F. (1997) Lipopolysaccharide-induced cytokine cascade and lethality in LT alpha/TNF alpha-deficient mice. *Mol. Med.* **3,** 864–875.
25. Koniaris, L. G., Wand, G., and Wright, T. M. (2001) TNF mediates a murine model of Addison's crisis. *Shock* **15,** 29–34.
26. Rothe, J., Lesslauer, W., Lotscher, H., et al. (1993) Mice lacking the tumour necrosis factor receptor 1 are resistant to TNF-mediated toxicity but highly susceptible to infection by *Listeria monocytogenes. Nature* **364,** 798–802.

27. Rothe, J., Mackay, F., Bluethmann, H., Zinkernagel, R., and Lesslauer, W. (1994) Phenotypic analysis of TNFR1-deficient mice and characterization of TNFR1-deficient fibroblasts in vitro. *Circ. Shock* **44,** 51–56.
28. Nowak, M., Gaines, G. C., Rosenberg, J., et al. (2000) LPS-induced liver injury in D-galactosamine-sensitized mice requires secreted TNF-alpha and the TNF-p55 receptor. *Am. J. Physiol. Regul. Integr. Comp. Physiol.* **278,** R1202–R1209.
29. Pfeffer, K., Matsuyama, T., Kundig, T. M., et al. (1993) Mice deficient for the 55 kd tumor necrosis factor receptor are resistant to endotoxic shock, yet succumb to *L. monocytogenes* infection. *Cell* **73,** 457–467.
30. Beck, G., Habicht, G. S., Benach, J. L., and Miller, F. (1986) Interleukin 1: a common endogenous mediator of inflammation and the local Shwartzman reaction. *J. Immunol.* **136,** 3025–3031.
31. Heremans, H., Van Damme, J., Dillen, C., Dijkmans, R., and Billiau, A. (1990) Interferon gamma, a mediator of lethal lipopolysaccharide-induced Shwartzman-like shock reactions in mice. *J. Exp. Med.* **171,** 1853–1869.
32. Matthys, P., Vermeire, K., Heremans, H., and Billiau, A. (2000) The protective effect of IFN-gamma in experimental autoimmune diseases: a central role of mycobacterial adjuvant-induced myelopoiesis. *J. Leukoc. Biol.* **68,** 447–454.
33. Cope, A. P. (1998) Regulation of autoimmunity by proinflammatory cytokines. *Curr. Opin. Immunol.* **10,** 669–676.
34. Grewal, I. S., Grewal, K. D., Wong, F. S., Picarella, D. E., Janeway, C. A., Jr., and Flavell, R. A. (1996) Local expression of transgene encoded TNF alpha in islets prevents autoimmune diabetes in nonobese diabetic (NOD) mice by preventing the development of auto-reactive islet-specific T cells. *J. Exp. Med.* **184,** 1963–1974.
35. Steinman, L. (1997) Some misconceptions about understanding autoimmunity through experiments with knockouts. *J. Exp. Med.* **185,** 2039–2041.
36. Fantuzzi, G. and Dinarello, C. A. (1998) Stem cell factor-deficient mice have a dysregulation of cytokine production during local inflammation. *Eur. Cytokine Netw.* **9,** 85–92.
37. Leon, L. R., Kozak, W., Peschon, J., and Kluger, M. J. (1997) Exacerbated febrile responses to LPS, but not turpentine, in TNF double receptor-knockout mice. *Am. J. Physiol.* **272,** R563–R569.
38. Fattori, E., Cappelletti, M., Costa, P., et al. (1994) Defective inflammatory response in interleukin 6-deficient mice. *J. Exp. Med.* **180,** 1243–1250.
39. Romano, M., Sironi, M., Toniatti, C., et al. (1997) Role of IL-6 and its soluble receptor in induction of chemokines and leukocyte recruitment. *Immunity* **6,** 315–325.
40. Baghai, M., Osmon, D. R., Wolk, D. M., Wold, L. E., Haidukewych, G. J., and Matteson, E. L. (2001) Fatal sepsis in a patient with rheumatoid arthritis treated with etanercept. *Mayo Clin. Proc.* **76,** 653–656.
41. Echtenacher, B., Falk, W., Mannel, D. N., and Krammer, P. H. (1990) Requirement of endogenous tumor necrosis factor/cachectin for recovery from experimental peritonitis. *J. Immunol.* **145,** 3762–3766.
42. van Enckevort, F. H., Sweep, C. G., Span, P. N., Demacker, P. N., Hermsen, C. C., and Hermus, A. R. (2001) Reduced adrenal response to bacterial lipopolysaccharide in interleukin-6-deficient mice. *J. Endocrinol. Invest.* **24,** 786–795.
43. Chesnokova, V., Auernhammer, C. J., and Melmed, S. (1998) Murine leukemia inhibitory factor gene disruption attenuates the hypothalamo-pituitary-adrenal axis stress response. *Endocrinology* **139,** 2209–2216.
44. Benigni, F., Faggioni, R., Sironi, M., et al. (1996) TNF receptor p55 plays a major role in centrally mediated increases of serum IL-6 and corticosterone after intracerebroventricular injection of TNF. *J. Immunol.* **157,** 5563–5568.
45. Annane, D. (2001) Corticosteroids for septic shock. *Crit. Care Med.* **29(Suppl. 7),** S117–S120.
46. Dhainaut, J. F., Yan, S. B., Cariou, A., and Mira, J. P. (2002) Soluble thrombomodulin, plasma-derived unactivated protein C, and recombinant human activated protein C in sepsis. *Crit. Care Med.* **30(5 suppl.),** S318–S324.
47. Libert, C., Brouckaert, P., and Fiers, W. (1994) Protection by alpha 1-acid glycoprotein against tumor necrosis factor-induced lethality. *J. Exp. Med.* **180,** 1571–1575.

2

The Use of Cytokine Knockouts to Study Host Defense Against Infection

Charles A. Dinarello

Summary

The sequencing of the human genome has revealed the existence of a large number of new members of the various cytokine families and has raised the perennial issue of how cytokines function to benefit human evolution. Usually duplication or redundancy of a gene suggests that it functions to assist the survival of the species. In the case of the proinflammatory cytokines, their role in the survival of the host is less clear since this class of cytokines is clearly implicated in host defense mechanisms against infection as well as the pathogenic processes of several diseases. The interleukin-1 (IL-1) and tumor necrosis factor (TNF) families of proinflammatory cytokines have been studied in great detail for their roles in disease; however, studies on their roles in host defense against infection are limited to a few organisms and models. However, it remains likely that these cytokines contribute to host defense mechanisms using the very same molecular and cellular pathways involved in chronic inflammation, tissue destruction, and tissue remodeling. How does one reconcile the existence of two opposing outcomes for the host—one clearly not in the interest of survival and another vital to the host in order to survive even a minor invasion by a microbe? In each case, identical molecular mechanisms are at work. For example, the processes for emigration of neutrophils into tissues to engulf microorganisms via an increase in endothelial adhesion molecules and chemokine production are the same for the host whether in infected tissue or an inflamed joint. On closer examination, the production and activity of proinflammatory cytokines reveal several levels of regulation, which may explain these seemingly discordant roles for the host. For routine infection or injury, cytokines such as IL-1β and TNF-α are transiently expressed and secreted, their activities are modulated by coproduction of naturally occurring antiinflammatory cytokines, and the levels of production fall rapidly. Thus, IL-1β and TNF-α turn on and off rapidly during infection. In contrast, the production of these same cytokines in chronic inflammatory diseases such as rheumatoid arthritis and inflammatory bowel disease fails to cease. Cytokine production in host defense is regulated, whereas in chronic disease it is dysregulated.

1. Introduction

More than 270,000 patients worldwide who have autoimmune diseases such as rheumatoid arthritis, psoriasis, or Crohn's disease are being treated with anti-cytokine-based therapies, and infections associated with anti-cytokine therapies, particularly anti-tumor necrosis factor-α (TNF-α) neutralizing antibodies, have increased. Therefore, the role of specific cytokines in host defense against infection has become a highly relevant area of investigation. Many experimental studies employ specific cytokine gene-targeted mice (knockouts). It must be stressed, however, that in the case of cytokine knockout mice, the effect of total deficiency of any particular cytokine or combination of cytokines in animal

From: *Contemporary Immunology: Cytokine Knockouts, 2nd Edition*
Edited by: Giamila Fantuzzi © Humana Press Inc., Totowa, NJ

models of live infection does not necessarily predict the human experience, particularly in patients treated with anti-cytokine therapies. It remains highly doubtful whether any anti-cytokine therapy can completely prevent or eliminate the action of a particular cytokine in host defense mechanisms. Even if a neutralizing antibody to a specific cytokine effectively prevented its action, the duration of the cytokine blockade using such an antibody is relatively transient, whereas in the knockout mouse, the deficiency is complete. In fact, the deficiency begins at conception and may affect developmental functions of cytokines.

The methodology of gene deletion requires the insertion of a cassette encoding a marker into the span of DNA encoding an early exon. During homologous recombination, the insertion may affect the function of adjacent genes. Such an event may explain why there can be differences in the phenotype of mice deficient for the same gene. Ligand and its specific receptor knockout gene can also result in different phenotypes. For example, when backcrossed to the nonobese diabetic mouse, the interferon-γ (IFN-γ) knockout mouse exhibits a phenotype different from that of the IFN-γ receptor α-chain knockout *(1)*. Therefore, studies on the effects of neutralizing antibodies to specific cytokines in animals are more relevant to human therapeutic interventions than data derived from knockout mice.

Can a cytokine knockout mouse be used to define the role of a particular cytokine in the host response to an infectious agent? When a cytokine knockout mouse fails to develop an inducible disease, one can conclude that such a cytokine probably plays a role in the pathogenesis of that disease. For example, the interleukin-1β (IL-1β) knockout mouse does not develop an inflammatory response to local tissue necrosis *(2)*. One can assume from these mouse studies that in a similar clinical setting, there may be a role for IL-1β in patients with local trauma injuries. In addition, when a cytokine knockout mouse fails to resist infection, one may conclude that a comparable clinical condition exists in humans. The best example is the IFN-γ receptor knockout mouse. This mouse is unusually susceptible to *Mycobacterium bovis* bacille Calmette-Guérin (BCG) infection *(3)*. Humans lacking a functional IFN-γ receptor are also susceptible to mycobacterial infections *(4)*.

2. Differences Between Infections in Patients Receiving Anticytokine Therapy and Infections in Chronically Immunosuppressed Patients

In HIV-1 patients with low CD4+ lymphocytes or in patients receiving immunosuppressive agents, the spectrum of opportunistic infections is well documented. Oral and esophageal *Candida* infections are prominent in both populations, and candidemia can be a cause of death in some patients. However, there are few reports of *Candida* infections in the estimated 170,000 patients who have been treated with infliximab (anti-human TNF-α monoclonal antibody) or in the approximately 110,000 patients treated with etanercept (soluble TNF receptor p75 linked to Fc). To date, there are no reports of systemic *Candida* infections in patients receiving anakinra. Herpes zoster infection is common in the older population and is believed to result from decreases in cell-mediated immunity. Zoster is frequently an infection in immunosuppressed patients; in fact, zoster is often the presenting complaint in patients unknowingly infected with HIV-1, yet reports of zoster are not prominent in patients treated with anti-cytokine therapies. *Mycobacterium avium-intracellulare* infection is also frequently found in HIV-1 patients with low CD4+ cell counts, but in the population receiving infliximab or etanercept, this is not a common diagnosis. These differences in infectious agents suggest that the nature of the impairment in host defense in the patient population receiving anti-cytokine therapies may be unique.

3. Advantages of Mice with Targeted Cytokine Gene Deletions in Models of Live Infection

The use of mice with specific cytokine or cytokine receptor gene deletion(s) (knockouts) offers several advantages, primarily because of an absolute absence of the gene product from conception to death. Compared with the use of cytokine inhibitors, when using knockout mice there are no questions concerning inadequate doses of neutralizing antibodies, low-affinity antibodies, poor antibody specificity, or the development of antibodies to foreign immunoglobulins; similar concerns exist for soluble receptors on binding proteins where ligand passing or a carrier function may occur. For example, some antibodies to IL-6 neutralize IL-6 in vitro but act as carriers of IL-6 in vivo and, in doing so, prolong the activity of IL-6 in models of disease *(5)*. Therefore, IL-6 knockout mice are preferred to address the role of IL-6 in models of disease.

With the use of knockout mice, there is also no concern about adequate drug penetration into tissues. In models of rheumatoid arthritis or autoimmune encephalomyelitis, however, penetration of the drug into joints or the brain by large molecules may be reduced, and dosing becomes a concern when assessing efficacy. Another advantage of the cytokine knockout models is the lack of an immune response to an antibody or a soluble receptor when either is exogenously administered over long periods. For example, when testing whether daily infusions of human IL-1 receptor antagonist (Ra) affect the development of a disease that evolves over several weeks, the animal will probably develop antibodies to the human IL-1Ra that reduce the effectiveness of the antagonist. In the BioBreeding rat, which develops spontaneous diabetes mellitus, treatment with human IL-1Ra reduced the disease for a few weeks, but later the rats developed antihuman IL-1Ra antibodies that limited the effectiveness of the IL-1Ra *(6)*.

4. Disadvantages of Using Knockout Mice

The primary disadvantage of using cytokine knockout mice is the lack of clinical relevance of total absence of cytokine activity in knockout mice compared with reduced cytokine activity when using anti-cytokine therapies. For example, the administration of any TNF inhibitor results in a peak of the inhibitor, followed by a nadir prior to the next injection. It is unlikely that complete and sustained neutralization of TNF-α occurs with any exogenous dosing, perhaps with the sole exception of a constant infusion. In the case of IL-1 inhibition, 24 h after an intravenous infusion of anakinra at 1 mg/kg in healthy volunteers, the blood levels of anakinra had fallen to levels of less than 1.0 ng/mL *(7)*. Therefore, to predict a clinically relevant defect in host defense during anti-cytokine therapy using data derived from cytokine knockout mice, one would have to sustain a high level of the anti-cytokine in the relevant body compartment to match the situation in the knockout mouse for the same cytokine. It is questionable whether that could be accomplished in the clinical setting.

Another widely held view is that the absence of a particular cytokine or cytokine receptor from conception into adult life results in other cytokines being overexpressed and compensating for the deleted signaling pathways. For example, in the IL-1β knockout mouse, the biologic response to IL-1-α is enhanced *(8)*, suggesting that, lacking receptor activation by IL-1β, the numbers of receptors or intracellular signaling by IL-1α have changed. These unusual responses have also been observed with other cytokine knockout

Table 1
Effect of Various Knockout Genes on Survival in Cecal Ligation and Puncture

Gene knockout	Survival	Ref.
TNF-α	↓ Survival	*22*
IFN-γR	No effect	*25*
TNFRp55/p75	↑ Survival	*81*
IL-6	No effect	*81*
IL-10	↓ Survival	*24*
STAT-4	↑ Survival	*10*
CD14	↓ Survival	*11*
C5a	↑ Survival (septic lung)	*16*
CD21/CD25	↓ Survival	*17*
Fas ligand	↑ Survival	*15*
iNOS	↑ Survival	*14*
iNOS	↓ Survival	*12,13*
E-selectin/P-selectin	↑ Survival	*18*
Mac-1	↓ Survival	*19*
SIgM	↓ Survival	*20*
PARP	↑ Survival	*21*

Abbreviations: IL, interleukin; iNOS, inducible nitric oxide synthase; IFN-γR, interferon-γ receptor; Mac-1, membrane attack complex-1; PARP, poly(adenosine diphosphate ribose) polymerase; sIgM, secreted immunoglobulin M; STAT-4, signal transducer and activator of transcription-4; TNF-α, tumor necrosis factor-α.

models. When mice deficient in TNF-receptor type II (RII) are challenged with bacterial endotoxin, TNF-α production is markedly enhanced *(9)*.

5. Polymicrobial Sepsis as a Model

Several studies have examined the role of cytokines using live infection, particularly cecal ligation and puncture. In this model, mice or rats undergo ligation of the cecum followed by a single or double puncture with a small or large needle. After the procedure, the peritoneal cavity is surgically closed. The rapidly evolving peritonitis varies in severity depending on the size and number of holes, but even with antibiotic treatment, death generally takes place in 2–10 d. Bacteria are found in the peritoneal cavity, in the liver, and occasionally in the lungs. Because of the surgical procedure, most studies employ rats, and hence cytokine knockout mice are used less frequently. Nevertheless, in addition to specific cytokine knockout mice, several studies have focused on knockout mice of genes related to cytokine production. For example, cecal ligation and puncture has been used in mice deficient in signal transducer and activation of transcription (STAT) 4 *(10)*, CD14 *(11)*, inducible nitric oxide synthase *(12–14)*, Fas ligand *(15)*, complement C5 *(16)* and complement receptors *(17)*, endothelial sections *(18)*, mast cells *(19)*, secretory IgM *(20)*, and poly (adenosine diphosphate ribose) polymerase (PARP) *(21)*. Survival data from cecal ligation and puncture in these various cytokine-related knockouts are given in Table 1.

In one study in mice deficient in TNF-α, increased mortality was observed *(22)*, consistent with other studies using the administration of antibodies to TNF-α (Table 1). However, in mice deficient in both the TNF receptors p55 and p75, increased survival was observed *(23)*. In IL-6 knockout mice, there was no difference in survival from wild-type mice *(23)*. Interestingly, in the IL-16 knockout mice, no fever was observed during cecal ligation and puncture, whereas fever was observed in the TNF double receptor knockout mice *(23)*. Mice deficient in IL-10 exhibit a 15-fold increase in serum TNF-α and IL-6 levels associated with decreased survival *(24)*.

Neutralization of either IL-12 or IFN-γ had no effect on survival, and similar results were reported in mice deficient in IFN-γ receptor *(25)*. Since STAT 4 is important for the activity of IL-12, mice deficient in STAT 4 were assessed for survival in the model; increased survival was observed compared with wild-type controls *(10)*. However, the lower mortality was associated with higher bacterial counts in tissues and in the blood. The administration of antibodies to IL-12 worsened mortality *(10)*.

CD14 is essential for cytokine production induced by endotoxins. In mice lacking CD14, decreased survival was observed even when mice were treated with antibiotics. However, when the size of the puncture needle was reduced, there were no differences in survival in the CD14-deficient mice compared with wild-type controls *(11)*. Regardless of the size of the puncture needle, there was a consistent reduction in IL-1β, TNF-α, IL-6, IL-1Ra, and IL-10 as well as chemokines in the CD14 knockout mice *(11)*. Complement is also required for optimal cytokine production. In mice lacking the complement receptors CD21/CD25, decreased survival associated with decreased TNF-α and decreased neutrophils was observed *(17)*. In contrast, in mice deficient in C5, mean survival time in a model of lethal lung sepsis was increased compared with mice producing C5a *(16)*. Fas ligand-deficient mice exhibit reduced lymphocyte apoptosis, and this is associated with increased survival in cecal ligation and puncture *(15)*.

Induction of inducible nitric oxide synthase (iNOS) is a property of IFN-γ, TNF-α, and to a lesser degree IL-1β. Also, nitric oxide (NO) inhibition usually decreases cytokine production *(26)*. Two reports have observed a decrease in survival in iNOS-deficient mice *(12, 13)*, whereas one study reported increased survival *(14)*. It is important to differentiate the studies. In the study showing an increase in survival, the mice were treated with fluids and antibiotics every 6 h *(14)*. In the studies reporting a decrease in survival in iNOS knockout mice, no resuscitation treatments were employed. Studies have also focused on the infiltration of neutrophils using mice deficient in endothelial selectins. In mice lacking E-selectin, P-selectin, or both, resistance to lethal cecal ligation and puncture was observed *(18)*. In these mice, IL-13 levels were higher than in wild-type controls, whereas chemokines were lower. In these studies, there were no differences in bacterial or leukocytes counts in the peritoneal cavity. In the model, the ability to form an abscess to contain the infection is critical for survival *(27)*. Neutrophils are also important in that attempts to decrease the numbers or the ability of neutrophils to emigrate and engulf bacteria worsen the infection.

Mice with reduced mast cells owing to knockout of membrane attack complex-1 (Mac-1; CD11b/CD18) exhibit decreased survival in the cecal ligation and puncture model *(19)*. This may be owing to a decrease in TNF-α production from mast cells. A deficiency in secretory IgM is also associated with decreased survival *(20)*. In those studies, there was a decrease in TNF-α and neutrophils but an increase in the bacterial counts. The lethality (70%) was reversed by the administration of IgM. Although decreased survival appears to be associated with decreased TNF-α or a total deficiency in TNF-α, in mice lacking the PARP gene, there is increased survival *(21)*, which is associated with decreased TNF-α, IL-6, IL-10, and myeloperoxidase. However, the effects of PARP can hardly be viewed as a model for assessing the role of cytokines in survival during polymicrobial sepsis. It is likely that cytokine production in PARP-deficient mice reflects cell survival, and the decrease in cytokines may reflect a decrease in the overall level of inflammation.

Endotoxemia is part of the cecal ligation and puncture model, but death is usually caused by a large bacterial burden. Therefore, increasing neutrophil function often results in increased survival. For example, the administration of chemokines such as the CC chemokine C10 increases survival *(28)*. Consistent with this observation, blocking TNF-α decreases the survival response to a mixed flora bacterial infection, but this appears to be dependent on the severity of the infectious challenge. For example, reducing the size of the needle used to puncture the cecum can produce a model with a modest mortality (approximately 10%). When endogenous TNF-α was neutralized in these mice using a monoclonal anti-mouse TNF-α antibody, mortality was dramatically increased *(27)*. Those studies revealed a requirement for TNF-α in order to form an abscess and sequester the infectious agents *(29)*. Increasing the size and/or number of the punctures increases the severity of the model to nearly 100% lethality; under those conditions, passive immunization against TNF-α alone produced no improvement in survival *(30–33)*.

In addition to suppressing TNFα and IL-1, IL-10 can be immunosuppressive, in part through its ability to block T-helper 1 (Th1) and promote Th2-mediated immune response. This has been most evident in models in which an endogenous IL-10 response to injury may contribute to the immunosuppression, leading to secondary infections. For example, following a burn injury, mice are more susceptible to lethal cecal ligation and puncture. However, this increase in susceptibility could be prevented by treating the mice with a monoclonal antibody against IL-10 in the interim between the burn injury and the cecal ligation and puncture *(34,35)*. Similarly, an endogenous IL-10 response following cecal ligation and puncture was responsible for the decreased antimicrobial response and increased mortality caused by lung exposure to *Pseudomonas aeruginosa (36)*.

The administration of recombinant IL-1Ra either alone *(37)* or with polyethylene glycol (PEG) soluble (s) TNF-RI *(38)* remarkably increased survival in rodent models with lethal cecal ligation and puncture. In the studies listed in Table 2, the protective effect of IL-1Ra compared with the decreased survival in animals given anti-TNF-α antibodies is a consistent finding. One possible mechanism for the survival benefit of IL-1Ra may be to reduce the inflammatory component of the disease while not impairing antimicrobial responses to the peritonitis.

6. Bacterial Pneumonia as a Model

Live *Streptococcus pneumoniae* can be instilled in the lungs of mice by natural inhalation. Bacterial pneumonia develops during the next 1.5–2 days and progresses over the next 3–4 days. The number of bacteria growing in the lung tissue can be determined using cultures of homogenized lungs. In addition, cytokines and cellular emigration can be measured in the homogenized lungs. The model has the advantage of live infection relevant to community-acquired pneumonia, which epidemiologically is a common cause of infectious death. Death can also be used as an endpoint in the mouse model. To date, whether studies

Table 2
Role of Cytokine Neutralization in Polymicrobial Sepsis using Cecal Ligation and Puncture[a]

Administration of:	Survival	Ref.
IL-1Ra to rats	↑ Survival	*37*
IL-1Ra + soluble TNFRI:PEG to mice	↑ Survival	*38*
Anti-TNF-α antibody to mice	↓ Survival	*27,82,83*
Anti-TNF-α antibody to mice	No effect	*30–33*
Anti-TNF-α antibody to rats	↑ Survival	*84*
Anti-IL-12 antibody to mice	↓ Survival	*85*
IL-12 to mice	↑ Survival	*86*
Anti-IL-10 antibody to mice	↓ Survival	*36,83*
IL-10 to mice	↑ Survival	*33*
CC chemokine C10	↑ Survival	*28*

[a]No effect indicates that the intervention did not increase or decrease survival to an extent different from that in control animals.

Abbreviations: IL-1Ra, interleukin-1 receptor antagonist; PEG, polyethylene glycol; TNF-α, tumor necrosis factor-α; TNFRI, TNF receptor type I.

Table 3
Cytokine Blockade in Models of Gram-Positive Infections

Experimental model	Result	Ref.
Pneumococcal pneumonia in IL-6-deficient mice	↓ Survival	*87*
Anti-TNF-α antibody in pneumococcal pneumonia	↓ Survival ↑ CFU in lung homogenates	*39–41*
Pneumococcal bacteremia in TNF-α-deficient mice	↑ Bacteremia	*44*
Pneumococcal peritonitis in TNFRI-deficient mice	↓ Survival	*41*
IL-1Ra administration in pneumococcal pneumonia	↑ Survival ↓ CFU in lung homogenates	*88*
Pneumococcal bacteremia in IL-1β-deficient mice	↓ Bacteremia	*44*
Staphylococcal catheter infection in IL-1RI-deficiency	↓ Infection	*43*
Anti-IL-10 in murine pneumococcal pneumonia	↑ Survival ↓ CFU; ↓ inflammation	*83*
Pneumococcal pneumonia in ICAM-1-deficient mice	↓ Survival	*89*

Abbreviations: ICAM-1, intercellular adhesion molecule-1.
For other abbreviations, see Tables 1 and 2 footnotes.

neutralized TNF-α or employed TNF-α knockout mice, an increase in the number of bacteria and an increase in mortality have been consistently observed *(39–41)* (Table 3).

P. aeruginosa pneumonia has also been studied. In IL-1RI knockout mice intranasally inoculated with live *P. aeruginosa*, there was a 2-log reduction in the number of live bacteria isolated from the lungs after 24 and 48 h compared with the control mice expressing the IL-1 receptor gene *(42)*. In that study, the influx of neutrophils was decreased in bronchoalveolar lavage (BAL) fluids in knockout mice compared with wild-type mice. Similarly, levels of cytokines (TNF-α and IL-6) and chemokines [macrophage inflammatory protein-2 (MIP-2)] in the lungs were lower in the knockout mice 24 h after inoculation. Consistent with these results, treatment of wild-type mice with recombinant IL-1Ra also resulted in a 2-log reduction in the number of bacteria that were grown from the infected lungs *(42)*. These findings demonstrate that an absence or reduction in endogenous IL-1 activity improves host defense against *Pseudomonas* pneumonia while suppressing the inflammatory response. A reduction in chemokine production following the administration of recombinant IL-1Ra, although reducing lung inflammation, would probably increase bacterial growth owing to reduced neutrophil emigration. However, the administration of recombinant IL-1Ra to mice with live *Pseudomonas* pneumonia reduces bacterial counts, suggesting a non-chemokine-mediated mechanism.

In a study by Boelens and colleagues *(43)*, the IL-1RI knockout mouse had a reduced number of *Staphylococcus epidermidis* bacteria growing around implanted catheters. In addition, IL-1β knockout mice have lower pneumococcal bacteremia compared with wild-type mice *(44)*. Table 3 lists the results of cytokine blockade in models of Gram-positive infections.

7. Models of Intracellular Killing

7.1. Listeria Infections

The most common models for cytokine-dependent host natural resistance to infection employ organisms that require intracellular killing. *Listeria monocytogenes* is an obligate intracellular Gram-positive bacterium that is frequently used. *Listeria* organisms live and multiply in macrophages, and the attempts of the host cell to contain the infection are modest. The organism itself mounts an effective battle against the host's killing processes, but this is apparently more effective in the absence of proinflammatory cytokines. As shown in Table 4, *Listeria* infection worsens and survival rates decrease in mice treated with antibodies against IL-1α and IL-1β, antibodies against IL-1RI, or antibodies against TNF-α. Nearly all cytokine knockout mice exhibit increased susceptibility to *Listeria* compared with wild-type control mice. Mice overexpressing IL-1Ra also are more vulnerable to death from *Listeria* organisms because of its inhibition of IL-1 activity. It is of interest that in IL-1RI knockout mice, the susceptibility to *Listeria* infection is mouse strain-dependent. In one particular genetic background with the knockout of the IL-1 receptor, there is decreased survival compared with control mice *(45)*. In contrast, mice of a different genetic background strain with the knockout gene were as resistant as wild-type mice to *L. monocytogenes (46)*.

The IL-10 knockout mouse, in contrast, exhibits increased resistance and a greater survival; this finding is interpreted to mean that production of IL-1 and TNF-α is increased in IL-10 knockout mice under conditions of this infection. Therefore, in the IL-10 knockout mouse, overproduction of IL-1 or TNF-α provides protection from *Listeria* infection. Hence, the findings in the *Listeria* model are highly consistent in that proinflammatory cytokines are needed for the intracellular killing of this organism. In patients receiving infliximab or etanercept, infections with *Listeria* have been reported. As of August, 2001, the Food and Drug Administration (FDA) lists 16 cases of listeriosis (with 4 deaths) in the infliximab population and 1 case (fatal) for etanercept. It should be noted that listeriosis in patients receiving infliximab occurs mostly in patients also taking an immunosuppressive agent such as methotrexate or low-dose prednisone.

Table 4
Proinflammatory Cytokines Are Needed for Defense Against Listeria[a]

Cytokine	Survival	Ref.
Anti-IL-1α + anti-IL-1β antibodies	↓ Survival	*90*
Anti-IL-1 receptor type I antibody	↓ Survival	*90,91*
IL-1β-deficient mice	No effect	*2*
IL-1Ra-deficient mice	↑ Survival	*92*
IL-1Ra overexpression	↓ Survival	*92*
IL-1R-activating kinase-deficient mice	No effect	*93*
IL-1RI-deficient mice	↓ Survival	*45*
IL-1RI-deficient C57BL6 mice	No effect	*46*
IL-10-deficient mice	↑ Survival	*94*
Anti-TNF-α antibody	↓ Survival	*95*
TNFRI-deficient mice	↓ Survival	*96,97*
IFN-γ R-deficient mice	↓ Survival	*98*

[a]No effect is used to indicate no difference from control mice.
For abbreviations, see Tables 1 and 2 footnotes.

Table 5
Decreased Survival in *Salmonella* Infections

Cytokine	Ref.
↓ Survival by anti-TNF-α antibody	*99*
↓ Survival by anti-TNF-α antibody	*100*
↓ Survival by anti-TNF-α antibody	*101*
↓ Survival by anti-IFN-γ antibody	*101*
↓ Survival in TNFRI-deficient mice	*47*
↓ Survival in TNF-α-deficient mice	*102*
↓ Survival by anti-IL-18 antibody	*103*
↓ Survival by anti-IL-12 antibody	*104*
↑ Survival by anti-IL-10 antibody	*105*

7.2. Salmonella *Infections*

Salmonella infection is a major disease in the United States and Europe as well as in developing countries. The most common *Salmonella* infection is gastroenteritis, which is often food-borne. Salmonellosis rarely advances to bacteremia, except in immunocompromised hosts. Typhoid fever (infection with *S. typhi*) is rare in the United States and Europe. There are several animal studies showing that a deficiency of TNF-α or TNF receptors or the neutralization of TNF-α results in increased mortality from *Salmonella* infection in mouse models (Table 5). The mechanism for increased infectivity and decreased survival associated with reduced TNF-α activity involves intracellular survival of the bacteria owing to a failure to kill the microorganism in the phagolysosome. This is partially, but not exclusively, secondary to reduced production of NO. TNF-α and IFN-γ are prominent in inducing NO. Not unexpectedly, mice treated with antibodies against IFN-γ as well as IFN-γ knockout mice are notably susceptible to Salmonella infection.

Although the failure to kill *Salmonella* organisms living in the phagolysosome of the macrophage is usually thought to be owing to TNF-α and IFN-γ induction of NO, some studies reveal that another mechanism may account for the defect, particularly in mice deficient in TNF-RI. TNF-RI knockout mice are profoundly susceptible to *Salmonella* infection. One day after peritoneal inoculation, TNF-RI knockout mice harbor 1000-fold more bacteria in the liver and spleen than wild-type mice, despite the formation of well-organized granulomas. Although macrophages from these deficient mice produce abundant quantities of reactive oxygen and NO in response to *Salmonella* infection, they nevertheless exhibit poor bactericidal activity. Peritoneal macrophages from TNF-RI knockout mice fail to localize NADPH oxidase-containing vesicles to *Salmonella*-containing vacuoles *(47)*. Thus, intracellular TNF-RI functions to deliver toxic reactive oxygen species to the phagosome via a common pathway of intracellular trafficking. In the absence of the localization of the NADPH to the *Salmonella*-containing phagosome, the bacteria survive the natural killing mechanism.

Despite several reports showing reduced host defense against *Salmonella* infections with various cytokine antagonists, no studies on the effect of administration of exogenous recombinant IL-1Ra have been reported. In addition, IL-1RI, IL-1β, or IL-1α knockout mice have not been reported to be unduly susceptible to *Salmonella* infections.

8. *Mycobacterium Tuberculosis* Infections

Granuloma formation is one of the host's most prominent defense mechanisms for containment of this intracellular microorganism. For example, granuloma formation in the liver of mice infected with bovine tuberculosis prevents the infection from spreading. However, when mice already infected with tuberculosis are then treated with anti-TNF-α antibodies, there is often a destabilization of the granulomas or a failure to form an organized granuloma *(48)*. As a result, there is an increase in bacterial burden in various tissues. Granuloma formation and stabilization of granulomas are critical functions for cytokines. In addition to cytokine-mediated NO production and reactive oxygen intermediates, granuloma formation is a primary host defense strategy against the spread of *M. tuberculosis*. In most of the studies described below, there is a highly consistent role for the formation of granulomas in the lung, liver, or spleen to contain the tuberculosis infection. The gradual formation of granulomas in the pulmonary parenchyma following the initial infection with *M. tuberculosis* is a fundamental host defense response. With persistence and maintenance of these granulomas, the host is provided with decades of protection against the spread of the infection.

Several cell types participate in granuloma formation, but macrophages play an essential role, as do CD4+ T-cells. In fact, granulomas are often characterized histologically as being tightly compacted epithelioid macrophages. Cytokines function in the migration of monocytes to initiate the formation of the granuloma as well as in the growth, stabilization, and maintenance of the containment mechanism. Reducing the activity of a particular cytokine results in a dissolution of the granuloma, an increase in the bacterial burden, and the systemic spread of the disease.

The formation of the tuberculous granuloma requires several growth factors for proliferation of the epithelioid macrophage-like cells as well as enzymes for tissue remodeling by collagen synthesis and breakdown. Metalloproteinases (MMPs) constitute a large family of such enzymes for remodeling of the extracellular matrix. Murine peritoneal macrophages infected with viable *M. tuberculosis* produce large amounts of MMP-9, which is dependent on TNF-α as well as IL-18 *(49)* IL-18 also induces IFN-γ production (as discussed below). In mice infected with *M. tuberculosis*, MMP-9 activity in infected tissues increases.

Granuloma formation around *M. tuberculosis* is associated with expression of iNOS. Pharmacologic inhibition of NO for up to 7 wk significantly exacerbated growth of *M. tuberculosis (50)*. In addition, the differences in the resistance to tuberculosis among mouse strains are reflected in the granulomatous reaction. For example, in C57BL/6 or A/J mice infected with a human isolate of *M. tuberculosis*, the A/J mice died sooner than the C57BL/6 mice. Furthermore, the lungs of A/J mice showed interstitial inflammation with widely disseminated mycobacteria without granuloma formation *(51)*. This was in distinct contrast to the lungs of C57BL/6 mice. Compared with the A/J mice, the C57BL/6 mice formation of granuloma coincided with a high induction of IL-6, IFN-γ, IL-1β, TNF-α, and NO.

Granuloma formation is not solely a property of human or bovine *M. tuberculosis* infection since it also occurs with *M. avium-intracellulare* infections. Following intravenous injection, the organism can be isolated from several tissues, and multiple granulomas also form with this organism. In mice deficient for TNF-RI, mycobacterial counts in the liver, spleen, and lung of these mice are similar to those in wild-type mice, but the formation of granulomata in the liver is significantly lower and delayed compared with the control mice *(52)*. Despite similar numbers of bacteria in both mouse strains, the lack of organized granuloma in the TNF-RI knockout mouse was also associated with hepatic necrosis *(52)*. In addition, the livers of mice infected with *M. avium-intracellulare* developed localized infiltrations of epithelioid macrophages, which were absent in the knockout mice. When depleted of CD4+ T cells, granuloma formation was also markedly abrogated and associated with a reduction in IFN-γ and TNF-α production. These and other studies support the concept that the CD4+ T-cell is a source of IFN-γ as well as TNF-α. Granuloma formation in the liver has also been studied 6 wk following infection with bovine tuberculosis. In mice deficient in CD40 ligand (a member of the TNF family), granuloma formation was reduced, and control of bacterial growth was impaired *(49)*.

Several components of mycobacteria such as the cell wall substance glycolipid trehalose contribute to the formation of granulomata. In the absence of live infection, microspheres coated with glycolipid trehalose induced local inflammatory reactions, with high production of IL-6, TNF-α, IFN-γ, and IL-12 *(53)*. NO production was elevated in cultures of bronchoalveolar lavage cells in these studies. It is thought that glycolipid trehalose facilitates recruitment of inflammatory cells and maintenance of the granulomatous process. Another mycobacterial component is a secreted 30-kDa antigen of *M. tuberculosis* that induces the production of Th1-type cytokines in vitro from T-cells in healthy tuberculinsensitive subjects; however, this is not observed in patients with active tuberculosis *(54)*. Lipoarabinomannan is a component of the cell wall of *M. tuberculosis* that induces the production of several cytokines and chemokines. In IL-1RI knockout mice given an intranasal dose of lipoarabinomannan, there were lower levels of neutrophilic infiltration into the lungs and lower production of TNF-α, IL-1β, IL-1α, and chemokines compared with wild-type mice *(55)*. These results suggest that IL-1 plays a role in the emigration of cells into infected sites.

8.1. Interferon-γ

Because patients with defects in the receptor for IFN-γ are unusually vulnerable to infections with mycobacteria *(4)*, we can conclude that this cytokine plays a particularly important

Table 6
Mycobacterial Infections in Mice with Altered Cytokine Activity

Mouse	Results	Ref.
IFN-γR-deficient mice	↓ Survival	*3,56,57*
Observations	↓ IL-1, ↓ TNF-α production; ↓ granuloma size	
IFN-γ-deficient mice	↑ Bacterial burden	*58*
TNF-α-deficient mice	↓ Survival	*76*
Observation	↓ Granuloma formation	
Overexpression of sol TNFp55	↓ Granuloma formation	*57*
TNFRp55 knockout mouse	↓ Survival	*75*
Anti-TNF-α in mice	↓ Survival	*74,75*
Observations	↑ Reactivation, dissemination	
IL-1RI-deficient mice	↓ Survival	*77*
Observations	↓ TNF-α, ↓ IFN-γ production	
IL-1α/β knockout mice	Survival equal to wild-type control	*78*
Observation	↑ Granuloma size	
IL-6 knockout mice	↓ Survival	*79*
Observation	↓ IFN-γ production	
IL-12 knockout mice	↑ Dissemination	*68*
IL-18 knockout mice	Nonnecrotic granulomas	*61*
Observations	↓ IFN-γ production; normal IL-12, normal nitric oxide	

[a]Indicates a finding (s) thought to be related to the decreased survival.
For abbreviations, see Tables 1 and 2 footnotes.

role in the pathogenesis of tuberculosis. Defects in the signaling receptor for IL-12 in humans also results in decreased IFN-γ levels, which may explain the increase in mycobacterial infections in these patients. In experimental models of tuberculosis, mice with gene knockouts for either IFN-γ itself or the IFN-γ receptor have been studied. As shown in Table 6, these mice exhibit increased infection or death when challenged with either *M. tuberculosis* or the bovine strain of the bacterium. In mice infected with the bovine strain, dissemination in the IFN-γ receptor knockout mouse is observed compared with the wild-type mouse *(56)*. Mice with the knockout of the IFN-γ receptor exhibited an enhanced susceptibility to BCG infection with small hepatic granulomas containing few differentiated macrophages *(57)*. It was concluded that during mycobacterial infections, IFN-γ plays a role in the development of protective granulomas containing highly differentiated macrophages, which kill ingested bacteria. When using a mouse with the IFN-γ receptor deficiency and also overexpressing the soluble form of the TNF-RI, the data suggest that the combination of IFN-γ plus TNF acts together to form the protective granuloma *(57)*. Using IFN-γ knockout mice rather than IFN-γ receptor knockout mice, similar findings have been reported. In these mice, bovine tuberculosis results in large bacterial burdens in the lungs within undifferentiated granulomas not expressing the gene for iNOS *(58)*.

8.2. Role of IL-18 in Mycobacterial Infection

IL-18 plays a major role in the production of IFN-γ; therefore, the role for IL-18 in models of mycobacterial disease should be interpreted for the probability of IL-18-dependent induction of IFN-γ. In humans infected with *M. tuberculosis*, cultured alveolar macrophages secrete IL-18 and IFN-γ spontaneously, and concentrations of these cytokines are higher in pleural fluid of patients than in pleural fluid of patients with nontuberculous diseases *(59)*. When DNA coding for IL-18 was injected into the skin of mice, cutaneous dermal cells transcribed IFN-γ mRNA. When these mice were subsequently infected with BCG, they exhibited a greater IFN-γ response to specific antigen challenge compared with mice injected with a control DNA *(60)*. IL-18 knockout mice infected with bovine tuberculosis developed nonnecrotic granulomas in the lungs and spleens compared with control mice expressing the IL-18 gene *(61)*. Not unexpectedly, the levels of IFN-γ were lower in the IL-18 knockout mice compared with wild-type control mice. However, IL-12 was at expected normal production levels. NO production from peritoneal macrophages was similar regardless of the presence of the IL-18 gene.

8.3. IL-12 and Tuberculosis

Humans born without the ability to express the IL-12Rβ chain experience recurrent infections with mycobacteria and *Salmonella* organisms *(62–66)*. Not unexpectedly, these patients also have reduced capacity to produce IFN-γ. IL-12, like several cytokines, is released from macrophages when they are infected by *M. tuberculosis* or stimulated by products of mycobacterial origin. Infection of mouse macrophages with live *M. tuberculosis* induces IL-12 and TNFα *(67)*. This induction of IL-12 has also been observed in macrophages from mice deficient in the IFN-γ receptor *(67)*. Mice inoculated with live bovine tuberculosis via the air-borne route had well-organized granulomatous lesions and effective control of infection in the lung. In contrast, mice lacking the gene for IL-12 did not produce IFN-γ or other Th1 cytokines and exhibited uncontrolled pulmonary growth and systemic spread of the mycobacteria *(68)*. Thus IL-12, similar to IFN-γ and TNFα, appears to play a critical role in containing the spread of the infection from the granulomatous phase.

8.4. Role of Nitric Oxide in IFN-γ Protection Against Mycobacteria

In general, the role of IFN-γ in host defense against intracellular organisms is attributed to its ability to induce NO production in macrophages. This is a prominent property of IFN-γ, and the combination of IFN-γ plus TNF-α is synergistic in inducing NO. In several models of inflammation, infection, and tumor killing, the beneficial role of IFN-γ has been shown to be dependent on induction of NO. NO is the principal mechanism by which macrophages kill intracellular organisms such as *M. tuberculosis* and *Salmonella*. For example, mouse macrophages infected with *M. tuberculosis* and treated with IFN-γ increase their production of NO and kill the bacteria *(69)*. During live infection with *M. tuberculosis*, products such as purified protein derivative (PPD) sensitize the CD4+ T-cell. Contact between the CD4+ T-cell and antigens such as PPD activate the production of IFN-γ by the T-cell as well as cytokines by the macrophages. The latter include TNF-α. PPD does not result in the induction of NO unless there is cell-to-cell contact between the CD4+ T-cells and antigen-presenting macrophages. The addition of neutralizing antibodies against TNF-α or IFN-γ abrogated the production of NO *(70)*.

Primarily a product of T-cells and natural killer (NK) cells, IFN-γ is induced by the combination of IL-12 plus IL-18. Although IL-12 is a well-known inducer of IFN-γ, IL-18 knockout mice challenged with bovine tuberculosis had normal levels of IL-12 but markedly reduced levels of IFN-γ *(71)*. Mice deficient in IL-12 have been injected with bovine tuberculosis; there was a reduced production of IFN-γ, although the Th1 response was intact *(71)*. When both genes are deleted (IL-12 and IL-18), there are impaired Th1 responses as well as NK cell activity. Therefore, one may conclude that both IL-12 and IL-18 are optimal for IFN-γ production and that IFN-γ then regulates NO production.

Mice deficient in inducible NO and infected with *M. tuberculosis* are unable to clear their infection and die from wasting and pneumonia, whereas wild-type control mice survive *(72)*. The absence of the inducible NO resulted in large splenic granulomas of caseous necrotic material. In addition, there was an *increase* in TNF-α production throughout the entire period of infection. However, in these NO-deficient mice, there was also an increase in the levels of soluble receptors for TNF *(72)*. Hence, the possibility exists that elevated soluble TNF receptors in these mice neutralized endogenous TNF-α. Nevertheless, the lack of the gene for inducible NO (an IFN-γ-inducible gene) is associated with failure to contain and kill bovine tuberculosis and the death of the mice. Other investigators have also examined the role of NO in tuberculosis. Using a low-dose aerosol-mediated infection model, *M. tuberculosis* infection was studied in the lungs of mice lacking the gene for inducible NO *(73)*. In contrast to systemic infection, the low-dose infection model via the lungs resulted in an infection that was contained nearly as well as the infection in wild-type mice. Of considerable interest, the lungs of the NO-deficient mice contained increased numbers of neutrophils compared with the infected wild-type mice, and the elevated number of infiltrating neutrophils may provide a mechanism for containing the mycobacteria in NO-deficient mice.

8.5. TNF Activity and Models of Tuberculosis

Mice overproducing sTNF-RI have been injected with either *M. tuberculosis* or BCG. With either infectious agent, there was overgrowth of the bacteria and evidence of reduced macrophage differentiation within granulomas *(57)*. In the case of infection with *M. tuberculosis*, extensive caseous necrosis was observed in the lungs. Using a low-inoculum model of infection with *M. tuberculosis*, neutralizing anti-mouse TNF-α was injected into mice after the establishment of the infection. This experimental design was performed to test the effect of neutralization of TNF-α in a model on reactivation of latent tuberculosis. Treatment with anti-TNFα leads to a lethal reactivation of the established disease, with an increase in the bacterial load and tissue destruction in the lungs *(74)*. In this low-inoculum model, NO synthase was decreased with the use of anti-TNF-α, although IL-12 and IFN-γ gene expression was not changed. Anti-TNF-α has also been tested in mice infected with *M. tuberculosis (74)*, resulting in decreased survival and higher bacterial burdens *(75)*. In addition, TNF-RI knockout mice also exhibited decreased survival with infection by *M. tuberculosis (75)*. In studies using either neutralizing anti-TNF-α antibodies or TNF-RI knockout mice, there was a decrease in NO from macrophages early in the infection that was thought to contribute to decreased host resistance *(75)*.

TNF-α deficient mice have been injected intravenously with either the Kurono strain of human *M. tuberculosis* or BCG. The Kurono strain is lethal in the TNF-α-deficient mice compared with wild-type mice, with 80% dead after 50 d compared with no deaths in wild-type mice *(76)*. In addition, in the TNF-α-deficient mice, granuloma formation was reduced, epithelioid cells surrounding necrotic lesions were absent, and numbers of bacteria were greatly increased compared with wild-type controls *(76)*. Administration of TNF-α to these deficient mice resulted in 50-d survival, which is comparable to that of the wild-type mice. Cytokine production from cultured spleen cells was evaluated in these studies. The levels of IFN-γ and IL-12 were higher in the wild-type mice, and the production of NO from peritoneal macrophages was similar in both strains of mice *(76)*. These studies reveal that the major impact of TNF-α deficiency in mice infected with virulent human Kurono *M. tuberculosis* is a failure to contain the infection, resulting in early death.

8.6. Role of IL-1 in Resistance to M. tuberculosis

Similar to mice lacking the gene for IFN-γ, IFN-γ receptor, TNF-α, TNF-RI, IL-6, or IL-12, mice lacking IL-1RI are more vulnerable to death from pulmonary *M. tuberculosis* infection compared with wild-type mice *(77)*. In the IL-1RI-deficient mouse, greater numbers of bacteria were isolated from the lungs and other organs, and defective granulomas were seen *(77)*. The decreased host response in these mice was thought to be caused by a reduced infiltration of lymphocytes into the infected tissues. In addition, there was a decrease in IFN-γ production from the spleen cells.

However, contrasting data have been reported in mice with the double knockout of both IL-1α and IL-1β genes *(78)*. In contrast to the findings with the IL-1RI knockout mice, all IL-1α/IL-1β double knockout mice survived after 100 d, as did the wild-type controls *(78)*. In that study, *M. tuberculosis* was administered by the air-borne route. Compared with wild-type controls, the IL-1 double knockout mice developed larger granulomas in the lungs compared with wild-type controls. IFN-γ and IL-12 production from spleen cells, as well as NO production by the alveolar macrophages of the knockout mice, were similar to those from wild-type mice. Although this study shows a dramatic difference between the host's ability to resist *M. tuberculosis* in mice deficient in TNF-α compared with mice deficient in IL-1α/IL-1β, it is not consistent with the studies in the IL-1 receptor knockout mouse *(77)*.

8.7. IL-6 and Tuberculosis

A causative role for IL-6 in resistance to tuberculosis has not been proved. In IL-6 knockout mice, infection with *M. tuberculosis* is lethal compared with the wild-type control mice expressing *(79)*. Spleen cells from *M. tuberculosis*-infected IL-6 knockout mice released less IFN-γ compared with the spleen cells from the control mouse strain. In that study, T-cell ratios were altered in the IL-6 knockout mice. However, the reduced production of IFN-γ may account for the reduced resistance of the IL-6 knockout mouse to infection with *M. tuberculosis*. Interestingly, infection with BCG was not affected by the lack of the IL-6 gene *(79)*.

The role of IL-6 in containment of infection with *M. tuberculosis* has been studied using mice deficient in the nuclear factor (NF) associated with IL-6 (NF-IL-6). NF-IL-6 is elevated, as are other nuclear factors such as NF-κB and IFN-γ regulatory factor, in macrophages stimulated by various microbial products via the Toll-like receptors. Using the air-borne infection route, NF-IL-6 knockout mice exhibited disseminated tuberculosis without granuloma formation *(80)*. Interestingly, the genes for IFN-γ, TNF-α, and IL-12 were expressed at the same level as in the wild-type mice. However, in mice deficient in NF-IL-6, there was a reduction in the generation of superoxide, important for killing of mycobacteria by neutrophils *(80)*.

8.8. Conclusions

The cytokines most essential for natural host defense against mycobacterial infection are IFN-γ and IL-12. Several cases of serious and often fatal mycobacterial infections in individuals with defects in IFN-γ, IL-12 receptors, or signaling mechanisms have been reported. Individuals with defective IL-12 or defective IL-12 receptors suffer from mycobacterial as well as *Salmonella* infections. This may be explained by defective IFN-γ production *(62–66)*. Interestingly, these patients as well as patients with IFN-γ receptor defects do not succumb to *Listeria* infections. Animal studies confirm the human experience.

Acknowledgments

This work was supported by NIH grant AI 15614.

References

1. Eizirik, D. L. and Mandrup-Poulsen. T. (2001) A choice of death—the signal transduction of immune-mediated beta-cell apoptosis. *Diabetologia* **44,** 2115–2133.
2. Zheng, H., Fletcher, D., Kozak, W., et al. (1995) Resistance to fever induction and impaired acute-phase response in interleukin-1β deficient mice. *Immunity* **3,** 9–19.
3. Kamijo, R., Le, J., Shapiro, D., et al. (1993) Mice that lack the interferon-gamma receptor have profoundly altered responses to infection with bacillus Calmette-Guerin and subsequent challenge with lipopolysaccharide. *J. Exp. Med.* **178,** 1435–1440.
4. Jouanguy, E., Altare, F., Lamhamedi, S., et al. (1996) Interferon-gamma-receptor deficiency in an infant with fatal bacille Calmette-Guerin infection. *N. Engl. J. Med.* **335,** 1956–1961.
5. Brochier, J., Liautard, J., Jacquet, C., Gaillard, J. P., and Klein, B. (2001) Optimizing therapeutic strategies to inhibit circulating soluble target molecules with monoclonal antibodies: example of the soluble IL-6 receptors. *Eur. J. Immunol.* **31,** 259–264.
6. Dayer-Metroz, M. D., Duhamel, D., Rufer, N., et al. (1992) IL-1ra delays the spontaenous auto-immune diabetes in the BB rat. *Eur. J. Clin. Invest.* **22,** A50 (abs).
7. Granowitz, E. V., Porat, R., Mier, J. W., et al. (1992) Pharmacokinetics, saftey, and immuno-modulatory effects of human recombinant interleukin-1 receptor antagonist in healthy humans. *Cytokine* **4,** 353–360.
8. Alheim, K., Chai, Z., Fantuzzi, G., et al. (1997) Hyperresponsive febrile reactions to interleukin (IL) 1alpha and IL-1beta, and altered brain cytokine mRNA and serum cytokine levels, in IL-1beta-deficient mice. *Proc. Natl. Acad. Sci. USA* **94,** 2681–2686.
9. Peschon, J. J., Torrance, D. S., Stocking, K. L., et al. (1998) TNF receptor-deficient mice reveal divergent roles for p55 and p75 in several models of inflammation. *J. Immunol.* **160,** 943–952.
10. Godshall, C. J., Lentsch, A. B., Peyton, J. C., Scott, M. J., and Cheadle, W. G. (2001) STAT4 is required for antibacterial defense but enhances mortality during polymicrobial sepsis. *Clin. Diagn. Lab. Immunol.* **8,** 1044–1048.
11. Ebong, S. J., Goyert, S. M., Nemzek, J. A., Kim, J., Bolgos, G. L., and Remick, D. G. (2001) Critical role of CD14 for production of proinflammatory cytokines and cytokine inhibitors during sepsis with failure to alter morbidity or mortality. *Infect. Immun.* **69,** 2099–2106.
12. Benjamim, C. F., Silva, J. S., Fortes, Z. B., Oliveira, M. A., Ferreira, S. H., and Cunha, F. Q. (2002) Inhibition of leukocyte rolling by nitric oxide during sepsis leads to reduced migration of active microbicidal neutrophils. *Infect. Immun.* **70,** 3602–3610.
13. Cobb, J. P., Hotchkiss, R. S., Swanson, P. E., et al. (1999) Inducible nitric oxide synthase (iNOS) gene deficiency increases the mortality of sepsis in mice. *Surgery* **126,** 438–442.
14. Hollenberg, S. M., Broussard, M., Osman, J., and Parrillo, J. E. (2000) Increased microvascular reactivity and improved mortality in septic mice lacking inducible nitric oxide synthase. *Circ. Res.* **86,** 774–778.
15. Chung, C. S., Wang, W., Chaudry, I. H., and Ayala, A. (2001) Increased apoptosis in lamina propria B cells during polymicrobial sepsis is FasL but not endotoxin mediated. *Am. J. Physiol. Gastrointest. Liver Physiol.* **280,** G812–G818.

16. Olson, L. M., Moss, G. S., Baukus, O., and Das Gupta, T. K. (1985) The role of C5 in septic lung injury. *Ann. Surg.* **202,** 771–776.
17. Gommerman, J. L., Oh, D. Y., Zhou, X., et al. (2000) A role for CD21/CD35 and CD19 in responses to acute septic peritonitis: a potential mechanism for mast cell activation. *J. Immunol.* **165,** 6915–6921.
18. Matsukawa, A., Lukacs, N. W., Hogaboam, C. M., et al. (2002) Mice genetically lacking endothelial selectins are resistant to the lethality in septic peritonitis. *Exp. Mol. Pathol.* **72,** 68–76.
19. Rosenkranz, A. R., Coxon, A., Maurer, M., et al. (1998) Impaired mast cell development and innate immunity in Mac-1 (CD11b/CD18, CR3)-deficient mice. *J. Immunol.* **161,** 6463–6467.
20. Boes, M., Prodeus, A. P., Schmidt, T., Carroll, M. C., and Chen, J. (1998) A critical role of natural immunoglobulin M in immediate defense against systemic bacterial infection. *J. Exp. Med.* **188,** 2381–2386.
21. Soriano, F. G., Liaudet, L., Szabo, E., et al. (2002) Resistance to acute septic peritonitis in poly (ADP-ribose) polymerase-1-deficient mice. *Shock* **17,** 286–292.
22. Calandra, T., Echtenacher, B., Roy, D. L., et al. (2000) Protection from septic shock by neutralization of macrophage migration inhibitory factor. *Nat. Med.* **6,** 164–170.
23. Leon, L. R., White, A. A., and Kluger, M. J. (1998) Role of IL-6 and TNF in thermoregulation and survival during sepsis in mice. *Am. J. Physiol.* **275,** R269–R277.
24. Latifi, S. Q., O'Riordan, M. A., and Levine, A. D. (2002) Interleukin-10 controls the onset of irreversible septic shock. *Infect. Immun.* **70,** 4441–4446.
25. Echtenacher, B., Freudenberg, M. A., Jack, R. S., and Mannel, D. N. (2001) Differences in innate defense mechanisms in endotoxemia and polymicrobial septic peritonitis. *Infect. Immun.* **69,** 7271–7276.
26. Mühl, H. and Dinarello, C. A. (1997) Macrophage inflammatory protein-1 alpha production in lipopolysaccharide-stimulated human adherent blood mononuclear cells is inhibited by the nitric oxide synthase inhibitor N(G)-monomethly-L-arginine. *J. Immunol.* **159,** 5063–5069.
27. Echtenacher, B., Falk, W., Mannel, D. N., and Krammer, P. H. (1990) Requirement of endogenous tumor necrosis factor/cachectin for recovery from experimental peritonitis. *J. Immunol.* **145,** 3762–3766.
28. Steinhauser, M. L., Hogaboam, C. M., Matsukawa, A., Lukacs, N. W., Strieter, R. M., and Kunkel, S. L. (2000) Chemokine C10 promotes disease resolution and survival in an experimental model of bacterial sepsis. *Infect. Immun.* **68,** 6108–6114.
29. Echtenacher, B., Weigl, K., Lehn, N., and Mannel, D. N. (2001) Tumor necrosis factor-dependent adhesions as a major protective mechanism early in septic peritonitis in mice. *Infect. Immun.* **69,** 3550–3555.
30. Remick, D., Manohar, P., Bolgos, G., Rodriguez, J., Moldawer, L., and Wollenberg, G. (1995) Blockade of tumor necrosis factor reduces lipopolysaccharide lethality, but not the lethality of cecal ligation and puncture. *Shock* **4,** 89–95.
31. Evans, G. F., Snyder, Y. M., Butler, L. D., and Zuckerman, S. H. (1989) Differential expression of interleukin-1 and tumor necrosis factor in murine septic shock models. *Circ. Shock* **29,** 279–290.
32. Eskandari, M. K., Bolgos, G., Miller, C., Nguyen, D. T., DeForge, L. E., and Remick, D. G. (1992) Anti-tumor necrosis factor antibody therapy fails to prevent lethality after cecal ligation and puncture or endotoxemia. *J. Immunol.* **148,** 2724–2730.
33. Kato, T., Murata, A., Ishida, H., et al. (1995) Interleukin 10 reduces mortality from severe peritonitis in mice. *Antimicrob. Agents Chemother.* **39,** 1336–1340.
34. Lyons, A., Kelly, J. L., Rodrick, M. L., Mannick, J. A., and Lederer, J. A. (1997) Major injury induces increased production of interleukin-10 by cells of the immune system with a negative impact on resistance to infection. *Ann. Surg.* **226,** 450–458.
35. Kelly, J., Lyons, A., Soberg, C. C., Mannick, J. A., and Lederer, J. A. (1997) Anti-interleukin-10 antibody restores burn-induced defects in T-cell function. *Surgery* **122,** 146–152.
36. Steinhauser, M. L., Hogaboam, C. M., Kunkel, S. L., Lukacs, N. W., Strieter, R. M., and Standiford, T. J. (1999) IL-10 is a major mediator of sepsis-induced impairment in lung antibacterial host defense. *J. Immunol.* **162,** 392–399.
37. Alexander, H. R., Doherty, G. M., Venzon, D. J., Merino, M. J., Fraker, D. L., and Norton, J. A. (1992) Recombinant interleukin-1 receptor antagonist (IL-1ra): effective therapy against gram-negative sepsis in rats. *Surgery* **112,** 188–194.

38. Remick, D. G., Call, D. R., Ebong, S. J., et al. (2001) Combination immunotherapy with soluble tumor necrosis factor receptors plus interleukin 1 receptor antagonist decreases sepsis mortality. *Crit. Care Med.* **29,** 473–481.
39. van der Poll, T., Keogh, C. V., Buurman, W. A., and Lowry, S. F. (1997) Passive immunization against tumor necrosis factor-alpha impairs host defense during pneumococcal pneumonia in mice. *Am. J. Respir. Crit. Care Med.* **155,** 603–608.
40. Takashima, K., Tateda, K., Matsumoto, T., Iizawa, Y., Nakao, M., and Yamaguchi, K. (1997) Role of tumor necrosis factor alpha in pathogenesis of pneumococcal pneumonia in mice. *Infect. Immun.* **65,** 257–260.
41. O'Brien, D. P., Briles, D. E., Szalai, A. J., Tu, A. H., Sanz, I., and Nahm, M. H. (1999) Tumor necrosis factor alpha receptor I is important for survival from *Streptococcus pneumoniae* infections. *Infect. Immun.* **67,** 595–601.
42. Schultz, M. J., Rijnveld. A. W., Floequin, S., Edwards, C. K., Dinarello, C. A., and van der Poll, T. (2002) The role of interleukin-1 in the pulmonary immune response during Pseudomonas aeruginosa pneumonia. *Am. J. Physiol. Lung Cell Mol. Physiol.* **2,** 285–290.
43. Boelens, J. J., van der Poll, T., Zaat, S. A., Murk, J. L., Weening, J. J., and Dankert, J. (2000) Interleukin-1 receptor type I gene-deficient mice are less susceptible to *Staphylococcus epidermidis* biomaterial-associated infection than are wild-type mice. *Infect. Immun.* **68,** 6924–6931.
44. Benton, K. A., VanCott, J. L., and Briles, D. E. (1998) Role of tumor necrosis factor alpha in the host response of mice to bacteremia caused by pneumolysin-deficient *Streptococcus pneumoniae*. *Infect. Immun.* **66,** 839–842.
45. Labow, M., Shuster, D., Zetterstrom, M., et al. (1997) Absence of IL-1 signaling and reduced inflammatory response in IL-1 type I receptor-deficient mice. *J. Immunol.* **159,** 2452–2461.
46. Glaccum, M. B., Stocking, K. L., Charrier, K., et al. (1997) Phenotypic and functional characterization of mice that lack the type I receptor for IL-1. *J. Immunol.* **159,** 3364–3371.
47. Vazquez-Torres, A., Fantuzzi, G., Edwards, C. K. 3rd, Dinarello, C. A., and Fang, F. C. (2001) Defective localization of the NADPH phagocyte oxidase to *Salmonella*-containing phagosomes in tumor necrosis factor p55 receptor-deficient macrophages. *Proc. Natl. Acad. Sci. USA* **98,** 2561–2565.
48. Kindler, V., Sappino, A. P., Grau, G. E., Piguet, P. F., and Vassalli, P. (1989) The inducing role of tumor necrosis factor in the development of bactericidal granulomas during BCG infection. *Cell* **56,** 731–740.
49. Hogan, L. H., Markofski, W., Bock, A., Barger, B., Morrissey, J. D., and Sandor, M. (2001) *Mycobacterium bovis* BCG-induced granuloma formation depends on gamma interferon and CD40 ligand but does not require CD28. *Infect. Immun.* **69,** 2596–2603.
50. Ehlers, S., Kutsch, S., Benini, J., et al. (1999) NOS2-derived nitric oxide regulates the size, quantity and quality of granuloma formation in *Mycobacterium avium*-infected mice without affecting bacterial loads. *Immunology* **98,** 313–323.
51. Actor, J. K., Olsen, M., Jagannath, C., and Hunter, R. L. (1999) Relationship of survival, organism containment, and granuloma formation in acute murine tuberculosis. *J. Interferon Cytokine Res.* **19,** 1183–1193.
52. Ehlers, S., Benini, J., Kutsch, S., Endres, R., Rietschel, E. T., and Pfeffer, K. (1999) Fatal granuloma necrosis without exacerbated mycobacterial growth in tumor necrosis factor receptor p55 gene-deficient mice intravenously infected with *Mycobacterium avium*. *Infect. Immun.* **67,** 3571–3579.
53. Lima, V. M., Bonato, V. L., Lima, K. M., et al. (2001) Role of trehalose dimycolate in recruitment of cells and modulation of production of cytokines and NO in tuberculosis. *Infect. Immun.* **69,** 5305–5312.
54. Song, C. H., Kim, H. J., Park, J. K., et al. (2000) Depressed interleukin-12 (IL-12), but not IL-18, production in response to a 30- or 32-kilodalton mycobacterial antigen in patients with active pulmonary tuberculosis. *Infect. Immun.* **68,** 4477–4484.
55. Juffermans, N. P., Verbon, A., Belisle, J. T., et al. (2000) Mycobacterial lipoarabinomannan induces an inflammatory response in the mouse lung. A role for interleukin-1. *Am. J. Respir. Crit. Care Med.* **162,** 486–489.

56. Kirman, J., Zakaria, Z., McCoy, K., Delahunt, B., and Le Gros, G. (2000) Role of eosinophils in the pathogenesis of *Mycobacterium bovis* BCG infection in gamma interferon receptor-deficient mice. *Infect. Immun.* **68,** 2976–2978.
57. Garcia, I., Miyazaki, Y., Marchal, G., Lesslauer, W., and Vassalli, P. (1997) High sensitivity of transgenic mice expressing soluble TNFR1 fusion protein to mycobacterial infections: synergistic action of TNF and IFN-gamma in the differentiation of protective granulomas. *Eur. J. Immunol.* **27,** 3182–3190.
58. Moreira, A. L., Tsenova, L., Murray, P. J., et al. (2000) Aerosol infection of mice with recombinant BCG secreting murine IFN-gamma partially reconstitutes local protective immunity. *Microb. Pathog.* **29,** 175–185.
59. Vankayalapati, R., Wizel, B., Weis, S. E., Samten, B., Girard, W. M., and Barnes, P. F. (2000) Production of interleukin-18 in human tuberculosis. *J. Infect. Dis.* **182,** 234–239.
60. Kremer, L., Dupre, L., Wolowczuk, I., and Locht, C. (1999) In vivo immunomodulation following intradermal injection with DNA encoding IL-18. *J. Immunol.* **163,** 3226–3231.
61. Sugawara, I., Yamada, H., Kaneko, H., Mizuno, S., Takeda, K., and Akira, S. (1999) Role of interleukin-18 (IL-18) in mycobacterial infection in IL-18-gene-disrupted mice. *Infect. Immun.* **67,** 2585–2589.
62. Verhagen, C. E., de Boer, T., Smits, H. H., et al. (2000) Residual type 1 immunity in patients genetically deficient for interleukin 12 receptor beta1 (IL-12Rbeta1): evidence for an IL-12Rbeta1-independent pathway of IL-12 responsiveness in human T cells. *J. Exp. Med.* **192,** 517–528.
63. Altare, F., Lammas, D., Revy, P., et al. (1998) Inherited interleukin 12 deficiency in a child with bacille Calmette-Guérin and *Salmonella enteritidis* disseminated infection. *J. Clin. Invest.* **102,** 2035–2040.
64. Altare, F., Durandy, A., Lammas, D., et al. (1998) Impairment of mycobacterial immunity in human interleukin-12 receptor deficiency. *Science* **280,** 1432–1435.
65. de Jong, R., Altare, F., Haagen, I. A., et al. (1998) Severe mycobacterial and *Salmonella* infections in interleukin-12 receptor-deficient patients. *Science* **280,** 1435–1438.
66. Sakai, T., Matsuoka, M., Aoki, M., Nosaka, K., and Mitsuya, H. (2001) Missense mutation of the interleukin-12 receptor beta1 chain-encoding gene is associated with impaired immunity against *Mycobacterium avium* complex infection. *Blood* **97,** 2688–2694.
67. Ladel, C. H., Szalay, G., Riedel, D., and Kaufmann, S. H. (1997) Interleukin-12 secretion by *Mycobacterium tuberculosis*-infected macrophages. *Infect. Immun.* **65,** 1936–1938.
68. Wakeham, J., Wang, J., Magram, J., et al. (1998) Lack of both types 1 and 2 cytokines, tissue inflammatory responses, and immune protection during pulmonary infection by *Mycobacterium bovis* bacille Calmette-Guérin in IL-12-deficient mice. *J. Immunol.* **160,** 6101–6111.
69. Sato, K., Akaki, T., and Tomioka, H. (1998) Differential potentiation of anti-mycobacterial activity and reactive nitrogen intermediate-producing ability of murine peritoneal macrophages activated by interferon-gamma (IFN-gamma) and tumour necrosis factor-alpha (TNF-alpha). *Clin. Exp. Immunol.* **112,** 63–68.
70. Saito, S. and Nakano, M. (1996) Nitric oxide production by peritoneal macrophages of *Mycobacterium bovis* BCG-infected or non-infected mice: regulatory role of T lymphocytes and cytokines. *J. Leukoc. Biol.* **59,** 908–915.
71. Takeda, K., Tsutsui, H., Yoshimoto, T., et al. (1998) Defective NK cell activity and Th1 response in IL-18-deficient mice. *Immunity* **8,** 383–390.
72. Garcia, I., Guler, R., Vesin, D., et al. (2000) Lethal *Mycobacterium bovis* bacillus Calmette-Guérin infection in nitric oxide synthase 2-deficient mice: cell-mediated immunity requires nitric oxide synthase 2. *Lab. Invest.* **80,** 1385–1397.
73. Cooper, A. M., Pearl, J. E., Brooks, J. V., Ehlers, S., and Orme, I. M. (2000) Expression of the nitric oxide synthase 2 gene is not essential for early control of *Mycobacterium tuberculosis* in the murine lung. *Infect. Immun.* **68,** 6879–6882.
74. Mohan, V. P., Scanga, C. A., Yu, K., et al. (2001) Effects of tumor necrosis factor alpha on host immune response in chronic persistent tuberculosis: possible role for limiting pathology. *Infect. Immun.* **69,** 1847–1855.

75. Flynn, J. L., Goldstein, M. M., Chan, J., et al. (1995) Tumor necrosis factor-alpha is required in the protective immune response against *Mycobacterium tuberculosis* in mice. *Immunity* **2,** 561–572.
76. Kaneko, H., Yamada, H., Mizuno, S., et al. (1999) Role of tumor necrosis factor-alpha in *Mycobacterium*-induced granuloma formation in tumor necrosis factor-alpha-deficient mice. *Lab. Invest.* **79,** 379–386.
77. Juffermans, N. P., Florquin, S., Camoglio, L., et al. (2000) Interleukin-1 signaling is essential for host defense during murine pulmonary tuberculosis. *J. Infect. Dis.* **182,** 902–908.
78. Yamada, H., Mizumo, S., Horai, R., Iwakura, Y., and Sugawara, I. (2000) Protective role of interleukin-1 in mycobacterial infection in IL-1 alpha/beta double-knockout mice. *Lab. Invest.* **80,** 759–767.
79. Ladel, C. H., Blum, C., Dreher, A., Reifenberg, K., Kopf, M., and Kaufmann, S. H. (1997) Lethal tuberculosis in interleukin-6-deficient mutant mice. *Infect. Immun.* **65,** 4843–4849.
80. Sugawara, I., Mizuno, S., Yamada, H., Matsumoto, M., and Akira, S. (2001) Disruption of nuclear factor-interleukin-6, a transcription factor, results in severe mycobacterial infection. *Am. J. Pathol.* **158,** 361–366.
81. Leon, L. R., Kozak, W., Peschon, J., Glaccum, M., and Kluger, M. J. (1997) Altered acute phase responses to inflammation in IL-1 and TNF receptor knockout mice. *Ann. NY Acad. Sci.* **813,** 244–254.
82. O'Riordain, M. G., O'Riordain, D. S., Molloy, R. G., Mannick, J. A., and Rodrick, M. L. (1996) Dosage and timing of anti-TNF-alpha antibody treatment determine its effect of resistance to sepsis after injury. *J. Surg. Res.* **64,** 95–101.
83. van der Poll, T., Marchant, A., Buurman, W. A., et al. (1995) Endogenous IL-10 protects mice from death during septic peritonitis. *J. Immunol.* **155,** 5397–5401.
84. Zamir, O., Hasselgren, P. O., Kunkel, S. L., Frederick, J., Higashiguchi, T., and Fischer, J. E. (1992) Evidence that tumor necrosis factor participates in the regulation of muscle proteolysis during sepsis. *Arch. Surg.* **127,** 170–174.
85. Steinhauser, M. L., Hogaboam, C. M., Lukacs, N. W., Strieter, R. M., and Kunkel, S. L. (1999) Multiple roles for IL-12 in a model of acute septic peritonitis. *J. Immunol.* **162,** 5437–5443.
86. O'Suilleabhain, C., O'Sullivan, S. T., Kelly, J. L., Lederer, J., Mannick, J. A., and Rodrick, M. L. (1996) Interleukin-12 treatment restores normal resistance to bacterial challenge after burn injury. *Surgery* **120,** 290–296.
87. van der Poll, T., Keogh, C. V., Guirao, X., Buurman, W. A., Kopf, M., and Lowry, S. F. (1997) Interleukin-6 gene-deficient mice show impaired defense against pneumococcal pneumonia. *J. Infect. Dis.* **176,** 439–444.
88. Wieland, C., Fantuzzi, G., Edwards, C. K., Dinarello, C. A., and van der Poll, T. (2001) Unpublished data.
89. Tan, T. Q., Smith, C. W., Hawkins, E. P., Mason, E. O. Jr., and Kaplan, S. L. (1995) Hematogenous bacterial meningitis in an intercellular adhesion molecule-1-deficient infant mouse model. *J. Infect. Dis.* **171,** 342–349.
90. Rogers, H. W., Sheehan, K. C., Brunt, L. M., Dower, S. K., Unanue, E. R., and Schreiber, R. D. (1992) Interleukin 1 participates in the development of anti-*Listeria* responses in normal and SCID mice. *Proc. Natl. Acad. Sci. USA* **89,** 1011–1015.
91. Havell, E. A., Moldawer, L. L., Helfgott, D., Kilian, P. L., and Sehgal, P. B. (1992) Type I IL-1 receptor blockade exacerbates murine listeriosis. *J. Immunol.* **148,** 1486–1492.
92. Hirsch, E., Irikura, V. M., Paul, S. M., and Hirsh, D. (1996) Functions of interleukin 1 receptor antagonist in gene knockout and overproducing mice. *Proc. Natl. Acad. Sci. USA* **93,** 11008–11013.
93. Thomas, J. A., Allen, J. L., Tsen, M., et al. (1999) Impaired cytokine signaling in mice lacking the IL-1 receptor-associated kinase. *J. Immunol.* **163,** 978–984.
94. Dai, W. J., Kohler, G., and Brombacher, F. (1997) Both innate and acquired immunity to *Listeria monocytogenes* infection are increased in IL-10-deficient mice. *J. Immunol.* **158,** 2259–2267.
95. Hauser, T., Frei, K., Zinkernagel, R. M., and Leist, T. P. (1990) Role of tumor necrosis factor in *Listeria* resistance of nude mice. *Med. Microbiol. Immunol.* **179,** 95–104.
96. Rothe, J., Mackay, F., Bluethmann, H., Zinkernagel, R., and Lesslauer, W. (1994) Phenotypic analysis of TNFR1-deficient mice and characterization of TNFR1-deficient fibroblasts in vitro. *Circ. Shock* **44,** 51–56.

97. Zhan, Y. and Cheers, C. (1998) Control of IL-12 and IFN-gamma production in response to live or dead bacteria by TNF and other factors. *J. Immunol.* **161,** 1447–1453.
98. Taylor, G. A., Collazo, C. M., Yap, G. S., et al. (2000) Pathogen-specific loss of host resistance in mice lacking the IFN-gamma-inducible gene IGTP. *Proc. Natl. Acad. Sci. USA* **97,** 751–755.
99. Mastroeni, P., Arena, A., Costa, G. B., Liberto, M. C., Bonina, L., and Hormaeche, C. E. (1991) Serum TNF alpha in mouse typhoid and enhancement of a *Salmonella* infection by anti-TNF alpha antibodies. *Microb. Pathog.* **11,** 33–38.
100. Nakano, T., Ohara, O. H. T., and Arita, H. (1990) Group II phospholipase A2 mRNA synthesis is stimulated by two distinct mechanisms in rat vascular smooth muscle cells. *FEBS Lett.* **261,** 171–174.
101. Nauciel, C. and Espinasse-Maes, F. (1992) Role of gamma interferon and tumor necrosis factor alpha in resistance to *Salmonella typhimurium* infection. *Infect. Immun.* **60,** 450–454.
102. Yamamoto, T., Sashinami, H., Takaya, A., et al. (2001) Disruption of the genes for ClpXP protease in *Salmonella enterica* serovar *Typhimurium* results in persistent infection in mice, and development of persistence requires endogenous gamma interferon and tumor necrosis factor alpha. *Infect. Immun.* **69,** 3164–3174.
103. Dybing, J. K., Walters, N., and Pascual, D. W. (1999) Role of endogenous interleukin-18 in resolving wild-type and attenuated *Salmonella typhimurium* infections. *Infect. Immun.* **67,** 6242–6248.
104. Kincy-Cain, T., Clements, J. D., and Bost, K. L. (1996) Endogenous and exogenous interleukin-12 augment the protective immune response in mice orally challenged with *Salmonella dublin*. *Infect. Immun.* **64,** 1437–1440.
105. Arai, T., Hiromatsu, K., Nishimura, H., et al. (1995) Effects of in vivo administration of anti-IL-10 monoclonal antibody on the host defence mechanism against murine *Salmonella* infection. *Immunology* **85,** 381–388.

3

The Use of Cytokine Knockouts in Animal Models of Autoimmune Disease

Alfons Billiau, Hubertine Heremans, and Patrick Matthys

Summary

This chapter overviews studies that have relied on knockout mice to elucidate the role of several cytokines in the pathogenesis of experimental autoimmune encephalomyelitis, collagen II-induced arthritis, insulin-dependent diabetes mellitus, myasthenia gravis, and autoimmune thyroiditis. A predominantly disease-promoting role of some cytokines (tumor necrosis factor, interferon-γ, interleukins-1, -4, -6, -12, and -18), and a predominantly disease-limiting role of other cytokines (interferon-β and interleukin-10) have been demonstrated. Thus, cytokine knockout mice have considerably helped to clarify the pathogenesis of models of autoimmune disease. Most strikingly, the mechanisms and the cell populations whose impacts were brought to light by these studies belong almost exclusively to the innate immunity compartment. This strengthens the view that disturbed recruitment of innate immunity mechanisms is at least as important in the pathogenesis of the autoimmune disease process as the antigen-specific reaction towards self.

Key words

tumor necrosis factor, interferon-β, interferon-γ, interleukin-1, interleukin-4, interleukin-6, interleukin-10, interleukin-12, interleukin-18, experimental autoimmune encephalomyelitis, collagen II-induced arthritis, myasthenia gravis, insulin-dependent diabetes mellitus, autoimmune thyroiditis

1. Introduction

Knockouts that eliminate the production or function of cytokines can provide information on pathogenesis in two ways: (1) by establishing that the cytokine does indeed play a role in the disease model under study, and (2) by showing what parameters of immunopathogenesis change in parallel with the disease manifestations, thus clarifying aspects of pathogenesis, e.g., the participation of certain cell populations. As to the first point, it is important to keep in mind that a "no effect" outcome does not always signify that the cytokine has no role to play in the disease. Indeed, genetic ablation of a single cytokine can in principle be compensated for by modified production of other functionally redundant cytokines *(1)*. As to the second point, the gene knockout approach suffers from the weakness that it does not always reveal the time point in pathogenesis at which the cytokine initiates its action. This issue is particularly important in the case of autoimmune diseases, which most often follow a protracted course. For both reasons, techniques of postgenetic knockout, such as the use of neutralizing antibodies or antisense oligonucleotides, are needed to provide complementary information.

From: *Contemporary Immunology: Cytokine Knockouts, 2nd Edition*
Edited by: Giamila Fantuzzi © Humana Press Inc., Totowa, NJ

For the discussion in this chapter, we selected a limited number of animal models because classically, they have been considered to have an autoimmune nature: experimental autoimmune encephalomyelitis (EAE), collagen-induced arthritis (CIA), type 1 diabetes mellitus in the NOD mouse, myasthenia gravis (MG), and experimental autoimmune thyroiditis (EAT). Assignment of an autoimmune nature to a disease implies that for one reason or another an important role is attributed to the formation of autoantigen-reactive antibodies and/or T-lymphocytes, i.e., failure of peripheral tolerance to be established or to function adequately. This is not to say that mechanisms of innate immunity are unimportant in such model diseases *(2,3)*. The initiation and shaping of antigen-specific immune reactions in general require early deployment of mechanisms of innate immunity, such as activation of phagocytes and dendritic cells following recognition of pathogen-associated molecular patterns (PAMPs), typically by Toll-like receptors. Most typically, this early involvement of innate immunity mechanisms determines whether an immune response will be of the T-helper (Th)1 or Th2 type, and this is only one example in which the cytokine network plays a crucial role. What is true for immune reactions in general also holds for reactions to autoantigens: maintenance and disruption of peripheral tolerance to autoantigens is generally considered to be a matter of adequate or inadequate functioning of innate immunity. Significantly, many animal models of autoimmune disease rely on the use of immunoadjuvants [complete Freund's adjuvant (CFA) lipopolysaccharide (LPS) and others] that address Toll-like receptors. Hence, the *primum movens* in models of autoimmune diseases may in fact be disturbances in innate immunity. When this is seemingly not the case, e.g., in models of spontaneous autoimmune disease or of self-perpetuating autoimmune disease primarily elicited by antibody, the role of PAMPs may be taken over by products released from damaged tissue, e.g., heat shock proteins (hsps). Human hsp60, in particular, binds to and activates the Toll-like receptor Tlr4, resulting in an LPS-like effect on mononuclear phagocytes *(4,5)*.

The cytokine network is an important instrument by which innate immunity regulates and directs the adaptive immune response. Therefore, experiments with cytokine knockouts should contribute considerably to the elucidation of both the primary causes and the further pathogenesis of autoimmune disease.

2. Experimental Autoimmune Encephalomyelitis

EAE is an inflammatory and demyelinating disease of the central nervous system (CNS) that serves as the prime animal model for multiple sclerosis (MS) *(6)*. In several animal species EAE can be induced actively by immunization with myelin components together with one or several immune adjuvants (Freund's adjuvant, *Mycobacterium tuberculosis*, *Bordetalla pertussis*) or adoptively by injection of encephalitogenic T-lymphocytes, T-cell lines, or T-cell clones sensitized to myelin basic protein or myelin proteolipid protein (for reviews, *see* refs. *7* and *8*). Depending on the animal species and the induction schedule, a (hyper)acute form of the disease or a chronic progressive and/or relapsing form (CREAE) of the disease develops *(9–11)*.

EAE lesions are proposed to originate as a result of the proliferation and activity of CNS antigen-specific CD4+ lymphocytes of the Th1 phenotype. One model of pathogenesis holds that any circulating activated T-cell, whether CNS antigen-specific or not, tends to cross the blood-brain barrier. In the CNS, these cells die by apoptosis, except if they encounter antigen-presenting cells (APCs) that present the cognate antigenic epitope. In that case they proliferate, secrete Th1 cytokines, and activate glial cells to produce tissue-destructive enzymes. Recently, involvement of CD8+ T-cells has become evident *(12,13)*. Analysis of cytokine profiles in the CNS of animals with EAE suggests that the onset of disease and subsequent spontaneous recovery are associated with a switch from an initial predominantly Th1-type response, with production of interleukin-2 (IL-2), IL-12, interferon-γ (IFN-γ), and tumor necrosis factor-α (TNF-α), to a subsequent more Th2-type response, with IL-4, IL-10, and TGF-β being produced within the inflammatory foci *(14–21)*. However, there is evidence that CNS-reactive Th2-type lymphocytes can have encephalitogenic potential *(22)* and that Th2-type cytokines can under certain circumstances worsen rather than ameliorate the clinical course of the disease *(23,24)*. Moreover, remission from EAE is not systematically associated with conversion to Th2-type responsiveness *(25)*. Instead, apoptosis of T-cells in the CNS is considered a main mechanism of disease termination *(26)*.

Finally, by what mechanisms spontaneous relapses occur in a more or less predictable way is not known at present.

2.1. TNF-α and LT-α Knockouts

As reviewed by Probert et al. *(27)*, a large body of evidence (other than that derived from studies of knockout mice) supports the notion that TNF-α and lymphotoxin-α (LT-α) play important, predominantly disease-promoting roles in the pathogenesis of EAE. Both cytokines affect CNS cellular components; both can be shown to be locally induced during disease, and ablation of either of them by antibody or other antagonists inhibits or attenuates disease.

In TNF-α knockout mice, EAE can still be induced *(28)*, albeit in a modified form *(29–32)*. The effect of the knockout mutation varies with the strain of mice and the induction schedule. However, in general, the early inflammatory phase of the disease is inhibited and the appearance of clinical signs is delayed. Later on, although demyelination is less pronounced, the inflammatory component is enhanced and disease signs tend to be more severe than in wild-type animals, suggesting that by some pathway TNF-α can exert a protective effect. In fact, in 129/Sv mice, which are naturally resistant to EAE, *(30)*, the TNF-α knockout mutation imparts susceptibility. The overall interpretation is that TNF-α, produced locally in the early disease phase, induces chemokines that account for the immigration of leukocytes. In the later phase, TNF-α is proposed to account for demyelination. Thus, knockout mice would be less prone to mount an early inflammatory response and to develop demyelination. The mechanism whereby knockouts mount more inflammation in the second phase could be by failing to eliminate T-cells by TNF-mediated apoptosis.

Whereas LT-α/TNF-α double knockout mice were found to display a phenotype similar to that of single TNF-α knockouts, single LT-α knockouts were found to be resistant to EAE *(33)*. Remarkably, however, these mice were highly susceptible to adoptive induction by T-cell lines or spleen cells from wild-type induced mice, again pointing at a protective pathway triggered by TNF-α and/or LT-α.

2.2. TNFR Knockouts

TNF receptor type II (TNFRII) single knockouts, as opposed to wild types, were found to develop more severe EAE associated with intense demyelination *(29)*. A possible explanation is that the TNFRII$^{-/-}$ mutation results in absence of both membrane-bound and soluble TNFRII, which, during inflammatory reactions, leads to excess levels of TNF-α and enhanced stimulation of TNF target cells through TNFRI.

TNFRI single and TNFRI and II double knockouts were found to develop modified EAE similar to that in TNF-α/LT-α knockouts, i.e., with a delayed but protracted course. In fact, a chronic progressive disease developed without a preceding acute phase, with little demyelination but intense inflammation in late-stage disease. A possible explanation for the intense inflammation in these TNFRI knockout mice is the reduction in apoptosis of T-cells *(34)*. Thus, these observations with TNFR knockout mice have allowed one to define the role of TNF in EAE as a mediator of (1) early inflammation, (2) late demyelination, and (3) late T-cell apoptosis and "terminator" of disease.

The use of TNFR knockout mice has also provided further supportive evidence for the notion that demyelination depends on TNF but is otherwise independent of the inflammatory reponse. This has been done by using TNF-transgenic mice that overexpress TNF-α in the CNS and thereby spontaneously develop demyelination. Backcrossing of such mice with TNFRI-deficient mice yielded strains that still overproduced TNF but failed to develop demyelinative disease *(35)*. A mechanism involving membrane-bound TNF and cell-cell contact has been proposed to account for in vivo demyelination *(27)*.

2.3. IFN-γ Knockouts

Both IFN-γ ligand and IFN-γ receptor knockout mice were found to be more sensitive to induction of EAE than their wild-type counterparts *(36–39)*. Also, in several variant models of the disease, treatment of the mice with neutralizing antibody against IFN-γ was found to result in augmented symptoms and mortality (reviewed in ref. *40*). Relapses of the disease, whether actively induced or occurring spontaneously, are facilitated by administration of anti-IFN-γ antibody in the disease-free interval *(41)*. Thus, although local CNS production of IFN-γ is maximal during the clinically active phases af the disease, the overall role of IFN-γ is to inhibit pathogenesis. These are rather unexpected and so far insufficiently explained observations. Indeed, IFN-γ is generally considered a proinflammatory and immunostimulatory cytokine, with strong activating effects on mononuclear phagocytes (MPCs). Furthermore, it is also a hallmark of Th1 activity and a promotor of such activity through upregulation of the transcription factor T-bet *(42)*.

Whereas IFN-γ that is present in the periphery and that produced in the CNS may affect EAE pathogenesis in opposite directions, neither the experiments with knockout mice nor those involving blockade of IFN-γ with neutralizing antibody allow dissociation of the effects at these two locations. Injection of exogenous IFN-γ were found to attenuate EAE *(43)*, suggesting that peripheral IFN-γ is protective. Local, intraventricular injection of IFN-γ in a rat model of EAE failed to affect primary induction of EAE but facilitated relapse induction, suggesting that local IFN-γ promotes disease development *(44)*. Contradicting these observations was a result obtained by Voorthuis et al. *(45)* showing no change in disease course following systemic administration of IFN-γ but complete suppression of symptoms following intraventricular administration. In mice overexpressing IFN-γ in oligodendrocytes, the incidence, severity, and histopathology of EAE were found to be similar to those in wild-type controls, but the transgenics did develop chronic neurologic deficits, whereas disease completely resolved in the controls *(46)*.

The cellular mechanism by which IFN-γ suppresses EAE also remains unclear. Several studies have documented a role for IFN-γ in the generation and action of MPC-like cells that can suppress proliferative responses of T-cells to mitogens (for reviews, see refs. *40* and *47*). Such cells were found to appear in the course of experimental infections with mycobacteria or trypanosomes, but also in a study involving delayed-type hypersensitivity (DTH) reactions toward haptenes *(48)*.

Another possible mechanism is by induction of apoptosis in T-lymphocytes. Blockage of IFN-γ inhibits cell death induced in effector T-cells by T-cell receptor (TCR) linkage in the absence of accessory cells *(49)*. Furthermore, in both normal and cultured malignant lymphocytes, IFN-γ has been shown to exert contrasting effects, i.e., apoptosis or proliferation, depending on the level of expression of IFN-γ receptors: high-level expression is associated with an apoptotic response, and low-level expression with a proliferative response *(50)*. Chu et al. *(51)* noted that, during EAE, IFN-γ knockout mice accumulate larger numbers of activated CD4 T-cells in their CNS than wild-type mice; the authors related this to increased proliferation and reduced apoptosis of these cells when exposed to antigen ex vivo. A similar situation was found to occur in mycobacterial infection of IFN-γ knockout and wild-type mice, and in this case it appeared that less proliferation and more apoptosis in the IFN-γ-competent mice was not a direct effect of IFN-γ but was rather mediated by IFN-γ-activated MPCs *(52)*.

2.4. IRF-1 Knockouts

Interferon-regulatory factor-1 (IRF-1) belongs to a seven-member family of transcription factors. It affects transcription of genes inducible by both type I and type II interferons but also intervenes in transcriptional control of the type I IFN gene itself, following induction by double-stranded RNA or viruses. IRF-1 is also induced by granulocyte colony-stimulating factor (G-CSF) *(53)*, prolactin *(54)*, and possibly other endogenous mediators. Aside from mediating transcription of IFN and IFN-controlled genes, IRF-1 behaves as a tumor suppressor factor, its inactivation being associated with hematologic malignancy in humans. Significantly, IRF-1 is required for the T-cell apoptosis that follows radiation-induced DNA damage, and there is evidence that IRF-1 mediates transcription of the gene coding for IL-1-converting enzyme (ICE), which is important in IL-1 secretion as well as in the process of apoptosis. Nitric oxide (NO) synthase induction in macrophages was shown to depend on IRF-1 *(55)*. Thus, IRF-1 is at the crossroads of several pathways triggered by endogenous mediators that act as danger signals and hence is likely to play a role in autoimmune diseases in which tissue damage may constitute such a signal.

IRF-1 deficiency was shown to be associated with reduced susceptibility to EAE. Crossbreeding of EAE-susceptible PL/J mice with IRF-1 knockout mice yielded homozygous IRF-$1^{-/-}$ offspring in which the incidence of actively induced EAE was less than in heterozygous littermates *(56)*. However, the severity of the disease in homozygous knockouts that did develop EAE was not reduced. One possible pathway by which IRF-1 may intervene in the EAE pathogenesis is by mediating NO synthase induction and NO production in the CNS. Of note, induction of NO synthase was detected in some of the homozygous IRF-1 knockout mice that did develop EAE, suggesting that NO synthase can be induced via IRF-1-independent signaling pathways.

2.5. IL-6 Knockouts

Studies using IL-6-deficient mice have been unanimous in reporting that such mice are virtually completely resistant against actively induced EAE *(57–61)*. T-cells recognizing the CNS antigen used for immunization could be obtained from both wild-type and IL-6 knockouts. Adoptively induced EAE could be induced in IL-6-deficient mice by infusion of activated T-cells from immunized wild-type congenic mice. In one study, the reverse, induction in wild-type mice by infusion of T-cells from IL-6 knockouts, was completely impossible, suggesting that endogenous IL-6 exerts most of its disease-promoting effect on events occurring during the induction phase *(58)*.

Production of antibody against CNS antigen was reduced in IL-6-deficient mice, but this was not considered relevant for the almost annihilated sensitivity to disease *(60,61)*.

Analysis of the cytokine profiles of T-cells from immunized IL-6-deficient mice indicated a failure to differentiate into either the Th1 or Th2 direction *(57)* or a more Th2-directed differentiation than in the wild types *(58)*.

A striking difference was the strongly upregulated expression of vascular cell adhesion molecule-1 (VCAM-1) and intercellular adhesion molecule-1 (ICAM-1) in the endothelial cells of the CNS of wild-type and absence of such upregulation in the CNS of IL-6-deficient mice. VCAM-1/very late activation antigen-1 (VLA-1) interaction was established as a crucial event for the transgression of activated T-cells through the blood-brain barrier *(62)*. There is, however, no evidence that IL-6 exerts any direct effect on VCAM-1 expression, so other cytokines must be secondarily involved.

2.6. IL-12 Knockouts

IL-12 knockout mice (C57BL/6 background) were reported to be completely resistant to MBP-induced EAE *(63)*. This is concordant with results from studies employing neutralizing anti-IL-12 antibodies and supports the notion that a Th1-type response is essential for EAE to develop.

2.7. IL-10 Knockouts

IL-10-deficient mice (C57BL/6 background) were reported to be more sensitive than wild types to myelin-oligodendrocyte glycoprotein (MOG) induction of EAE, and T-cells from such mice developed stronger proliferative responses and higher cytokine yields when stimulated with encephalitogenic peptides *(64)*. Concordantly, C57BL/10 IL-10-deficient mice were reported to have a higher incidence of MBP-induced EAE *(63)*, and, similarly, C57BL/6-strain IL-10-deficient mice were found to have accelerated MOG-induced EAE with no spontaneous recovery *(65)*.

Together with data from studies employing IL-10-overexpressing mice, or administration of IL-10 or anti-IL-10 antibody, these data establish a protective role for endogenous IL-10 during EAE. The source of IL-10 seems to be a population of antigen-nonspecific CD4+ T-cells *(63)*. Stimulation of the innate immune system by mycobacterial adjuvant in the EAE immunization procedure is postulated to result in production of several cytokines, whereby the balance between the amounts of IL-12 and IL-10 is crucial in determining disease course.

3. Collagen-Induced Arthritis

CIA in rats *(66)* or mice *(67)* is only one of a large panoply of more or less representative animal models for human rheumatoid arthritis (RA). Among these, CIA is by far the best studied. An important point is that the classical induction schedule of CIA comprises the use of complete or incomplete Freund's adjuvant (CFA or IFA). In DBA/1 mice, immunization with collagen II in CFA results in a much higher incidence and severity of disease than IFA-assisted immunization *(67,68)*.

In certain strains of rats, treatment with IFA or CFA, without any joint-specific antigen, can cause arthritis *(69)*. Such arthritis induced by IFA only is called oil-induced arthritis (OIA); it is an acute and self-limited affection *(70)*. Other oils such as pristane *(71)* and squalene *(72)*, the latter being a normal body component, have also been found to induce arthritis in susceptible rats or mice *(73)*. Adjuvant-induced arthritis (AIA), inducible by CFA (without added autoantigen) in rats, is a chronic disease *(74)*. In Lewis rats it develops in two phases, an acute periarticular inflammation being followed by a phase of bone involvement *(75)*. Arthritogenic T-cell clones have been isolated that recognize epitopes of the mycobacterial heat shock protein hsp65, and this has led to the assumption that the pathogenesis is closely linked to the immune response to these mycobacterial antigens. Antibodies and specific T-cells against hsp65 epitopes do crossreact with epitopes on host HSP. The pathogenesis of oil-induced and adjuvant-induced arthritis are closely related. Both diseases are CD4+ T-cell-dependent *(73,76)*, and both are associated with an immune response to HSP. However, the overall in vivo effect of the anti-HSP response is protective rather than disease-promoting *(77)*. In addition, injection of IFA can prevent induction by CFA *(71)*.

It would seem that certainly not all these models are to be considered autoimmune diseases in the stricter sense of being primarily caused by emergence of autoantibodies or specifically auto-reactive T-cells directed against joint-specific antigens. The mere fact that systemic administration of aspecifically active adjuvants is a constant element in the induction protocols suggests that these diseases are basically generalized inflammatory conditions with a tendency to express themselves preferentially in joint tissues. The role of collagen II in the induction schedule of CIA may consist of generating DTH-reactive T-cells and autoantibodies, thereby enhancing the sensitivity of the joints. Disease susceptibility is restricted by the class II MHC locus I-A, indicating strong involvement of CD4 T-cells. However, in contrast to EAE, no evidence is available that collagen-specific T-cells can by themselves induce the disease in transfer experiments.

3.1. TNF-α Knockouts

There is now abundant evidence that TNF-α plays an important role in the pathogenesis of inflammatory joint diseases, including rheumatoid arthritis (RA). Many properties of TNF-α, such as induction of cartilage and bone resorption, induction of collagenase by synovial cells, and inhibition of the synthesis of proteoglycan and collagen in cartilage, are consistent with a disease-promoting role in RA. In cell cultures prepared from rheumatoid joint tissue, the production of several proinflammatory cytokines such as IL-1, IL-6, and granulocyte/macrophage (GM)-CSF can be inhibited by neutralization of TNF, and this finding has led to the view that TNF is the proximal trigger of the cytokine cascade that results in destruction of the joints. In vivo, a pathogenic role of endogenous TNF-α in arthritis was first demonstrated by a study conducted with mice carrying a human TNF-α transgene. These animals developed a chronic inflammatory polyarthritis that could be prevented by anti-TNF antibody treatment *(78)*. In several other studies using CIA as a model of RA, the administration of TNF-α-inhibitors before or after the onset of arthritis was found to reduce the severity of the disease (reviewed in ref. *79*).

These and other studies have provided the rationale for initiating clinical trials with TNF-α inhibitors in RA patients. However, in the past few years, studies assessing the role of TNF-α in CIA by the gene knockout approach were not in all instances consistent with a simple disease-promoting role of TNF-α. In a study by Mori et al. *(80)*, although the incidence and severity of arthritis in TNFR1 knockout mice were reduced, once the disease was established in a given joint, it progressed in severity in a fashion similar to that seen in wild-type mice. More recently, Tada et al. *(81)* reported unaltered incidence and severity in TNFRI-deficient mice and suggested that this discordant result may be accounted for by differences in the induction protocol of CIA. Indeed, Mori et al. *(80)* used live *Mycobacterium bovis* bacillus Calmette-Guérin (BCG) as a supplementary adjuvant at the time of injection of collagen type II in CFA, which is an unusual procedure. BCG is well known to induce granuloma formation. Since this is abrogated by anti-TNF antibody treatment *(82)* and since granuloma formation might be necessary for development of arthritis, the decreased incidence and severity of arthritis in TNFRI-deficient mice, as reported by Mori et al. *(80)*, may be explained by the failure to develop granuloma formation.

CIA has also been evaluated in TNF knockout mice of B6 genetic background. These mice showed delayed disease onset, lower disease incidence, and reduced disease severity, but none of these differences were statistically significant *(83)*. Histologic examination revealed the mutant mice to have a significantly greater percentage of joints with a normal appearance. However, severe arthritis was still evident in more than half of the affected joints in spite of the impaired humoral but not cellular response to collagen type II. TNF knockout mice also developed lymphadenopathy and splenomegaly associated with increased numbers of activated and memory CD4+ T-cells. The increased accumulation of activated T-cells can be found in unmanipulated TNF- or TNFRI-deficient mice and has to be seen as a result of impaired T-cell apoptosis *(84)*. Thus, with the use of the knockout approach, a pathway has been exposed in which TNF-α exhibits immune-suppressive properties that might be important in the pathogenesis of autoimmune arthritis, as has also been reported for EAE. In addition, the results call into doubt the concept that TNF-α acts only or mainly as a trigger of the proinflammatory cytokine cascade and suggest the involvement of TNF-independent pathways in arthritis.

3.2. IL-1 and IL-1Ra Knockouts

IL-1α and -β are generally recognized as strong proinflammatory and immunopotentiating agents and can therefore be expected to play a disease-promoting role in autoimmune diseases. Actions of IL-1 that are specifically pertinent to its possible role in CIA are its ability to induce production of matrix-degrading enzymes and to cause cartilage destruction. Importantly, the biologic actions of IL-1 produced during inflammatory responses are mitigated by simultaneous production of the IL-1 receptor antagonist (IL-1Ra). Mice that are deficient in IL-1Ra were reported to develop a chronic inflammatory arthropathy spontaneously, resembling RA *(85)*. Also, IL-1α/β double knockout DBA/1 mice were found to be completely resistant against CIA *(86)*. The absence of arthritis was associated with a reduced production of IL-6 mRNA, but not of TNF mRNA, as analyzed by Northern blot hybridization on joints of mice. The proliferative response of lymph node cells to collagen type II was defective in the IL-1α/β knockout mice, whereas the humoral autoantibody response was comparable with that of wild-type mice. These data suggest that, beside its function on cartilage destruction and inhibition of proteoglycan synthesis, IL-1 acts on cellular immunity, which is crucial for the development of autoimmune arthritis; the data also provide strong evidence for IL-1 as a valuable target in chronic arthritis.

3.3. Interferon-γ Knockouts

Classical CIA, induced in DBA1 mice by immunization with collagen type II in CFA, was found to develop more rapidly and to reach a higher cumulative incidence in IFN-γR knockout mice than in wild-type mice *(87,88)*. Concordantly, IFN-γ ligand knockout mice of a normally nonsusceptible strain (C57/Black) were found to be susceptible *(89)*. These findings also corroborated previous findings that treatment of wild-type susceptible mice with neutralizing monoclonal antibodies against IFN-γ, followed by immunization with collagen type II in CFA, resulted in more rapidly developing and more severe disease. Together, these data were seen as evidence for a pathway by which endogenous IFN-γ can provide protection against classical CIA. Significantly, when CIA was induced by an IFA-assisted immunization schedule, IFN-γR ablation or treatment with anti-IFN-γ antibody inhibited disease progression, thus revealing a disease-promoting role of endogenous IFN-γ *(90)*. Apparently, under the influence of mycobacteria from the CFA, a pathogenic pathway becomes dominant that is counteracted by endogenous IFN-γ, resulting in conversion from a normally disease-promoting to a disease-mitigating effect of IFN-γ.

This inhibition of CIA by ablation of IFN-γR in mice immunized without assistance of mycobacteria was associated with suppression of both anti-collagen type II-antibody formation and collagen type II-elicited DTH reactivity at the time of arthritis development. In principle, therefore, the disease-promoting component of IFN-γ's action may be mediated by enhancement of either cellular or humoral immunity effector mechanisms. On the other hand, the protective effect of endogenous IFN-γ in mice given the CFA-assisted immunization schedule appeared to be associated with mitigation of DTH. Indeed, in the IFN-γR knockout mice, disease scores being increased, DTH reactivity was also augmented, whereas antibody formation was suppressed *(90)*.

The mechanisms underlying the protective effect of IFN-γ in classical CIA might be the same as those proposed in the case of EAE, i.e., inhibition of T-cell proliferation and/or stimulation of apoptosis (see above). However, cogent evidence for this is not available. By contrast, there is evidence that a myeloid cell population is the target of IFN-γ. CIA in IFN-γR knockout mice immunized by the CFA-assisted schedule was associated with pronounced splenomegaly, extramedullary hematopoiesis, and overexpansion of a Mac-1-positive cell population. In these IFN-γR-deficient mice, the splenic Mac-1+ cell population not only reached a higher maximal level than in wild-type mice, but also did so at an earlier time point that coincided with the time of disease onset. In wild-type mice, the expansion of the Mac-1+ cell population was less pronounced and also followed a biphasic time-course. Remarkably, the second peak coincided with the later time of disease onset in these mice. Of note, increased expansion of Mac-1+ cells in IFN-γR knockout mice was found to occur irrespective of whether collagen type II is given simultaneously *(91)*. Therefore, increased expansion can reasonably be assumed to take place also and to play a similar role in IFN-γR knockout mice challenged to develop EAE.

What might this role be? Cells of the monocyte/macrophage lineage play an important role as producers of cytokines and other inflammatory mediators. However, they are functionally heterogeneous, being able to develop into tissue-destructive macrophage-like cells, but under other circumstances, to become suppressors of T-cells, two pathways that affect disease scores in an opposite sense. IFN-γ seems to be necessary for maximal development of both activities. Hence, endogenous IFN-γ acts at at least three sites: *de novo* generation of Mac-1+ cells and their differentiation into suppressor and regulator cells *(91,92)*.

In contrast to the reports that IFN-γR knockout mice are more sensitive than wild types to induction of CIA by collagen type II in CFA, Kageyama et al. *(93)* found opposite effects. However, in this study, the IFN-$\gamma R^{-/-}$ 129 mice were crossed only once with DBA/1 mice, and then the (129sv/$Ev^{-/-}$ x DBA/1)F_1 mice were intercrossed to yield heterogeneous F_2 offspring. Within this F_2 offspring, sensitivity to CIA was compared among IFN-$\gamma R^{-/-}$, IFN-$\gamma R^{+/-}$, and IFN-$\gamma R^{+/+}$ mice that were homozygous or heterozygous for the H-2 allele (either H-2^q or H-2^b). Thus, the F_2 mice contained a mixture of the 129 and the DBA/1 genome, which is skewed toward the 129 genes in the IFN-$\gamma R^{-/-}$ mice, owing to co-segregation with the 129-specific deleted IFN-γR allele. Arguably, 129 genes that are loosely linked to the mutated 129 IFN-γR locus, and are therefore lost in IFN-$\gamma R^{-/-}$ DBA/1 mice obtained by classical successive backcrossing, might have contributed to the low CIA sensitivity in the F_2 IFN-$\gamma R^{-/-}$ mice.

Controlling for MHC type, as the authors did, may not be sufficient to avoid this bias. Indeed, although the susceptibility of mice to CIA is known to be genetically determined by the MHC locus, mice bearing the H-2^q allele being highly susceptible and those bearing the H-2^b being resistant, genes not linked to the MHC locus have also been shown to interfere with the susceptibility to CIA. For instance, B10.Q, SWR, and AU/ssJ mice, which have the same MHC haplotype (H-2^q) as the highly susceptible DBA/1 mice, develop CIA at only a very low incidence *(94–97)*. Interestingly, the resistance to CIA of B10.Q mice (H-2^q) was found to be associated with a failure of IL-12 to increase the collage type II-specific antibody response *(97)*. The importance of non-MHC-related genes in the induction of CIA was in fact supported by the data of Kageyama et al. *(93)*, although it was not discussed. Indeed, the study reports a significantly lower incidence of arthritis in the F_2 wild-type offspring bearing H-$2^{q/q}$ than in the parental wild-type DBA/1 (H-$2^{q/q}$) mice (53% versus 75%). This result points to a protective role of non-MHC 129 background genes that could interfere with the disease-promoting effects of the IFN-$\gamma R^{-/-}$ and H-2^q alleles. Conversely, $F_2^{b/b}$ mice exhibited a higher incidence of arthritis (including the IFN-$R^{-/-}$ mice) than parental 129 $H^{b/b}$ mice, indicating that genes other than MHC-restricted genes from the DBA/1 mouse render F_2 offspring more susceptible to CIA.

3.4. IRF-1 Knockouts

In homozygous IRF-$1^{-/-}$, compared with heterozygous $IRF^{+/-}$ mice, the incidence and severity of CIA was found to be significantly decreased *(56)*. There was also a delay in disease onset, and the arthritis index, i.e., the mean score of arthritis in affected mice only, was about half of that in the heterozygous mice. That arthritis was milder in the IRF-1 knockout mice was confirmed by histologic examination. Levels of anti-collagen type II IgG antibodies were similar in the two groups of mice. IRF-1 knockout mice exhibited decreased IFN-γ production in lymph node cells after stimulation with collagen type II, whereas the production of IL-1α, IL-1β, and TNF-α by lipopolysaccharide (LPS)-stimulated macrophages was comparable to that in heterozygous mice. In order to bypass effects on primary immune responses against collagen type II, the authors adoptively transferred the disease by injection of IRF-1 homozygous or heterozygous knockout mice with collagen type II-specific T-cell lines together with sera from arthritic mice. In these experiments, disease development in IRF-1 knockout mice was still impaired, suggesting that IRF-1 acts through other than collage type II-specific T-cells. The authors also considered the possibility that IRF-1 acts by augmenting iNOS expression and NO production. Although inducible nitric oxide synthase (iNOS) expression was less frequently observed in joints of IRF-1 knockout mice, some iNOS-negative joints did show symptoms of arthritis, indicating that the iNOS pathway may not be the most important one by which IRF-1 affected the disease course.

3.5. IL-6 Knockouts

Aside from its complex regulatory effects on inflammation in general, IL-6 exerts effects that can be presumed to be specifically pertinent to inflammation and degenerative changes in joints. Thus, IL-6 potentiates induction of collagenase in chondrocyte cultures by IL-1 and TNF-α, but on the other hand induces tissue inhibitor of metalloproteinase-1 (TIMP-1) production in chondrocyte or fibroblast cultures *(98,99)*. IL-6 also stimulates formation of osteoclast-like cells in long-term human bone marrow cultures, although this effect seemed to require induction of IL-1 *(100)*. A murine in vitro system for induction of osteoclasts consists of coculture of bone marrow (containing the osteoclast progenitors) with osteoblasts. For IL-6 to induce osteoclast formation in this sytem, addition of soluble IL-6 receptor or treatment with dexamethasone, which induces expression of IL-6R mRNA in the osteoblasts, is required. Signal transduction mediated by IL-6R on the osteoblasts, but not on the osteoclast progenitors, is crucial for the effect *(101)*. Finally, IL-6 applied in conjunction with its soluble receptor has been reported to induce proliferation of fibroblastoid synovial cells from an RA patient *(102)*. Influx of leukocytes into joints is considered to be of particular importance in arthritis. IL-6 may favor this process as, again in conjunction with soluble receptor, it has the ability to stimulate endothelial cells to produce chemokines *(103)*.

IL-6 knockouts were described to be either completely or partially resistant to induction of CIA. Alonzi et al. *(104)* used IL-6-deficient mice obtained by backcrossing for five generations with susceptible DBA/1 mice. These mice were found to be completely resistant to induction of CIA. Sasai et al. *(105)* used mice obtained by an eight-generation backcrossing and reported development of arthritis with a delayed onset and reduced scores, but with an incidence similar to that of wild-type mice. An explanation for the difference between the two studies may be the presence of more non-DBA genes (carrying alleles conveying CIA resistance) physically linked to the IL-6 locus in the mice that were backcrossed for only five generations. However, an alternative explanation may be the difference in the immunization procedure between the two studies, in particular the dose of heat-killed mycobacteria present in Freund's adjuvant. Indeed, as is known from studies investigating the role of IFN-γ, an important factor in CIA pathogenesis is the myelopoiesis induced by the Freund's adjuvant, and anti-IL-6 antibodies can suppress this myelopoiesis *(90,91)*. In the study by Alonzi et al., mice received a fourfold higher dose of mycobacteria; hence, it may be argued that, under these circumstances, myelopoiesis becomes a dominant factor in the pathogenesis and IL-6 knockout mice are therefore completely resistant. Further investigation of the role of IL-6 will have to take these effects into account.

3.6. IL-12 Knockouts

IL-12 levels have been reported to be detectable in synovial fluids of RA patients and to correlate with disease activity. IL-12-deficient mice of DBA/1 genetic background (backcrossed for five generations) were demonstrated to have a reduced incidence and severity of arthritis *(106)*. The reduction was associated with an impaired Th1 response, as was evident from the decreased serum levels of collagen type II-specific IgG2a antibodies and collagen-induced secretion of IFN-γ. However, some of the IL-12-deficient mice developed severe disease in a single paw in spite of the highly diminished Th1 response, indicating that neither IL-12 nor a shift in Th1 response is absolutely required for development of CIA. One pathway by which IL-12 promotes CIA could be by stimulating myelopoiesis, as is suggested by the observation that anti-IL-12 antibody completely prevented the establishment of CIA and the associated myelopoiesis in IFN-γR knockout mice *(90)*. IL-12 has also been shown to be able to replace the need for mycobacterial adjuvant in the immunization protocol of CIA, as it markedly augments the incidence of arthritis in DBA/1 mice.

3.7. IL-18 Knockouts

Expression of IL-18 has been observed in synovial tissue from patients with RA at significantly higher levels than in osteoarthritis patients. The role of endogenous IL-18 in CIA has been investigated in IL-18 knockout mice obtained by backcrossing for five generations into DBA/1 background *(107)*. Compared with wild-type DBA/1 mice, these IL-18 knockout mice had a reduced incidence and severity of arthritis, reduced serum anti-CII IgG2a antibody levels, and a reduced collagen type II-specific proliferative response of lymph node and spleen cells. In association with this reduced proliferative responsiveness, collagen type II-stimulated spleen and draining lymph node cells produced less TNF-α, IL-6, and IL-12 than those of wild types. The fact that some IL-18 knockout mice still developed CIA suggests the involvement of other cytokines in the pathogenesis.

3.8. GM-CSF Knockouts

GM-CSF is known for its role as a regulator of leukopoiesis. However, GM-CSF also affects the function of mature mononuclear and polynuclear phagocytes. Both actions may have an impact on the pathogenesis of autoimmune diseases. GM-CSF knockout mice on a C57BL/6 ($H2^b$) genetic background were employed to test the requirement for endogenous GM-CSF in CIA *(108)*. Mice of this background are less susceptible than DBA/1 mice to classically induced CIA; however, this relative resistance can be bypassed by increasing the dose of killed mycobacteria in the Freund's adjuvant. Using this immunization schedule, arthritis was found to be induced in 70% of the wild-type mice, versus only 13% in GM-CSF-deficient mice. Moreover, clinical symptoms were very mild in these affected mice. The anti-collagen type II antibody responses of the mutant and wild-type mice were not different. In contrast, the cell-mediated immunity, as determined by the cutaneous DTH response to collagen type II, was significantly reduced in the GM-CSF knockout mice. Whether this reduction is sufficient to account for the reduced arthritis symptoms remains uncertain. Given the importance of GM-CSF in myelopoiesis and since these mice were injected with enormous amounts of mycobacteria, it is remarkable that the authors did not investigate the levels of circulating monocytes and granulocytes.

3.9. IL-10 Knockouts

IL-10-deficient mice have been used to investigate the role of endogenous IL-10 in the pathogenesis of CIA *(109)*. A technical problem with such mice is that they spontaneously develop colitis in a non-specific pathogen-free (SPF) environment. The authors succeeded in circumventing this problem by using IL-10-deficient mice bred on a C57BL/10Q background, which appear to be less sensitive to such colitis, and by treating the mice with antibiotics. Following immunization with collage type II in CFA, the mice developed more frequent and more severe arthritis than their heterozygous IL-10-producing littermates. IL-10 deficiency did not affect the antibody response to collage type II and also failed to alter proliferative responsiveness of antigen-stimulated draining lymph node cells. The authors also investigated the susceptibility of IL-10-deficient mice to another type of experimental arthritis, i.e., arthritis induced by injection of anti-collagen type II antibodies and subsequent LPS challenge. In contrast to the higher sensitivity to CIA, the IL-10-deficient mice were rather protected against this alternative form of arthritis: only 30% showed sign of arthritis compared with 90% of the littermates.

Cuzzocrea et al. *(110)* have also used IL-10 knockout mice to investigate the role of endogenous IL-10 in the pathogenesis of CIA. These authors did not mention colitis and did not treat the mice with antibiotics. Nevertheless, the knockout mice demonstrated higher scores of arthritis and more bone erosion than wild-type controls. The production of the chemokines macrophage inflammatory protein (MIP)-1α and MIP-2, as assessed by enzyme-linked immunosorbent assay (ELISA) on aqueous joint extracts, was increased in the mutant mice; plasma levels of TNF, IL-1β, and IL-6 were increased. Immunohistochemical analysis of joints sections revealed increased staining for two enzymes known to be involved in the arthritis, i.e., poly-ADP-ribose synthase (PARS) and cyclooxygenase 2 (COX-2). The authors propose that the antiinflammatory effects of IL-10 in CIA may be owing to the prevention of the production or activation of these mediators.

4. Type 1 Diabetes Mellitus: The NOD Mouse

Mice of the nonobese diabetic (NOD) strain spontaneously develop autoimmune disorders, in particular a mononuclear infiltration of pancreatic islets (insulitis) appearing from age 4 wk, followed from age wk 20 by type 1 diabetes mellitus in about three of four males and one of three females. Other exocrine glands such as the salivary gland are also affected.

4.1. IFN-γ and IFN-γ Receptor Knockouts

Breeding of a null mutation of the IFN-γ receptor α-chain (IFN-γRα) from strain 129 mice into the NOD mice resulted in a drastic reduction of spontaneous insulitis and diabetes *(111)*. However, a subsequent study showed that this reduction had been caused by cotransfer from strain 129 to NOD mice of a gene closely linked to that of the IFN-γRα gene and carrying an autoimmune-diabetes resistance allele. In a subsequent study, more extended backcrossing yielded an IFN-γRα knockout NOD strain whose sensitivity to spontaneous diabetes was similar to that of wild-type NOD mice *(112)*. Similar transfer from strain 129 to NOD mice of a null-mutant gene of the IFN-γRα-chain resulted in a knockout NOD strain that again did not differ in susceptibility to spontaneous diabetes *(113)*. Significantly, T-cells of these mice did produce larger amounts of IL-4. In conclusion, it would seem that endogenous IFN-γ is of little influence in the pathogenesis of the pure spontaneous autoimmune diabetes of the NOD mouse, which is also the conclusion of an early study on IFN-γ ligand knockout mice that were found to retain susceptibility, although the incubation period was prolonged *(114)*.

The situation appears to be different in "manipulated" NOD mice. Anti-IFN-γ antibody pretreatment was found to reduce the incidence and severity of diabetes in NOD mice in which occurrence of diabetes is boosted by cyclophosphamide *(115,116)*. Counter to expectation, administration of IFN-γ in this model did not affect blood glucose profiles. In fact, in combination with TNF-α, IFN-γ treatment was associated with a reduction in severity of islet inflammation, although this treatment caused moderate to severe pancreatitis and several other pathologic changes *(117)*.

Another manipulation of the NOD model consists of treatment with CFA or BCG at young age, prior to development of diabetes. Such treatment results in a dormant state of the autoimmune process, as is evident from (1) inhibition of spontaneous development of the disease, (2) prevention of recurrence of the disease in treated recipients of islet transplants, and (3) prevention of adoptive induction of the disease by spleen lymphocytes of diabetic mice *(118–120)*.

The mechanism whereby CFA and BCG exert this unexpected immunosuppressive effect has been a subject of investigation, using various approaches including the use of cytokine knockout mice. A "suppressor" Mac-1+ cell population was identified in the spleens of treated mice. These cells could inhibit transfer of disease by splenocytes of diabetic donors to unaffected recipients and could also suppress T-cell responses of untreated diabetic mice to mitogens or anti-CD3 antibody. On the other hand, BCG-infected NOD mice, although protected against diabetes, were found to develop lupus-like disease *(121)*. Also, protection by CFA or BCG treatment was found to be associated with skewing of the cytokine production pattern of B-cell-reactive T-cells toward a Th2-type profile. However, a study using IFN-γ-, IL-4-, and IL-10 deficient mice led to the conclusion that this association is not a causal one *(122)*. In fact, the ability of BCG and of CFA to protect the mice was found to be dependent on an intact IFN-γ gene function. A possibility not considered by the authors is that IFN-γ mediates this protective effect by influencing the induction by the mycobacterial adjuvants of the suppressor Mac-1+ cell population. Mycobacteria and mycobacterial adjuvant have been described to act as strong stimulators of medullary and extramedullary myelopoiesis, particularly affecting Mac-1+ myeloid cell populations *(91, 92)*. In the absence of a functional IFN-γ system, the effect is quantitatively more pronounced and the cells have a less mature appearance. Conceivably they may assume a pathogenic rather than an immune-suppressive phenotype.

4.2. IRF-1 Knockouts

IRF-1 knockout NOD mice were found to be completely resistant against the development of insulitis and diabetes *(123)*. The proliferative response of splenocyte cultures stimulated with concanavalin A (ConA) or the peptide GAD65 (one of the β-cell autoantigens) was found to be stronger in the IRF-1 knockout than in wild-type mice, and the ratio of IFN-γ production versus IL-10 production was decreased. Furthermore, the proportion of Mac-1+ cells was increased, whereas that of CD3+ cells was decreased. The decreased IFN-γ/IL-10 ratio was interpreted by the authors as being suggestive of a Th2-directed deviation of the autoimmune response in the knockout mice. A factor not taken into consideration is the possible role of the increased proportion of Mac-1+ cells, which, in other systems of autoimmune disease, have been shown to suppress disease manifestations of autoimmune responses *(91,92)*.

4.3. IL-4 Knockouts

The IL-4 null mutation introduced in the NOD mouse, did not accelerate or intensify insulitis and did not affect timing or frequency of transition to overt diabetes. Apparently IL-4 is not required for adequate control of this murine autoimmune disease *(124)*. It is of interest to note that IL-$4^{-/-}$ NOD mice do differ from congenic wild types in that they fail to develop xerostomia, a manifestation suggested to be related to the production of autoantibodies against the acetylcholine muscarinic receptor (M3R) *(125)*.

5. Myasthenia Gravis

Myasthenia gravis is caused by a loss of functional acetylcholine receptors (AChRs) at the postsynaptic membrane of motoneurons, owing to the formation of anti-AChR autoantibodies. A model disease can be induced experimentally in rodents by immunization with *Torpedo* AChR in complete Freund's adjuvant.

5.1. IL-12 and IFN-γ

On the basis of the Th1 dependency of autoantibody formation, it was expected that endogenous IL-12 and IFN-γ would favor disease development. Direct evidence for such a role of IFN-γ came from experiments showing that IFN-γ gene knockout mice, in contrast to wild-type ones, failed to develop AChR autoantibodies and were protected against clinical expression of the disease *(126)*. Remarkably, however, the IFN-γ gene knockout mice did generate anti-AChR autoreactive T-cells. Moreover, the antibody response to a coadministered non-self-antigen, keyhole limpet hemocyanin (KLH), was found to be the same as in wild-type animals. The authors felt this result indicated that, in IFN-γ gene knockout mice, the autoantibody response was too weak to interfere in vivo with AChR function. They proposed that, as a general rule, IFN-γ is indispensable for efficient T-B-cell interaction in the case of antigens, such as autoantigens, for which, owing to negative thymic selection, only low-affinity T-cell receptors are available. The role of IFN-γ was speculated to consist of ensuring sufficient expression of costimulatory molecules.

In a subsequent similar study *(127)* IFN-γ gene knockout mice were found to develop myasthenia with the same frequency as wild-type mice, but differences were noted in the isotype distribution of the autoantibodies (loss of IgG2b). In contrast, IL-12 knockout mice were completely resistant to disease induction and, in this case, more profound alterations in isotype were noted (loss of both IgG2b and IgG2c). Moreover, capture of complement in the muscle correlated with disease occurrence, leading to speculation that the formation of autoantibodies of complement-fixing isotypes is critical.

5.2. IL-4

As the autoantibodies responsible for myasthenia gravis are of the complement-fixing isotypes and therefore probably promoted by Th1-type responsiveness, the expectation was that IL-4 deficiency would promote the disease. In a first study, this expectation was only partially borne out, as IL-4 knockout mice were found not to differ from their wild-type counterparts in terms of susceptibility to the disease, although a shift in antibody isotype from IgG1 to IgG2a was observed *(128)*.

6. Thyroiditis

Experimental autoimmune thyroiditis (EAT) is operationally similar to EAE, or CIA. It can be actively induced in sensitive strains by immunization with thyroglobulin in adjuvant. The disease can also be induced by adoptive immunization using splenocytes taken from thyroglobulin-immunized donors and cultivated in vitro in the presence of the antigen.

6.1. IFN-γ Knockouts

In IFN-γR knockout mice (CBA/J strain, $H2^k$ haplotype) actively induced disease manifestations occurred earlier but also subsided earlier, after having reached lower peak levels *(129)*. Thus, in this case, there is a mixed disease-promoting and -inhibitory effect of IFN-γ. The main mechanism of tissue damage in this model seems to derive from the presence of large numbers of thyroglobulin-specific CD8+ cytolytic cells and high levels of anti-thyroglobulin antibody. Both were reduced in anti-IFN-γ antibody-treated or IFN-γR knockout mice. This may explain the lower overall severity. However, the earlier onset should derive from another mechanism, possibly related to the use of CFA and a role for myelopoiesis *(91)*.

Deletion of the IFN-γ ligand gene in $H2^q$-haplotype mice resulted in a more severe thyroiditis, with granulomatous lesions and eosinophil infiltrations *(130)*. On the other hand, anti-IFN-γ antibody was found to inhibit actively induced disease *(131)*, but to enhance disease manifestations in an adoptive transfer model, if used to treat donor splenocytes in vitro or recipient mice in vivo *(132)*.

7. Concluding Remarks

Cytokine knockout mice have helped considerably to clarify the pathogenesis of models of autoimmune disease. Results obtained by other approaches were readily confirmed, and new information was gathered at an increased pace. Also, new pathways of pathogenesis emerged, as these pathways appeared to be more prominent in cytokine knockout than wild-type mice, for example, the CFA-stimulated extramedullary myelopoiesis that is more prominent in IFN-γR knockout mice. Most strikingly, the mechanisms and the cell populations whose impact was brought to light by this rapid progress belong exclusively to the innate immunity system. Some typical examples are TNF-mediated apoptosis of T-cells in the CNS, local chemokine induction and recruitment of leukocytes to affected organs, and the extramedullary myelopoiesis already mentioned.

This strengthens the view that recruitment of innate immunity mechanisms is much more than just a complement to the autoimmune disease process. In fact, the opposite may be true: whereas disruption of peripheral tolerance was long considered to be the essence of autoimmune diseases, the reaction toward autoantigens may in fact intervene only as a collateral mechanism. To simplify matters: the origin of autoimmune disease may lie in a disturbed distinction between dangerous and innocent, rather than in a disturbed distinction between self and non-self. Hence, diseases classically categorized as chronic inflammatory, e.g., inflammatory bowel diseases, may in essence not differ so much from those considered autoimmune, e.g., type 1 diabetes or MS. Whether this is good news for the patient remains to be seen. The approach consisting of manipulating the cytokine network has met with some success, e.g., anti-TNF-α therapy in some forms of rheumatoid arthritis or IFN-β therapy in MS. Perhaps a combination of cytokine/anticytokine therapy with antigen-specific intervention, e.g., T-cell vaccination, is the ultimate answer.

Research relying on the use of cytokine knockouts has not been devoid of pitfalls. Indeed, discordance in results has shown that the generation of knockout mice from any particular strains by crossbreeding with a cytokine-mutant strain needs to be done with great care so as to ensure that other genes (which independently control pathogenesis pathways) are not inadvertently cotransferred with the mutated cytokine gene.

References

1. Steinman, L. (1997) Some misconceptions about understanding autoimmunity through experiments with knockouts. *J. Exp. Med.* **185,** 2039–2041.
2. Bachman, M. F. and Kopf, M. (2001) On the role of the innate immunity in autoimmune disease (Commentary). *J. Exp. Med.* **193,** F47–F50.
3. Corr, M. and Firestein, G. S. (2002) Innate immunity as a hired gun: but is it rheumatoid arthritis (Commentary). *J. Exp. Med.* **195,** F33–F35.
4. Kol, A., Lichtman, A. H., Finberg, R. W., Libby, P., and Kurt-Jones, E. A. (2000) Heat shock protein (HSP) 60 activates the innate immune response: CD14 is an essential receptor for HSP60 activation of mononuclear cells. *J. Immunol.* **164,** 13–17.
5. Ohashi, K., Burkart, V., Flohé, S., and Kolb, H. (2000) Heat shock protein 60 is a putative endogenous ligand of the toll-like receptor-4 complex. *J. Immunol.* **164,** 558–561.
6. Owens, T. and Sriram, S. (1995) The immunology of multiple sclerosis and its animal model, experimental allergic encephalomyelitis. *Neurol. Clin.* **13,** 51–73.
7. Zamvil, S. S. and Steinman, L. (1990) The T lymphocyte in experimental allergic encephalomyelitis. *Annu. Rev. Immunol.* **8,** 579–621.
8. Martin, R., McFarland, H. F., and McFarlin, D. E. (1992) Immunological aspects of demyelinating diseases. *Annu. Rev. Immunol.* **10,** 153–187.
9. Brown, A. M. and McFarlin, D. E. (1981) Relapsing experimental allergic encephalomyelitis in the SJL/J mouse. *Lab. Invest.* **45,** 278–284.
10. Mokhatarian, M. K., McFarlin, D. E., and Raine, C. S. (1984) Adoptive transfer of myelin basic protein-sensitized T cells produces chronic relapsing demyelinating disease in mice. *Nature* **309,** 356–358.
11. Baker, D., O'Neill, J. K., Gschmeissner, S. E., Wilcox, S. E., Butter, C., and Turk, J. L. (1990) Induction of chronic relapsing experimental allergic encephalomyelitis in *Biozzi* mice. *J. Neuroimmunol.* **28,** 261–270.
12. Sun, D., Whitaker, D., Huang, Z., et al. (2001) Myelin antigen-specific CD8+ T cells are encephalitogenic and produce severe disease in C57BL/6 mice. *J. Immunol.* **166,** 7579–7587.
13. Huseby, E. S., Liggitt, D., Brabb, T., Schnabel, B., Öhlen, C., and Goverman, J. (2001) A pathogenic role for myelin-specific CD8+ cells in a model for multiple sclerosis. *J. Exp. Med.* **194,** 669–676.
14. Khoury, S. J., Hancock, W. W., and Weiner, H. L. (1992) Oral tolerance to myelin basic protein and natural recovery from experimental autoimmune encephalomyelitis are associated with downregulation of inflammatory cytokines and differential upregulation of transforming growth factor β, interleukin 4, and prostaglandin E expression in the brain. *J. Exp. Med.* **176,** 1355–1364.
15. Kennedy, M. K., Torrance, D. S., Picha, K. S., and Mohler, K. M. (1992) Analysis of cytokine mRNA expression in the central nervous system of mice with experimental autoimmune encephalomyelitis reveals that IL-10 mRNA expression correlates with recovery. *J. Immunol.* **149,** 2496–2505.
16. Merrill, J. E., Kono, D. H., Clayton, J., Ando, D. G., Hinton, D. R., and Hofman, F. M. (1992) Inflammatory leukocytes and cytokines in the peptide-induced disease of experimental allergic encephalomyelitis in SJL/J and B10.PL mice. *Proc. Natl. Acad. Sci. USA* **89,** 574–578.
17. Issazadeh, S., Navikas, V., Schaub, M., Sayegh, M., and Khoury, S. (1998) Kinetics of expression of costimulatory molecules and their ligands in murine relapsing experimental autoimmune encephalomyelitis in vivo. *J. Immunol.* **161,** 1104–1112.

18. Issazadeh, S., Lorentzen, J. C., Mustafa, M. I., Hojeberg, B., Mussener, A., and Olsson, T. (1996) Cytokines in relapsing experimental autoimmune encephalomyelitis in DA rats: persistent mRNA expression of proinflammatory cytokines and absent expression of interleukin-10 and transforming growth factor-β. *J. Neuroimmunol.* **69,** 103–115.
19. Issazadeh, S., Ljungdahl, A., Hojeberg, B., Mustafa, M., and Olsson, T. (1995) Cytokine production in the central nervous system of Lewis rats with experimental autoimmune encephalomyelitis: dynamics of mRNA expression for interleukin-10, interleukin-12, cytolysin, tumor necrosis factor α and tumor necrosis factor β. *J. Neuroimmunol.* **61,** 205–212.
20. Bright, J. J., Musuro, B. F., Du, C., and Sriram, S. (1998) Expression of IL-12 in CNS and lymphoid organs of mice with experimental allergic encephalitis. *J. Neuroimmunol.* **82,** 22–30.
21. Tanuma, N., Kojima, T., Shin, T., et al. (1997) Competitive PCR quantification of pro- and anti-inflammatory cytokine mRNA in the central nervous system during autoimmune encephalomyelitis. *J. Neuroimmunol.* **73,** 197–206.
22. Lafaille, J. J., Van de Keere, F., Hsu, A. L., et al. (1997) Myelin basic protein-specific T helper 2 (Th2) cells cause experimental autoimmune encephalomyelitis in immunodeficient hosts rather than protect them from the disease. *J. Exp. Med.* **186,** 307–312.
23. Steinman, L. (1996) A few autoreactive cells in an autoimmune infiltrate control a vast population of nonspecific cells: a tale of smart bombs and the infantry. *Proc. Natl. Acad. Sci. USA* **93,** 2253–2256.
24. Cannella, B., Gao, Y., Brosnan, C., and Raine, C. S. (1996) IL-10 fails to abrogate experimental autoimmune encephalomyelitis. *J. Neurosci. Res.* **45,** 735–746.
25. Di Rosa, F., Francesconi, A., Di Virgilio, A., Finocchi, L., Santilio, I., and Barnaba, V. (1998) Lack of Th2 cytokine increase during spontaneous remission of experimental allergic encephalomyelitis. *Eur. J. Immunol.* **28,** 3893–3903.
26. Schmied, M., Breitschopf, H., Gold, R., Zischer, H., Rothe, G., and Wekerle, H. (1993) Apoptosis of T lymphocytes in experimental autoimune encephalomyelitis. Evidence for programmed cell death as a mechanism to control inflammation in the brain. *Am. J. Pathol.* **143,** 446–452.
27. Probert, L., Eugster, H. P., Akassoglou, K., et al. (2000) TNFR1 signalling is critical for the development of demyelination and the limitation of T-cell responses during immune-mediated CNS disease. *Brain* **123,** 2005–2019.
28. Frei, K., Eugster, H.-P., Bopst, M., Constantinescu, C. S., Lavi, E., and Fontana, A. (1997) Tumor necrosis factor-α and lymphotoxin-α are not required for induction of acute experimental autoimmune encephalomyelitis. *J. Exp. Med.* **185,** 2177–2182.
29. Eugster, H.-P., Frei, K., Bachman, R., Bluethmann, H., Lassman, H., and Fontana, A. (1999) Severity of symptoms and demyelination in MOG-induced EAE depends on TNFR1. *Eur. J. Immunol.* **29,** 626–632.
30. Liu, J., Marino, M. W., Wong, G., et al. (1998) TNF is a potent anti-inflammatory cytokine in autoimmune-mediated demyelination. *Nature Med.* **4,** 78–83.
31. Körner, H., Riminton, D. S., Strickland, D. H., Lemckert, F. A., Pollard, J. D., and Sedgwick, J. D. (1997) Critical points of tumor necrosis factor action in central nervous system autoimmune inflammation defined by gene targeting. *J. Exp. Med.* **186,** 1585–1590.
32. Riminton, D. S., Körner, H., Strickland, D. H., Lemckert, F. A., Pollard, J. D., and Sedgwick, J. D. (1998) Challenging cytokine redundancy: inflammatory cell movement and clinical course of experimental autoimmune encephalomyelitis are normal in lymphotoxin-deficient, but not tumor necrosis factor-deficient mice. *J. Exp. Med.* **187,** 1517–1528.
33. Suen, W. E., Bergman, C. M., Hjelmstrom, P., and Ruddle, N. H. (1997) A critical role for lymphotoxin in experimental allergic encephalomyelitis. *J. Exp. Med.* **186,** 1233–1240.
34. Bachman, R., Eugster, H.-P., Frei, K., Fontana, A., and Lassman, H. (1999) Impairment of TNF-receptor-1 signalling but not Fas signalling diminishes T-cell apoptosis in myelin oligodendrocyte glycoprotein peptide-induced chronic demyelinating autoimmune encephalomyelitis in mice. *Am. J. Pathol.* **154,** 1417–1422.
35. Akassoglou, K., Bauer, J., Kassiotis, G., et al. (1998) Oligodendrocyte apoptosis and primary demyelination induced by local TNF/p55TNF receptor signaling in the central nervous system of transgenic mice: models for multiple sclerosis with primary oligodendrogliopathy. *Am. J. Pathol.* **153,** 801–813.

36. Ferber, I. A., Brocke, S., Taylor-Edwards, C., et al. (1996) Mice with a disrupted IFN-γ gene are susceptible to the induction of experimental autoimmune encephalomyelitis (EAE). *J. Immunol.* **156,** 5–7.
37. Krakowski, M. and Owens, T. (1996) Interferon-γ confers resistance to experimental allergic encephalomyelitis. *Eur. J. Immunol.* **26,** 1641–1646.
38. Willenborg, D. O., Fordham, S. A., Staykova, M. A., Ramshaw, I. A., and Cowden, W. B. (1999) IFN-γ is critical to the control of murine autoimmune encephalomyelitis and regulates both in the periphery and in the target tissue: a possible role for nitric oxide. *J. Immunol.* **163,** 5278–5286.
39. Willenborg, D. O., Fordham, S., Bernard, C. C. A., Cowden, W. B., and Ramshaw, I. A. (1996) IFN-γ plays a critical down-regulatory role in the induction and effector phase of myelin oligodendrocyte glycoprotein-induced autoimmune encephalomyelitis. *J. Immunol.* **157,** 3223–3227.
40. Billiau, A. (1996) Interferon-γ: biology and role in pathogenesis. *Adv. Immunol.* **62,** 61–130.
41. Heremans, H., Dillen, C., Groenen, M., Martens, E., and Billiau, A. (1996) Chronic relapsing experimental autoimmune encephalomyelitis (CREAE) in mice: enhancement by monoclonal antibodies against IFN-γ. *Eur. J. Immunol.* **26,** 2393–2398.
42. Lighvani, A. A., Frucht, D. M., Jankovic, D., et al. (2001) T-bet is rapidly induced by interferon-γ in lymphoid and myeloid cells. *Proc. Natl. Acad. Sci. USA* **98,** 15137–15142.
43. Billiau, A., Heremans, H., Vandekerckhove, F., et al. (1988) Enhancement of experimental allergic encephalomyelitis in mice by antibodies against IFN-γ. *J. Immunol.* **140,** 1506–1510.
44. Tanuma, N., Shin, M. L., Shin, T., Koga, T., Kogure, K., and Matsumoto, Y. (1999) Differential role of TNF-α and IFN-γ in the brain of rats with chronic relapsing autoimmune encephalomyelitis. *J. Neuroimmunol.* **96,** 73–79.
45. Voorthuis, J. A. C., Uitdehaag, B. M. J., De Groot, C. J. A., Goede, P. H., Van der Meide, P. H., and Dijkstra, C. D. (1990) Suppression of experimental allergic encephalomyelitis by intraventricular administration of interferon-γ in rats. *Clin. Exp. Immunol.* **81,** 183–188.
46. Renno, T., Taupin, V., Bourbonniere, L., et al. (2000) Interferon-γ in progression to chronic demyelination and neurological deficit following acute EAE. *Mol. Cell. Neurosci.* **12,** 376–389.
47. Billiau, A., Heremans, H., and Matthys, P. (2000) The role of interferon-γ in experimental autoimmune disease. In: Bona, C. A. and Revillard, J.-P., eds. *Cytokines and Cytokine Receptors. Physiology and Pathological Disorders.* Harwood Academic Publishers, New York, NY, pp. 300–315.
48. Noma, T. and Dorf, M. E. (1985) Modulation of suppressor T cell induction with γ-interferon. *J. Immunol.* **135,** 3655–3660.
49. Liu, Y. and Janeway, C. A. Jr. (1990) Interferon γ plays a critical role in induced cell death of effector T cell: a possible third mechanism of self-tolerance. *J. Exp. Med.* **172,** 1735–1739.
50. Novelli, F., Di Pierro, F., Di Celle, P. F., et al. (1994) Environmental signals influencing expression of the IFN-γ receptor on human T cells control whether IFN-γ promotes proliferation or apoptosis. *J. Immunol.* **152,** 496–504.
51. Chu, C.-Q., Wittmer, S., and Dalton, D. K. (2000) Failure to suppress the expansion of the activated CD4 T cell population in interferon γ-deficient mice leads to exacerbation of experimental autoimmune encephalomyelitis. *J. Exp. Med.* **192,** 123–128.
52. Dalton, D. K., Haynes, L., Chu, C.-Q., Swain, S. L., and Wittmer, S. (2000) Interferon γ eliminates responding CD4 T cells during mycobacterial infection by inducing apoptosis of activated CD4 T cells. *J. Exp. Med.* **192,** 117–122.
53. Coccia, E. M., Stellaci, E., Valtieri, M., et al. (2001) Ectopic expression of interferon regulatory factor-1 potentiates granulocytic differentiation. *Biochem. J.* **360,** 285–294.
54. Yu-Lee, L. (2001) Stimulation of interferon-regulatory factor-1 by prolactin. *Lupus* **10,** 691–699.
55. Kamijo, R., Harada, H., Matsuyama, T., et al. (1994) Requirement for transcription factor IRF-1 in NO synthase induction in macrophages. *Science* **263,** 1612–1615.
56. Tada, Y., Ho, A., Matsuyama, T., and Mak, T. W. (1997) Reduced incidence and severity of antigen-induced autoimmune diseases in mice lacking interferon regulatory factor-1. *J. Exp. Med.* **185,** 231–238.
57. Samoilova, E. B., Horton, J. L., Hilliard, B., Liu, T. T., and Chen, Y. (1998) IL-6-deficient mice are resistant to experimental autoimmune encephalomyelitis: roles of IL-6 in the activation and differentiation of autoreactive T cells. *J. Immunol.* **161,** 6480–6486.

58. Okuda, Y., Sakoda, S., Fujimura, H., Saeki, Y., Kishimoto, T., and Yanagihara, T. (1999) IL-6 plays a crucial role in the induction phase of myelin oligodrendrocyte glycoprotein 35-55 induced experimental autoimmune encephalomyelitis. *J. Neuroimmunol.* **101,** 188–196.
59. Okuda, Y., Sakoda, S., Bernard, C. C., et al. (1998) IL-6-deficient mice are resistant to the induction of experimental autoimmune encephalomyelitis provoked by myelin oligodendrocyte glycoprotein. *Int. Immunol.* **10,** 703–708.
60. Mendel, I., Katz, A., Kozak, N., Ben-Nun, A., and Revel, M. (1998) Interleukin-6 functions in autoimmune encephalomyelitis: a study in gene-targeted mice. *Eur. J. Immunol.* **28,** 1727–1737.
61. Eugster, H.-P., Frei, K., Kopf, M., Lassman, H., and Fontana, A. (1998) IL-6-deficient mice resist myelin oligodendrocyte glycoprotein-induced autoimmune encephalomyelitis. *Eur. J. Immunol.* **28,** 2178–2187.
62. Baron, J. L., Madri, J. A., Ruddle, N. H., Hashim, G., and Janeway, C. A. Jr. (1993) Surface expression of α4 integrin by CD4 T cells is required for their entry into brain parenchyma. *J. Exp. Med.* **177,** 57–68.
63. Segal, B. M., Dwyer, B. K., and Shevach, E. M. (1998) An interleukin (IL)-10/IL-12 immunoregulatory circuit controls susceptibility to autoimmune disease. *J. Exp. Med.* **187,** 537–546.
64. Bettelli, E., Das, M. P., Howard, E. D., Weiner, H. L., Sobel, R. A., and Kuchroo, V. K. (1998) IL-10 is critical in the regulation of autoimmune encephalomyelitis as demonstrated by studies of IL-10- and IL-4-deficient and transgenic mice. *J. Immunol.* **161,** 3299–3306.
65. Samoilova, E. B., Horton, J. L., and Chen, Y. (1998) Acceleration of experimental autoimmune encephalomyelitis in interleukin-10-deficient mice: roles of interleukin-10 in disease progression and recovery. *Cell Immunol.* **188,** 118–124.
66. Trentham, D. E., Townes, A. S., and Kang, A. H. (1977) Autoimmunity to type II collagen: an experimental model of arthritis. *J. Exp. Med.* **145,** 857–868.
67. Courtenay, J. S., Dallman, M. J., Dayan, A. D., Martin, A., and Mosedale, B. (1980) Immunisation against heterologous type II collagen induces arthritis in mice. *Nature* **283,** 666–668.
68. Matthys, P., Vermeire, K., Mitera, T., et al. (1999) Enhanced autoimmune arthritis in IFN-γ receptor-deficient mice is conditioned by mycobacteria in Freund's adjuvant and by increased expansion of Mac-1$^+$ myeloid cells. *J. Immunol.* **163,** 3503–3510.
69. Joe, B. and Wilder, R. L. (1999) Animal models of rheumatoid arthritis. *Mol. Med. Today* **5,** 367–369.
70. Holmdahl, R. and Kvick, C. (1992) Vaccination and genetic experiments demonstrate that adjuvant-oil-induced arthritis and homologous type II collagen-induced arthritis in the same rat strain are different diseases. *Clin. Exp. Immunol.* **88,** 96–100.
71. Zhang, L., Mia, M. Y., Zheng, C. L., et al. (1999) The preventive effects of incomplete Freund's adjuvant and other vehicles on the development of adjuvant-induced arthritis in Lewis rats. *Immunology* **98,** 267–272.
72. Carlson, B. C., Jansson, A. M., Larsson, A., Bucht, A., and Lorentzen, J. C. (2000) The endogenous adjuvant squalene can induce a chronic T-cell-mediated arthritis in rats. *Am. J. Pathol.* **156,** 2057–2065.
73. Stasiuk, L. M., Ghoraishian, M., Elson, C. J., and Thompson, S. J. (1997) Pristane-induced arthritis is CD4+ T cell-dependent. *Immunology* **90,** 81–86.
74. Pearson, C. M. (1956) Development of arthritis, periarthritis and periostitis in rats given adjuvants. *Proc. Soc. Exp. Biol. Med.* **91,** 95–101.
75. Jacobson, P. B., Morgan, S. J., Wilcox, D. M., et al. (1999) A new spin on an old model: in vivo evaluation of disease progression by magnetic resonance imaging with respect to standard inflammatory parameters and histopathology in the adjuvant arthritic rat. *Arthritis Rheum.* **42,** 2060–2073.
76. Svelander, L., Mussener, A., Erlandsson-Harris, H., and Kleinau, S. (1997) Polyclonal T cells transfer oil-induced arthritis. *Immunology* **91,** 260–265.
77. van Eeden, W., van der Zee, R., Paul, A. G. A., et al. (1998) Do heat shock proteins control the balance of T-cell regulation in inflammatory diseases? *Immunol. Today* **19,** 303–307.
78. Keffer, J., Probert, L., Cazlaris, H., et al. (1991) Transgenic mice expressing human tumour necrosis factor: a predictive genetic model of arthritis. *EMBO J.* **10,** 4025–4031.
79. Feldmann, M., Brennan, F. M., and Maini, R. N. (1996) Role of cytokines in rheumatoid arthritis. *Annu. Rev. Immunol.* **14,** 397–440.

80. Mori, L., Iselin, S., De Libero, G., and Lesslauer, W. (1996) Attenuation of collagen-induced arthritis in 55-kDa TNF receptor type 1 (TNFR1)-IgG1-treated and TNFR1-deficient mice. *J. Immunol.* **157,** 3178–3182.
81. Tada, Y., Ho, A., Koarada, S., et al. (2001) Collagen-induced arthritis in TNF receptor-1-deficient mice: TNF receptor-2 can modulate arthritis in the absence of TNF receptor-1. *Clin. Immunol.* **99,** 325–333.
82. Kindler, V., Sappino, A.-P., Grau, G., Piguet, P.-F., and Vassalli, P. (1989) The inducing role of tumor necrosis factor in the development of bactericidal granulomas during BCG infection. *Cell* **56,** 731–740.
83. Campbell, I. K., O'Donnell, K., Lawlor, K. E., and Wicks, I. P. (2001) Severe inflammatory arthritis and lymphadenopathy in the absence of TNF. *J. Clin. Invest.* **107,** 1519–1527.
84. Lenardo, M., Chan, K. M., Hornung, F., et al. (1999) Mature T lymphocyte apoptosis—immune regulation in a dynamic and unpredictable antigenic environment. *Annu. Rev. Immunol.* **17,** 221–253.
85. Horai, R., Saijo, S., Tanioka, H., et al. (2000) Development of chronic inflammatory arthropathy resembling rheumatoid arthritis in interleukin 1 receptor antagonist-deficient mice. *J. Exp. Med.* **191,** 313–320.
86. Saijo, S., Asano, M., Horai, R., Yamamoto, H., and Iwakura, Y. (2002) Suppression of autoimmune arthritis in interleukin-1-deficient mice in which T cell activation is impaired due to low levels of CD40 ligand and OX40 expression on T cells. *Arthritis Rheum.* **46,** 533–544.
87. Vermeire, K., Heremans, H., Vandeputte, M., Huang, J., Billiau, A., and Matthys, P. (1997) Accelerated collagen-induced arthritis in interferon-γ receptor-deficient mice. *J. Immunol.* **158,** 5507–5513.
88. Manoury-Schwartz, B., Chiocchia, G., Bessis, N., et al. (1997) High susceptibility to collagen-induced arthritis in mice lacking IFN-γ receptors. *J. Immunol.* **158,** 5501–5506.
89. Guedez, Y. B., Whittington, K. B., Clayton, J. L., et al. (2001) Genetic ablation of interferon-γ up-regulates interleukin-1β expression and enables the elicitation of collagen-induced arthritis in a nonsusceptible mouse strain. *Arthritis Rheum.* **44,** 2413–2424.
90. Matthys, P., Vermeire, K., Heremans, H., and Billiau, A. (2000) The protective effect of IFN-γ in experimental autoimmune diseases: a central role of mycobacterial adjuvant-induced myelopoiesis. *J. Leukoc. Biol.* **68,** 447–454.
91. Matthys, P., Vermeire, K., and Billiau, A. (2001) Mac-1$^+$ myelopoiesis induced by complete Freund's adjuvant (CFA): a clue to the paradoxical effects of IFN-γ in autoimmune disease models. *Trends Immunol.* **22,** 367–371.
92. Billiau, A. and Matthys, P. (2001) Modes of action of Freund's adjuvants in experimental models of autoimmune diseases. *J. Leukoc. Biol.* **70,** 849–860.
93. Kageyama, Y., Koide, Y., Yoshida, A., et al. (1998) Reduced susceptibility to collagen-induced arthritis in mice deficient in IFN-γ receptor. *J. Immunol.* **161,** 1542–1548.
94. Holmdahl, R., Jansson, L., Andersson, M., and Larsson, E. (1988) Immunogenetics of type II collagen autoimmunity and susceptibility to collagen arthritis. *Immunology* **65,** 305–310.
95. Haqqi, T. M., Banerjee, S., Jones, W. L., et al. (1989) Identification of another T-cell receptor Vβ deletion mutant mouse strain AU/ssJ (H-2q) which is resistant to collagen-induced arthritis. *Immunogenetics* **29,** 180–185.
96. Seki, N., Sudo, Y., Yoshioka, T., et al. (1988) Type II collagen-induced murine arthritis: induction and perpetuation of arthritis require synergy between humoral and cell-mediated immunity. *J. Immunol.* **140,** 1477–1484.
97. Szeliga, J., Hess, H., Rude, E., Schmitt, E., and Germann, T. (1996) IL-12 promotes cellular but not humoral type II collagen-specific Th1-type responses in C57BL/6 and B10.Q mice and fails to induce arthritis. *Int. Immunol.* **8,** 1221–1227.
98. Sato, T., Ito, A., and Mori, Y. (1990) Interleukin 6 enhances the production of tissue inhibitor of metalloproteinases (TIMP) but not that of metalloproteinases by human fibroblasts. *Biochem. Biophys. Res. Commun.* **170,** 824–829.
99. Shingu, M., Miyauchi, S., Nagai, Y., Yasutake, C., and Horie, K. (1995) The role of IL-4 and IL-6 in IL-1-dependent cartilage matrix degradation. *Br. J. Rheumatol.* **34,** 101–106.

100. Kurihara, N., Bertolini, D., Suda, T., Akiyama, Y., and Roodman, G. D. (1990) IL-6 stimulates osteoclast-like multinucleated cell formation in long-term human marrow cultures by inducing IL-1 release. *J. Immunol.* **144,** 4226–4230.
101. Udagawa, T., Takahashi, N., Katagiri, T., et al. (1995) Interleukin (IL)-6 induction of osteoclast differentiation depends on IL-6 receptors expressed on osteoblastic cells but not osteoclast progenitors. *J. Exp. Med.* **182,** 1461–1468.
102. Mihara, M., Moriya, Y., Kishimoto, T., and Ohsugi, Y. (1995) Interleukin-6 (IL-6) induces the proliferation of synovial fibroblastic cells in the presence of soluble IL-6 receptor. *Br. J. Rheumatol.* **34,** 321–325.
103. Romano, M., Sironi, M., Toniatti, C., et al. (1995) Role of IL-6 and its soluble receptor in induction of chemokines and leukocyte recruitment. *Immunity* **6,** 315–325.
104. Alonzi, T., Fattori, E., Lazzaro, D., et al. (1998) Interleukin 6 is required for the development of collagen-induced arthritis. *J. Exp. Med.* **187,** 461–468.
105. Sasai, M., Saeki, Y., Ohshima, S., et al. (1999) Delayed onset and reduced severity of collagen-induced arthritis in interleukin-6-deficient mice. *Arthritis Rheum.* **42,** 1635–1643.
106. McIntyre, K. W., Shuster, D. J., Gillooly, K. M., et al. (1996) Reduced incidence and severity of collagen-induced arthritis in interleukin-12-deficient mice. *Eur. J. Immunol.* **26,** 2933–2938.
107. Wei, X. Q., Leung, B. P., Arthur, H. M. L., McInness, I. B., and Liew, F. Y. (2001) Reduced incidence and severity of collagen-induced arthritis in mice lacking IL-18. *J. Immunol.* **166,** 517–521.
108. Campbell, I. K., Rich, M. J., Bischof, R. J., Dunn, A. R., Grail, D., and Hamilton, J. A. (1998) Protection from collagen-induced arthritis in granulocyte-macrophage colony-stimulating factor-deficient mice. *J. Immunol.* **161,** 3639–3644.
109. Johansson, A. C. M., Hansson, A.-S., Nandukumar, K. S., Backlund, J., and Holmdahl, R. (2001) IL-10-deficient B10.Q mice develop more severe collagen-induced arthritis, but are protected from arthritis induced with anti-type II collagen antibodies. *J. Immunol.* **167,** 3505–3512.
110. Cuzzocrea, S., Mazzon, E., Dugo, L., et al. (2001) Absence of endogeneous interleukin-10 enhances the evolution of murine type-II collagen-induced arthritis. *Eur. Cytokine Netw.* **12,** 568–580.
111. Wang, B., Andre, I., Gonzalez, A., et al. (1997) Interferon-γ impacts at multiple points during the progression of autoimmune diabetes. *Proc. Natl. Acad. Sci. USA* **94,** 13844–13849.
112. Kanagawa, O., Xu, G., Tevaarwerk, A., and Vaupel, B. A. (2000) Protection of nonobese diabetic mice from diabetes by gene(s) closely linked to IFN-γ receptor loci. *Immunology* **164,** 3919–3923.
113. Serreze, D. V., Post, C. M., Chapman, H. D., Johnson, E. A., and Rothman, P. B. (2000) Interferon-γ receptor signalling is dispensable in the development of autoimmune type 1 diabetes in NOD mice. *Diabetes* **49,** 2007–2011.
114. Hultgren, B., Huang, X., Dybdal, N., and Stewart, T. A. (1996) Genetic absence of γ-interferon delays but does not prevent diabetes in NOD mice. *Diabetes* **45,** 812–817.
115. Campbell, I. L., Kay, T. W. H., Oxbrow, L., and Harrison, L. C. (1991) Essential role for interferon-γ and interleukin-6 in autoimmune insulin-dependent diabetes in NOD/Wehi mice. *J. Clin. Invest.* **87,** 739–742.
116. Debraye-Sachs, M., Carnaud, C., Boitard, C., et al. (1991) Prevention of diabetes in NOD mice treated with antibody to murine IFNγ. *J. Autoimmun.* **4,** 237–248.
117. Campbell, I. L., Oxbrow, L., and Harrison, L. C. (1991) Reduction in insulitis following administration of IFN-γ and TNF-α in the NOD mouse. *J. Autoimmun.* **4,** 249–262.
118. Ulaeto, D., Lacy, P. E., Kipnis, D. M., Kanagawa, O., and Unanue, E. R. (1992) A T-cell dormant state in the autoimmune process of nonobese diabetic mice treated with complete Freund's adjuvant. *Proc. Natl. Acad. Sci. USA* **89,** 3927–3931.
119. McInerney, M. F., Pek, S. B., and Thomas, D. W. (1991) Prevention of insulitis and diabetes onset by treatment with complete Freund's adjuvant in NOD mice. *Diabetes* **40,** 715–725.
120. Yagi, H., Matsumoto, C., Suzuki, S., et al. (1991) Possible mechanisms of the preventive effect of BCG against diabetes mellitus in NOD mouse. I. Generation of suppressor macrophages in spleen cells of BCG-vaccinated mice. *Cell. Immunol.* **138,** 130–141.
121. Baxter, A. G., Healey, D., and Cooke, A. (1994) Mycobacteria precipitate autoimmune rheumatic disease in NOD mice via an adjuvant-like activity. *Scand. J. Immunol.* **39,** 602–606.

122. Serreze, D. V., Chapman, H. D., Post, C. M., Johnson, E. A., Suarez-Pinzon, W. L., and Rabinovitch, A. (2001) Thl to Th2 cytokine shifts in nonobese diabetic mice: sometimes an outcome, rather than the cause of, diabetes resistance elicited by immunostimulation. *J. Immunol.* **166,** 1352–1359.
123. Nakazawa, T., Satoh, J., Takahashi, K., et al. (2001) Complete suppression of insulitis and diabetes in NOD mice lacking interferon-regulatory factor-1. *J. Autoimmun.* **17,** 119–125.
124. Wang, B., Gonzalez, A., Hoglund, P., Katz, J., Benoist, C., and Mathis, D. (1998) Interleukin-4 deficiency does not exacerbate disease in NOD mice. *Diabetes* **47,** 1207–1211.
125. Brayer, J. B., Cha, S., Nagashima, H., et al. (2001) IL-4-dependent effector phase in autoimmune exocrinopathy as defined by the NOD.IL-4-gene knockout mouse model of Sjögren's syndrome. *Scand. J. Immunol.* **54,** 133–140.
126. Balasa, B., Deng, C., Lee, J., et al. (1997) Interferon-γ (IFN-γ) is necessary for the genesis of acetylcholine receptor-induced clinical experimental autoimmune *myasthenia gravis* in mice. *J. Exp. Med.* **186,** 385–391.
127. Karachunski, P. I., Ostlie, N. S., Monfardini, C., and Conti-Fine, B. M. (2000) Absence of IFN-γ or IL-12 has different effects on experimental myasthenia gravis. *J. Immunol.* **164,** 5236–5244.
128. Balasa, B., Deng, C., Lee, J., Christadoss, P., and Sarvetnick, N. (1998) The Th2 cytokine IL-4 is not required for the progression of autobody-dependent autoimmune myasthenia gravis. *J. Immunol.* **161,** 2856–2862.
129. Alimi, E., Huang, S., Brazillet, M. P., and Charreire, J. (1998) Experimental autoimmune thyroiditis (EAT) in mice lacking the IFN-γ receptor gene. *Eur. J. Immunol.* **28,** 201–208.
130. Tang, H., Sharp, G. C., Peterson, K. P., and Braley-Mullen, H. (1998) IFN-γ-deficient mice develop severe granulomatous experimental autoimmune thyroiditis with eosinophil infiltration in thyroids. *J. Immunol.* **160,** 5105–5112.
131. Tang, H., Mignon-Godefroy, K., Meroni, P. L., Garotta, G., Charreire, J., and Nicoletti, F. (1993) The effects of a monoclonal antibody to interferon-γ on experimental autoimmune thyroiditis (EAT): prevention of disease and decrease of EAT-specific T cells. *Eur. J. Immunol.* **23,** 275–278.
132. Stull, S. J., Sharp, G. C., Kyriakos, M., Bickel, J. T., and Braley-Mullen, H. (1992) Induction of granulomatous experimental autoimmune thyroiditis in mice with in vitro activated effector T cells and anti-IFN-γ antibody. *J. Immunol.* **149,** 2219–2226.

4

The Use of Cytokine Knockout Mice in Cancer Research

Robert H. Wiltrout, Jon M. Wigginton, and William J. Murphy

Summary

The immune system is regulated by a complex network of cytokines that have unique, redundant, or complementary effects on various facets of innate and adaptive responses to tumors, infectious agents, and in the bone marrow transplant setting. The use of appropriate cytokine knockout mice provides an invaluable approach to understanding the key elements of response and nonresponse in various settings. This mechanistic insight is vital for developing and fine-tuning the preclinical hypotheses that serve as a key translational component in the ultimate clinical application of exciting new strategies for cancer treatment. This chapter reviews important insights, provided by the role of cytokine knockout mice, into the role of Th1 cytokines in regulation of development and progression of neoplasia, and their potential use as cancer therapeutics.

1. Introduction

The interaction between a developing cancer and the immune system is complex and may vary greatly based on the tumor histotype, the nature of organ microenvironment, the expression of unique tumor-associated antigens, and the nature of immune-modifying substances produced by the tumor. These factors contribute to a dynamic interaction between neoplastic cells and local or systemic components of the interdependent innate and adaptive arms of the immune system *(1,2)*. This balance in communication between tumor and host can be skewed in favor of a productive immune response when the host/tumor interaction results in local production of T-helper (Th)1-type cytokines that can initiate and/or amplify nascent immune responses against the tumor. The frequency with which such beneficial cytokine-driven endogenous responses occur against tumors and the efficiency with which they may actually eliminate developing tumors or impair their progression is unclear. However, in several settings in which oncogenes or carcinogens act to stimulate tumor growth, immune mechanisms can modify the incidence and efficiency with which tumors develop and progress *(3)*. Such observations have provided a conceptual foundation for many reports demonstrating that the exogenous administration of Th1 cytokines or inducers of Th1 cytokines can have potent antitumor effects against a variety of tumor histotypes in both mice *(4–6)* and in human cancer patients *(7,8)*. In particular, Th1 cytokines that have central roles

From: *Contemporary Immunology: Cytokine Knockouts, 2nd Edition*
Edited by: Giamila Fantuzzi © Humana Press Inc., Totowa, NJ

in both innate and adaptive responses hold considerable promise as antitumor agents. However, the mechanisms by which these agents mediate antitumor effects are still not completely understood, and the degree to which the effectiveness of cytokine-based immunotherapeutics can be improved remains unclear.

Approaches that allow the selective neutralization/elimination of specific cytokines provide a powerful tool for identifying critical roles for these proteins in endogenously arising or exogenously induced antitumor responses. The targeted inactivation of individual, specific cytokine genes can provide information on direct mechanisms of antitumor activity and (because cytokines function in a complex interdependent network) may also provide new insight into the role of downstream mediators whose production and functions may be regulated by that particular cytokine. It must be noted that the interpretation of results obtained from cytokine knockout mice can be complicated because there can be considerable redundancy of function between different cytokines. Also, removal of a particular cytokine and its downstream effects may chronically perturb the immune system to a broader degree than would be expected in the context of various acute immune responses.

An additional limitation to the more rapid application of this technology to experimental tumor models is the fact that much initial gene targeting has been done in either the 129 or FVB strains of mice, whereas most transplantable tumor models are on the C57BL/6, BALB/c, or C3H backgrounds. This means that considerable additional time is needed to backcross the dysregulated genes onto mouse strains in which the impact of gene loss on tumor progression and cytokine therapy can be determined. The development of technology to target cytokine genes directly in a variety of widely used inbred strains would have great practical benefit.

The overall focus of this chapter is on the use of cytokine knockout mice to understand pathways by which Th1-type cytokines inhibit tumor development, the mechanisms by which they can activate antitumor responses, and their roles in therapeutic transplant procedures.

2. Role of Interferons in Cancer Immunosurveillance and Tumor Treatment

Various members of the interferon family, including both type 1 interferons (IFN; α and β) and IFN-γ, are known to play critical regulatory roles in a variety of innate and adaptive responses *(1,9,10)*. To date the use of gene-targeted mice has mostly contributed to the understanding of IFN-γ's contribution to tumor growth and treatment. Mice lacking either the IFN-γ ligand *(11)* or its receptor *(12,13)* have been produced. These mice have been instrumental in demonstrating central roles for IFN-γ in detection and elimination of nascent tumors, as well as antitumor responses induced by several highly active IFN-γ-inducing Th1 cytokines.

2.1. Role of IFN-γ in Endogenous Responses Against Transplanted or Spontaneously Arising Tumors

A central role for IFN-γ in monitoring and limiting tumor growth was revealed when tumors were induced with methylcholanthrene (MCA) in wild-type or IFN-γ receptor $(R)^{-/-}$ mice *(14)*. Under these conditions, the IFN-γ$R^{-/-}$ mice developed tumors more rapidly and with a greater incidence than did identically treated wild-type mice. This finding was confirmed by the complementary approach taken by Street et al. *(15)*, who showed that mice with a dysregulated IFN-γ gene also had decreased resistance to metastasis formation in mice transplanted with several different syngeneic tumor types. Thus, dysregulation of IFN-γ function through gene targeting of either the IFN-γ receptor or ligand provided dramatic, parallel documentation of the importance of IFN-γ in the regulation of tumor incidence and progression. This paradigm of targeting both ligands and receptors for a cytokine is a valuable approach that can provide redundancy and complementarity to demonstrate a vital role for that cytokine in various biologic processes, in this case carcinogen-induced tumorigenesis/progression or resistance to metastasis formation. However, it remains unclear whether immune perturbations arising in these mice predisposed them to tumorigenesis or whether interferon itself was providing selective pressures on the tumor.

A variant of the approach outlined above has also been used to demonstrate a central role for IFN-γ in mice lacking a functional p53 tumor suppressor gene *(14)*. In this study, mice lacking p53 function were crossed with IFN-γ$R^{-/-}$ mice; such mice developed spontaneous tumors more quickly than did mice exhibiting only a dysregulated p53 gene. This approach demonstrates how mice with inactivated cytokine genes can be used to study the relevance of those genes in the overall, complex process of oncogenesis. The results may also indicate an ability to detect facilitating interactions between the loss of selected immunoregulatory events and oncogenic stimuli.

2.2. Central Role of IFN-γ in Powerful Th1-Initiated Antitumor Responses

Several IFN-γ-inducing cytokines, including interleukin (IL)-12 *(5,16,17)* and IL-18 *(18)* have been shown to mediate potent antitumor effects against a variety of tumor types in mice. Further studies have shown that the antitumor effects of both IL-12 *(17,19)* and IL-18 *(20)* can be critically dependent on IFN-γ, since the antitumor effects of these cytokines were largely lost in mice with a dysregulated IFN-γ gene. The central role of IFN-γ in Th1-cytokine driven therapeutic effects has recently been reemphasized in settings in which IL-12 or IL-18 have been shown to synergize with IL-2 for antitumor activity *(6,21)*. Wigginton et al. *(6)* have shown that the combination of IL-12 + IL-2 has an enhanced ability to induce IFN-γ production and yields greater antitumor activity against both spontaneously developing breast cancer in C(3)1-TAg transgenic mice *(22)* and advanced metastatic renal cell carcinoma in BALB/c mice *(6)*. The enhanced antitumor effects of IL-12 + IL-2 are completely lost in IFN-$\gamma^{-/-}$ mice. Similarly, the combination of IL-18 + IL-2 also shows enhanced antitumor activity against both metastatic renal cell carcinoma and the 3LL Lewis lung carcinoma *(6)*, and these enhanced antitumor effects are also lost in IFN-$\gamma^{-/-}$ mice. Overall, these results demonstrate that IFN-$\gamma^{-/-}$ mice are a powerful tool for defining a central intermediate role of downstream IFN-γ in the complex process of Th-1-type cytokine-driven antitumor responses.

2.3. Use of IFN-$\gamma^{-/-}$ Mice to Define the Cellular and Molecular Mechanisms of Th1 Cytokine-Driven Antitumor Responses

The availability of IFN-$\gamma^{-/-}$ mice provides a valuable tool for illustrating the vital role of IFN-γ in the setting of cytokine-induced tumor regression. These mice also provide opportunities to dissect the mechanisms by which IFN-γ-dependent antitumor responses occur, and to determine whether the effects are predominantly dependent on host responses or direct reactivity of the tumor to IFN-γ. In this regard, our laboratory has been able to critically associate a dependency on IFN-γ of IL-12 + IL-2-induced antitumor effects with rapidly induced IFN-γ-dependent damage to the tumor-associated neovasculature *(6)*. When IL-12

+ IL-2 was given to IFN-$\gamma^{-/-}$ mice, this rapid destruction of tumor-associated endothelium and the inhibition of further neovascularization seen in wild-type mice were lost.

These IFN-γ-dependent antitumor and antiangiogenic effects are closely linked to the activation of IFN-γ-inducible genes, most notably the CXC chemokines Mig and IP-10. Although some studies have shown that neutralization of Mig and IP-10 blunts IL-12-induced antitumor effects *(23,24)*, the exact mechanism(s) for CXC chemokine-mediated antitumor activity remains unclear. Recent reports of successful knockout of these genes *(25)* will provide a new opportunity to dissect these antitumor activities further. In particular, studies performed in mice lacking either of these functional ligands or their common CXCR3 receptor *(26)* will provide a powerful tool for studying these molecules in the context of immune response, leukocyte recruitment and function, and angiogenesis.

Recently, Smyth and colleagues *(27)* have used IFN-$\gamma^{-/-}$ mice in a series of elegant studies to show that the antitumor effects of the immunomodulator αGalCer are dependent on IFN-γ production by natural killer (NK)T cells. In this novel approach, purified NKT cells from IFN-$\gamma^{-/-}$ mice were transferred into mice in which the host NKT cells had been deleted by gene targeting (Jα281$^{-/-}$ mice). Under these conditions the NKT cells from wild-type mice, but not IFN-$\gamma^{-/-}$ mice, were able to mediate antitumor effects after treatment with αGalCer. Thus, the use of IFN-$\gamma^{-/-}$ mice as a source of effector cells provided a unique experimental platform for delineating the linkage between IFN-γ and a discrete population of innate effector cells in an antitumor response.

Overall, although the availability of both IFN-γ R$^{-/-}$ and IFN-$\gamma^{-/-}$ mice has already provided great insight into the importance of IFN-γ in innate and adaptive immune responses, many additional questions remain to be addressed using these unique reagents such as effects on immune cell development and function in these deficient mice not related to effector functions of the cytokine.

3. Mice with Dysregulated TNF Superfamily Components Have Abnormal Immunologic Responses and Impaired Responses to Cytokine Therapy

The tumor necrosis factor (TNF) superfamily is composed of many structurally related cytokines that have diverse effects on both innate and adaptive immune responses through binding to various receptors that are ubiquitously or differentially expressed on various hematopoietic and nonhematopoietic cells. The members of this family have some redundant biologic activities as well as many unique immunologic functions. Some members of the TNF superfamily also have direct apoptosis-inducing activities for a variety of normal and neoplastic cell types when they bind to various TNF family receptors (TNFRs) that contain a cytoplasmic death domain. The creation of mouse strains with selected inactivation of TNF superfamily ligands and receptors has provided much new information about the mechanisms by which various cytokines induce regression of cancer, or mechanisms of endogenous resistance to tumor formation and progression.

3.1. Role of TNF-α and LT Mutant Mice in Understanding the Structure/Function of the Immune System

Several research groups have used knockout technology to demonstrate important roles for these cytokines in the function of immune cells and the development of lymphoid tissue. TNF-α plays a complex and broad role in regulating inflammation and immunity *(28,*

29). Mice with a dysregulated TNF-α gene develop normally and do not display gross physiologic abnormalities *(29)*. However, their host defenses to infectious agents and cancer are markedly impaired. Smyth and colleagues *(30)* have noted that TNF-$\alpha^{-/-}$ mice exhibit a decreased response to RMA-S tumor cell growth in the peritoneal cavity, and the mechanism for this impaired response includes a diminished migration capacity of NK cells into the peritoneum. The specific mechanisms by which TNF-α can contribute to antitumor responses are illustrated by additional studies showing that mice treated with antibodies specific for TNF-α had an impaired capacity for recruitment of NK cells to the liver in response to administration of immunomodulators *(28)*. In contrast, TNF-α has been reported to play a promoting role in skin carcinogenesis. Moore and colleagues have shown that TNF-$\alpha^{-/-}$ mice exhibit an increased resistance to the formation of both benign and malignant TPA-induced skin tumors, and this effect coincided with a reduction in dermal inflammation that is thought to contribute to tumor promotion in this model *(31)*.

Lymphotoxin-α (LT-α) has also been implicated as a regulator of tumor growth through the use of LT-$\alpha^{-/-}$ mice. Mice deficient in this gene exhibit impaired NK cell function, although the specific aspects of NK cell dysregulation may differ somewhat. Smyth et al. *(32)* have noted that LT-$\alpha^{-/-}$ mice show a reduced number of NK cells in various hematopoietic and immunologic organs that and these mice also show a reduction in the lytic activity of the NK cells that correlates with an impaired resistance to metastasis. Similar findings have been reported by Ito et al. *(33)*, who showed that LT-$\alpha^{-/-}$ mice have depressed NK cell-dependent antimetastatic activity in the lungs that corresponded to an impaired recruitment of NK cells into the lungs and liver. This group also noted that bone marrow from LT-$\alpha^{-/-}$ mice was not efficient in producing NK cells in response to IL-2 or IL-15, suggesting that the loss of antimetastatic efficiency could relate to both impaired NK cell maturation and recruitment. However, LT-$\alpha^{-/-}$ mice also present with significant defects in lymph node architecture *(34)*, and TNFR$^{-/-}$ (p55) mice have deficiencies in T-cell activation *(35)*, suggesting that these cytokines like, IFN-γ, have multiple and complex roles in immune development and function.

Overall, these studies using appropriate gene-targeted mice support a critical role for TNF-α and LT-α in the regulation of NK cell functions and show that a decrease in those functions correlates with a decrease in host resistance to tumor growth and metastasis.

3.2. Mice with Dysregulated FasL and Fas Genes Have Impaired Immune Systems and Diminished Cytokine-Mediated Antitumor Responses

The engagement of the Fas receptor by its naturally occurring ligand (FasL) or agonist Fas antibodies usually results in rapid induction of apoptosis *(36)*. There are naturally occurring, loss-of-function mutations for both the FasR (*lpr*) and the FasL (*gld*) genes *(37)*. In both cases, the mutant mice exhibit a lymphoproliferative syndrome and development of autoimmune disease. A central immunotherapeutic role for the Fas/FasL pathway has also been demonstrated through several approaches using *lpr* and *gld* mice. In particular, *gld* mice, which lack a functional FasL gene, have been used to investigate the cytotoxic and antitumor contributions of FasL+ effector cells, such as NK cells and activated T-cells *(37,38)*. The mechanisms for these effects can be direct destruction of Fas+ tumor cells by FasL-expressing effector cells *(38,39)*, or destruction of Fas+ tumor-associated neovascular endothelial cells by FasL+ leukocytes *(6)*. These antitumor capacities of endogenous *(39)* or cytokine-induced host responses *(6)* were lost when tumors were implanted into *gld* mice. Thus, the transfer of naturally occurring mutations in both the FasR and FasL genes to the BALB/c and C57BL/6 backgrounds has allowed the performance of a variety of studies illustrating the central role of the Fas pathway in several immunologic events critical for cancer detection or treatment.

3.3. Use of TRAIL-Deficient Mice in Models of Cancer Development and Immunotherapy

TNF-related apoptosis-inducing ligand (TRAIL) is a type II membrane member of the TNF superfamily *(40)* that induces apoptosis in a variety of normal and neoplastic cells. The recent development of TRAIL mutant mice (J. J. Peschon and M. Galccum, unpublished observations), and their subsequent backcross to both C57BL/6 and BALB/c backgrounds *(41)*, have provided unique mouse models to study the role of this potent apoptosis-inducing factor in tumor progression and therapy. Takeda et al. *(42)* have reported that treatment of tumor-bearing mice with an antibody specific for TRAIL increased the development of both MCA-induced fibrosarcomas and spontaneous tumors in $p53^{+/-}$ mice. The recent development of the C57BL/6 and BALB/c $TRAIL^{-/-}$ mice described above has allowed Cretney et al. *(41)* to show a vital role for functional TRAIL in NK-mediated resistance to formation of experimental Renca metastases in the liver and for the ability of αGalCer to induce regression of preexisting Renca micrometastases. Similarly, primary tumor growth and spontaneous metastases of the 4TJ mammary carcinoma were also enhanced in syngeneic $TRAIL^{-/-}$ BALB/c mice *(42)*, as was MCA-induced fibrosarcoma formation. Overall, the use of these novel $TRAIL^{-/-}$ mice has provided new information on the mechanisms by which NK cells contribute resistance against the formation of new primary tumors, as well as to resistance to metastatic spread. Further studies will use these mutant mice to determine the contributions of TRAIL to a variety of cytokine-based therapeutic approaches and thereby provide new insight into additional strategies for the immunotherapy of cancer.

4. Use of IL-12 and IL-18 Knockout Mice in Preclinical Tumor Studies

IL-12 and IL-18 are potent immunoregulatory cytokines that play key roles in linking nonspecific innate immune responses with the engagement of specific adaptive T-cell-mediated immunoregulatory mechanisms *(5,18)*. As such, substantial interest has focused on the potential use of these cytokines as components of immunotherapeutic approaches for the treatment of cancer.

IL-12 is a heterodimeric protein composed of covalently linked p35 and p40 subunits that enhances several aspects of T- and/or NK cell function including proliferation, cytokine production, and cytolytic activity *(5)*; it has demonstrated substantial therapeutic activity in a wide variety of murine tumor models *(5,16,17,19,43)*. Cell populations that produce the IL-12 p70 heterodimer may also synthesize and secrete free single-chain p40 as well as p40 homodimers *(44,45)*. These homodimers may serve as antagonists of the biologic effects of IL-12 p70 under certain circumstances *(45)*, although the overall role of p40 homodimers in the physiologic regulation of IL-12 function remains to be defined. IL-12 interacts with target cells via binding to receptors composed of β_1 and β_2 subunits *(46)*. Although the IL-12 p40 subunit may bind with low affinity to the β_1 subunit of the IL-12 receptor, high-affinity binding and functional signaling requires the concurrent presence of both the β_1 and β_2 subunits in the receptor complex.

Mice with targeted disruption of the genes encoding the p35 or p40 subunits of IL-12 *(47,48)*, as well as the respective β_1 *(49)* and β_2 *(50)* subunits of the IL-12 receptor complex, have now been generated. Interestingly, patients with well-characterized mutations in the genes encoding IL-12 p40 or the IL-12 receptor β_1 subunit have also been described *(51)*. Affected patients and mice with targeted disruption (–/–) of the respective components of the IL-12 pathway have a variety of immunologic impairments and increased susceptibility to a spectrum of infectious disorders, further emphasizing the central role of IL-12 in the immune response *(5,47–51)*. Various IL-12 and IL-12R$^{-/-}$ strains will be quite useful for detailed investigation of the role of the IL-12 pathway in the endogenous antitumor response and in the antitumor mechanisms engaged by other immune-based therapies.

Studies using gene targeted mice have to date focused on the role of IL-12 itself, and there have been no reports investigating the role of the respective IL-12 receptor subunits in mediating endogenous or therapeutically- induced antitumor immune responsiveness. A recent study by Smyth et al. *(52)* compared the role of T, NKT, and NK cell populations, perforin, and IL-12 in endogenous mechanisms of tumor control, using a panel of class I deficient tumors (YAC-1, RM-1, and EL4-S3). In these models, tumor rejection was similar in wild-type, IL-12 p40$^{-/-}$, and B6.Jα281$^{-/-}$ mice (lacking in Vα14Jα281+ NKT cells) or in mice depleted of T-cells with anti-Thy1 but was significantly attenuated in perforin$^{-/-}$ mice or in mice depleted of NK cells with NK1.1. Thus, endogenous IL-12 production does not play a role in tumor control in these models. In contrast, in mice treated with MCA, new fibrosarcoma tumors emerge more frequently and earlier in B6.Jα281$^{-/-}$ and IL-12p40$^{-/-}$ mice compared with wild-type control mice. These observations suggest a linkage between the participation of NKT cell populations and endogenous IL-12 production in mechanisms of tumor surveillance. In a syngeneic orthotopic model of murine MB49 bladder carcinoma, IL-12 p35$^{-/-}$ mice succumb to MB49 tumor inocula much more rapidly than age-matched wild-type control mice *(53)*. Similarly, we have observed that transplantable 3LL lung carcinoma tumors grow more rapidly in IL-12 p40$^{-/-}$ mice compared with 3LL-bearing wild-type mice (J. M. Wigginton, unpublished observations). Collectively, these studies suggest that IL-12 production plays a key role in the endogenous antitumor immune response in a variety of murine solid tumor models.

IL-12 also mediates therapeutic induction of the host antitumor response through immune-based mechanisms. In the immunogenic RMA murine lymphoma model, vaccination of mice with a single dose of irradiated tumor cells protects against a subsequent challenge with live tumor cells *(54)*. In contrast, IL-12p35$^{-/-}$ mice were unable to reject a subsequent live tumor challenge after a single vaccination with irradiated RMA tumor cells. Furthermore, ex vivo generation of cytotoxic T-lymphocyte (CTL) responses using splenocytes restimulated with tumor cells post vaccination was consistently more effective using splenocytes from wild-type mice compared with those from IL-12p35$^{-/-}$ mice. In this model, the induction of antigen-specific CTL responses also appears to be dependent on the presence of endogenous IL-12 produced by antigen-presenting cells (APCs). The induction of CTL responses by peptide-loaded bone marrow-derived dendritic cells (DCs) is significantly reduced when DCs from IL-12p35$^{-/-}$ mice are used as APCs compared with DCs derived from wild-type mice *(54)*. Intravesical administration of bacillus Calmette-Guérin (BCG) induces local secretion of cytokines including IL-12 in the bladders of treated patients *(55)* and significantly prolongs the survival of mice bearing MB49 bladder carcinoma *(53)*. In turn, the antitumor efficacy of intravesical BCG is ablated in IL-12 p35 knockout mice, and although administration of BCG induces a marked local infiltration of CD4+ and CD8+ T-cells and NK cells into MB49 tumors, enhancement of the infiltration of CD8+ T-cells by BCG is not observed in IL-12p35$^{-/-}$ mice *(53)*.

The observation that IL-18 and IL-12 both potently enhance the production of IFN-γ *(5,18)* and possess substantial single agent antitumor activity *(5,16,17,19,20,43,56)*, led to the proposal that IL-12 might mediate the antitumor activity of IL-18. Although CL8-1 melanoma tumors grow more rapidly in IL-12 p40$^{-/-}$ mice than in wild-type mice, the antitumor activity of IL-18 against this tumor is mediated via mechanisms that are independent of endogenous IL-12 production *(20)*. Notably, IL-12 actually induces the production of IL-18, and the induction of IFN-γ by IL-12 occurs via mechanisms that are dependent of caspase-1-mediated cleavage of pro-IL-18 into mature IL-18 *(57)*. These studies suggest that IL-18 can under some circumstances mediate at least some of the potent antitumor mechanisms engaged by IL-12.

IL-18 is a potent immunoregulatory cytokine, which was initially described as interferon-γ-inducing factor (IGIF) *(58,59)*. IL-18 enhances T and/or NK cell cytokine production, proliferation, and cytolytic activity *(18,60)*, as well as the expression of FasL and FASL or perforin-mediated cytotoxicity *(61–63)*; systemic administration of IL-18 protein has demonstrated considerable therapeutic activity in murine tumor models *(20,56)*. The biology of IL-18 has been reviewed previously in detail *(5,18)*. IL-18 is synthesized as a pro-IL-18 precursor that lacks a signal peptide and is processed to mature, biologically active IL-18 via cleavage mediated by IL-1β-converting enzyme (ICE). In turn, IL-18 binds to a specific receptor on target cells consisting of a cytokine-binding receptor chain [originally described as IL-1R-related protein (IL-1Rrp)] and an accessory protein-like chain (AcPL). Binding of IL-18 leads to the recruitment and activation of IL-1R-associated kinase (IRAK), TNF receptor-associated factor-6 (TRAF-6), nuclear factor (NF)-κB, and c-Jun N-terminal kinase (JNK) *(5,18)*. MyD88, originally isolated as a myeloid differentiation factor, interacts with IRAK, and appears to play a role in mediating IL-18-induced activation of NF-κB and JNK *(64)*. Mice with targeted disruption of IL-18 *(65)*, caspase-1/ICE *(66)*, IL-1Rrp *(67)*, IRAK *(68)*, and MyD88 *(64)* have been reported; a number of specific impairments in immune function, and in some instances increased susceptibility to infection, have been observed in these mice *(18,64–68)*. Despite the central role of IL-18 as a link between innate and adaptive immune responses *(5,18)* and the potent antitumor activity of IL-18 *(20,56)*, there have been no studies reported to date using IL-18$^{-/-}$ mice to investigate the role of IL-18 as a mediator of either endogenous or therapeutically induced antitumor immune responses.

5. Cytokine Knockout Mice and Experimental Bone Marrow Transplantation

The use of hematopoietic stem cell transplantation (HSCT) has dramatically risen since the mid-1980s and has become a widely used approach for cancer treatment. Although the number of autologous transplants has declined in the last few years owing to the reduction in the use of this treatment for breast cancer (International Bone Marrow Transplant Registry, 2002) and the number of allogeneic transplants per year has leveled off, these procedures were performed on an estimated 40–50,000 persons worldwide in 2001. In autologous HSCT, the patient is also the donor for the transplant. Hematopoietic stem cells, in the form of either blood or bone marrow, are collected and cryopreserved prior to high-dose radio- and/or chemotherapy to treat the underlying cancer. The thawed cells are returned to the patient to rescue the hematopoietic system destroyed in the cancer therapy. In contrast, in allogeneic HSCT a donor provides the source of hematopoietic stem cells that are infused into the patient after conditioning regimens that can utilize either chemo- or radiotherapy or both. The donor graft is intended to provide both hematopoietic rescue and antitumor activity. It is still unclear whether the antitumor activity is specific to the tumor or represents a more generalized allogeneic response. Experimental models of allogeneic murine bone marrow transplantation (alloBMT) have given investigators the tools to dissect the mechanisms of both antitumor responses (graft-versus-tumor; GvT) and anti-host (graft-versus-host disease, GvHD) responses. Induction of the first and avoidance of the second is key to successful treatment of cancer with alloBMT. The use of various cytokine knockout mice has allowed great insight into the complex roles of various effector and immunoregulatory molecules in these processes.

5.1. Study of Effector Mechanisms in Experimental BMT

Availability of various genetically disparate strains has resulted in the development of several commonly employed models of alloBMT, each with distinct advantages and limitations. Although they may sometimes provide conflicting results, careful analysis of the experimental data can lead to a better understanding of how various effector molecules and cell types contribute to complex cellular interactions involved in T-cell activation, expansion, and inflammatory processes. One example of disparate results from various investigators studying GvHD and GvT involves the use of mice with deficiencies in effector mechanisms that resulted from spontaneous mutations (*gld* and *lpr*) or were genetically engineered (perforin knockouts; pfp$^{-/-}$). It has been reported that perforin is one mechanism by which allogeneic T-cells affect GHvD pathology *(69–72)*, whereas other laboratories claim that perforin does not play an important role in GvHD *(73,74)* but is a critical component of effective GvT responses *(72,74–77)*. Conversely, through the use of *gld* mice, it has been shown that FasL appears to be an important mediator of GvHD but not GvT *(72,74,78)*, although some investigators have shown a role for FasL-dependent GvT mediated by CD4+ T-cells *(77)*.

The conflicting reports can be explained, in part, by the differences and complexities in the various models employed for these studies and, importantly, by the tumor cell lines used to assess GvT effects. Several factors can influence the outcome of GvHD. Some are intrinsic to the model; the amount of conditioning can cause tissue damage and initiate inflammatory processes, and it is an important mechanism to reduce host resistance. Also, both the type and degree of MHC incompatibility and other genetic differences in the strains can affect outcome. Jiang and colleagues *(73)* have shown that mutations resulting in diminished FasL activity (*gld*) can result in delayed GvHD when the transplant is performed under conditions that preserve a greater portion of host resistance. When host resistance is ablated with higher doses of conditioning, T-cells from *gld* mice are as effective as T-cells from wild-type mice in the induction of GvHD. Similarly, two groups found that perforin was a major contributor to CD8+ T-cell mediated GvHD but disagreed on the role of perforin in CD4+ T-cell-mediated GvHD *(69,71)*. Differences in the amount of conditioning and tissue targets of GvHD could account for the discordance.

These results illustrate the value and challenges of using mice with dysregulated lytic mechanisms to dissect the complex mechanisms involved in GvHD and GvT. Additionally, some tumor types are more susceptible to a particular lytic pathway (i.e., Fas, perforin) and by a particular effector population (i.e., NK or T-cells).

5.2. Cytokines and GvHD

Differences in conditioning regimens can alter patterns of cytokine expression that can ultimately influence the outcome of GvHD and GvT at various stages of disease pathophysiology. These stages include an initiation phase of allogeneic recognition, followed by the alloreactive T-cell expansion phase and concurrent cytokine storm and finally the effector phase *(79)*. IL-12 *(80)* and IL-18 *(81)* have been shown to be important inducers of Fas, resulting in donor T-cell apoptosis and ultimately amelioration of GvHD. Administration of either of these cytokines reduced GvHD, and the activity was lost when Fas-deficient donor T-cells were employed. For IL-18 and presumably IL-12 administration, induction of IFN-γ by donor T-cells is a critical event *(14)*.

Acute GvHD has been associated with the type 1 pattern of cytokine expression. High levels of inflammatory cytokines such as IL-12, IFN-γ, IL-1, and TNF-α are observed during the early phase of allogeneic T-cell expansion. However, the use of cytokine$^{-/-}$ mice has demonstrated that the classic paradigm does not always clearly fit. The pleotropic and often redundant activity of the cytokines and the complexity of biologic systems has often resulted in unexpected findings when cytokine$^{-/-}$ mice were employed. Specifically, loss of IFN-γ expression in donor T-cells resulted in an unexpected acceleration in acute lethal GvHD in mice that received high-dose radiotherapy for pretransplant conditioning, whereas loss of IL-4 expression in donor T-cells ameliorated disease *(82)*. Accelerated disease in IFN-γ$^{-/-}$ mice was associated with increased production of IL-2 *(82)*. The studies of Reddy and colleagues *(81)* provided information showing that IFN-γ is important in autocrine upregulation of Fas and control of alloreactive T-cell proliferation. However, lack of IFN-γ expression by donor T-cells does not always result in exacerbation of GvHD. When the intensity of the conditioning regimen is lowered, IFN-γ expression in donor T-cells is associated with accelerated GvHD *(83,84)*. In these models, Fas-dependent cytotoxicity may be the major mechanism for GvHD-associated tissue injury, and loss of IFN-γ would result in diminished or protracted disease.

Overall, these disparate conclusions regarding the mechanisms of GvHD and GvT illustrate the complexity of the biologic responses and the limitations of individual genetically altered experimental mice but illustrate the power to clarify complex events when multiple different gene-modified mouse models are studied in concert.

Conclusion

The use of cytokine knockout mice has proven to be a unique and highly informative resource for untangling the complex web of Th1-cytokine mediated contributions to prevention and treatment of cancer. Unique gene-targeted mice have allowed the scientific community to gain new insight into the critical role of IFN-γ in regulating tumor development, progression, and immune-mediated rejection. Similarly, IFN-γ targeted mice have also been central to dissecting the contributions of NK, NKT, and T cells in these processes. The use of mice with targeted deletions in various members of the TNF superfamily of genes has also been vital for implicating specific family members in the structure and function of the immune system, as well as the key role of family members in antitumor effector mechanisms. Many recent conclusions about the interplay between innate and adaptive components of the immune system for immune response development and antitumor effects have been provided by experiments performed in mice lacking functional IL-12 or IL-18 genes. Finally, cytokine knockout mice have been used to identify and exploit complex cytokine-cytokine interferons in the setting of BMT and GvHD. Overall, the use of existing cytokine gene-targeted mice, and the development of new ones, will continue to provide vital information on the functions and therapeutic applications of these powerful immune regulators for years to come.

Acknowledgments

The content of this publication does not necessarily reflect the views or policies of the Department of Health and Human Services, nor does mention of trade names, commercial products, or organizations imply endorsement by the U.S. Government. Animal care was provided in accordance with the procedures outlined in the *Guide for the Care and Use of Laboratory Animals* (NIH Pub. No. 86-23, 1985).

This publication was funded in whole or in part with Federal funds from the National Cancer Institute, National Institutes of Health, under contract no. N01-CO-12400.

References

1. Belardelli, F. and Ferrantini, M. (2002) Cytokines as a link between innate and adaptive antitumor immunity. *Trends Immunol.* **23,** 201–208.
2. Fearon, D. T. and Locksley, R. M. (1996) The instructive role of innate immunity in the acquired immune response. *Science* **272,** 50–53.
3. Smyth, M. J., Godfrey, D. I., and Trapani, J. A. (2001) A fresh look at tumor immunosurveillance and immunotherapy. *Nat. Immunol.* **2,** 293–299.
4. Coughlin, C. M., Salhany, K. E., Wysocka, M., et al. (1998) Interleukin-12 and interleukin-18 synergistically induce murine tumor regression which involves inhibition of angiogenesis. *J. Clin. Invest.* **101,** 1441–1452.
5. Trinchieri, G. (1998) Interleukin-12: a cytokine at the interface of inflammation and immunity. *Adv. Immunol.* **70,** 83–243.
6. Wigginton, J. M., Gruys, E., Geiselhart, L., et al. (2001) IFN-gamma and Fas/FasL are required for the antitumor and antiangiogenic effects of IL-12/pulse IL-2 therapy. *J. Clin. Invest.* **108,** 51–62.
7. Fyfe, G., Fisher, R. I., Rosenberg, S. A., Sznol, M., Parkinson, D. R., and Louie, A. C. (1995) Results of treatment of 255 patients with metastatic renal cell carcinoma who received high-dose recombinant interleukin-2 therapy. *J. Clin. Oncol.* **13,** 688–696.
8. Atkins, M. B., Lotze, M. T., Dutcher, J. P., et al. (1999) High-dose recombinant interleukin 2 therapy for patients with metastatic melanoma: analysis of 270 patients treated between 1985 and 1993. *J. Clin Oncol.* **17,** 2105–2116.
9. Biron, C. A. (2001) Interferons alpha and beta as immune regulators—a new look. *Immunity* **14,** 661–664.
10. Ikeda, H., Old, L. J., and Schreiber, R. D. (2002) The roles of IFNgamma in protection against tumor development and cancer immunoediting. *Cytokine Growth Factor Rev.* **13,** 95–109.
11. Dalton, D. K., Pitts-Meek, S., Keshav, S., Figari, I. S., Bradley, A., and Stewart, T. A. (1993) Multiple defects of immune cell function in mice with disrupted interferon-gamma genes. *Science* **259,** 1739–1742.
12. Huang, S., Hendriks, W., Althage, A., et al. (1993) Immune response in mice that lack the interferon-gamma receptor. *Science* **259,** 1742–1745.
13. Lu, B., Ebensperger, C., Dembic, Z., et al. (1998) Targeted disruption of the interferon-gamma receptor 2 gene results in severe immune defects in mice. *Proc. Natl. Acad. Sci. USA* **95,** 8233–8238.
14. Kaplan, D. H., Shankaran, V., Dighe, A. S., et al. (1998) Demonstration of an interferon gamma-dependent tumor surveillance system in immunocompetent mice. *Proc. Natl. Acad. Sci. USA* **95,** 7556–7561.

15. Street, S. E., Cretney, E., and Smyth, M. J. (2001) Perforin and interferon-gamma activities independently control tumor initiation, growth, and metastasis. *Blood* **97,** 192–197.
16. Brunda, M. J., Luistro, L., Warrier, R. R., et al. (1993) Antitumor and antimetastatic activity of interleukin 12 against murine tumors. *J. Exp. Med.* **178,** 1223–1230.
17. Nastala, C. L., Edington, H. D., McKinney, T. G., et al. (1994) Recombinant IL-12 administration induces tumor regression in association with IFN-gamma production. *J. Immunol.* **153,** 1697–1706.
18. Dinarello, C. A. (1999) IL-18: A TH1-inducing, proinflammatory cytokine and new member of the IL-1 family. *J. Allergy Clin. Immunol.* **103,** 11–24.
19. Coughlin, C. M., Salhany, K. E., Gee, M. S., et al. (1998) Tumor cell responses to IFNgamma affect tumorigenicity and response to IL-12 therapy and antiangiogenesis. *Immunity* **9,** 25–34.
20. Osaki, T., Peron, J. M., Cai, Q., et al. (1998) IFN-gamma-inducing factor/IL-18 administration mediates IFN-gamma-and IL-12-independent antitumor effects. *J. Immunol.* **160,** 1742–1749.
21. Wigginton, J. M., Lee, J.-K., Wiltrout, T. A., et al. (2002) Synergistic engagement of an ineffective endogenous antitumor immune response and induction of IFN-gamma and FAS-L-dependent tumor irradication by combined administration of interleukin-18 and interleukin-2. *J. Immunol.* **8,** 4467–4474.
22. Wigginton, J. M., Park, J. W., Young, H. A., et al. (2001) Complete regression of established spontaneous mammary carcinoma, and therapeutic prevention of genetically-programmed neoplastic transition by IL-12/pulse IL-2: induction of local T cell infiltration, Fas/FasL gene expression and mammary epithelial apoptosis. *J. Immunol.* **166,** 1156–1168.
23. Tannenbaum, C. S., Tubbs, R., Armstrong, D., Finke, J. H., Bukowski, R. M., and Hamilton, T. A. (1998) The CXC chemokines IP-10 and Mig are necessary for IL-12-mediated regression of the mouse RENCA tumor. *J. Immunol.* **161,** 927–932.
24. Kanegane, C., Sgadari, C., Kanegane, H., et al. (1998) Contribution of the CXC chemokines IP-10 and Mig to the antitumor effects of IL-12. *J. Leukoc. Biol.* **64,** 384–392.
25. Dufour, J. H., Dziejman, M., Liu, M. T., Leung, J. H., Lane, T. E., and Luster, A. D. (2002) IFN-gamma-inducible protein 10 (IP-10; CXCL10)-deficient mice reveal a role for IP-10 in effector T cell generation and trafficking. *J. Immunol.* **168,** 3195–3204.
26. Hancock, W. W., Lu, B., Gao, W., et al. (2000) Requirement of the chemokine receptor CXCR3 for acute allograft rejection. *J. Exp. Med.* **192,** 1515–1520.
27. Smyth, M. J., Crowe, N. Y., Pellicci, D. G., et al. (2002) Sequential production of interferon-gamma by NK1.1(+) T cells and natural killer cells is essential for the antimetastatic effect of alpha-galactosylceramide. *Blood* **99,** 1259–1266.
28. Pilaro, A. M., Taub, D. D., McCormick, K. L., et al. (1994) TNF-alpha is a principal cytokine involved in the recruitment of NK cells to liver parenchyma. *J. Immunol.* **153,** 333–342.
29. Marino, M. W., Dunn, A., Grail, D., et al. (1997) Characterization of tumor necrosis factor-deficient mice. *Proc. Natl. Acad. Sci. USA* **94,** 8093–8098.
30. Smyth, M. J., Kelly, J. M., Baxter, A. G., Korner, H., and Sedgwick, J. D. (1998) An essential role for tumor necrosis factor in natural killer cell-mediated tumor rejection in the peritoneum. *J. Exp. Med.* **188,** 1611–1619.
31. Arnott, C. H., Scott, K. A., Moore, R. J., et al. (2002) Tumour necrosis factor-alpha mediates tumour promotion via a PKCalpha- and AP-1-dependent pathway. *Oncogene* **21,** 4728–4738.
32. Smyth, M. J., Johnstone, R. W., Cretney, E., et al. (1999) Multiple deficiencies underlie NK cell inactivity in lymphotoxin-alpha gene-targeted mice. *J. Immunol.* **163,** 1350–1353.
33. Ito, D., Back, T. C., Shakhov, A. N., Wiltrout, R. H., and Nedospasov, S. A. (1999) Mice with a targeted mutation in lymphotoxin-alpha exhibit enhanced tumor growth and metastasis: impaired NK cell development and recruitment. *J. Immunol.* **163,** 2809–2815.
34. Alimzhanov, M. B., Kuprash, D. V., Kosco-Vilbois, M. H., et al. (1997) Abnormal development of secondary lymphoid tissues in lymphotoxin beta-deficient mice. *Proc Natl Acad Sci USA* **94,** 9302–9307.
35. Hill, G. R., Teshima, T., Rebel, V. I., et al. (2000) The p55 TNF-alpha receptor plays a critical role in T cell alloreactivity. *J. Immunol* **164,** 656–663.
36. Nagata, S. (1997) Apoptosis by death factor. *Cell* **88,** 355–365.
37. Nagata, S. and Suda, T. (1995) Fas and Fas ligand: lpr and gld mutations. *Immunol. Today* **16,** 39–43.

38. Sayers, T. J., Brooks, A. D., Lee, J. K., et al. (1998) Molecular mechanisms of immune-mediated lysis of murine renal cancer: differential contributions of perforin-dependent versus Fas-mediated pathways in lysis by NK and T cells. *J. Immunol.* **161,** 3957–3965.
39. Lee, J. K., Sayers, T. J., Brooks, A. D., et al. (2000) IFN-gamma-dependent delay of in vivo tumor progression by Fas overexpression on murine renal cancer cells. *J. Immunol.* **164,** 231–239.
40. Wiley, S. R., Schooley, K., Smolak, P. J., et al. (1995) Identification and characterization of a new member of the TNF family that induces apoptosis. *Immunity* **3,** 673–682.
41. Cretney, E., Takeda, K., Yagita, H., Glaccum, M., Peschon, J. J., and Smyth, M. J. (2002) Increased susceptibility to tumor initiation and metastasis in TNF-related apoptosis-inducing ligand-deficient mice. *J. Immunol.* **168,** 1356–1361.
42. Takeda, K., Smyth, M. J., Cretney, E., et al. (2002) Critical role for tumor necrosis factor-related apoptosis-inducing ligand in immune surveillance against tumor development. *J. Exp. Med.* **195,** 161–169.
43. Colombo, M. P. and Trinchieri, G. (2002) Interleukin-12 in anti-tumor immunity and immunotherapy. *Cytokine Growth Factor Rev.* **13,** 155–168.
44. D'Andrea, A., Rengaraju, M., Valiante, N. M., et al. (1992) Production of natural killer cell stimulatory factor (interleukin 12) by peripheral blood mononuclear cells. *J. Exp. Med.* **176,** 1387–1398.
45. Gillessen, S., Carvajal, D., Ling, P., et al. (1995) Mouse interleukin-12 (IL-12) p40 homodimer: a potent IL-12 antagonist. *Eur. J. Immunol.* **25,** 200–206.
46. Gately, M. K., Renzetti, L. M., Magram, J., et al. (1998) The interleukin-12/interleukin-12-receptor system: role in normal and pathologic immune responses. *Annu. Rev. Immunol.* **16,** 495–521.
47. Mattner, F., Magram, J., Ferrante, J., et al. (1996) Genetically resistant mice lacking interleukin-12 are susceptible to infection with Leishmania major and mount a polarized Th2 cell response. *Eur. J. Immunol.* **26,** 1553–1559.
48. Magram, J., Connaughton, S. E., Warrier, R. R., et al. (1996) IL-12-deficient mice are defective in IFN gamma production and type 1 cytokine responses. *Immunity* **4,** 471–481.
49. Wu, C., Ferrante, J., Gately, M. K., and Magram, J. (1997) Characterization of IL-12 receptor beta1 chain (IL-12Rbeta1)-deficient mice: IL-12Rbeta1 is an essential component of the functional mouse IL-12 receptor. *J. Immunol.* **159,** 1658–1665.
50. Wu, C., Wang, X., Gadina, M., O'Shea, J. J., Presky, D. H., and Magram, J. (2000) IL-12 receptor beta 2 (IL-12R beta 2)-deficient mice are defective in IL-12-mediated signaling despite the presence of high affinity IL-12 binding sites. *J. Immunol.* **165,** 6221–6228.
51. Dorman, S. E. and Holland, S. M. (2000) Interferon-gamma and interleukin-12 pathway defects and human disease. *Cytokine Growth Factor Rev.* **11,** 321–333.
52. Smyth, M. J., Thia, K. Y., Street, S. E., et al. (2000) Differential tumor surveillance by natural killer (NK) and NKT cells. *J. Exp. Med.* **191,** 661–668.
53. Riemensberger, J., Bohle, A., and Brandau, S. (2002) IFN-gamma and IL-12 but not IL-10 are required for local tumour surveillance in a syngeneic model of orthotopic bladder cancer. *Clin. Exp. Immunol.* **127,** 20–26.
54. Grufman, P. and Karre, K. (2000) Innate and adaptive immunity to tumors: IL-12 is required for optimal responses. *Eur. J. Immunol.* **30,** 1088–1093.
55. Schamhart, D. H., de Boer, E. C., de Reijke, T. M., and Kurth, K. (2000) Urinary cytokines reflecting the immunological response in the urinary bladder to biological response modifiers: their practical use. *Eur. Urol.* **37(Suppl. 3),** 16–23.
56. Hashimoto, W., Osaki, T., Okamura, H., et al. (1999) Differential antitumor effects of administration of recombinant IL-18 or recombinant IL-12 are mediated primarily by Fas-Fas ligand. *J. Immunol.* **163,** 583–589.
57. Fantuzzi, G., Reed, D. A., and Dinarello, C. A. (1999) IL-12-induced IFN-gamma is dependent on caspase-1 processing of the IL-18 precursor. *J. Clin. Invest.* **104,** 761–767.
58. Nakamura, K., Okamura, H., Wada, M., Nagata, K., and Tamura, T. (1989) Endotoxin-induced serum factor that stimulates gamma interferon production. *Infect. Immun.* **57,** 590–595.
59. Okamura, H., Tsutsi, H., Komatsu, T., et al. (1995) Cloning of a new cytokine that induces IFN-gamma production by T cells. *Nature* **378,** 88–91.
60. Okamura, H., Tsutsui, H., Kashiwamura, S., Yoshimoto, T., and Nakanishi, K. (1998) Interleukin-18: a novel cytokine that augments both innate and acquired immunity. *Adv. Immunol.* **70,** 281–312.

61. Tsutsui, H., Nakanishi, K., Matsui, K., et al. (1996) IFN-gamma-inducing factor up-regulates Fas ligand-mediated cytotoxic activity of murine natural killer cell clones. *J. Immunol.* **157,** 3967–3973.
62. Dao, T., Ohashi, K., Kayano, T., Kurimoto, M., and Okamura, H. (1996) Interferon-gamma-inducing factor, a novel cytokine, enhances Fas ligand-mediated cytotoxicity of murine T helper 1 cells. *Cell. Immunol.* **173,** 230–235.
63. Dao, T., Mehal, W. Z., and Crispe, I. N. (1998) IL-18 augments perforin-dependent cytotoxicity of liver NK-T cells. *J. Immunol.* **161,** 2217–2222.
64. Adachi, O., Kawai, T., Takeda, K., et al. (1998) Targeted disruption of the MyD88 gene results in loss of IL-1- and IL-18-mediated function. *Immunity* **9,** 143–150.
65. Takeda, K., Tsutsui, H., Yoshimoto, T., et al. (1998) Defective NK cell activity and Th1 response in IL-18-deficient mice. *Immunity* **8,** 383–390.
66. Kuida, K., Lippke, J. A., Ku, G., et al. (1995) Altered cytokine export and apoptosis in mice deficient in interleukin-1 beta converting enzyme. *Science* **267,** 2000–2003.
67. Hoshino, K., Tsutsui, H., Kawai, T., et al. (1999) Cutting edge: generation of IL-18 receptor-deficient mice: evidence for IL-1 receptor-related protein as an essential IL-18 binding receptor. *J. Immunol.* **162,** 5041–5044.
68. Thomas, J. A., Allen, J. L., Tsen, M., et al. (1999) Impaired cytokine signaling in mice lacking the IL-1 receptor-associated kinase. *J. Immunol.* **163,** 978–984.
69. Blazar, B. R., Taylor, P. A., and Vallera, D. A. (1997) CD4+ and CD8+ T cells each can utilize a perforin-dependent pathway to mediate lethal graft-versus-host disease in major histocompatibility complex-disparate recipients. *Transplantation* **64,** 571–576.
70. Braun, M. Y., Lowin, B., French, L., Acha-Orbea, H., and Tschopp, J. (1996) Cytotoxic T cells deficient in both functional fas ligand and perforin show residual cytolytic activity yet lose their capacity to induce lethal acute graft-versus-host disease. *J. Exp. Med.* **183,** 657–661.
71. Graubert, T. A., DiPersio, J. F., Russell, J. H., and Ley, T. J. (1997) Perforin/granzyme-dependent and independent mechanisms are both important for the development of graft-versus-host disease after murine bone marrow transplantation. *J. Clin. Invest.* **100,** 904–911.
72. Tsukada, N., Kobata, T., Aizawa, Y., Yagita, H., and Okumura, K. (1999) Graft-versus-leukemia effect and graft-versus-host disease can be differentiated by cytotoxic mechanisms in a murine model of allogeneic bone marrow transplantation. *Blood* **93,** 2738–2747.
73. Jiang, Z., Podack, E., and Levy, R. B. (2001) Major histocompatibility complex-mismatched allogeneic bone marrow transplantation using perforin and/or Fas ligand double-defective CD4(+) donor T cells: involvement of cytotoxic function by donor lymphocytes prior to graft-versus-host disease pathogenesis. *Blood* **98,** 390–397.
74. Schmaltz, C., Alpdogan, O., Horndasch, K. J., et al. (2001) Differential use of Fas ligand and perforin cytotoxic pathways by donor T cells in graft-versus-host disease and graft-versus-leukemia effect. *Blood* **97,** 2886–2895.
75. Pan, L., Teshima, T., Hill, G. R., et al. (1999) Granulocyte colony-stimulating factor-mobilized allogeneic stem cell transplantation maintains graft-versus-leukemia effects through a perforin-dependent pathway while preventing graft-versus-host disease. *Blood* **93,** 4071–4078.
76. Hsieh, M. H. and Korngold, R. (2000) Differential use of FasL- and perforin-mediated cytolytic mechanisms by T-cell subsets involved in graft-versus-myeloid leukemia responses. *Blood* **96,** 1047–1055.
77. Hsieh, M. H., Patterson, A. E., and Korngold, R. (2000) T-cell subsets mediate graft-versus-myeloid leukemia responses via different cytotoxic mechanisms. *Biol. Blood Marrow Transplant.* **6,** 231–240.
78. Lan, F., Zeng, D., Huie, P., Higgins, J. P., and Strober, S. (2001) Allogeneic bone marrow cells that facilitate complete chimerism and eliminate tumor cells express both CD8 and T-cell antigen receptor-alphabeta. *Blood* **97,** 3458–3465.
79. Ferrara, J. L., Cooke, K. R., Pan, L., and Krenger, W. (1996) The immunopathophysiology of acute graft-versus-host-disease. *Stem Cells* **14,** 473–489.
80. Dey, B. R., Yang, Y. G., Szot, G. L., Pearson, D. A., and Sykes, M. (1998) Interleukin-12 inhibits graft-versus-host disease through a Fas-mediated mechanism associated with alterations in donor T-cell activation and expansion. *Blood* **91,** 3315–3322.

81. Reddy, P., Teshima, T., Kukuruga, M., et al. (2001) Interleukin-18 regulates acute graft-versus-host disease by enhancing Fas-mediated donor T cell apoptosis. *J. Exp. Med.* **194,** 1433–1440.
82. Murphy, W. J., Welniak, L. A., Taub, D. D., et al. (1998) Differential effects of the absence of interferon-gamma and IL-4 in acute graft-versus-host disease after allogeneic bone marrow transplantation in mice. *J. Clin. Invest.* **102,** 1742–1748.
83. Welniak, L. A., Blazar, B. R., Anver, M. R., Wiltrout, R. H., and Murphy, W. J. (2000) Opposing roles of interferon-gamma on CD4+ T cell-mediated graft-versus-host disease: effects of conditioning. *Biol. Blood Marrow Transplant.* **6,** 604–612.
84. Ellison, C. A., Fischer, J. M., HayGlass, K. T., and Gartner, J. G. (1998) Murine graft-versus-host disease in an F1-hybrid model using IFN-gamma gene knockout donors. *J. Immunol.* **161,** 631–640.

5

The Use of Cytokine Knockout Mice in Neuroimmunology

Giamal N. Luheshi, Emmanuel Pinteaux, and Hervé Boutin

Summary

In this chapter, we have attempted to provide a synopsis of current work being performed using cytokine knockout or transgenic animals in neuroimmunology research. This is a fast-growing area that is expanding dramatically as genetically modified animals for cytokines, their receptors, or signalling components become available. We have focused primarily on the best-known cytokines (IL-1, IL-6, TNF-α, IL-10 & IL-4) simply to highlight the contribution so far of this tool to research into cytokines and neuroimmunology. In addition and as a reflection of the growing areas of research using this technology, we were limited to focusing on the use of genetically modified animals in two areas, namely, fever as a model of infection and stroke following middle cerebral artery occlusion as an approach to study brain injury and inflammation.

Key words

interleukins-1, 4, 6, and 10, tumor necrosis factor, fever, stroke, primary cultures, infection, injury, inflammation

1. Introduction

The last decade has seen an explosion in the area of cytokine research, in particular the role of cytokines as neuroimmune modulators of central nervous system (CNS)-mediated responses to infection, inflammation or injury. The importance of these mediators became increasingly apparent as the extent of their actions and influence on these events became better understood. These discoveries have been aided by an array of new technologies and advances that have facilitated the unravelling of the role of these molecules. The development of genetically modified organisms represents possibly the greatest advance in this and other areas of research. The notion of developing a genetically designed mouse that has the gene of a particular cytokine, either deleted or modified such that it could be overexpressed, presented a tool that has already had significant impact on many areas of research. Not surprisingly, researchers in the cytokine field have taken full advantage of this technology, especially since genetically modified mice are now available for most proinflammatory cytokines and in some cases their immediate family members, including their receptors, signaling peptides, and in the case of interleukin (IL)-1 its endogenously occurring receptor antagonist. More recently animals have also been developed to study some of the antiinflammatory cytokines, the importance of which is becoming more recognizable in neuroimmunology research.

From: *Contemporary Immunology: Cytokine Knockouts, 2nd Edition*
Edited by: Giamila Fantuzzi © Humana Press Inc., Totowa, NJ

For the purposes of this chapter we focus primarily on the relatively more important or at least more recognizable proinflammatory cytokines, such as IL-1, IL-6, and tumor necrosis factor (TNF)-α, and two antiinflammatory cytokines, namely, IL-4 and IL-10. In addition, we concentrate only on the use of these genetically modified animals in areas involving studies of systemic infection/inflammation (as represented by research on fever) and their role in neurodegenerative processes, by focusing mainly on cerebral ischemia.

2. Interleukin-1

IL-1 is the first discovered and by far the best studied member of the cytokine family. It is not surprising therefore that a great deal of effort has been expended in the development of genetically modified animals for all the components of the IL-1 system, including the enzyme caspase-1 (which cleaves the 32-kDa proform of IL-1 into its mature 17-kDa form), the IL-1 type I receptor (IL-1RI), IL-1 receptor accessory protein (IL-1RAcP), the two ligands (IL-1α, IL-1β), and the endogenous IL-1 receptor antagonist (IL-1Ra) *(1–4)*. In fact, the only component of the IL-1 family for which a knockout mouse is not available is the IL-1 type II receptor (IL-1RII). This 68-kDa receptor has a short intracellular domain and does not initiate signal transduction, acting instead as a decoy soluble receptor.

IL-1 was the first discovered endogenous pyrogen (for review, *see* ref. *5*), and most of the early work on IL-1 was conducted on its role in fever. The availability of knockout animals facilitated research into its function as an endogenous mediator of the febrile response to infection or inflammation. Despite the established role of IL-1 in fever, studies on genetically modified animals proved contradictory, and to a large extent did not reproduce data obtained using pharmacologic means of neutralizing action, i.e., antibodies or the receptor antagonist IL-1Ra *(6,7)*. For example, one of the earlier studies using IL-1RI knockout mice demonstrated identical fevers in the knockout compared with wild-type mice in response to low and high doses of bacterial lipopolysaccharide (LPS) administered intraperitoneally (ip) *(8)*, a potent exogenous pyrogen and inducer of cytokines both in vivo and in vitro. Interestingly, in the same study, the febrile response was totally abolished in the knockout compared with wild-type mice when the animals received a single intramuscular (im) injection of the local inflammatory stimulus turpentine instead of LPS. Similar experiments, using the IL-1 knockouts again produced contradictory data following a single injection of LPS but clear-cut data when turpentine was used instead. Kozak and colleagues *(9)* demonstrated that IL-1β knockout and wild-type mice responded to a single dose of LPS in an identical manner, whereas Alheim et al. *(10)* demonstrated a hyperresponsiveness of IL-1β to a single injection of LPS in IL-1β knockout mice. In contrast, and similar to the findings obtained from the IL-1RI knockout studies, injection of turpentine in IL-1β knockout mice failed to produce a fever *(4,11)*. In the same studies, injection of turpentine, this time into IL-1α knockout mice, produced normal febrile responses, indicating that in models of localized inflammation, IL-1β is the main mediator of fever.

On the whole, these data are rather confusing given that if IL-1β is an essential component of the fever response to LPS, one would expect that fever generated in response to LPS by mice not expressing the genes for IL-1 or its functional receptor (IL-1RI) should at the very least be attenuated. These observations are even more puzzling given the absence of a fever response in turpentine-treated IL-1β and IL-1RI knockout animals, especially since fevers in response to both exogenous stimuli (LPS and turpentine) are significantly attenuated by ip injection of IL-1Ra in rats *(7,12)*. One possibility for the differences between

LPS and turpentine could be direct actions of LPS on the brain. Alternatively, LPS could still be inducing a febrile response in these animals via the induction of another circulating cytokine, most likely IL-6 (for excellent reviews of this area, *see* ref. *13–15*), or another functional receptor.

Apart from their use in fever studies, IL-1 family knockouts and transgenics are being increasingly used in other areas of research such as neurodegeneration. The role of endogenous cytokines, in particular IL-1, in chronic and acute neurodegenerative diseases is well established (for reviews, *see* ref. *16*) *(17–19)*. The involvement of IL-1 in neurodegeneration was first confirmed in cerebral ischemia *(20–23)*. These studies showed that in rodents that have undergone middle cerebral artery occlusion (MCAO; a recognized rodent model for human stroke), addition of IL-1 exacerbated ischemic damage whereas addition of IL-1Ra dramatically reduced this damage, as assessed by the size of the infarct (for review, *see* ref. *24*). Similar studies, this time utilizing genetically modified mice, have since confirmed these findings and added significantly to our understanding of how IL-1 is involved in ischemic-neuronal death. Most of these studies were conducted using a well-established model of cerebral ischemia in mice; MCAO was induced by insertion of a thread in the carotid up to the bifurcation between the middle cerebral artery and the circle of Willis *(25)*. Following permanent focal cerebral ischemia in mice expressing a dominant negative form of caspase-1 (the enzyme responsible for cleaving the inactive proform to the active mature form of IL-1β), Friedlander et al. *(26)* demonstrated a significant reduction in infarct size in transgenic mice compared with wild-type mice (66 ± 11 mm^3 versus 125 ± 5 mm^3). This study demonstrated that inhibition in production of mature IL-1β is correlated with a significant decrease in infarct size (–50% versus wild-type), as well as an improvement in neurologic score, 24 h post MCAO. Similarly, Hara et al. *(27)* demonstrated a decrease in labeling of immunoreactive IL-1β (–77%) and infarct size (–44% to –46%), in transgenic mice following transient (3-h) focal ischemia, compared with their wild-type littermates. Moreover, Schielke et al. *(28)* demonstrated that this reduction in infarct size was not caused by an increased cerebral blood flow in the caspase-1 deficient mice. Following neonatal hypoxia/ischemia (HI), similar neuroprotection (–53 ± 41% and –40 ± 29% in cortex and striatum infarct volumes, respectively) has been reported in mice deficient in caspase-1 *(29,30)*. Although it cannot be excluded that inhibition of the proapoptotic activity of caspase-1 may have a beneficial role following ischemic insults in transgenic mice, other studies suggest that the neuroprotection observed in caspase-1 knockout mice are primarily due to inhibition of the proinflammatory actions of IL-1β, such as decrease in adhesion molecules and other proinflammatory cytokines expression, leukocyte and monocyte infiltration, and lipid peroxydation *(30–32)*.

More recently, the availability of mice deficient for the ligands of the IL-1 system, namely, IL-1α, IL-1β, and IL-1Ra *(4)*, made it possible for us to study their contribution to brain damage following temporary focal cerebral ischemia *(33,34)*. Twenty-four hours after 30 min MCAO, IL-1α and IL-1β knockout mice exhibited similar infarct volumes as those observed in wild-type animals, whereas IL-1α/β double knockout mice had a –70 to –85% reduction in infarct size (Fig. 1). These data suggest that inhibition of both forms of IL-1 agonist is required to obtain optimal neuroprotection. Because acute inhibition of IL-1β by an antibody or IL-1Ra reduced ischemic cell death, whereas deletion of the IL-1β gene did not, we investigated whether compensatory changes in the expression of one of the agonists (namely, upregulation of IL-1α in IL-1β knockout mice and of IL-1β in IL-1α

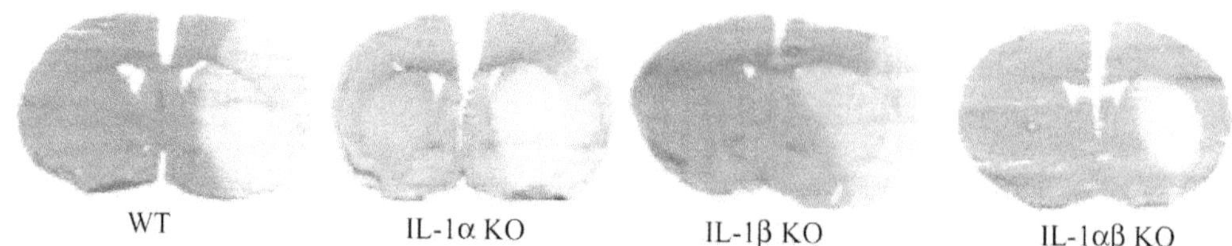

Fig. 1. Representative coronal brain sections (20 μm) of wild-type (WT), interleukin (IL)-1α knockout, IL-1β knockout, and IL-1αβ knockout mice 24 h after 30 min of middle cerebral artery occlusion.

knockout mice) occurred using reverse transcriptase polymerase chain reaction (RT-PCR). No compensation in mRNA synthesis could be observed in either IL-1α knockout or IL-1β knockout mice. In the same study, IL-1Ra induced neuroprotection in wild-type and IL-1α knockout (–32% and –56%), but not in IL-1β knockout animals, suggesting that IL-1Ra might not be able to block the effect of IL-1α fully on cell death *(33)*. This last result seems to indicate that potential compensatory processes within the IL-1 system, or other proinflammatory cytokines, might take place in IL-1α and IL-1β knockout mice.

More recently, using a model of global ischemia induced by transient cardiac arrest, Mizushima et al. *(35)* demonstrated reduced neuronal death in IL-1α/β knockout mice, which correlated with a reduction in nitrite and nitrate production, indicating that reduced nitric oxide (NO) production in these animals could contribute partially to the reduced ischemic damage. In parallel to the neuroprotection observed by deletion of both forms of IL-1 agonists, deletion of the endogenous antagonist IL-1Ra conferred a high susceptibility to cerebral ischemia in these mice. Indeed, IL-1Ra knockout mice exhibited a sevenfold increase in cortical infarct volume compared with wild-type mice, suggesting a strong neuroprotective action of endogenous IL-1Ra *(34)*. Since IL-1Ra is the endogenous antagonist for IL-1β, the first hypothesis to explain the hypersensitivity to focal ischemia observed in IL-1Ra knockout mice is the lack of IL-1Ra to antagonize the endogenous IL-1β, but further investigations in such mice should be undertaken to determine whether other intracellular processes are implicated.

More recently, our own studies *(36)* demonstrated that, in contrast to experiments on caspase-1 knockout mice *(26–29)* and on IL-1αβ knockout mice *(33)*, the IL-1RI knockout mice exhibit similar damage to their wild-type controls following temporary MCAO. In addition, we reported that IL-1Ra did not confer any neuroprotection in these animals. Perhaps most interestingly, and despite the lack of effect of IL-1Ra, we showed that intracerebroventricular (icv) administration of IL-1β to the IL-1RI knockout mice after experimental stroke still significantly increases ischemic damage. These observations led us to hypothezise that IL-1β is inducing this effect by interacting with a functional receptor other than IL-1RI in the brain *(36)*. Although strong, this evidence has yet to be confirmed with further studies aimed at identification of this new receptor and/or signaling pathways.

Another key component of the IL-1 signaling pathway is the accessory protein (IL-1RAcP), which upon ligand binding forms a complex with IL-1RI that shows increased affinity for IL-1α and IL-1β and allows signal transduction *(3,37)*. Mice lacking the gene for IL-1RAcP have now been generated *(3)*, and early studies indicate that this component of the IL-1 signaling pathway is required for IL-1 actions on food intake *(38)*. To date there have been no studies investigating neurodegeneration in these mice.

Overall, these studies using mice deficient for one or more of the components of the IL-1 system have shown that IL-1 plays a major role in neurodegenerative disease following cerebral ischemia. Moreover, they have shown that partial inhibition of IL-1 is not sufficient and that potential yet unidentified receptors or ligands could be involved in this response. Support for this hypothesis has recently been added with the discovery of potential new ligands (such as IL-1F5-F10) and IL-1 receptor-related proteins (IL-1Rrp2, IL-1RAPL) *(39)*. Future studies using transgenic mice for these new members of the expanding IL-1 family, as well as for IL-1RII, should further increase our knowledge of the mechanisms of action of the IL-1 family in neurodegeneration following cerebral ischemia.

Finally, the role of IL-18, another ligand of the IL-1 superfamily (initially named IL-1γ because of its homology with IL-1β) has been recently studied following cerebral ischemia *(40)* or HI brain injury in neonate mice *(41)*. In the latest study *(41)*, using IL-18-deficient mice, these workers demonstrated that not only IL-18 is strongly induced after HI brain injury in microglial cells but that infarct volumes (–21%) and neuropathologic scores (–22% to –35%) were slightly, but significantly, reduced in IL-18 knockout mice compared with wild-type, suggesting a potential role for IL-18 in HI brain damage.

In addition to the in vivo studies investigating the role of IL-1 as a neuroimmune modulator in sickness behavior (e.g., fever) and in ischemic neuronal death, the actions of IL-1 and its family at the cellular level are being intensely investigated. Extensive in vitro studies conducted during the last 20 years have significantly contributed to our understanding of the role and functions of the different cell types of the brain during physiologic and pathologic conditions. These techniques have been particularly useful in unravelling the actions of cytokines in the brain. In particular, using cultured cells (either immortalized or primary cells prepared from tissues) have resulted in the unravelling of the sequence of events during brain inflammation and have identified the different cell types and molecular mediators that trigger extensive neuronal cell death. The use of knockout technology has been a major asset in this type of research. Mixed glial or neuronal cultures prepared from the brain of mice lacking the gene for IL-1, its receptor(s), and its associated signal components have provided a powerful tool to help elucidate the function of this cytokine.

Our current understanding of the inflammatory processes in the brain indicate that early stages of brain injury/infection are followed by rapid activation of microglial cells, which are the primary immune cells of the brain. This activation is characterized by a change of morphology and migration of microglial cells to the site of injury accompanied by release of an array of cytokines including IL-1α and -β *(42,43)*. In vitro studies have used LPS extensively as a model of infection/inflammation. Activation of microglial cells by LPS, for example, has been demonstrated to occur via the Toll-like receptor-4 (TLR-4), since LPS fails to induce activation of microglial cells isolated from C3H/HeJ mice, which bear loss-of-function mutation in the *tlr4* gene *(44)*. A recent study has demonstrated that LPS induction of IL-1 is limited to the synthesis of the inactive 32-kDa pro-IL-1β in microglial cells *(45)*. This proform, however, lacks a classical signal peptide, and its mechanism of processing and release is largely unknown. The 32-kDa pro-IL-1β is known to be cleaved to a 17-kDa mature IL-1β by caspase-1. Mice deficient in this enzyme lack the capability of producing the mature active form of IL-1β, demonstrating therefore that this enzyme is essential in the processing/release of functional IL-1β *(46)*.

In addition, neurons isolated from the dorsal root ganglion of mice with a mutant caspase-1 gene (C285G), which acts as a dominant negative caspase-1 inhibitor, were resistant to trophic factor withdrawal-induced apoptosis accompanied by reduced mature IL-1β production *(26)*.

More recent studies have shown that this mechanism is dependent on activation of caspase-1 by adenosine triphosphate (ATP) via the purinergic $P2X_7$ receptor expressed on the surface membrane of microglial cells and is accompanied by cell death. This has since been confirmed since ATP failed to induce cell death and IL-1β release from microglial cell cultures isolated from $P2X_7$ knockout mice *(45)*. The same study showed that the rate of cell death observed in these conditions is, however, independent of IL-1β release since ATP induced rates of cell death in LPS-primed IL-1β knockout microglial cells similar to those of LPS-primed wild-type microglia.

IL-1β released by activated microglial cells is known to act on astrocytes to activate distinct intracellular signaling pathways. These culminate in the activation of the nuclear factor-κB (NF-κB) and mitogen-activated protein kinase (MAPK) p38, the extracellular signal-regulated kinase p42/44 (ERK1/2), and the c-Jun-N-terminal kinase (JNK) and to drive the transcription of genes for other inflammatory mediators such as TNF-α and IL-6, resulting in their release. These mechanisms occur via binding of IL-1β to IL-1RI, which then associates with IL-1RAcP. The generation of IL-1RI- and IL-1RAcP-deficient knockout mice has proved extremely useful in studying the cellular mechanisms of actions of this cytokine and the signaling pathways that it triggers. For example, in vitro studies using cultures from these mice helped to identify accurately the function of these two receptor subunits in the signal transduction induced by IL-1β in brain cells. Our own recent study showed that IL-1β induced the release of IL-6 and prostaglandin E_2 (PGE_2), and induced the activation of the MAPKs and NF-κB in wild-type mixed glial cultures, but failed to induce any of these responses in glial cells isolated from IL-1RI knockout mice *(47)*.

In addition, recombinant human IL-1β was shown to activate the neural sphingomyelinase in the P(2) fraction of wild-type mice but not in that from IL-1RI knockout mice *(48)*, suggesting that activation of the sphingomyelin signaling pathway might be an essential component of IL-1 signaling in the brain that requires IL-1RI. Similarly, IL-1RAcP has been shown to be an essential component of the IL-1 signaling pathway, since IL-1β failed to induce activation of NF-κB in primary astrocyte cultures from IL-1RAcP knockout mice *(49)* and also failed to induce the release of IL-6 from IL-1RAcP knockout fibroblast cultures *(3)*. Upon ligand binding to the IL-1RI/IL/1RAcP complex, downstream signaling elements are rapidly activated, including the adaptor MyD88, the IL-1 receptor associated kinase (IRAK), and the TNF receptor-associated-factor-6 (TRAF-6). In vitro experiments using available mice lacking MyD88 or IRAK have shown that these signaling elements are essential in IL-1β responses since cells isolated from MyD88, IRAK, or TRAF-6 knockout mice showed reduced responses to IL-1β *(50–52)*. A more recent study showed severe impairment of IL-1 signaling pathways in mice lacking IRAK-4 *(53)*. Finally, mice deficient in downstream elements for the IL-1 signaling cascade have also been generated (i.e., MEKK-1, -3, and -4, ERK1/2, p50 NF-κB), but to date none of these have been used to study their role in IL-1 actions in the brain. Figure 2 summarizes all the signaling elements of the IL-1 transduction pathways for which deficient mice are available and have been used to study actions of IL-1 in brain cells.

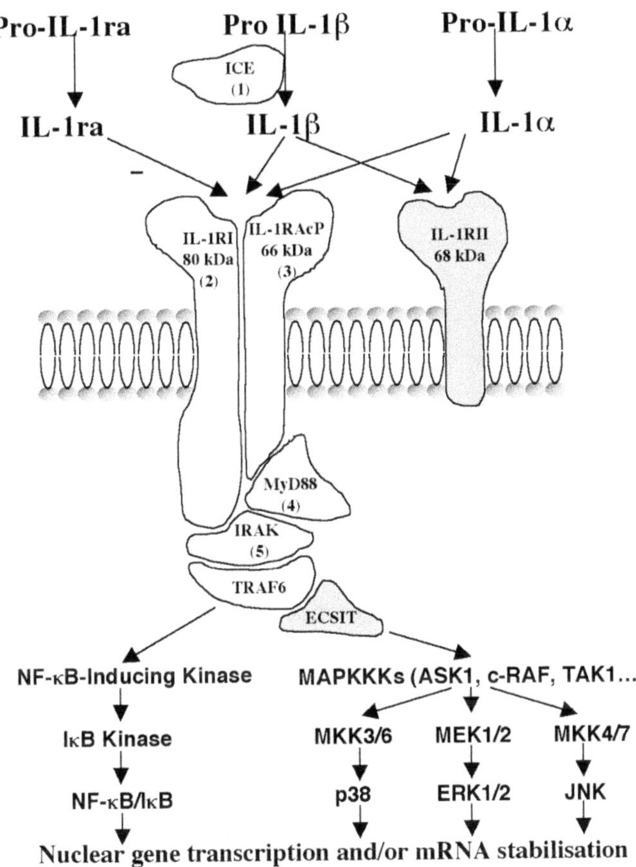

Fig. 2. Interleukin (IL)-1 signaling components for which knockout mice are available (in white), and those not yet generated (gray). (1), ref. *46*; (2), ref. *21*; (3), ref. *3*; (4), ref. *50*; (5), ref. *51*. Evolutionarily Conserved Signaling Intermediate in toll pathways (ECSIT), ERK1/2, extracellular signal-regulated kinase p42/44; ICE, IL-1-converting enzyme; IκB, inhibitory κB; IL-1ra, interleukin-1 receptor antagonist; IL-1RAcP, IL-1 receptor accessory protein; IL-1RI, IL-1 receptor type I; IRAK, IL-1 receptor-associated kinase; JNK, c-Jun-N-terminal kinase; MAPKKK, mitogen-activated protein kinase kinase kinase; MKK, MAPK kinase; NF-κB, nuclear factor-κB; TRAF6, tumor necrosis factor-associated factor 6.

Our recent observations that a functional receptor other than IL-1RI may exist *(36)* has prompted us to perform other studies using IL-1RI knockout mixed glial cell cultures in order to identify which signaling pathway might be activated by IL-1β in the absence of IL-1RI. Interestingly, none of the classical IL-1 signalling pathways have been found to be activated in IL-1RI knockout mixed glial cell cultures, suggesting that alternative pathways are involved *(47)* (Fig. 3). A more recent study has shown a significant reduction in the number of activated microglial cells following stab wound-induced brain injury in IL-1RI deficient mice compared with wild-type controls and showed that leukocyte infiltration, as well as astrogliosis, was also reduced in IL-1RI knockout mice *(43)*. These alterations were accompanied by reduced production of vascular cell adhesion molecule (VCAM-1), cyclooxygenase-2 (COX-2), IL-6, TNF-α, transforming growth factor-β (TGF-β), and

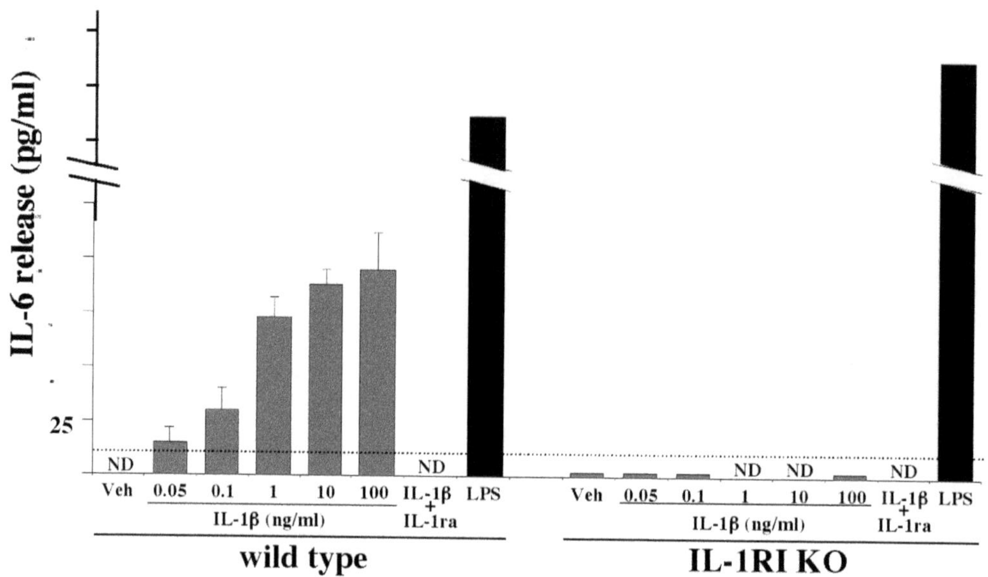

Fig. 3. Interleukin (IL)-1β- or lipopolysaccharide (LPS)-induced IL-6 from mixed glial cultures prepared from wild-type and IL-1rI knockout (KO) mice. Cells were treated with LPS (1 μg/mL), IL-1β (0.05–100 ng/mL), and/or IL-receptor antagonist (IL-1ra; 1 μg/mL) for 24 h. The supernatant was assayed for IL-6. Data are mean ± SEM. ND indicates that the concentration was below the detection limit (dotted line of the assay).

IL-1β. These results strongly demonstrate that IL-1 plays a pivotal role in the development of inflammatory responses to brain injury.

During the last decade interest has developed in the role of IL-1 in chronic neurodegenerative diseases. One example is Alzheimer's disease, a progressive neurodegenerative disorder characterized by an accumulation of neurofibrillary tangles and senile plaques, which are surrounded by activated microglia and astrocytes. The principal component of these plaques is β-amyloid (βA) derived from proteolytic cleavage of the amyloid precursor protein (APP). Several studies have shown increased expression of IL-1 associated with accumulation of necrotic plaques in the brain of patients who died from Alzheimer's disease *(54)*. Furthermore, βA 1–42 and 25–35 peptides have been previously shown to induce IL-1β production in astrocytes and microglial cell cultures *(55)*. Further studies using IL-1RI$^{-/-}$ mice showed that βA 25–35-induced increase of IL-1α expression was higher, whereas IL-6 expression was lower in astrocyte cultures from IL-1RI$^{-/-}$ mice compared with wild-type mice. APP-deficient mice have also been produced, and using these, Perez et al. *(56)* demonstrated that hippocampal neuronal cell cultures exhibited diminished viability and retarded development whereas no differences in susceptibility to βA toxicity were found between APP$^{-/-}$ and wild-type cortical and cerebellar neuronal cultures *(57)*. A more recent study showed delayed and limited local microglial activation (a cell type associated with IL-1 production in the brain) and a significant increase in neuron survival in response to distal axotomy of the substantia nigra compacta in APP-deficient mice *(58)*. These results suggest that endogenous APP plays a major role in neuron development, whereas APP neurotoxicity is associated with microglial activation in brain injury.

In conclusion, these results strongly suggest that increased expression of IL-1β plays an important role in the progression of inflammation in the brains of patients with Alzheimer's disease.

3. Interleukin-6

IL-6, like IL-1, has received a great deal of attention and has been studied extensively using genetically modified mice. The role of this cytokine as a neuroimmune modulator has been surrounded by some controversy, with some authors suggesting that it acts as a proinflammatory cytokine and others showing evidence for an antiinflammatory role (for reviews, *see* refs. *5* and *59*). In fever, for example, the evidence that IL-6 is a proinflammatory signal is overwhelming. The circulating as well as brain concentrations of this cytokine increase dramatically following administration of an exogenous pyrogen such as LPS or turpentine in rodents *(6,7,12)*, and direct administration of this cytokine into the brain induces a robust fever *(60,61)*. Recently we have demonstrated that neutralization of endogenous IL-6 using an anti IL-6 antiserum delivered systemically almost totally abolishes the febrile response to LPS, confirming earlier observations that this cytokine is an essential circulating mediator of fever. One such observation was made by Chai et al. *(62)* using IL-6-deficient mice. In elegant experiments, these workers demonstrated that IL-6-deficient mice failed to generate a fever in response to systemic administration of LPS or IL-1 [also shown to induce fever via induction of IL-6 *(7,63)*], compared with their wild-type littermates. The same mice, however, exhibited a fever following an icv injection of IL-6. Collectively, these data indicate an important role for IL-6 as a mediator of fever at both systemic (circulating) and brain levels.

Despite evidence for a proinflammatory role, other studies have shown antiinflammatory actions for IL-6. Experiments investigating the role of IL-6 in neurodegeneration have shown that this cytokine may have neuroprotective effects, reducing, for example, the infarct size following permanent focal cerebral ischemia *(64)*, possibly via induction of IL-1Ra or the TNF soluble receptor p55 *(65)*. More recently, studies using transgenic mice overexpressing IL-6 suggested that IL-6 might have neurotoxic and proinflammatory roles in the brain. These studies showed that such mice developed neurologic and motor disorders at different postnatal times ranging from 3 wk to 6 mo, leading to death probably as a result of seizures *(66)*. Some of the transgenic mice survived longer but finally developed the same type of disorder, such as ataxia, tremor, and seizures at 6 mo of age. Interestingly, the homozygous offspring of these mice also developed similar disorders at 1 mo of age.

Immunohistochemical studies of the brains of these animals demonstrated a decrease (–32%) in MAP-2 immunostaining in the hippocampus, reduced dendritic processes of the neurons of the hippocampal CA1 area and Purkinje cells, and atrophy of the molecular layer in the cerebellum, in parallel with a dramatic astrogliosis *(66)*. In addition, these mice also exhibited blood-brain barrier (BBB) abnormalities, with incomplete development and significant disruption of the BBB as early as 1 mo of age, accompanied by intense astrocytic and endothelial abnormalities *(67)*. Another group *(68)* reported that overexpression of IL-6, under the control of the neuron-specific enolase promoter, induced a significant increase in the expression of proinflammatory cytokines such as TNF and IL-1β. These molecular and morphologic changes in the CNS were strongly correlated with behavioral and motor disorders, as well as electrophysiologic perturbations *(69)*.

Overall, these studies showed that overexpression of IL-6 leads to spontaneous neurodegeneration, suggesting a deleterious action of IL-6 in the brain. Conversely, other studies using IL-6-deficient mice showed that IL-6 could also contribute to the recovery and healing processes. Swartz et al. *(70)* reported reduced gliosis and revascularization in IL-6 knockout mice correlated with slower recovery and healing following cryogenic cerebral injury. Similarly, Penkowa et al. *(71)* showed that following traumatic injury induced by a cortical freeze lesion, IL-6 knockout mice had a significantly increased number of apoptotic cells and reduced reactive astrogliosis and microgliosis and that regeneration was delayed compared with wild-type controls. These observations could be correlated with a decrease in expression of antioxidant and antiapoptotic factors such as metallothionein I and II. The results obtained in IL-6 knockout mice seem to indicate that IL-6 could have a beneficial action in the brain following acute brain injury. However following cerebral ischemia *(72)*, no difference was observed in infarct volumes or in neurologic function between IL-6 knockout and wild-type mice. Although infarct volumes reported in this publication were variable, the authors demonstrated that proinflammatory cytokine levels were decreased by 50% in the serum and cerebrospinal fluid of IL-6 knockout mice compared with wild-type mice.

At the cellular level, IL-6 has been shown to promote the viability of neurons in culture via expression of brain-derived neurotrophic factor (BDNF). This was confirmed in studies showing that induction of BDNF in dorsal root ganglion neurons after nerve injury is severely attenuated in mice with a null mutation of the IL-6 gene *(73)*. In contrast, IL-6 deficiency led to significant decrease in astrogliosis and moderate reduction in microglial activation in response to axotomy or brain injury *(71,74)*. These studies suggest that basal expression of brain IL-6 is important for development and survival of neurons, whereas IL-6 promotes inflammation via glial activation in the injured brain.

Overall, studies using acute administration of IL-6 following cerebral ischemia *(64,75)*, or using IL-6 treatment on cultured cells *(76)*, as well as studies using IL-6 knockout mice, have shown that IL-6 may have neuroprotective/antiinflammatory actions, reducing the acute expression of proinflammatory cytokines. Conversely, use of IL-6 transgenic mice suggested that this cytokine may have neurotoxic effects when constitutively expressed. IL-6 may effectively have this dual action in the brain, but potential compensation in the expression of other pro- or antiinflammatory cytokines should be taken into account in mice that have been genetically modified.

4. Tumor Necrosis Factor-α

Like IL-6, the role of TNF-α as a neuroimmune mediator remains rather controversial. In fever, a number of experiments performed by Kluger and colleagues demonstrated an antipyretic role for this cytokine. These workers showed that TNF-α attenuated the febrile response to pyrogenic stimuli such as LPS *(77,78)* and that antiserum to TNF-α enhances LPS fever and stress hyperthermia *(79,80)* in rats. Others, including ourselves, demonstrated the converse by showing a pyrogenic effect of TNF-α after icv injection in rats *(81)* or rabbits *(82)* and that TNF-α antiserum inhibits turpentine-induced fever in rats *(12)*. To a large extent, studies performed on knockout mice seem to support an antipyretic role for TNF in fever, or no role at all. Most of these studies used TNF receptor knockout mice. TNF-α elicits its biologic activity by binding to two distinct receptors, TNFRI or p55 and TNFRII or p75 TNF receptor. Studies by Leon et al. *(83)* demonstrated that TNFRI/TNFRII double knockouts exhibited an enhanced fever after a high dose (2.5 mg/kg) but not a low dose (50 μg/kg) of LPS and failed to respond any differently from their wild-type littermates when injected with turpentine. These data suggest that TNF is not involved in mediating turpentine-induced changes in temperature in mice.

Similar observations were shown after sepsis in TNF receptor double knockout mice that had undergone cecal ligation and puncture (CLP). These animals exhibited an identical fever to their corresponding wild-type controls. These studies therefore provide a strong indicator that at least when a strong inflammatory stimulus is used, TNF-α can play an anti-pyretic role, acting to limit the ensuing fever. Further investigations are needed to reconcile these observations with others obtained from studies in other species.

Similar to studies on fever, the role of TNF-α in neurodegenerative disease has also benefited from the use of knockout mice. Several reports in this area have demonstrated both a neuroprotective and detrimental role for TNF-α in neurodegeneration *(84–90)*. The generation of mice with the gene for TNF-α or one or both of its receptors *(91–94)* has helped significantly in resolving this question. Interestingly, Stahel et al. *(91)* showed that TNF-α knockout mice had a higher mortality rate compared with their wild-type controls following traumatic brain injury, whereas the neurologic recovery was slightly better in TNF-α knockout mice than in wild-type. This indicated a possible dual role for TNF-α, such that it can be neuroprotective in the acute phase of trauma and detrimental during long-term recovery; no difference in terms of BBB permeability or number of apoptotic cells were observed in this study.

Similarly to mice overexpressing IL-6, mice overexpressing TNF-α developed spontaneous neurologic disorder. In one study *(94)*, chronic CNS inflammation, correlated with depletion in nerve growth factor (NGF) production in the hippocampus, which seemed to lead to a decrease in choline acetyltransferase immunoreactivity of the septal cholinergic neurons, suggesting potential implications for TNF-α in chronic neurodegenerative diseases, such as Alzheimer's disease *(95)*. Conversely, studies using TNF-α receptor knockout mice showed quite unequivocally that TNF-α may be neuroprotective following cerebral ischemia and neurotoxic brain damage *(93,96)*.

These studies demonstrated an increase in oxidative stress and cell death and a decrease in antioxidant enzymes in TNF-α knockout mice, indicating that TNF-α could exert its acute neuroprotective effects by reducing oxidative stress following stroke. This hypothesis is similar to the one made using IL-6 knockout mice, and results obtained by Benigni et al. *(92)*, showing a decrease in IL-6 production following LPS in TNFRI knockout mice, may suggests that neuroprotective effects of TNF-α could be mediated by IL-6. Interestingly, it seems that mainly p55 is involved in this neuroprotective action and that the suppression of TNFRII has having little effect on either cell death or oxidative stress *(92,93, 96)*. Thus, the studies conducted on TNF-α transgenic animals support the concept that this cytokine plays a dual progressive role, which potentially can make it either neuroprotective during the acute phase of excitotoxic neurodegeneration or cytotoxic in chronic neurodegenerative diseases.

Perhaps a better understanding of a possible dual function for TNF-α can be obtained by studying its actions at the level of the cell. Neuronal cell cultures prepared from TNF-α-deficient embryos show a higher survival rate than those prepared from wild-type embryos *(97)*. In addition, exogenous TNF-α has been shown to trigger reduced outgrowth and branching of neuritis in wild-type neuronal cultures but had no effect on cultures prepared from TNFRI/TNFRII double knockout mice *(98)*. This suggests that TNF-α can strongly compromise the development of neurons in cultures by exhibiting neurotoxic actions. TNF-α has also been found to participate in IFN-γ actions since microglial cells isolated from TNF-α-deficient mice showed altered responses to IFN-γ *(99)*. In addition, TNF-α is believed to exert proinflammatory properties in synergy with IL-1β, and it has recently been hypothesized that TNF-α could be a serious candidate in compensation mechanisms that occur in IL-1RI-deficient mice *(100)*.

The two TNF receptors differ in structure, since TNFRI exclusively contains an intracellular death domain (DD), suggesting that they may trigger different signaling pathways and therefore play specific functions. Recently, Yang et al. *(101)* have shown that TNF-α has little or no neurotoxic effect on neurons isolated from mice lacking TNFRI, whereas neurons prepared from TNFRII knockout mice are vulnerable to TNF-α, even at low doses. They further demonstrated that binding of TNF-α to TNFRI triggers cell death via an NF-κB-dependent mechanism. In addition, a recent study conducted using TNFRI or TNFRII knockout astrocyte cultures showed that TNF-α-induced inducible nitric oxide synthase (iNOS) expression was exclusively mediated through TNFRI *(102)*. Furthermore, the neurotoxic effect of TNF-α mediated by TNFRI has been further confirmed since increased susceptibility to TNF-α-induced apoptosis was observed in astrocyte cultures prepared from PEA-15-deficient mice, an endogenous protein that inhibits Fas and TNFRI-mediated apoptosis *(103)*. In contrast, TNFRII has been found to trigger neurotrophic actions via activation of the p38 MAPK *(102)*, and analysis of mice lacking TNFRI or TNFRII showed that TNFRII exclusively is critical for oligodendrocyte regeneration *(104)*, confirming the neurotrophic function of TNFRII.

5. Interleukin-10

This cytokine belongs to a subgroup of the interleukin family that is increasingly being investigated as a potential therapeutic target in the treatment of inflammatory disease. Studies on these cytokines have already demonstrated that they are by in large produced by and act on brain cells to render protection by counterbalancing the effects of the proinflammatory cytokines such as IL-1 and TNF-α (for review, *see* ref. *105*). IL-10 is the best studied member of this subgroup. Like many other cytokines, a substantial amount of early research into IL-10 and neuroimmunology focused on its role in fever. Early studies on this cytokine demonstrated that it acts by inhibiting the production of proinflammatory "pyrogenic" cytokines by both peripheral macrophages and glial cells in the brain *(106–108)*. In addition, other studies have shown that IL-10 inhibits LPS-induced fever in rats *(109)* through a site-specific action depending on the site of inflammation *(110)*. The antipyretic actions of IL-10 were confirmed in studies using IL-10 knockout mice. Using these animals, Leon et al. *(111)* injected LPS or turpentine and demonstrated that they responded with an exacerbated and prolonged fever. Furthermore, these workers showed that these responses correlated closely with enhanced levels of IL-6, indicating that actions of endogenous IL-10 are related to regulation of IL-6 production in fever.

More recently the role of IL-10 in neurodegeneration was examined in stroke following experimental cerebral ischemia in mice deficient in this cytokine *(112)*. This study showed that IL-10 knockout mice had a larger infarct volume (21.8 ± 1.2 mm^3 versus 16.9 ± 1.0 mm^3, mean ± SEM, IL-10 knockout and wild-type, respectively). These authors

(112) also studied neuronal death in cell cultures from both wild-type and IL-10 knockout mice. Cell death induced by *N*-methyl-D-aspartate or oxygen/glucose deprivation was significantly higher in IL-10 knockout mice compared with primary neuronal cultures from wild-type mice. Interestingly, exogenous recombinant IL-10 was able to revert neuronal cell death in both wild-type and IL-10 knockout mice. The results of this study agreed with those another report *(113)* showing a combined antiinflammatory/neuroprotective role for IL-10. Another study, this time using primary glial cultures prepared from the brains of these mice, further confirmed the role of IL-10 as an antiinflammatory mediator in the brain *(114)*. This study showed that LPS induced a dose-dependent increase in NO and PGE_2 release in wild-type mixed glial cultures, which was severely attenuated in cultures prepared from IL-10 knockout mice. Furthermore addition of exogenous IL-10 inhibited the LPS-induced NO (–30%) and PGE_2 responses (–50%), and dose-dependently reduced the LPS-induced IL-1β and TNF-α release in wild-type cultures but completely abolished all these responses in IL-10 knockout cultures, demonstrating that IL-10 deficiency induces reduced responses to LPS and increases sensitivity to exogenous IL-10.

6. Interleukin-4

IL-4 is believed to exert antiinflammatory/neuroprotective actions similar to those of IL-10 in the brain. Mice deficient in IL-4 have been generated *(115)*; however, very little work has been conducted to study the role of this cytokine in inflammation leading to sickness-type behaviors such as fever or in chronic or acute neurodegeneration. Experimental allergic demyelination processes have been studied with these mice as a model of autoimmune demyelination disease in humans. Controversial results have been obtained, showing reduced *(116)* or increased *(115)* extension of autoimmune neuropathology. In parallel, we have recently investigated the effect of 30 min of MCAO in IL-4 knockout mice. A slight neuroprotection seemed to be induced by IL-4 gene deletion, since in IL-4 knockout mice the total infarct size was reduced by –27%, whereas cortical infarct volume was not significantly modified (Fig. 4).

Like IL-10, IL-4 has been demonstrated to attenuate IL-1β-induced NF-κB activation and Akt phosphorylation in vitro using mouse astrocytes cultures *(107)*. IL-4, however, has specific actions on glial cells by binding to a distinct plasma membrane receptor complex composed of the IL-4 receptor α/β-chain (IL-4Rα/β), which dimerizes with the common γ-chain (γ c) that is also found associated with other cytokine receptors, such as IL-2, IL-7, IL-9, and IL-15. Cells isolated from γ c-deficient mice failed to respond to IL-4 *(117)*. Interestingly the IL-4 receptor α-chain is also an essential component of the IL-13 receptor since cells isolated from IL-4Rα-chain-deficient mice failed to respond to either IL-4 or IL-13 *(118)*. Binding of IL-4 to its receptor complex leading to signal transduction involving the insulin receptor substrate-2 (IRS-2) has been observed, which then activates downstream signaling elements such as signal transducer and activator of infection-6 (STAT-6). In vitro experiments using cells isolated from IRS-2, STAT-6, or IRS-2/STAT-6 double knockout mice have been conducted and showed that both IRS-2 and especially STAT-6 are critically involved in IL-4 signal transduction. IL-4-deficient mice have been generated *(119)*, and the use of these animals in in vivo experiments has confirmed the antiinflammatory properties of this cytokine in the brain (see above). In contrast, this field of research has not yet benefited from studies using neuronal or glial cultures prepared from these knockout mice.

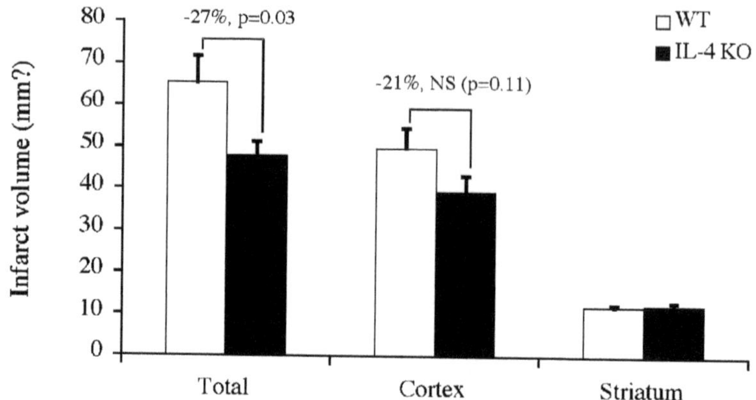

Fig. 4. Effect of 30 min of middle cerebral artery in wild-type (WT) versus interleukin (IL-4) knockout (KO) mice ($n = 9$ per group). Infarct volumes are represented as mean ± SEM; p values from unpaired t-test.

Conclusion

As was discussed above, many of the results obtained using genetically modified animals do not correlate well with earlier observations using pharmacological approaches. This could to a large extent could be a reflection of compensatory mechanisms known to operate by reflecting the cascade nature of cytokine function. Thus it is important that, as with any new technology, caution is used when tampering with such approaches, because the majority of genetically modified animals in cytokine research exhibit a normal phenotype when compared to their wild type equivalents. Therefore, constitutive compensatory adaptations, potentially unrelated to the system studied, may occur and could alter the responses observed, whether in vivo or in vitro. Nevertheless, genetically modified animals provide an extremely important tool, which has already been extensively utilized in neuroimmunology research leading to significant advances in this field.

References

1. Li, P., Allen, H., Banerjee, S., and Seshadri, T. (1997) Characterization of mice deficient in interleukin-1 beta converting enzyme. *J. Cell Biochem.* **64,** 27–32.
2. Glaccum, M. B., Stocking, K. L., Charrier, K., et al. (1997) Phenotypic and functional characterization of mice that lack the type I receptor for IL-1. *J. Immunol.* **159,** 3364–3371.
3. Cullinan, E. B., Kwee, L., Nunes, P., et al. (1998) IL-1 receptor accessory protein is an essential component of the IL-1 receptor. *J. Immunol.* **161,** 5614–5620.
4. Horai, R., Asano, M., Sudo, K., et al. (1998) Production of mice deficient in genes for interleukin (IL)-1alpha, IL-1beta, IL-1alpha/beta, and IL-1 receptor antagonist shows that IL-1beta is crucial in turpentine-induced fever development and glucocorticoid secretion. *J. Exp. Med.* **187,** 1463–1475.
5. Dinarello, C. A. (1999) Cytokines as endogenous pyrogens. *J. Infect. Dis.* **179(Suppl. 2),** S294–S304.
6. Klir, J. J., McClellan, J. L., and Kluger, M. J. (1994) Interleukin-1 beta causes the increase in anterior hypothalamic interleukin-6 during LPS-induced fever in rats. *Am. J. Physiol.* **266,** R1845–R1848.
7. Luheshi, G., Miller, A. J., Brouwer, S., Dascombe, M. J., Rothwell, N. J., and Hopkins, S. J. (1996) Interleukin-1 receptor antagonist inhibits endotoxin fever and systemic interleukin-6 induction in the rat. *Am. J. Physiol.* **270,** E91–E95.
8. Leon, L. R., Conn, C. A., Glaccum, M., and Kluger, M. J. (1996) IL-1 type I receptor mediates acute phase response to turpentine, but not lipopolysaccharide, in mice. *Am. J. Physiol.* **271,** R1668–R1675.

9. Kozak, W., Kluger, M. J., Soszynski, D., et al. (1998) IL-6 and IL-1 beta in fever. Studies using cytokine-deficient (knockout) mice. *Ann. NY Acad. Sci.* **856,** 33–47.
10. Alheim, K., Chai, Z., Fantuzzi, G., et al. (1997) Hyperresponsive febrile reactions to interleukin (IL) 1alpha and IL-1beta, and altered brain cytokine mRNA and serum cytokine levels, in IL-1beta-deficient mice. *Proc. Natl. Acad. Sci. USA* **94,** 2681–2686.
11. Zheng, H., Fletcher, D., Kozak, W., et al. (1995) Resistance to fever induction and impaired acute-phase response in interleukin-1 beta-deficient mice. *Immunity* **3,** 9–19.
12. Luheshi, G. N., Stefferl, A., Turnbull, A.V., et al. (1997) Febrile response to tissue inflammation involves both peripheral and brain IL-1 and TNF-alpha in the rat. *Am. J. Physiol.* **272,** R862–R868.
13. Leon, L. R. (2002) Invited review: cytokine regulation of fever: studies using gene knockout mice. *J. Appl. Physiol.* **92,** 2648–2655.
14. Fantuzzi, G. (2001) Lessons from interleukin-deficient mice: the interleukin-1 system. *Acta Physiol. Scand.* **173,** 5–9.
15. Kluger, M. J., Kozak, W., Leon, L. R., and Conn, C. A. (1998) The use of knockout mice to understand the role of cytokines in fever. *Clin. Exp. Pharmacol. Physiol.* **25,** 141–144.
16. Zhao, B. and Schwartz, J. P. (1998) Involvement of cytokines in normal CNS development and neurological diseases: recent progress and perspectives. *J. Neurosci. Res.* **52,** 7–16.
17. Munoz-Fernandez, M. A. and Fresno, M. (1998) The role of tumour necrosis factor, interleukin 6, interferon-gamma and inducible nitric oxide synthase in the development and pathology of the nervous system. *Prog. Neurobiol.* **56,** 307–340.
18. Rothwell, N. J. and Luheshi, G. N. (2000) Interleukin 1 in the brain: biology, pathology and therapeutic target. *Trends Neurosci.* **23,** 618–625.
19. Neumann, H. (2001) Control of glial immune function by neurons. *Glia* **36,** 191–199.
20. Minami, M., Kuraishi, Y., Yabuuchi, K., Yamazaki, A., and Satoh, M. (1992) Induction of interleukin-1 beta mRNA in rat brain after transient forebrain ischemia. *J. Neurochem.* **58,** 390–392.
21. Relton, J. K. and Rothwell, N. J. (1992) Interleukin-1 receptor antagonist inhibits ischaemic and excitotoxic neuronal damage in the rat. *Brain Res. Bull.* **29,** 243–246.
22. Liu, T., McDonnell, P. C., Young, P. R., et al. (1993) Interleukin-1 beta mRNA expression in ischemic rat cortex. *Stroke* **24,** 1746–1750.
23. Yamasaki, Y., Matsuura, N., Shozuhara, H., Onodera, H., Itoyama, Y., and Kogure, K. (1995) Interleukin-1 as a pathogenetic mediator of ischemic brain damage in rats. *Stroke* **26,** 676–680.
24. Touzani, O., Boutin, H., Chuquet, J., and Rothwell, N. (1999) Potential mechanisms of interleukin-1 involvement in cerebral ischaemia. *J. Neuroimmunol.* **100,** 203–215.
25. Clark, W. M., Lessov, N. S., Dixon, M. P., and Eckenstein, F. (1997) Monofilament intraluminal middle cerebral artery occlusion in the mouse. *Neurol. Res.* **19,** 641–648.
26. Friedlander, R. M., Gagliardini, V., Hara, H., et al. (1997) Expression of a dominant negative mutant of interleukin-1 beta converting enzyme in transgenic mice prevents neuronal cell death induced by trophic factor withdrawal and ischemic brain injury. *J. Exp. Med.* **185,** 933–940.
27. Hara, H., Fink, K., Endres, M., et al. (1997) Attenuation of transient focal cerebral ischemic injury in transgenic mice expressing a mutant ICE inhibitory protein. *J. Cereb. Blood Flow Metab.* **17,** 370–375.
28. Schielke, G. P., Yang, G. Y., Shivers, B. D., and Betz, A. L. (1998) Reduced ischemic brain injury in interleukin-1 beta converting enzyme-deficient mice. *J. Cereb. Blood Flow Metab.* **18,** 180–185.
29. Liu, X. H., Kwon, D., Schielke, G. P., Yang, G. Y., Silverstein, F. S., and Barks, J. D. E. (1999) Mice deficient in interleukin-1 converting enzyme are resistant to neonatal hypoxic-ischemic brain damage. *J. Cereb. Blood Flow Metab.* **19,** 1099–1108.
30. Xu, H., Barks, J. D., Schielke, G. P., and Silverstein, F. S. (2001) Attenuation of hypoxia-ischemia-induced monocyte chemoattractant protein-1 expression in brain of neonatal mice deficient in interleukin-1 converting enzyme. *Brain Res. Mol. Brain Res.* **90,** 57–67.
31. Yang, G. Y., Schielke, G. P., Gong, C., et al. (1999) Expression of tumor necrosis factor-alpha and intercellular adhesion molecule-1 after focal cerebral ischemia in interleukin-1beta converting enzyme deficient mice. *J. Cereb. Blood Flow Metab.* **19,** 1109–1117.
32. Koedel, U., Winkler, F., Angele, B., Fontana, A., Flavell, R. A., and Pfister, H. W. (2002) Role of Caspase-1 in experimental pneumococcal meningitis: evidence from pharmacologic Caspase inhibition and Caspase-1-deficient mice. *Ann. Neurol.* **51,** 319–329.

33. Boutin, H., LeFeuvre, R. A., Horai, R., Asano, M., Iwakura, Y., and Rothwell, N. J. (2001) Role of IL-1alpha and IL-1beta in ischemic brain damage. *J. Neurosci.* **21,** 5528–5534.
34. Boutin, H. and Rothwell, N. (2001) Endogenous IL-1 receptor antagonist is neuroprotective after cerebral ischaemia in mice. *Soc. Neurosci. Abstr.* 27:329.2.
35. Mizushima, H., Zhou, C. J., Dohi, K., et al. (2002) Reduced postischemic apoptosis in the hippocampus of mice deficient in interleukin-1. *J. Comp Neurol.* **448,** 203–216.
36. Touzani, O., Boutin, H., Lefeuvre, R. A., et al. (2002) Interleukin-1 influences ischemic brain damage in the mouse independently of the interleukin-1 type I receptor. *J. Neurosci.* **22,** 38–43.
37. Greenfeder, S. A., Nunes, P., Kwee, L., Labow, M., Chizzonite, R. A., and Ju, G. (1995) Molecular cloning and characterization of a second subunit of the interleukin 1 receptor complex. *J. Biol. Chem.* **270,** 13757–13765.
38. Laye, S., Liege, S., Li, K. S., Moze, E., and Neveu, P. J. (2001) Physiological significance of the interleukin 1 receptor accessory protein. *Neuroimmunomodulation* **9,** 225–230.
39. Sims, J. E., Nicklin, M. J., Bazan, J. F., et al. (2001) A new nomenclature for IL-1-family genes. *Trends Immunol.* **22,** 536–537.
40. Jander, S., Schroeter, M., and Stoll, G. (2002) Interleukin-18 expression after focal ischemia of the rat brain: association with the late-stage inflammatory response. *J. Cereb. Blood Flow Metab.* **22,** 62–70.
41. Hedtjarn, M., Leverin, A. L., Eriksson, K., Blomgren, K., Mallard, C., and Hagberg, H. (2002) Interleukin-18 involvement in hypoxic-ischemic brain injury. *J. Neurosci.* **22,** 5910–5919.
42. Yao, J., Keri, J. E., Taffs, R. E., and Colton, C. A. (1992) Characterization of interleukin-1 production by microglia in culture. *Brain Res.* **591,** 88–93.
43. Basu, A., Krady, J. K., O'Malley, M., Styren, S. D., DeKosky, S. T., and Levison, S. W. (2002) The type 1 interleukin-1 receptor is essential for the efficient activation of microglia and the induction of multiple proinflammatory mediators in response to brain injury. *J. Neurosci.* **22,** 6071–6082.
44. Lehnardt, S., Lachance, C., Patrizi, S., et al. (2002) The toll-like receptor TLR4 is necessary for lipopolysaccharide-induced oligodendrocyte injury in the CNS. *J. Neurosci.* **22,** 2478–2486.
45. Brough, D., Le Feuvre, R. A., Iwakura, Y., and Rothwell, N. J. (2002) Purinergic (P2X7) receptor activation of microglia induces cell death via an interleukin-1-independent mechanism. *Mol. Cell Neurosci.* **19,** 272–280.
46. Fantuzzi, G., Ku, G., Harding, M. W., et al. (1997) Response to local inflammation of IL-1 beta-converting enzyme- deficient mice. *J. Immunol.* **158,** 1818–1824.
47. Parker, L. C., Luheshi, G. N., Rothwell, N. J., and Pinteaux, E. (2002) IL-1beta signalling in glial cells in wildtype and IL-1RI deficient mice. *Br. J. Pharmacol.* **136,** 312–320.
48. Nalivaeva, N. N., Rybakina, E. G., Pivanovich, I. Y., Kozinets, I. A., Shanin, S. N., and Bartfai, T. (2000) Activation of neutral sphingomyelinase by IL-1beta requires the type 1 interleukin 1 receptor. *Cytokine* **12,** 229–232.
49. Zetterstrom, M., Lundkvist, J., Malinowsky, D., Eriksson, G., and Bartfai, T. (1998) Interleukin-1-mediated febrile responses in mice and interleukin-1 beta activation of NFkappaB in mouse primary astrocytes, involves the interleukin-1 receptor accessory protein. *Eur. Cytokine Netw.* **9,** 131–138.
50. Kawai, T., Adachi, O., Ogawa, T., Takeda, K., and Akira, S. (1999) Unresponsiveness of MyD88-deficient mice to endotoxin. *Immunity* **11,** 115–122.
51. Thomas, J. A., Allen, J. L., Tsen, M., et al. (1999) Impaired cytokine signaling in mice lacking the IL-1 receptor-associated kinase. *J. Immunol.* **163,** 978–984.
52. Kanakaraj, P., Schafer, P. H., Cavender, D. E., et al. (1998) Interleukin (IL)-1 receptor-associated kinase (IRAK) requirement for optimal induction of multiple IL-1 signaling pathways and IL-6 production. *J. Exp. Med.* **187,** 2073–2079.
53. Suzuki, N., Suzuki, S., Duncan, G. S., et al. (2002) Severe impairment of interleukin-1 and Toll-like receptor signalling in mice lacking IRAK-4. *Nature* **416,** 750–756.
54. Cacabelos, R., Alvarez, X. A., Fernandez-Novoa, L., et al. (1994) Brain interleukin-1 beta in Alzheimer's disease and vascular dementia. *Methods Find. Exp. Clin. Pharmacol.* **16,** 141–151.
55. Del Bo, R., Angeretti, N., Lucca, E., De Simoni, M. G., and Forloni, G. (1995) Reciprocal control of inflammatory cytokines, IL-1 and IL-6, and beta-amyloid production in cultures. *Neurosci. Lett.* **188,** 70–74.

56. Perez, R. G., Zheng, H., Van der Ploeg, L. H., and Koo, E. H. (1997) The beta-amyloid precursor protein of Alzheimer's disease enhances neuron viability and modulates neuronal polarity. *J. Neurosci.* **17,** 9407–9414.
57. White, A. R., Zheng, H., Galatis, D., et al. (1998) Survival of cultured neurons from amyloid precursor protein knock-out mice against Alzheimer's amyloid-beta toxicity and oxidative stress. *J. Neurosci.* **18,** 6207–6217.
58. DeGiorgio, L. A., Shimizu, Y., Chun, H. S., et al. (2002) APP knockout attenuates microglial activation and enhances neuron survival in substantia nigra compacta after axotomy. *Glia* **38,** 174–178.
59. Gadient, R. A. and Otten, U. H. (1997) Interleukin-6 (IL-6)—a molecule with both beneficial and destructive potentials. *Prog. Neurobiol.* **52,** 379–390.
60. LeMay, L. G., Vander, A. J., and Kluger, M. J. (1990) Role of interleukin 6 in fever in rats. *Am. J. Physiol.* **258,** R798–R803.
61. Rothwell, N. J., Busbridge, N. J., LeFeuvre, R. A., Hardwick, A. J., Gauldie, J., and Hopkins, S. J. (1991) Interleukin-6 is a centrally acting endogenous pyrogen in the rat. *Can. J. Physiol. Pharmacol.* **69,** 1465–1469.
62. Chai, Z., Gatti, S., Toniatti, C., Poli, V., and Bartfai, T. (1996) Interleukin (IL)-6 gene expression in the central nervous system is necessary for fever response to lipopolysaccharide or IL-1 beta: a study on IL-6-deficient mice. *J. Exp. Med.* **183,** 311–316.
63. LeMay, L. G., Otterness, I. G., Vander, A. J., and Kluger, M. J. (1990) In vivo evidence that the rise in plasma IL 6 following injection of a fever-inducing dose of LPS is mediated by IL 1 beta. *Cytokine* **2,** 199–204.
64. Loddick, S. A., Turnbull, A. V., and Rothwell, N. J. (1998) Cerebral interleukin-6 is neuroprotective during permanent focal cerebral ischemia in the rat. *J. Cereb. Blood Flow Metab.* **18,** 176–179.
65. Tilg, H., Trehu, E., Atkins, M. B., Dinarello, C. A., and Mier, J. W. (1994) Interleukin-6 (IL-6) as anti-inflammatory cytokines: induction of circulating IL-1 receptor antagonist and soluble tumor necrosis factor receptor p55. *Blood* **83,** 113–118.
66. Campbell, I. L., Abraham, C. R., Masliah, E., et al. (1993) Neurologic disease induced in transgenic mice by cerebral overexpression of interleukin 6. *Proc. Natl. Acad. Sci. USA* **90,** 10061–10065.
67. Brett, F. M., Mizisin, A. P., Powell, H. C., and Campbell, I. L. (1995) Evolution of neuropathologic abnormalities associated with blood-brain barrier breakdown in transgenic mice expressing interleukin-6 in astrocytes. *J. Neuropathol. Exp. Neurol.* **54,** 766–775.
68. Di Santo, E., Alonzi, T., Fattori, E., et al. (1996) Overexpression of interleukin-6 in the central nervous system of transgenic mice increases central but not systemic proinflammatory cytokine production. *Brain Res.* **740,** 239–244.
69. Steffensen, S. C., Campbell, I. L., and Henriksen, S. J. (1994) Site-specific hippocampal pathophysiology due to cerebral overexpression of interleukin-6 in transgenic mice. *Brain Res.* **652,** 149–153.
70. Swartz, K. R., Liu, F., Sewell, D., et al. (2001) Interleukin-6 promotes post-traumatic healing in the central nervous system. *Brain Res.* **896,** 86–95.
71. Penkowa, M., Giralt, M., Carrasco, J., Hadberg, H., and Hidalgo, J. (2000) Impaired inflammatory response and increased oxidative stress and neurodegeneration after brain injury in interleukin-6-deficient mice. *Glia* **32,** 271–285.
72. Clark, W. M., Rinker, L. G., Lessov, N. S., et al. (2000) Lack of interleukin-6 expression is not protective against focal central nervous system ischemia. *Stroke* **31,** 1715–1720.
73. Murphy, P. G., Borthwick, L. A., Altares, M., Gauldie, J., Kaplan, D., and Richardson, P. M. (2000) Reciprocal actions of interleukin-6 and brain-derived neurotrophic factor on rat and mouse primary sensory neurons. *Eur. J. Neurosci.* **12,** 1891–1899.
74. Klein, M. A., Moller, J. C., Jones, L. L., Bluethmann, H., Kreutzberg, G. W., and Raivich, G. (1997) Impaired neuroglial activation in interleukin-6 deficient mice. *Glia* **19,** 227–233.
75. D'Arcangelo, G., Tancredi, V., Onofri, F., D'Antuono, M., Giovedi, S., and Benfenati, F. (2000) Interleukin-6 inhibits neurotransmitter release and the spread of excitation in the rat cerebral cortex. *Eur. J. Neurosci.* **12,** 1241–1252.
76. Ali, C., Nicole, O., Docagne, F., et al. (2000) Ischemia-induced interleukin-6 as a potential endogenous neuroprotective cytokine against NMDA receptor-mediated excitotoxicity in the brain. *J. Cereb. Blood Flow Metab.* **20,** 956–966.

77. Klir, J. J., McClellan, J. L., Kozak, W., Szelenyi, Z., Wong, G. H., and Kluger, M. J. (1995) Systemic but not central administration of tumor necrosis factor-alpha attenuates LPS-induced fever in rats. *Am. J. Physiol.* **268,** R480–R486.
78. Long, N. C., Otterness, I., Kunkel, S. L., Vander, A. J., and Kluger, M. J. (1990) Roles of interleukin 1 beta and tumor necrosis factor in lipopolysaccharide fever in rats. *Am. J. Physiol.* **259,** R724–R728.
79. Long, N. C., Vander, A. J., Kunkel, S. L., and Kluger, M. J. (1990) Antiserum against tumor necrosis factor increases stress hyperthermia in rats. *Am. J. Physiol.* **258,** R591–R595.
80. Long, N. C., Kunkel, S. L., Vander, A. J., and Kluger, M. J. (1990) Antiserum against tumor necrosis factor enhances lipopolysaccharide fever in rats. *Am. J. Physiol.* **258,** R332–R337.
81. Kettelhut, I. C. and Goldberg, A. L. (1988) Tumor necrosis factor can induce fever in rats without activating protein breakdown in muscle or lipolysis in adipose tissue. *J. Clin. Invest.* **81,** 1384–1389.
82. Nakamura, H., Seto, Y., Motoyoshi, S., Kadokawa, T., and Sunahara, N. (1988) Recombinant human tumor necrosis factor causes long-lasting and prostaglandin-mediated fever, with little tolerance, in rabbits. *J. Pharmacol. Exp. Ther.* **245,** 336–341.
83. Leon, L. R., Kozak, W., Peschon, J., and Kluger, M. J. (1997) Exacerbated febrile responses to LPS, but not turpentine, in TNF double receptor-knockout mice. *Am. J. Physiol.* **272,** R563–R569.
84. Nawashiro, H., Tasaki, K., Ruetzler, C. A., and Hallenbeck, J. M. (1997) TNF-alpha pretreatment induces protective effects against focal cerebral ischemia in mice. *J. Cereb. Blood Flow Metab.* **17,** 483–490.
85. Wang, X., Li, X., Erhardt, J. A., Barone, F. C., and Feuerstein, G. Z. (2000) Detection of tumor necrosis factor-alpha mRNA induction in ischemic brain tolerance by means of real-time polymerase chain reaction. *J. Cereb. Blood Flow Metab.* **20,** 15–20.
86. Feuerstein, G., Wang, X., and Barone, F. C. (1998) Cytokines in brain ischemia—the role of TNF alpha. *Cell Mol. Neurobiol.* **18,** 695–701.
87. Liu, T., Clark, R. K., McDonnell, P. C., et al. (1994) Tumor necrosis factor-alpha expression in ischemic neurons. *Stroke* **25,** 1481–1488.
88. Yang, G. Y., Gong, C., Qin, Z., Liu, X. H., and Lorris, B. A. (1999) Tumor necrosis factor alpha expression produces increased blood-brain barrier permeability following temporary focal cerebral ischemia in mice. *Brain Res. Mol. Brain Res.* **69,** 135–143.
89. Shohami, E., Ginis, I., and Hallenbeck, J. M. (1999) Dual role of tumor necrosis factor alpha in brain injury. *Cytokine Growth Factor Rev.* **10,** 119–130.
90. Rothwell, N. J. and Luheshi, G. N. (1996) Brain TNF: damage limitation or damaged reputation? *Nat. Med.* **2,** 746–747.
91. Stahel, P. F., Shohami, E., Younis, F. M., et al. (2000) Experimental closed head injury: analysis of neurological outcome, blood-brain barrier dysfunction, intracranial neutrophil infiltration, and neuronal cell death in mice deficient in genes for pro-inflammatory cytokines. *J. Cereb. Blood Flow Metab.* **20,** 369–380.
92. Benigni, F., Faggioni, R., Sironi, M., et al. (1996) TNF receptor p55 plays a major role in centrally mediated increases of serum IL-6 and corticosterone after intracerebroventricular injection of TNF. *J. Immunol.* **157,** 5563–5568.
93. Bruce, A. J., Boling, W., Kindy, M. S., et al. (1996) Altered neuronal and microglial responses to excitotoxic and ischemic brain injury in mice lacking TNF receptors. *Nat. Med.* **2,** 788–794.
94. Akassoglou, K., Probert, L., Kontogeorgos, G., and Kollias, G. (1997) Astrocyte-specific but not neuron-specific transmembrane TNF triggers inflammation and degeneration in the central nervous system of transgenic mice. *J. Immunol.* **158,** 438–445.
95. Aloe, L., Fiore, M., Probert, L., Turrini, P., and Tirassa, P. (1999) Overexpression of tumour necrosis factor alpha in the brain of transgenic mice differentially alters nerve growth factor levels and choline acetyltransferase activity. *Cytokine* **11,** 45–54.
96. Gary, D. S., Bruce-Keller, A. J., Kindy, M. S., and Mattson, M. P. (1998) Ischemic and excitotoxic brain injury is enhanced in mice lacking the p55 tumor necrosis factor receptor. *J. Cereb. Blood Flow Metab.* **18,** 1283–1287.
97. Barker, V., Middleton, G., Davey, F., and Davies, A. M. (2001) TNFalpha contributes to the death of NGF-dependent neurons during development. *Nat. Neurosci.* **4,** 1194–1198.

98. Neumann, H., Schweigreiter, R., Yamashita, T., Rosenkranz, K., Wekerle, H., and Barde, Y. A. (2002) Tumor necrosis factor inhibits neurite outgrowth and branching of hippocampal neurons by a rho-dependent mechanism. *J. Neurosci.* **22,** 854–862.
99. Nguyen, V. T. and Benveniste, E. N. (2002) Critical role of tumor necrosis factor-alpha and NF-kappa B in interferon-gamma-induced CD40 expression in microglia/macrophages. *J. Biol. Chem.* **277,** 13796–13803.
100. Parnet, P., Kelley, K. W., Bluthe, R. M., and Dantzer, R. (2002) Expression and regulation of interleukin-1 receptors in the brain. Role in cytokines-induced sickness behavior. *J. Neuroimmunol.* **125,** 5–14.
101. Yang, L., Lindholm, K., Konishi, Y., Li, R., and Shen, Y. (2002) Target depletion of distinct tumor necrosis factor receptor subtypes reveals hippocampal neuron death and survival through different signal transduction pathways. *J. Neurosci.* **22,** 3025–3032.
102. Da Silva, J., Pierrat, B., Mary, J. L., and Lesslauer, W. (1997) Blockade of p38 mitogen-activated protein kinase pathway inhibits inducible nitric-oxide synthase expression in mouse astrocytes. *J. Biol. Chem.* **272,** 28373–28380.
103. Kitsberg, D., Formstecher, E., Fauquet, M., et al. (1999) Knock-out of the neural death effector domain protein PEA-15 demonstrates that its expression protects astrocytes from TNFalpha-induced apoptosis. *J. Neurosci.* **19,** 8244–8251.
104. Arnett, H. A., Mason, J., Marino, M., Suzuki, K., Matsushima, G. K., and Ting, J. P. (2001) TNF alpha promotes proliferation of oligodendrocyte progenitors and remyelination. *Nat. Neurosci.* **4,** 1116–1122.
105. Vitkovic, L., Maeda, S., and Sternberg, E. (2001) Anti-inflammatory cytokines: expression and action in the brain. *Neuroimmunomodulation* **9,** 295–312.
106. Ledeboer, A., Breve, J. J., Poole, S., Tilders, F. J., and Van Dam, A. M. (2000) Interleukin-10, interleukin-4, and transforming growth factor-beta differentially regulate lipopolysaccharide-induced production of pro-inflammatory cytokines and nitric oxide in co-cultures of rat astroglial and microglial cells. *Glia* **30,** 134–142.
107. Pousset, F., Cremona, S., Dantzer, R., Kelley, K., and Parnet, P. (1999) Interleukin-4 and interleukin-10 regulate IL1-beta induced mouse primary astrocyte activation: a comparative study. *Glia* **26,** 12–21.
108. de Waal, M. R., Abrams, J., Bennett, B., Figdor, C. G., and de Vries, J. E. (1991) Interleukin 10 (IL-10) inhibits cytokine synthesis by human monocytes: an autoregulatory role of IL-10 produced by monocytes. *J. Exp. Med.* **174,** 1209–1220.
109. Nava, F., Calapai, G., Facciola, G., et al. (1997) Effects of interleukin-10 on water intake, locomotory activity, and rectal temperature in rat treated with endotoxin. *Int. J. Immunopharmacol.* **19,** 31–38.
110. Ledeboer, A., Binnekade, R., Breve, J. J., Bol, J. G., Tilders, F. J., and Van Dam, A. M. (2002) Site-specific modulation of LPS-induced fever and interleukin-1 beta expression in rats by interleukin-10. *Am. J. Physiol. Regul. Integr. Comp. Physiol.* **282,** R1762–R1772.
111. Leon, L. R., Kozak, W., Rudolph, K., and Kluger, M. J. (1999) An antipyretic role for interleukin-10 in LPS fever in mice. *Am. J. Physiol.* **276,** R81–R89.
112. Grilli, M., Barbieri, I., Basudev, H., et al. (2000) Interleukin-10 modulates neuronal threshold of vulnerability to ischaemic damage. *Eur. J. Neurosci.* **12,** 2265–2272.
113. Spera, P. A., Ellison, J. A., Feuerstein, G. Z., and Barone, F. C. (1998) IL-10 reduces rat brain injury following focal stroke. *Neurosci. Lett.* **251,** 189–192.
114. Molina-Holgado, F., Grencis, R., and Rothwell, N. J. (2001) Actions of exogenous and endogenous IL-10 on glial responses to bacterial LPS/cytokines. *Glia* **33,** 97–106.
115. Falcone, M., Rajan, A. J., Bloom, B. R., and Brosnan, C. F. (1998) A critical role for IL-4 in regulating disease severity in experimental allergic encephalomyelitis as demonstrated in IL-4-deficient C57BL/6 mice and BALB/c mice. *J. Immunol.* **160,** 4822–4830.
116. Keogh, B., Atkins, G. J., Mills, K. H., and Sheahan, B. J. (2002) Avirulent Semliki Forest virus replication and pathology in the central nervous system is enhanced in IL-12-defective and reduced in IL-4-defective mice: a role for Th1 cells in the protective immunity. *J. Neuroimmunol.* **125,** 15–22.

117. Andersson, A., Grunewald, S. M., Duschl, A., Fischer, A., and DiSanto, J. P. (1997) Mouse macrophage development in the absence of the common gamma chain: defining receptor complexes responsible for IL-4 and IL-13 signaling. *Eur. J. Immunol.* **27,** 1762–1768.
118. Mohrs, M., Ledermann, B., Kohler, G., Dorfmuller, A., Gessner, A., and Brombacher, F. (1999) Differences between IL-4- and IL-4 receptor alpha-deficient mice in chronic leishmaniasis reveal a protective role for IL-13 receptor signaling. *J. Immunol.* **162,** 7302–7308.
119. Wurster, A. L., Withers, D. J., Uchida, T., White, M. F., and Grusby, M. J. (2002) Stat6 and IRS-2 cooperate in interleukin 4 (IL-4)-induced proliferation and differentiation but are dispensable for IL-4-dependent rescue from apoptosis. *Mol. Cell. Biol.* **22,** 117–126.

II

Cytokine Knockout Mice

6

The Role of IL-1 in the Immune System

**Susumu Nakae, Reiko Horai, Yutaka Komiyama,
Aya Nambu, Masahide Asano, Akio Nakane, and Yoichiro Iwakura**

1. Introduction

Interleukin-1 (IL-1) is a proinflammatory cytokine that plays an important role in inflammation and host responses to infection (for reviews, *see* refs. *1–3*). The original identification of IL-1 as an endogenous pyrogen, lymphocyte-activating factor, hemopoietin-1, and osteoclast-activating factor, serves to demonstrate its pleiotropic activity *(4)*. IL-1, produced by cell types such as macrophages, monocytes, and synovial lining cells, induces inflammation by activating synovial cells, endothelial cells, lymphocytes, and macrophages. Upon activation, these cells produce a variety of chemokines, cytokines, and inflammatory mediators *(5)*, including IL-1 itself, IL-6, tumor necrosis factor-α (TNF-α), IL-8, and cyclooxygenase (COX)-2; these molecules cause infiltration of leukocytes into inflammatory sites, increase the permeability of blood vessel walls, and induce fever *(1,2,6)*.

IL-1 consists of two molecular species, IL-1α and IL-1β, derived from two distinct genes separated by 50 kb on chromosome 2 of the mouse genome *(7,8)*. Despite only a 25% amino acid sequence identity between these molecules *(4)*, both species exert similar, but not completely overlapping, biologic activities through binding to the IL-1 type I receptor (IL-1RI) *(9)*. Although an IL-1 type II receptor (IL-1RII) also exists, this receptor does not function in signal transduction *(10)*. Another member of the IL-1 gene family, the IL-1 receptor antagonist (Ra), binds IL-1 receptors without exerting an agonistic activity *(11,12)*. Thus, IL-1Ra can inhibit IL-1 activity as a decoy. IL-18 possesses some structural similarity to IL-1α and IL-1β *(13)*. Recently, six additional members of the IL-1 family have been reported, although their function has not yet been elucidated completely *(14,15)*.

IL-1β knockout (IL-1$\beta^{-/-}$) mice were first reported by Zheng et al. in 1995 *(16)*; they are resistant to fever induction and have impaired acute-phase responses to turpentine. Shornick et al. *(17)* also reported on IL-1$\beta^{-/-}$ mice, showing that contact hypersensitivity (CHS) responses are also impaired in these mice. IL-1$\alpha^{-/-}$ and IL-1α/$\beta^{-/-}$ mice as well as IL-1$\beta^{-/-}$ mice were reported by Horai et al. *(18)*. As the IL-1α and IL-1β loci are too close to produce double knockout mice by intercrossing single gene knockout mice, IL-1α/$\beta^{-/-}$ mice were produced by two sequential knockout procedures. These knockout mice demonstrated that induction of IL-1α in the brain upon turpentine treatment is largely dependent on IL-1β and that IL-1β is crucial in fever development and the stimulation of glucocorticoid

From: *Contemporary Immunology: Cytokine Knockouts, 2nd Edition*
Edited by: Giamila Fantuzzi © Humana Press Inc., Totowa, NJ

secretion from the adrenal cortex. Knockout mice of the IL-1Ra gene were reported by Hirsch et al. *(19)*, Horai et al. *(18,20)*, and Nicklin et al. *(21)*; they exhibited early mortality, spontaneously developing arthritis, and arteritis, respectively. These knockout mice are described in greater detail in Chapter 7. IL-1RI$^{-/-}$ mice were reported by Labow et al. *(22)* and Glaccum et al. *(23)* to lack responses against IL-1α and IL-1β, indicating that IL-1RI alone mediates the signaling of these molecules. IL-1RII$^{-/-}$ mice have not yet been reported, nor have knockout mice deficient for the six additional IL-1 family genes. In this review, we describe the roles of IL-1 in the immune system revealed by the use of IL-1 knockout mice.

2. The Role of IL-1 in Innate Immunity

2.1. LPS-Induced Septic Shock

IL-1 is thought to be the major mediator inducing septic shock following lipopolysaccharide (LPS) exposure *(24,25)*. IL-1β-converting enzyme (Caspase-1)-deficient mice, which produce no mature IL-1β and only low levels of IL-1α, are resistant to LPS *(26)*. IL-1α$^{-/-}$, IL-1β$^{-/-}$, and IL-1α/β$^{-/-}$ mice exhibit normal sensitivity to LPS-induced shock *(16,27)* (Asano, Horai, and Iwakura, unpublished data), suggesting that IL-1 is not the principal mediator of endotoxic shock. Consistent with these observations, IL-1RI$^{-/-}$ mice were not protected from LPS-induced toxicity *(23)*. IL-1Ra$^{-/-}$ mice were more sensitive to the lethal effects of LPS *(19)* (Asano et al., unpublished data). These observations suggest that either excess IL-1 signaling by IL-1Ra deficiency is toxic or endotoxic shock is mediated by additional cytokines antagonized by IL-1Ra. In contrast to the crucial role of Toll-like receptors in LPS responses, IL-1 is not required for endotoxin-induced lethality.

2.2. Listeria Infection

Listeria monocytogenes, a Gram-positive bacterium, infects both humans and rodents. The mechanisms of host defense against this bacterium have been well studied in the mouse, in which macrophages and hepatocytes are infected. Neutralization of IL-1 activity using a mixture of monoclonal antibodies (MAbs) against IL-1α, IL-1β, and IL-1RI in vivo decreased resistance to *L. monocytogenes* infection *(28)*. Administration of IL-1 enhanced resistance to this pathogen *(29)*. IL-1RI$^{-/-}$ mice are more sensitive to *L. monocytogenes* infection than control mice *(22)*. Deletion of the IL-1Ra gene increased host survival and reduced the numbers of bacteria resident in infected organs, whereas IL-1Ra overexpression exhibited the converse results *(19,30)*. IL-1β$^{-/-}$ mice, however, were as sensitive to *L. monocytogenes* infection as wild-type mice *(16)*. The mouse strains 129 and C57BL/6 vary significantly in susceptibility to *L. monocytogenes* owing to a genetic difference on chromosome 2 *(31)*, and IL-1RI$^{-/-}$ mice backcrossed to the C57BL/6 strain were more resistant to *L. monocytogenes* infection compared with IL-1RI$^{-/-}$ mice from a 129 × C57BL/6 hybrid strain, but C57BL/6-IL-1RI$^{-/-}$ mice were as sensitive as C57BL/6 wild-type mice *(23)*. Thus, it will be important to use well-defined genetic backgrounds to assess the role of IL-1 in *L. monocytogenes* infection.

We examined the roles of IL-1 and IL-1Ra in response to sublethal infection with *Listeria* organisms using IL-1$^{-/-}$ and IL-1Ra$^{-/-}$ mice backcrossed to the C57BL/6 strain for more than eight generations. We found that IL-1α$^{-/-}$ and IL-1α/β$^{-/-}$ mice were highly susceptible to the bacteria (Fig. 1A), and IL-1Ra$^{-/-}$ mice were more resistant (Fig. 1B). In contrast, IL-1β$^{-/-}$ mice showed similar susceptibility to wild-type mice (Fig. 1A). These

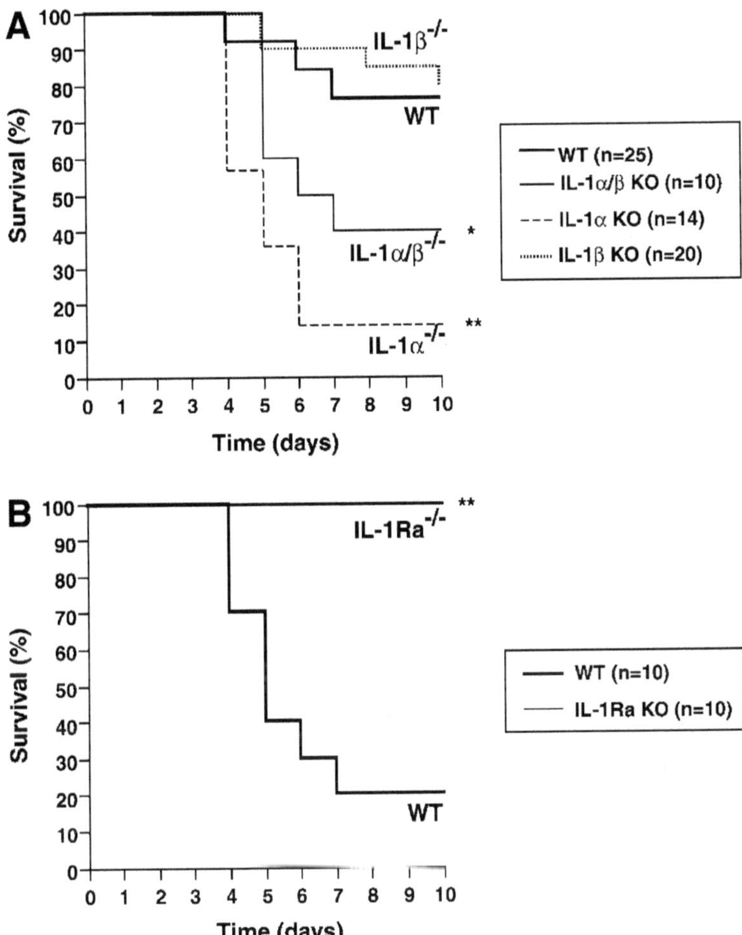

Fig. 1. Survival ratio of interleukin (IL-1)$^{-/-}$ and IL-1Ra$^{-/-}$ mice after *Listeria monocytogenes* infection. IL-1α$^{-/-}$, IL-1β$^{-/-}$, IL-1α/β$^{-/-}$, and IL-1 receptor antagonist (IL-1Ra)$^{-/-}$ mice backcrossed more than eight generations to the C57BL/6 strain were infected intravenously with sublethal doses of *L. monocytogenes*. The numbers of mice that survived were monitored every day, and survival ratios (%) were compared with C57BL/6 wild-type (WT) mice infected with the same doses of the bacteria. (**A**) Survival (%) of WT, IL-1α$^{-/-}$, IL-1β$^{-/-}$, and IL-1α/β$^{-/-}$ mice infected with 2×10^5 CFU of *L. monocytogenes*. (**B**) Survival (%) of WT and IL-1Ra$^{-/-}$ mice infected with 1×10^6 CFU of *L. monocytogenes*. *, $p < 0.05$; **, $p < 0.01$. KO, knockout mice.

observations demonstrate that IL-1 plays an important role in the host defense mechanisms against *L. monocytogenes* infection, in which IL-1α, but not IL-1β, is crucial for the protection against the bacterium.

3. The Role of IL-1 in Humoral Immune Response

IL-1, originally identified as a murine thymocyte proliferative factor, is thought to act as an activator of T-cells *(1,4)*. IL-1 exhibits an adjuvant effect, enhancing antibody production *(32,33)*. It breaks tolerance of T- and B-cells to certain antigens *(34–36)*. IL-1 promotes proliferation and differentiation of B-cells and potentiates antibody production

(37,38). Production of antibodies specific for sheep red blood cells (SRBCs) was reduced in IL-1β$^{-/-}$, IL-1α/β$^{-/-}$, and IL-1RI$^{-/-}$ mice, but not in IL-1α$^{-/-}$ mice, and was enhanced in IL-1Ra$^{-/-}$ mice *(39,40)*. IL-1 promotes antigen-specific T-cell priming and antibody production by inducing the cosignaling molecules CD40L and OX40 on T-cells in a manner independent of the CD28/CTLA-4-CD80/CD86 system *(39)*.

Antigen-specific serum antibody levels, however, are normal in IL-1RI$^{-/-}$ mice following immunization with trinitrophenyl/keyhole limpet hemocyanin (TNP/KLH) and either alum or complete Freund's adjuvant (CFA) *(23,41)*. As CFA can induce various cytokines, these inflammatory mediators may substitute for IL-1 function. Another explanation for this discrepancy may be differences in the molecular mechanisms that govern the production of antibodies against SRBCs and TNP/KLH. Antibody production against SRBCs depends on the follicular dendritic cell (FDC) network, whereas TNP-KLH with adjuvant does not *(42,43)*.

IL-1α/β$^{-/-}$ mice also exhibit reduced antibody production after exposure to the T-cell-independent antigen TNP/Ficoll *(39)*, which stimulates an immune response independent of MHC class II and most costimulatory molecules including CD28, CD40, and OX40 *(44–48)*. Thus, IL-1 may be involved in this response by inducing previously unidentified molecules.

4. The Role of IL-1 in Cellular Immune Response

4.1. Contact Hypersensitivity

CHS is a T-cell-mediated cellular immune response against contact allergens resulting from repeated epicutaneous exposure. After the first epicutaneous sensitization, Langerhans cells capture allergens and migrate from the skin to draining lymph nodes. There, naive T-cells are primed against allergens by the T-cell-Langerhans cell interaction *(49)*. In the elicitation phase, allergen-specific T-cells in lymph nodes are activated upon rechallenge with the same allergen. The activated T-cells then migrate from lymph nodes to the site of allergen challenge, resulting in local inflammation *(49)*.

CHS was markedly reduced by intradermal administration with anti-IL-1β MAb but not with anti-IL-1α MAb *(50)*. Using IL-1β$^{-/-}$ mice, however, IL-1β did not appear to be involved in oxazolone-induced CHS *(16,17)*. Low-dose trinitrochlorobenzone (TNCB)-induced CHS was suppressed in IL-1β$^{-/-}$ mice, whereas high-dose responses were not *(17)*. Using mice on the C57BL/6 background, both low- and high-dose TNCB-induced CHS responses were normal in IL-1β$^{-/-}$ mice, whereas those in IL-1α$^{-/-}$ mice as well as those in IL-1α/β$^{-/-}$ and IL-1RI$^{-/-}$ mice were significantly reduced *(51)*. The reason for the apparent discrepancies is not known completely, but the different genetic backgrounds of the mice may be involved *(51)*. These observations indicate that IL-1α, rather than IL-1β, leads to the development of CHS in C57BL/6 mice.

Skin Langerhans cell (LC) migration into lymph nodes is impaired both in IL-1α$^{-/-}$ and IL-1β$^{-/-}$ mice *(51)*. The enhancement of Langerhans cell migration by IL-1, however, may not be critical in CHS, as only IL-1α deficiency suppresses CHS responses *(51)*. The proliferation of TNP-specific T-cells is specifically reduced in IL-1α$^{-/-}$ mice. Furthermore, adoptive transfer of TNP-conjugated IL-1-deficient antigen-presenting cells (APCs) into wild-type mice indicates that only IL-1α, not IL-1β, can prime allergen-specific T-cells. Thus, the production of IL-1α, but not IL-1β, by Langerhans cells plays a crucial role in sensitizing naive T-cells against contact allergens.

Although the transfer of wild-type TNCB-sensitized T-cells could not elicit CHS in IL-1α/β$^{-/-}$ mice, this response could be recovered in tumor necrosis factor-α (TNF-α) injection. Moreover, CHS was exacerbated in IL-1Ra$^{-/-}$ mice, an effect suppressed by TNF-α-deficiency (Nakae et al., unpublished observations). Thus, the induction of TNF-α production by IL-1 plays a crucial role in inducing local inflammation during the elicitation phase of CHS.

4.2. Delayed-Type Hypersensitivity

In contrast to CHS, which is mediated by CD8$^+$ T-cells, delayed-type hypersensitivity (DTH) is believed to be mediated by CD4$^+$ T-helper (Th)1 cells *(49)*. DTH to methylated BSA (mBSA) develops normally in both IL-1β$^{-/-}$ *(16)* and IL-1α$^{-/-}$ mice (Nambu, Nakae, and Iwakura, unpublished observation). In contrast, DTH is suppressed in IL-1α/β$^{-/-}$ (Nambu et al., unpublished observation) and IL-1RI$^{-/-}$ mice *(22)* and is markedly exacerbated in IL-1Ra$^{-/-}$ mice (Nambu et al., in preparation). These observations indicate that both IL-1α and IL-1β are involved in DTH induction, whereas either are sufficient to induce the response. The use of IL-1α/β$^{-/-}$ mice suggested a critical role for IL-1 in antigen-specific Th1 cell activation rather than in the induction of local inflammation (Nambu et al., unpublished observation). Interestingly, DTH in IL-1R-associated kinase (IRAK-1)$^{-/-}$ mice developed normally, suggesting that IL-1 signaling in DTH reaction is mediated by other members of the IRAK families, such as IRAK-2 or IRAK-4 *(52)*.

5. The Role of IL-1 in Th1/Th2 Development

Th1 cells producing interferon-γ (IFN-γ) are involved in cellular immune responses, whereas Th2 cells producing IL-4, IL-5, and IL-13 generate humoral immune responses *(53)*. IL-1α is required for IL-12-dependent IFN-γ production by Th1 cells derived from BALB/c mice *(54)*. In human T-cells, IL-1β induces IFN-γ synergistically with IL-12 *(55)*. IL-1 also functions in Th2 activation, acting through mechanisms both dependent and independent of IL-4 *(56,57)*, through activation of Lck *(58)*. IFN-γ and IL-4 production by IL-1α/β$^{-/-}$ mouse T-cells cultured under either Th1 (+IL-12, +anti-IL-4) or Th2 (+IL-4, +anti-IFN-γ) conditions, however, were not significantly different from wild-type cells (Nakae et al., unpublished observation), indicating that T-cell-derived IL-1 is dispensable in Th1/Th2 polarization. Upon bacille Calmette-Guérin (BCG) injection, conditions known to evoke strong Th1 responses, the numbers of IFN-γ-positive CD4+ and CD8+ cells did not differ among IL-1α/β$^{-/-}$, IL-1RI$^{-/-}$, IL-1Ra$^{-/-}$, and wild-type mice on either the C57BL/6 or BALB/c backgrounds (Fig. 2 and data not shown). It was reported that Th2 cytokine production upon infection with *Leishmania major* is higher in IL-1RI$^{-/-}$ mice (129 × B6 F1) than in wild-type mice *(41)*. Thus, IL-1 is not essential for Th1/Th2 development but is required for activation, as described in Th1- and Th2-cell-mediated immune responses.

6. The Role of IL-1 in Diseases

6.1. Asthma

Allergic asthma is a Th2-type cytokine-mediated inflammatory response in the lungs, characterized by hypersecretion of mucus, airway inflammation, and airway hyperresponsiveness (AHR) to spasmogenic stimuli *(59)*. IL-1, detectable in alveolar macrophages

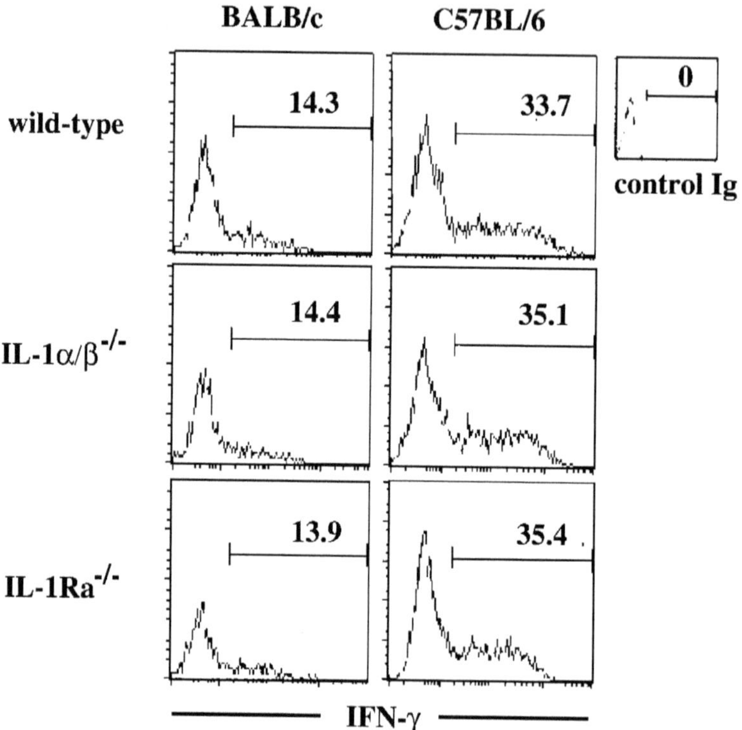

Fig. 2. Normal Th1 cell develpoment in interleukin (IL-1)$^{-/-}$ mice after bacille Calmette-Guérin (BCG) injection. Mice were immunized with 1 mg of BCG intravenously. One week after injection, splenic T-cells were stimulated with 10 μg/mL of plate-coated anti-CD3 MAb in the presence of 2 m*M* monensin for 6 h. Then, intracellular IFN-γ in $CD4^+$ cells was stained with fluorescein isothiocyanate (FITC)-anti-mouse IFN-γ Ab (XMG1.1).

from asthmatic patients *(60)*, enhances eosinophil infiltration *(61)*, mast cell activation, and production of Th2-type cytokines *(62,63)*.

Neutralization of IL-1 activity by anti-IL-1β Abs or recombinant IL-1Ra (rIL-1Ra) effectively suppresses asthmatic reactions *(64–67)*. Eosinophil infiltration following sensitization with ovalbumin (OVA)/alum was markedly reduced in IL-1RI$^{-/-}$ mice (129 × B6 F1) owing to the reduced expression of vascular cell adhesion molecule-1 (VCAM-1) *(68)*. AHR in IL-1α/β$^{-/-}$ mice (BALB/c) sensitized with OVA/alum was normal (Umeda, Nakae, and Iwakura, unpublished observations). When sensitized to OVA in the absence of adjuvant [OVA/phosphate-buffered saline (PBS)], AHR was markedly reduced in IL-1α/β$^{-/-}$ mice and greatly exacerbated in IL-1Ra$^{-/-}$ mice (Nakae et al., unpublished observation). This OVA/PBS-induced AHR was similarly suppressed in both IL-1α$^{-/-}$ and IL-1β$^{-/-}$ mice to the levels seen in IL-1α/β$^{-/-}$ mice. It seems likely that high levels of inflammatory cytokines are induced in the presence of alum, which may substitute for IL-1 function in AHR. It should be noted that OVA/alum induces IgE- and mast cell-independent AHR *(69,70)*, whereas AHR induction by OVA/PBS is dependent on mast cells *(71)*. Thus, IL-1 is critical in both eosinophilia and AHR induction.

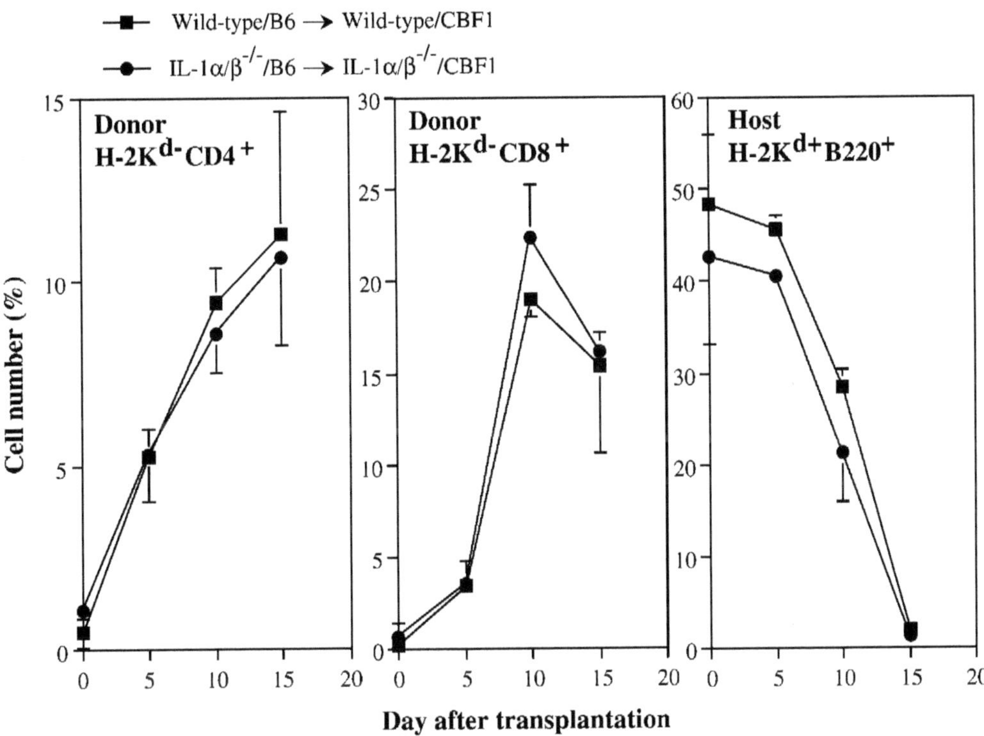

Fig. 3. Normal acute graft-versus-host reaction in interleukin (IL)-$1^{-/-}$ mice. Spleen cells from wild-type or IL-$1\alpha/\beta^{-/-}$ mice on the C57BL/6 background (H-$2K^{b/b}$) were intravenously transferred into wild-type or IL-$1\alpha/\beta^{-/-}$ mice on the CBF1 (C57BL/6J × BALB/cA F1: H-$2K^{b/d}$) background. At the indicated time points, the spleens of the recipient mice were removed, and H-$2K^{d-}CD4^{+}$ or H-$2K^{d-}CD8^{+}$ cells from the donor mice and H-$2K^{d+}B220^{+}$ cells of the recipient mice were analyzed by fluorescence-activated sorting. Symbols represent the average of four mice and SD.

6.2. Graft-Versus-Host Reaction

Incompatibility of histocompatibility antigens between transplanted bone marrow cells and recipient tissues results in severe acute and/or chronic graft-versus-host (GvH) diseases *(72,73)*. Acute GvH features mononuclear cell infiltration and injury to target organs mediated by IFN-γ-producing donor T-cells *(74)*. IL-1 is present in the affected GvH target organs *(75)*; administration of rIL-1Ra and soluble IL-1R prolonged the survival of allografts *(76–78)*. It has also been reported that IL-1Ra treatment is not effective for the treatment of GvH *(79)*.

Acute GvH is induced upon the transfer of C57BL/6 mouse-derived spleen cells into CBF1 (C57BL/6 × BALB/c F1) mice (B6 ⇒ CBF1). When IL-$1\alpha/\beta^{-/-}$ spleen cells are transferred into IL-$1\alpha/\beta^{-/-}$ mice (IL-$1\alpha/\beta^{-/-}$ B6 ⇒ IL-$1\alpha/\beta^{-/-}$ CBF1), the expansion of donor $CD4^{+}$ and $CD8^{+}$ T-cells was comparable with that of wild-type cells (Fig. 3). The reduction of host H-$2K^{d}$ + B-cells was also similar between the mice (Fig. 3). No differences were observed in the cytotoxic T-cell activity to H-2^{d}-specific P815 target cells between wild-type and IL-$1\alpha/\beta^{-/-}$ B6 $CD8^{+}$ T-cells (data not shown).

Chronic GvH, mediated by Th2 cells, is characterized by autoantibody production by hyperactivated host B-cells. This inappropriate activation leads to a pathology of immune complex deposition and glomerulonephritis resembling systemic lupus erythematosus *(80–82)*. Chronic GvH can be induced by transferring BALB/c spleen cells into CBF1 mice (BALB ⇒ CBF1). Serum levels of anti-dsDNA Ig are similar between wild-type (BALB ⇒ CBF1) and IL-1α/$\beta^{-/-}$ (BALB ⇒ CBF1) mice (data not shown). No differences were observed between wild-type (BALB ⇒ CBF1) and IL-1α/$\beta^{-/-}$ (BALB ⇒ CBF1) mice in the composition of donor and host $CD4^+$, $CD8^+$, and $B220^+$ cells in the spleen (data not shown). These results indicate that IL-1 does not play an important role in the development of either acute or chronic GvH responses.

6.3. Experimental Autoimmune Encephalomyelitis

Experimental autoimmune encephalomyelitis (EAE) is an antigen-specific T-cell-mediated autoimmune response in the nervous system, recognizing autoantigens such as myelin basic protein (MBP) *(83)*. EAE is exacerbated by rIL-1α injection and ameliorated by the administration of soluble IL-1R or rIL-1Ra *(84–86)*. The induction of MBP-specific T-cell anergy is inhibited by rIL-1β *(87)*. Administration of rIL-1, however, led to elevated corticosterone levels, subsequently suppressing the development of EAE *(88)*. Although EAE is markedly suppressed in IL-$1RI^{-/-}$ mice *(89)*, the molecular mechanism of this suppression remains unknown.

6.4. Inflammatory Bowel Disease

The multiple forms of inflammatory bowel disease (IBD), including ulcerative colitis and Crohn's disease, are characterized by bowel lesions containing accumulating inflammatory cells *(90)*. Dysregulation of Th1 cells, resulting in the secretion of inflammatory cytokines and chemokines and the activation of macrophages and neutrophils, is critical in the pathogenesis of IBD *(91)*.

Dextran sulfate sodium (DSS)-induced colitis in mice is a well-accepted model of human ulcerative colitis. DSS-induced colitis is suppressed by the administration of either anti-IL-1β Ab, soluble IL-1R, or rIL-1Ra *(92,93)*, although other reports have suggested the beneficial effects of IL-1 *(94)*. Although DSS-induced colitis in caspase-$1^{-/-}$ mice was suppressed *(93)*, this suppression may involve the absence of both IL-1 and IL-18. Thus, the role of IL-1 in IBD remains controversial.

6.5. Rheumatoid Arthritis

Rheumatoid arthritis (RA) is a typical autoimmune disease characterized by chronic inflammation of the synovial tissues that leads to joint destruction. The etiopathogenesis of this disease has not yet been completely elucidated. High levels of IL-1 expression have been observed in the joints of RA patients *(95–101)*, and plasma IL-1 levels have been correlated with disease activity *(102)*. In addition, the association of juvenile RA with an IL-1α polymorphism further supports the possible role of IL-1 in disease induction *(103)*. Recently, the role of IL-1 in the development of arthritis in animal models has been reviewed *(104)*.

Collagen-induced arthritis (CIA) is one of the most well-established models of RA *(105, 106)*. CIA can be induced in susceptible rodents by intradermal injections of homologous or heterologous native type II collagen. The development of CIA was severely suppressed in IL-1-deficient mice; 68% of wild-type mice developed arthritis 10 wk after type II collagen immunization, whereas none (0%) of the IL-1α/$\beta^{-/-}$ mice developed any pathology

(107). It has also been reported that local expression of IL-1Ra protein can prevent murine CIA *(108,109)*. These results support the crucial role of IL-1 in the development of CIA.

Disruption of either the IL-1α or IL-1β gene significantly suppressed CIA, suggesting the synergistic action of these molecules. Treatment with anti-IL-1α/β or anti-IL-1β Abs ameliorated CIA in mice *(110,111)*. In these reports, however, treatment with anti-IL-1α Ab did not demonstrate any protection. Ab production following type II collagen immunization in the presence of CFA was normal in IL-1α/β$^{-/-}$ mice. T-cell proliferative responses against type II collagen, however, were greatly reduced in the CIA model, indicating that T-cell priming is inefficient in the absence of IL-1 *(107)*. Recently, the importance of IL-1 in the development of arthritis was also shown in an anti-type II collagen Ab-induced arthritis model using IL-1RI$^{-/-}$ mice *(112)*. Suppression of the development of arthritis in IL-1RI$^{-/-}$ mice was also reported in the K/BxN model, a T-cell receptor transgenic mouse producing Abs to glucose-6-phosphate isomerase *(113)*.

Human T-lymphotropic virus-I (HTLV-I) is the causative agent of adult T-cell leukemia *(114,115)*. The HTLV-I Tax protein serves as a transcriptional transactivator, which activates transcription from both the cognate viral promoter and endogenous cellular genes, including those for IL-1 or IL-6. Previously, we found that transgenic mice carrying the HTLV-1 *tax* gene (HTLV-I Tg mice) develop chronic inflammatory polyarthropathy resembling RA at a high incidence *(116,117)*. Multiple proinflammatory cytokine genes, including IL-1α, IL-1β, IL-6, and TNF-α, are activated in the joints of these mice *(118)*. The development of arthritis was suppressed in IL-1α/β$^{-/-}$ mice; incidence of arthritis was 60 and 80% at 3 and 6 mo of age, respectively, in IL-1α/β$^{+/+}$ HTLV-I Tg mice on the BALB/c background, whereas only 10 and 30% of IL-1α/β$^{-/-}$ mice developed disease at the same time points. The severity score of arthritic IL-1α/β$^{-/-}$ HTLV-I Tg mice, however, did not differ from that of their wild-type counterparts. Thus, although these IL-1 activities may be required to initiate the development of inflammation, they are not necessarily required during the effecter phase *(107)*. T-cell proliferative responses against type II collagen were also greatly reduced in IL-1α/β$^{-/-}$ HTLV-I Tg mice, indicating inefficient T-cell priming *(107)*.

IL-1Ra$^{-/-}$ mice spontaneously develop chronic inflammatory arthropathy *(20)*. The incidence of arthritis differs between different genetic backgrounds; incidence is high on the BALB/c background, but low on the C57BL/6 background, similar to the results observed for HTLV-I-induced arthritis, suggesting the involvement of BALB/c-specific host genes. Total immunoglobulin levels as well as autoantibody levels against immunoglobulin, type II collagen, and dsDNA are elevated in these IL-1Ra$^{-/-}$ mice *(20)*. When IL-1Ra$^{-/-}$ mice were crossed to *scid/scid* mice, the development of arthritis was completely suppressed (Horai et al., unpublished observation). Furthermore, the transfer of T-cells from IL-1Ra$^{-/-}$ mice into *nu/nu* mice resulted in the development of arthritis (Horai et al., unpublished observation). These observations indicate that excessive IL-1 signaling resulting from a deficiency in IL-1Ra causes autoimmunity, joint-specific inflammation, and subsequent bone destruction. IL-1Ra$^{-/-}$ mice also develop arteritis *(21)* or die early *(19)* on a MF1 × 129/Ola background or C57BL/6 background, respectively.

IL-1α, IL-1β, and IL-1Ra are constitutively expressed in the joints of normal wild-type mice. The expression of IL-1β, but not IL-1α, increased two- to threefold in IL-1Ra$^{-/-}$ mice in comparison with wild-type controls *(20)*. The expression of other inflammatory cytokines, including TNF-α and IL-6, was also elevated, indicating a regulatory role for IL-1Ra in the cytokine network. Thus, in the absence of IL-1Ra, physiologic levels of IL-1 result in the development of autoimmunity. The development of arthritis is suppressed in mice deficient for either TNF-α or IL-17, but not IL-6. Thus, these downstream cytokines of IL-1 are suggested to play important roles in the effector phase (Horai et al. and Nakae et al., unpublished observation). Similar effects of TNF-α and IL-6 deficiency were also observed in an anti-type II collagen Ab-induced arthritis and a K/BxN models *(112, 113)*. Although *Staphylococcus aureus*-induced arthritis was worsened in IL-1RI$^{-/-}$ mice, this is because IL-1 plays an important role for the protection against *S. aureus* infection, and higher numbers of bacteria are detected in the circulation of the knockout mice *(119)*.

These results suggest a link between excess IL-1 signaling and autoimmunity and support the existence of a crucial balance between IL-1 and IL-1Ra in the maintenance of immune system homeostasis.

7. Conclusions

Clearly, IL-1 is crucial for host defense mechanisms, not only in the activation of innate immunity but also in the activation of acquired immunity. This cytokine is also involved in the host defense mechanisms through regulation of the neuronal and endocrine systems. IL-1 knockout mice as well as IL-1Ra knockout mice should play critical roles in analyzing the functions of these molecules within the body.

References

1. Dinarello, C. A. (1996) Biologic basis for interleukin-1 in disease. *Blood* **87,** 2095–2147.
2. Tocci, M. J. and Schmidt, J. A. (1997) Interleukin-1: structure and function. In: Remick, D. G. and Friedland, J. S., eds. *Cytokines in Health and Disease*, 2nd ed. Marcel Dekker, New York, pp. 1–27.
3. Durum, S. K. and Oppenheim, J. J. (1993) Proinflammatory cytokines and immunity. In: Paul, W. E., ed. *Fundamental Immunology,* 3rd ed. Raven, New York, pp. 801–835.
4. Dinarello, C. A. (1991) Interleukin-1 and interleukin-1 antagonism. *Blood* **77,** 1627–1652.
5. Feldmann, M., Brennan, F. M., and Maini, R. N. (1996) Role of cytokines in rheumatoid arthritis. *Annu. Rev. Immunol.* **14,** 397–440.
6. Davis, P. and MacIntyre, D. E. (1992) Prostaglandins and inflammation. In: Gallin, J. I., Goldstein, I. M., and Snyderman, R., eds. *Inflammation: Basic Principles and Clinical Correlates.* Raven, New York, pp. 123–137.
7. Silver, A. R., Masson, W. K., George, A. M., Adam, J., and Cox, R. (1990) The IL-1 alpha and beta genes are closely linked (less than 70 kb) on mouse chromosome 2. *Somat. Cell Mol. Genet.* **16,** 549–556.
8. D'Eustachio, P., Jadidi, S., Fuhlbrigge, R. C., Gray, P. W., and Chaplin, D. D. (1987) Interleukin-1 alpha and beta genes: linkage on chromosome 2 in the mouse. *Immunogenetics* **26,** 339–343.
9. Sims, J. E., Gayle, M. A., Slack, J. L., et al. (1993) Interleukin 1 signaling occurs exclusively via the type I receptor. *Proc. Natl. Acad. Sci. USA* **90,** 6155–6159.
10. Colotta, F., Re, F., Muzio, M., et al. (1993) Interleukin-1 type II receptor: a decoy target for IL-1 that is regulated by IL-4. *Science* **261,** 472–475.
11. Carter, D. B., Deibel, M. R. Jr., Dunn, C. J., et al. (1990) Purification, cloning, expression and biological characterization of an interleukin-1 receptor antagonist protein. *Nature* **344,** 633–638.
12. Hannum, C. H., Wilcox, C. J., Arend, W. P., et al. (1990) Interleukin-1 receptor antagonist activity of a human interleukin-1 inhibitor. *Nature* **343,** 336–340.
13. Bazan, J. F., Timans, J. C., and Kastelein, R. A. (1996) A newly defined interleukin-1? *Nature* **379,** 591.
14. Dunn, E., Sims, J. E., Nicklin, M. J., and O'Neill, L. A. (2001) Annotating genes with potential roles in the immune system: six new members of the IL-1 family. *Trends Immunol.* **22,** 533–536.
15. Sims, J. E., Nicklin, M. J., Bazan, J. F., et al. (2001) A new nomenclature for IL-1-family genes. *Trends Immunol.* **22,** 536–537.

16. Zheng, H., Fletcher, D., Kozak, W., et al. (1995) Resistance to fever induction and impaired acute-phase response in interleukin-1 beta-deficient mice. *Immunity* **3,** 9–19.
17. Shornick, L. P., De Togni, P., Mariathasan, S., et al. (1996) Mice deficient in IL-1beta manifest impaired contact hypersensitivity to trinitrochlorobenzone. *J. Exp. Med.* **183,** 1427–1436.
18. Horai, R., Asano, M., Sudo, K., et al. (1998) Production of mice deficient in genes for interleukin (IL)-1alpha, IL- 1beta, IL-1alpha/beta, and IL-1 receptor antagonist shows that IL-1beta is crucial in turpentine-induced fever development and glucocorticoid secretion. *J. Exp. Med.* **187,** 1463–1475.
19. Hirsch, E., Irikura, V. M., Paul, S. M., and Hirsh, D. (1996) Functions of interleukin 1 receptor antagonist in gene knockout and overproducing mice. *Proc. Natl. Acad. Sci. USA* **93,** 11008–11013.
20. Horai, R., Saijo, S., Tanioka, H., et al. (2000) Development of chronic inflammatory arthropathy resembling rheumatoid arthritis in interleukin 1 receptor antagonist-deficient mice. *J. Exp. Med.* **191,** 313–320.
21. Nicklin, M. J., Hughes, D. E., Barton, J. L., Ure, J. M., and Duff, G. W. (2000) Arterial inflammation in mice lacking the interleukin 1 receptor antagonist gene. *J. Exp. Med.* **191,** 303–312.
22. Labow, M., Shuster, D., Zetterstrom, M., et al. (1997) Absence of IL-1 signaling and reduced inflammatory response in IL-1 type I receptor-deficient mice. *J. Immunol.* **159,** 2452–2461.
23. Glaccum, M. B., Stocking, K. L., Charrier, K., et al. (1997) Phenotypic and functional characterization of mice that lack the type I receptor for IL-1. *J. Immunol.* **159,** 3364–3371.
24. Ohlsson, K., Bjork, P., Bergenfeldt, M., Hageman, R., and Thompson, R. C. (1990) Interleukin-1 receptor antagonist reduces mortality from endotoxin shock. *Nature* **348,** 550–552.
25. Alexander, H. R., Doherty, G. M., Buresh, C. M., Venzon, D. J., and Norton, J. A. (1991) A recombinant human receptor antagonist to interleukin 1 improves survival after lethal endotoxemia in mice. *J. Exp. Med.* **173,** 1029–1032.
26. Li, P., Allen, H., Banerjee, S., et al. (1995) Mice deficient in IL-1beta-converting enzyme are defective in production of mature IL-1beta and resistant to endotoxic shock. *Cell* **80,** 401–411.
27. Fantuzzi, G., Zheng, H., Faggioni, R., et al. (1996) Effect of endotoxin in IL-1beta-deficient mice. *J. Immunol.* **157,** 291–296.
28. Rogers, H. W., Tripp, C. S., Schreiber, R. D., and Unanue, E. R. (1994) Endogenous IL-1 is required for neutrophil recruitment and macrophage activation during murine listeriosis. *J. Immunol.* **153,** 2093–2101.
29. Czuprynski, C. J., Brown, J. F., Young, K. M., Cooley, A. J., and Kurtz, R. S. (1988) Effects of murine recombinant interleukin 1 alpha on the host response to bacterial infection. *J. Immunol.* **140,** 962–968.
30. Irikura, V. M., Hirsch, E., and Hirsh, D. (1999) Effects of interleukin-1 receptor antagonist overexpression on infection by *Listeria monocytogenes*. *Infect. Immun.* **67,** 1901–1909.
31. Cheers, C. and McKenzie, I. F. C. (1980) A single gene (*Lr*) controlling resistance to murine listeriosis. In: Skamene, E., Kongshavn, P. A. L., and Landy, M., eds. *Genetic Control of Natural Resistance to Infection and Malignancy*. Academic, New York, p. 141.
32. Staruch, M. J. and Wood, D. D. (1983) The adjuvanticity of interleukin 1 in vivo. *J. Immunol.* **130,** 2191–2194.
33. Reed, S. G., Pihl, D. L., Conlon, P. J., and Grabstein, K. H. (1989) IL-1 as adjuvant. Role of T cells in the augmentation of specific antibody production by recombinant human IL-1 alpha. *J. Immunol.* **142,** 3129–3133.
34. Nakata, Y., Matsuda, K., Uzawa, A., Nomura, M., Akashi, M., and Suzuki, G. (1995) Administration of recombinant human IL-1 by *Staphylococcus* enterotoxin B prevents tolerance induction in vivo. *J. Immunol.* **155,** 4231–4235.
35. Gahring, L. C. and Weigle, W. O. (1990) The regulatory effects of cytokines on the induction of a peripheral immunologic tolerance in mice. *J. Immunol.* **145,** 1318–1323.
36. Duan, J. M. and Habicht, G. S. (1989) Effect of interleukin 1 on the induction and maintenance of B cell tolerance in vitro. *J. Leukoc. Biol.* **45,** 329–335.
37. Lipsky, P. E., Thompson, P. A., Rosenwasser, L. J., and Dinarello, C. A. (1983) The role of interleukin 1 in human B cell activation: inhibition of B cell proliferation and the generation of immunoglobulin-secreting cells by an antibody against human leukocytic pyrogen. *J. Immunol.* **130,** 2708–2714.

38. Maliszewski, C. R., Sato, T. A., Vanden Bos, T., et al. (1990) Cytokine receptors and B cell functions. I. Recombinant soluble receptors specifically inhibit IL-1- and IL-4-induced B cell activities in vitro. *J. Immunol.* **144,** 3028–3033.
39. Nakae, S., Asano, M., Horai, R., Sakaguchi, N., and Iwakura, Y. (2001) IL-1 enhances T cell-dependent antibody production through induction of CD40 ligand and OX40 on T cells. *J. Immunol.* **167,** 90–97.
40. Nakae, S., Asano, M., Horai, R., and Iwakura, Y. (2001) Interleukin-1β, but not interleukin-1α, is required for T-cell-dependent antibody production. *Immunology* **104,** 402–409.
41. Satoskar, A. R., Okano, M., Connaughton, S., Raisanen-Sokolwski, A., David, J. R., and Labow, M. (1998) Enhanced Th2-like responses in IL-1 type 1 receptor-deficient mice. *Eur. J. Immunol.* **28,** 2066–2074.
42. Matsumoto, M., Lo, S. F., Carruthers, C. J., et al. (1996) Affinity maturation without germinal centres in lymphotoxin-alpha-deficient mice. *Nature* **382,** 462–466.
43. Fu, Y. X., Molina, H., Matsumoto, M., Huang, G., Min, J., and Chaplin, D. D. (1997) Lymphotoxin-alpha (LTalpha) supports development of splenic follicular structure that is required for IgG responses. *J. Exp. Med.* **185,** 2111–2120.
44. Gosgrove, D., Gray, D., Dierich, A., et al. (1991) Mice lacking MHC class II molecules. *Cell* **66,** 1051–1066.
45. Sethna, M. P., van Parijs, L., Sharpe, A. H., Abbas, A. K., and Freeman, G. J. (1994) A negative regulatory function of B7 revealed in B7-1 transgenic mice. *Immunity* **1,** 415–421.
46. Xu, J., Foy, T. M., Laman, J. D., et al. (1994) Mice deficient for the CD40 ligand [published erratum appears in Immunity 1994;1:following 613]. *Immunity* **1,** 423–431.
47. Stuber, E. and Strober, W. (1996) The T cell-B cell interaction via OX40-OX40L is necessary for the T cell-dependent humoral immune response. *J. Exp. Med.* **183,** 979–989.
48. Pippig, S. D., Pena-Rossi, C., Long, J., et al. (1999) Robust B cell immunity but impaired T cell proliferation in the absence of CD134 (OX40) [In Process Citation]. *J. Immunol.* **163,** 6520–6529.
49. Grabbe, S. and Schwarz, T. (1998) Immunoregulatory mechanisms involved in elicitation of allergic contact hypersensitivity [see comments]. *Immunol. Today* **19,** 37–44.
50. Enk, A. H., Angeloni, V. L., Udey, M. C., and Katz, S. I. (1993) An essential role for Langerhans cell-derived IL-1 beta in the initiation of primary immune responses in skin. *J. Immunol.* **150,** 3698–3704.
51. Nakae, S., Naruse-Nakajima, C., Sudo, K., Horai, R., Asano, M., and Iwakura, Y. (2001) IL-1α, but not IL-1β, is required for contact-allergen-specific T cell activation during the sensitization phase in contact hypersensitivity. *Int. Immunol.* **13,** 1471–1478.
52. Thomas, J. A., Allen, J. L., Tsen, M., et al. (1999) Impaired cytokine signaling in mice lacking the IL-1 receptor-associated kinase. *J. Immunol.* **163,** 978–984.
53. Constant, S. L. and Bottomly, K. (1997) Induction of Th1 and Th2 CD4+ T cell responses: the alternative approaches. *Annu. Rev. Immunol.* **15,** 297–322.
54. Shibuya, K., Robinson, D., Zonin, F., et al. (1998) IL-1 alpha and TNF-alpha are required for IL-12-induced development of Th1 cells producing high levels of IFN-gamma in BALB/c but not C57BL/6 mice. *J. Immunol.* **160,** 1708–1716.
55. Tominaga, K., Yoshimoto, T., Torigoe, K., et al. (2000) IL-12 synergizes with IL-18 or IL-1beta for IFN-gamma production from human T cells. *Int. Immunol.* **12,** 151–160.
56. Kurt-Jones, E. A., Hamberg, S., Ohara, J., Paul, W. E., and Abbas, A. K. (1987) Heterogeneity of helper/inducer T lymphocytes. I. Lymphokine production and lymphokine responsiveness. *J. Exp. Med.* **166,** 1774–1787.
57. Huber, M., Beuscher, H. U., Rohwer, P., Kurrle, R., Rollinghoff, M., and Lohoff, M. (1998) Costimulation via TCR and IL-1 receptor reveals a novel IL-1alpha-mediated autocrine pathway of Th2 cell proliferation. *J. Immunol.* **160,** 4242–4247.
58. al-Ramadi, B. K., Welte, T., Fernandez-Cabezudo, M. J., et al. (2001) The Src-protein tyrosine kinase Lck is required for IL-1-mediated costimulatory signaling in Th2 cells. *J. Immunol.* **167,** 6827–6833.
59. Wills-Karp, M. (1999) Immunologic basis of antigen-induced airway hyperresponsiveness. *Annu. Rev. Immunol.* **17,** 255–281.

60. Borish, L., Mascali, J. J., Dishuck, J., Beam, W. R., Martin, R. J., and Rosenwasser, L. J. (1992) Detection of alveolar macrophage-derived IL-1 beta in asthma. Inhibition with corticosteroids. *J. Immunol.* **149,** 3078–3082.
61. Godding, V., Stark, J. M., Sedgwick, J. B., and Busse, W. W. (1995) Adhesion of activated eosinophils to respiratory epithelial cells is enhanced by tumor necrosis factor-alpha and interleukin-1 beta. *Am. J. Respir. Cell. Mol. Biol.* **13,** 555–562.
62. Hultner, L., Kolsch, S., Stassen, M., et al. (2000) In activated mast cells, IL-1 up-regulates the production of several Th2-related cytokines including IL-9. *J. Immunol.* **164,** 5556–5563.
63. Stassen, M., Arnold, M., Hultner, L., et al. (2000) Murine bone marrow-derived mast cells as potent producers of IL-9: costimulatory function of IL-10 and kit ligand in the presence of IL-1. *J. Immunol.* **164,** 5549–5555.
64. Okada, S., Inoue, H., Yamauchi, K., et al. (1995) Potential role of interleukin-1 in allergen-induced late asthmatic reactions in guinea pigs: suppressive effect of interleukin-1 receptor antagonist on late asthmatic reaction. *J. Allergy Clin. Immunol.* **95,** 1236–1245.
65. Hakonarson, H., Herrick, D. J., Serrano, P. G., and Grunstein, M. M. (1997) Autocrine role of interleukin 1beta in altered responsiveness of atopic asthmatic sensitized airway smooth muscle. *J. Clin. Invest.* **99,** 117–124.
66. Hakonarson, H., Maskeri, N., Carter, C., Chuang, S., and Grunstein, M. M. (1999) Autocrine interaction between IL-5 and IL-1beta mediates altered responsiveness of atopic asthmatic sensitized airway smooth muscle. *J. Clin. Invest.* **104,** 657–667.
67. Selig, W. and Tocker, J. (1992) Effect of interleukin-1 receptor antagonist on antigen-induced pulmonary responses in guinea pigs. *Eur. J. Pharmacol.* **213,** 331–336.
68. Broide, D. H., Campbell, K., Gifford, T., and Sriramarao, P. (2000) Inhibition of eosinophilic inflammation in allergen-challenged, IL-1 receptor type 1-deficient mice is associated with reduced eosinophil rolling and adhesion on vascular endothelium. *Blood* **95,** 263–269.
69. Korsgren, M., Erjefalt, J. S., Korsgren, O., Sundler, F., and Persson, C. G. (1997) Allergic eosinophil-rich inflammation develops in lungs and airways of B cell-deficient mice. *J. Exp. Med.* **185,** 885–892.
70. Takeda, K., Hamelmann, E., Joetham, A., et al. (1997) Development of eosinophilic airway inflammation and airway hyperresponsiveness in mast cell-deficient mice. *J. Exp. Med.* **186,** 449–454.
71. Williams, C. M. and Galli, S. J. (2000) Mast cells can amplify airway reactivity and features of chronic inflammation in an asthma model in mice. *J. Exp. Med.* **192,** 455–462.
72. Blazar, B. R., Korngold, R., and Vallera, D. A. (1997) Recent advances in graft-versus-host disease (GVHD) prevention. *Immunol. Rev.* **157,** 79–109.
73. Marcellus, D. C. and Vogelsang, G. B. (1997) Graft-versus-host disease. *Curr. Opin. Oncol.* **9,** 131–138.
74. Ellison, C. A., Fischer, J. M., HayGlass, K. T., and Gartner, J. G. (1998) Murine graft-versus-host disease in an F1-hybrid model using IFN-gamma gene knockout donors. *J. Immunol.* **161,** 631–640.
75. Abhyankar, S., Gilliland, D. G., and Ferrara, J. L. (1993) Interleukin-1 is a critical effector molecule during cytokine dysregulation in graft versus host disease to minor histocompatibility antigens. *Transplantation* **56,** 1518–1523.
76. McCarthy, P. L. Jr., Abhyankar, S., Neben, S., et al. (1991) Inhibition of interleukin-1 by an interleukin-1 receptor antagonist prevents graft-versus-host disease. *Blood* **78,** 1915–1918.
77. Antin, J. H., Weinstein, H. J., Guinan, E. C., et al. (1994) Recombinant human interleukin-1 receptor antagonist in the treatment of steroid-resistant graft-versus-host disease. *Blood* **84,** 1342–1348.
78. McCarthy, P. L. Jr., Williams, L., Harris-Bacile, M., et al. (1996) A clinical phase I/II study of recombinant human interleukin-1 receptor in glucocorticoid-resistant graft-versus-host disease. *Transplantation* **62,** 626–631.
79. Vallera, D. A., Taylor, P. A., Vannice, J. L., Panoskaltsis-Mortari, A., and Blazar, B. R. (1995) Interleukin-1 or tumor necrosis factor-alpha antagonists do not inhibit graft-versus-host disease induced across the major histocompatibility barrier in mice. *Transplantation* **60,** 1371–1374.
80. Gleichmann, E., Van Elven, E. H., and Van der Veen, J. P. (1982) A systemic lupus erythematosus (SLE)-like disease in mice induced by abnormal T-B cell cooperation. Preferential formation of autoantibodies characteristic of SLE. *Eur. J. Immunol.* **12,** 152–159.

81. Via, C. S. and Shearer, G. M. (1988) T-cell interactions in autoimmunity: insights from a murine model of graft-versus-host disease. *Immunol. Today* **9,** 207–213.
82. Goldman, M., Druet, P., and Gleichmann, E. (1991) TH2 cells in systemic autoimmunity: insights from allogeneic diseases and chemically-induced autoimmunity. *Immunol. Today* **12,** 223–227.
83. Kuchroo, V. K., Anderson, A. C., Waldner, H., Munder, M., Bettelli, E., and Nicholson, L. B. (2002) T cell response in experimental autoimmune encephalomyelitis (EAE): role of self and cross-reactive antigens in shaping, tuning, and regulating the autopathogenic T cell repertoire. *Annu. Rev. Immunol.* **20,** 101–123.
84. Jacobs, C. A., Baker, P. E., Roux, E. R., et al. (1991) Experimental autoimmune encephalomyelitis is exacerbated by IL-1 alpha and suppressed by soluble IL-1 receptor. *J. Immunol.* **146,** 2983–2989.
85. Martin, D. and Near, S. L. (1995) Protective effect of the interleukin-1 receptor antagonist (IL-1ra) on experimental allergic encephalomyelitis in rats. *J. Neuroimmunol.* **61,** 241–245.
86. Badovinac, V., Mostarica-Stojkovic, M., Dinarello, C. A., and Stosic-Grujicic, S. (1998) Interleukin-1 receptor antagonist suppresses experimental autoimmune encephalomyelitis (EAE) in rats by influencing the activation and proliferation of encephalitogenic cells. *J. Neuroimmunol.* **85,** 87–95.
87. Bourdoulous, S., Beraud, E., Le Page, C., et al. (1995) Anergy induction in encephalitogenic T cells by brain microvessel endothelial cells is inhibited by interleukin-1. *Eur. J. Immunol.* **25,** 1176–1183.
88. del Rey, A., Klusman, I., and Besedovsky, H. O. (1998) Cytokines mediate protective stimulation of glucocorticoid output during autoimmunity: involvement of IL-1. *Am. J. Physiol.* **275,** R1146–R1151.
89. Schiffenbauer, J., Streit, W. J., Butfiloski, E., LaBow, M., Edwards, C. 3rd and Moldawer, L. L. (2000) The induction of EAE is only partially dependent on TNF receptor signaling but requires the IL-1 type I receptor. *Clin. Immunol.* **95,** 117–123.
90. Fiocchi, C. (1998) Inflammatory bowel disease: etiology and pathogenesis. *Gastroenterology* **115,** 182–205.
91. Dohi, T., Fujihashi, K., Kiyono, H., Elson, C. O., and McGhee, J. R. (2000) Mice deficient in Th1- and Th2-type cytokines develop distinct forms of hapten-induced colitis. *Gastroenterology* **119,** 724–733.
92. Arai, Y., Takanashi, H., Kitagawa, H., and Okayasu, I. (1998) Involvement of interleukin-1 in the development of ulcerative colitis induced by dextran sulfate sodium in mice. *Cytokine* **10,** 890–896.
93. Siegmund, B., Lehr, H. A., Fantuzzi, G., and Dinarello, C. A. (2001) IL-1β-converting enzyme (caspase-1) in intestinal inflammation. *Proc. Natl. Acad. Sci. USA* **98,** 13249–13254.
94. Kojouharoff, G., Hans, W., Obermeier, F., et al. (1997) Neutralization of tumour necrosis factor (TNF) but not of IL-1 reduces inflammation in chronic dextran sulphate sodium-induced colitis in mice. *Clin. Exp. Immunol.* **107,** 353–358.
95. Nouri, A. M., Panayi, G. S., and Goodman, S. M. (1984) Cytokines and the chronic inflammation of rheumatic disease. I. The presence of interleukin-1 in synovial fluids. *Clin. Exp. Immunol.* **55,** 295–302.
96. Firestein, G. S., Alvaro-Gracia, J. M., Maki, R., and Alvaro-Garcia, J. M. (1990) Quantitative analysis of cytokine gene expression in rheumatoid arthritis. *J. Immunol.* **144,** 3347–3353.
97. MacNaul, K. L., Hutchinson, N. I., Parsons, J. N., Bayne, E. K., and Tocci, M. J. (1990) Analysis of IL-1 and TNF-alpha gene expression in human rheumatoid synoviocytes and normal monocytes by in situ hybridization. *J. Immunol.* **145,** 4154–4166.
98. Miyasaka, N., Sato, K., Goto, M., et al. (1988) Augmented interleukin-1 production and HLA-DR expression in the synovium of rheumatoid arthritis patients. Possible involvement in joint destruction. *Arthritis Rheum.* **31,** 480–486.
99. Fontana, A., Hengartner, H., Weber, E., Fehr, K., Grob, P. J., and Cohen, G. (1982) Interleukin 1 activity in the synovial fluid of patients with rheumatoid arthritis. *Rheumatol. Int.* **2,** 49–53.
100. Buchan, G., Barrett, K., Turner, M., Chantry, D., Maini, R. N., and Feldmann, M. (1988) Interleukin-1 and tumour necrosis factor mRNA expression in rheumatoid arthritis: prolonged production of IL-1 alpha. *Clin. Exp. Immunol.* **73,** 449–455.
101. Wood, N. C., Dickens, E., Symons, J. A., and Duff, G. W. (1992) In situ hybridization of interleukin-1 in CD14-positive cells in rheumatoid arthritis. *Clin. Immunol. Immunopathol.* **62,** 295–300.

102. Eastgate, J. A., Symons, J. A., Wood, N. C., Grinlinton, F. M., di Giovine, F. S., and Duff, G. W. (1988) Correlation of plasma interleukin 1 levels with disease activity in rheumatoid arthritis. *Lancet* **2,** 706–709.
103. McDowell, T. L., Symons, J. A., Ploski, R., Forre, O., and Duff, G. W. (1995) A genetic association between juvenile rheumatoid arthritis and a novel interleukin-1 alpha polymorphism. *Arthritis Rheum.* **38,** 221–228.
104. Iwakura, Y. (2002) Roles of IL-1 in the development of rheumatoid arthritis: consideration from mouse models. *Cytokine Growth Factor Rev.* **13,** 341–355.
105. Trentham, D. E., Townes, A. S., and Kang, A. H. (1977) Autoimmunity to type II collagen an experimental model of arthritis. *J. Exp. Med.* **146,** 857–868.
106. Holmdahl, R., Andersson, M., Goldschmidt, T. J., Gustafsson, K., Jansson, L., and Mo, J. A. (1990) Type II collagen autoimmunity in animals and provocations leading to arthritis. *Immunol. Rev.* **118,** 193–232.
107. Saijo, S., Asano, M., Horai, R., Yamamoto, H., and Iwakura, Y. (2002) Suppression of autoimmune arthritis in interleukin-1-deficient mice in which T cell activation is impaired due to low levels of CD40 ligand and OX40 expression on T cells. *Arthritis Rheum.* **46,** 533–544.
108. Bakker, A. C., Joosten, L. A., Arntz, O. J., et al. (1997) Prevention of murine collagen-induced arthritis in the knee and ipsilateral paw by local expression of human interleukin-1 receptor antagonist protein in the knee. *Arthritis Rheum.* **40,** 893–900.
109. van de Loo, F. A. and van den Berg, W. B. (2002) Gene therapy for rheumatoid arthritis. Lessons from animal models, including studies on interleukin-4, interleukin-10, and interleukin-1 receptor antagonist as potential disease modulators. *Rheum. Dis. Clin. North Am.* **28,** 127–149.
110. van den Berg, W. B., Joosten, L. A., Helsen, M., and van de Loo, F. A. (1994) Amelioration of established murine collagen-induced arthritis with anti-IL-1 treatment. *Clin. Exp. Immunol.* **95,** 237–243.
111. Joosten, L. A., Helsen, M. M., van de Loo, F. A., and van den Berg, W. B. (1996) Anticytokine treatment of established type II collagen-induced arthritis in DBA/1 mice. A comparative study using anti-TNF alpha, anti-IL-1 alpha/beta, and IL-1Ra. *Arthritis Rheum.* **39,** 797–809.
112. Kagari, T., Doi, H., and Shimozato, T. (2002) The importance of IL-1 beta and TNF-alpha, and the noninvolvement of IL-6, in the development of monoclonal antibody-induced arthritis. *J. Immunol.* **169,** 1459–1466.
113. Ji, H., Pettit, A., Ohmura, K., et al. (2002) Critical roles for interleukin 1 and tumor necrosis factor alpha in antibody-induced arthritis. *J. Exp. Med.* **196,** 77–85.
114. Yoshida, M. (1993) HTLV-1 Tax: regulation of gene expression and disease. *Trends Microbiol.* **1,** 131–135.
115. Sugamura, K. and Hinuma, Y. (1993) Human retroviruses: HTLV-I and HTLV-II. In: Levy, A., ed. *The Retroviridae,* vol. 2. Plenum, New York, pp. 399–435.
116. Iwakura, Y., Tosu, M., Yoshida, E., et al. (1991) Induction of inflammatory arthropathy resembling rheumatoid arthritis in mice transgenic for HTLV-I. *Science* **253,** 1026–1028.
117. Habu, K., J, Y., Asano, M., Saijo, S., et al. (1999) The HTLV-I-tax gene is responsible for the development of both inflammatory polyarthropathy resembling rheumatoid arthritis and non-inflammatory ankylotic in transgenic mice. *J. Immunol.* **162,** 2956–2963.
118. Iwakura, Y., Saijo, S., Kioka, Y., et al. (1995) Autoimmunity induction by human T cell leukemia virus type 1 in transgenic mice that develop chronic inflammatory arthropathy resembling rheumatoid arthritis in humans. *J. Immunol.* **155,** 1588–1598.
119. Hultgren, O. H., Svensson, L., and Tarkowski, A. (2002) Critical role of signaling through IL-1 receptor for development of arthritis and sepsis during *Staphylococcus aureus* infection. *J. Immunol.* **168,** 5207–5212.

7

IL-1 Receptor Antagonist-Deficient Mice

Martin J. H. Nicklin and Joanna Shepherd

1. Introduction

Interleukin-1 receptor antagonist (IL-1Ra) is unique among primary inflammatory cytokines because its molecular activity is entirely passive and negative *(1–3)*. Because it is a pure antagonist of the inflammatory cytokine IL-1, a deficiency of IL-1Ra not only reveals processes for which IL-1Ra is essential but highlights pathologies that involve overactivity of IL-1. IL-1Ra deficiency is not associated with developmental pathology. To some extent IL-1Ra knockouts resemble transgenics that overexpress inflammatory cytokines (*see*, for example, refs. *4* and *5*) in that both types of mice develop site-specific inflammatory diseases because of localized excessive inflammatory responses. The remarkable feature of the inflammatory diseases that we observe in IL-1Ra-deficient mice is that they are tissue-specific without any intention on the part of the investigators to target the hyperactivity of IL-1. The disturbed balance of activity of the IL-1 system, even though it is part of the innate immune system, appears to feed into the activity of the adaptive immune response, creating autoimmune conditions. Investigating the mechanism for this specificity may well yield important insights into the nature of chronic inflammatory diseases.

1.1. The Genetic Environment of the IL-1Ra Gene, Il1rn

Mouse *Il1rn* is the terminal gene in a cluster of IL-1-like genes. The ancestral gene cluster, which is retained in the human genome, contains nine IL-1 family members and is 380 kb in length in humans *(6)*. In the mouse genome, it has become split into two fragments that reside 106 Mb apart on mouse chromosome 2 *(7)*, creating two IL-1 clusters of similar physical size. Only one mouse IL-1 family gene, the most divergent, encoding IL-18, is not located within these clusters. All but one (*IL1F7*) of the remaining human IL-1 family genes have orthologs within the mouse IL-1 clusters, and multiple alignments indicate that all the protein products are composed of a single highly characteristic protein domain, which has been revealed in the X-ray crystal structures of IL-1α *(8)*, IL-1β *(9)*, and IL-1Ra *(10)*. The molecular functions of IL-1α, IL-1β, IL-1Ra, and IL-18 are well understood, but those of the products of the five other mouse IL-1 family genes are only beginning to be investigated *(11,12)*. High-affinity receptors for them have not been found, and there is no evidence for any biologic overlap between these new molecules and IL-1Ra that might complicate interpretation of the phenotype of IL-1Ra knockout mice. The IL-1F5

From: *Contemporary Immunology: Cytokine Knockouts, 2nd Edition*
Edited by: Giamila Fantuzzi © Humana Press Inc., Totowa, NJ

protein is most similar to IL-1Ra, sharing approx. 50% sequence identity, and has been described as "an IL-1Ra," yet, importantly, IL-1F5 has no functional IL-1Ra activity *(13)*. Only IL-1F10 has been reported to have some weak affinity for the signaling type I IL-1 receptor *(14)*.

In the mouse genome *(7)*, one of the IL-1 cluster fragments contains *Il1a* and *Il1b (15)*; the other contains the novel family members and *Il1rn*. From a practical point of view, there is very weak genetic linkage between the two clusters *(16)*, making it simple to recombine alleles (such as null alleles) of the two clusters through breeding. This is not possible in any species that carries its IL-1 cluster in the ancestral form. Perhaps coincidentally, the human type I IL-1 receptor gene, *IL1R1*, also lies fairly close (11 Mb) to the IL-1 cluster, but in the mouse *Il1r1* is located on a separate chromosome, permitting mendelian reassortment of alleles of the *Il1r1* and the two IL-1 clusters. On the other hand, the extremely tight linkage (<70 kb) between mouse *Il1a* and *Il1b* is retained, and this makes recombination of alleles of these two genes experimentally impractical. To overcome this, Horai et al. *(17)* have generated double knockouts by performing two cycles of homologous recombination on a single cell line. A similar approach would be needed to make double knockouts of *Il1rn* and any of the other newly found members, *Il1f5,-6, -8, -9, or -10*.

1.2. *The Mouse* **Il1rn** *Gene*

This gene appears to be functionally identical to the human gene, and the sequence identity of the processed secreted proteins is 77%. The core of the gene is compact, and the functional protein is encoded in approx. 6 kb of genomic sequence *(18)*, but an alternative, tissue-specific exon (b1) lies 10 kb distal (Fig. 1) in both species. Two predominant, tissue-specific types of product have been unambiguously identified in the mouse and correspond precisely to the human sIL-1Ra and icIL-1Ra *(16,19)*, which are the *secreted* and *intracellular* forms, respectively. A second form of mouse icIL-1Ra, corresponding to human icIL-1Ra3 has been identified with some confidence in the mouse too *(20)*.

sIL-1Ra (in human or mouse) is produced from a transcript that originates from the downstream promoter that precedes exon a1 (Fig. 1). The initiator codon is followed by a conventional secretion signal sequence, and sIL-1Ra is exceptional among the IL-1 family because it can be secreted through a conventional pathway and is generally glycosylated. In humans, an alternative 144-amino acid polypeptide, icIL-1Ra3, can be translated from the same mRNA. The protein product is abundant in neutrophils and monocytes *(21)*. Translation is initiated at the second rather than the first AUG, and this codon and its environment are conserved in the mouse sIL-1Ra mRNA *(20)*. icIL-1Ra3 is produced without a signal sequence and is expected to be retained in the cytoplasm. Its biochemical properties resemble those of the processed sIL-1Ra, but with slightly reduced affinity for IL-1R1, probably because of the loss of some of the contacts between the first β-sheet of IL-1Ra and receptor. A protein of the corresponding molecular weight has been reported recently in the mouse *(20)* and appears to derive from the same transcript as sIL-1Ra, as would be expected.

The second major mRNA, which has been well demonstrated in the mouse, originates from the distal promoter of exon b1 (Fig. 1), which encodes little more than the translational start. Exon b1 is spliced to the short exon b2, which represents the 3' part of exon a1. This splicing skips the signal sequence of exon a1, and icIL-1Ra appears to be retained within the cytoplasm. The icIL-1Ra protein is 159 amino acids and its activity, and its affinity for IL-1R1 cannot be distinguished from sIL-1Ra *(22)*.

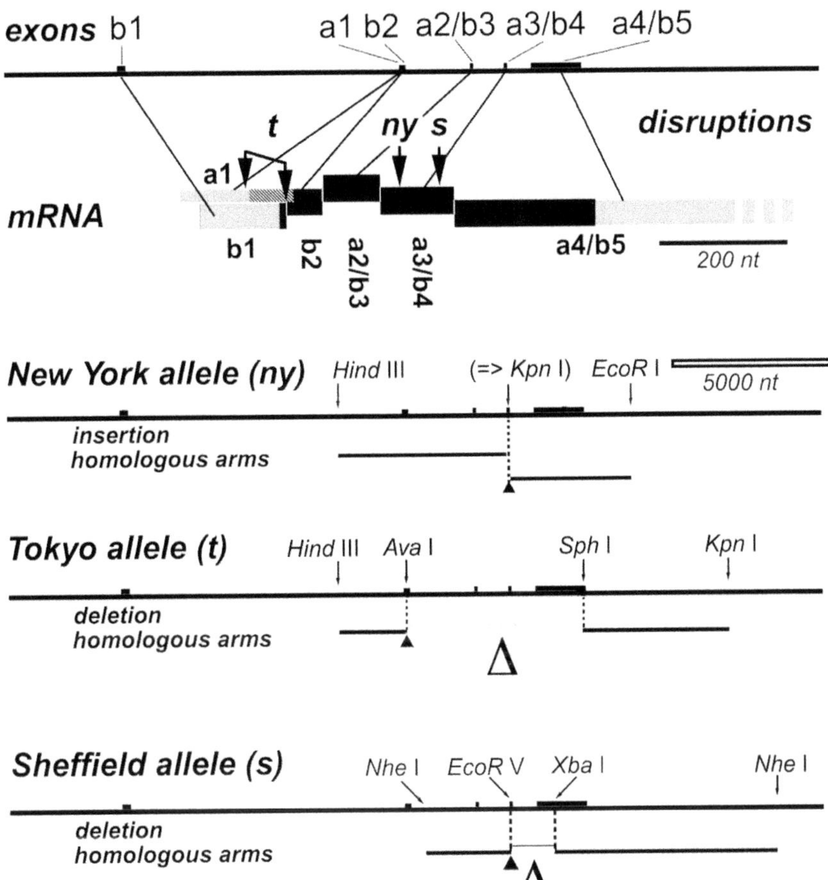

Fig. 1. The structure of the mouse interelukin-1 receptor antagonist gene and a summary of the null alleles. The map is based on the current publicly available contig of the IL-1Ra gene from the C57BL/6 mouse (*http://www.ensembl.org/Mus_musculus/*) The top line illustrates the five major exons of the gene, to scale (indicated above the third line). Tissue-specific promoters precede exons a1 and b1. The two major gene products are produced from the following exon combinations. sIL-1ra mRNA contains a1-a2/b3-a3/b4-a4/b5, and icIL-1ra contains b1-b2-a2/b3-a3/b4-a4/b5. Exon b2 is nested in exon a1, which contains an internal splice acceptor. The second line indicates the assembly of the two mRNAs from the different exons (*16,18,19*; accessions M74294 and AF001795) and the engineered points where the transcript is disrupted in the three alleles, illustrated below. Gray boxes represent untranslated regions, and the hatched box in exon a1 marks the signal sequence, which is removed by processing of sIL-1ra. *t (17)* indicates the points at which any surviving transcript from the *t* allele would fail to encode sIL-1ra (left) or icIL-1ra (right). *ny* indicates the New York alele *(54)*, which has its ORF interrupted after roughly one-third of the mature protein sequence, and *s* indicates the site of disruption of the Sheffield allele *(55)*, which encodes the first half of the mature protein. In fact, there is no evidence that either the *ny* or *s* alleles are translated. The next three lines show, to scale, an overview of the constructs used to disrupt the genes in the three laboratories. Restriction sites flanking the homologous arms are indicated. In the case of the *ny* allele, no sequence was deleted, but a *Kpn*I site was introduced by a single base mutation (=> *Kpn* I), and a disruptive insertion was made. Inserted sequences are discussed in the text.

An extra form of human IL-1Ra, *(23)* is produced from the upstream promoter by inclusion of an additional exon (c2) that lies in the interval between b1 and b2 and encodes a glycine-rich peptide of 21 amino acids. Exon c2 does not seem to exist in the mouse, and there is no evidence for this variant of icIL-1Ra in the mouse.

1.3. The Molecular Function and Cell Distribution of IL-1Ra

IL-1Ra was originally identified as an activity in human urine *(24,25)* and from monocytes *(1,2)* that inhibited IL-1 in various bioassays. Purification, sequencing, and cloning of the macrophage protein revealed that IL-1Ra is a structural homolog of IL-1α and IL-1β *(1,2)*. The subsequent discovery and functional characterization of the IL-1 receptor accessory protein (IL-1RacP) *(26,27)*, and a comparison of the structures of the complexes between the extracellular portion of IL-1R1 with IL-1Ra or IL-1β *(28,29)* has suggested that IL-1Ra functions as an agonist because it does not engage the third (membrane-proximal) domain of IL-1R1, which is responsible for recruiting, or altering, the conformation of IL-1RacP. The affinity of IL-1Ra for the type I receptor is in the 0.1-n*M* range and is comparable with the two forms of IL-1. IL-1Ra appears to be a purely competitive antagonist and is often expressed in massive excess over the concentration of IL-1α or IL-1β, which accords with this interpretation. The second "receptor" for IL-1, the type II IL-1 receptor (IL-1RII), does not have any detectable function in signal transduction and is now regarded both as a decoy for IL-1 (particularly IL-1β) and IL-1RAcP *(30,31)*. IL-1RII is the only other known extracellular inhibitor of the IL-1 system, apart from IL-1Ra. The relative importance of IL-1Ra and IL-1RII in controlling IL-1 signaling is yet to be investigated, and the IL-1RII gene has not yet been knocked out. IL-1Ra has only relatively weak affinity ($K_d \geq 0.1\ \mu M$), of dubious physiologic significance, for IL-1RII *(32)*, as might be expected if IL-1RII, like IL-1Ra, is an antagonistic regulator of the response to IL-1 and is therefore required only to compete for the agonistic ligands of IL-1RI.

There is little evidence that IL-1Ra has any other function, apart from blocking type I IL-1 receptors. At least two groups have tested whether IL-1Ra blocks IL-18 signaling, with negative results (J. Symons, M. Nicklin. and J. Barton, unpublished data; J. Sims, personal communication). Although evidence was presented in 1995 for a cytoplasmic function of the icIL-1Ra protein in the regulation of IL-1β mRNA stability, there has been no further investigation of this activity, as far as we are aware *(33)*.

mRNA for the secreted form of IL-1Ra (sIL-1Ra), like IL-1β mRNA, has now been reported in many cell types, including monocytes *(1)*, macrophages *(34)*, dendritic cells *(35)*, neutrophils *(36,37)*, endothelial cells *(38)*, mast cells *(39)*, fibroblasts *(40,41)*, and hepatocytes *(42,43)*. Whereas IL-1β protein export appears to be dependent on regulated processing of pro-IL-1β *(44)* and a secretion pathway that appears to be tissue-specific and to require activation *(45)*, sIL-1Ra is conventionally secreted. Thus cells that synthesize sIL-1Ra presumably secrete it too. sIL-1Ra mRNA, like IL-1β, is strongly inducible by proinflammatory stimuli in cells of the monocyte/macrophage lineage, but some signals either activate the gene independently of activation of IL-1 expression *(46)* or seem to modulate the ratio of secreted IL-1 to IL-1Ra *(47–49)* that results from a proinflammatory stimulus.

The intracellular form of IL-1Ra *(22)*, icIL-1Ra, is predominantly a product of epithelia, although it has also been reported in other cells, notably vascular smooth muscle *(50)*. It is not conventionally secreted, and specific secretion pathways have not been identified. The function of an apparently nonsecreted ligand for a cell surface receptor has seemed perplexing, but it is now known to be a feature that is shared with all the novel IL-1 family genes as well as IL-1α. The most plausible explanation is that icIL-1Ra may serve as a depot that can be released on cell rupture or necrosis. It is also possible, although not demonstrated, that icIL-1Ra, like IL-1β, might be released from cells by a specialized secretory pathway. Although it has been suggested that disruption might be required to cause release of icIL-1Ra from epithelia *(51)*, evidence has also been presented that icIL-1Ra is secreted *(52)*.

In studies of tissue-specific expression of mouse IL-1Ra mRNA and protein *(19,20)*, high levels of icIL-1Ra mRNA are seen constitutively in skin of mice, but sIL-1Ra is not observed in the unstimulated animal. After challenge with endotoxin, however, the latter mRNA appears in lung (presumably in macrophages), spleen, and liver. Protein products have also been demonstrated. icIL-1Ra protein is constitutively present in the skin, whereas sIL-1Ra is produced in the liver of challenged animals. Evidence was also presented, based on gel mobility, for the inducible production of icIL-1Ra3 protein, alongside sIL-1Ra *(20)*. IL-1α and IL-1β are also reported to be present constitutively in human skin *(53)*.

2. The Null Alleles of Il1rn

Standard knockout techniques have been used to create all of the three null alleles of *Il1rn* described below, and each group of investigators has disrupted the gene with a construct containing a selectable *E. coli* aminoglycoside phosphotransferase gene (*aph*, Neo^R, $G418^R$) under a strong eukaryotic promoter. Horai et al. *(17)* placed the selectable marker in the same orientation as the gene, whereas Hirsch et al. *(54)* and Nicklin et al. *(55)* reversed it. The disruptive insertion made by Nicklin et al. also contained the entire pUC13-based plasmid vector. Appropriately sceptical reviewers have questioned the effects that the insertion of the selectable marker might have on transcription of other genes within the *Il1f8*-*Il1rn* cluster. This criticism has not been rigorously addressed for the spontaneous tissue-specific inflammatory phenotypes, but one of the comforting aspects of the fact that three independent laboratories created different "null" disruptions of the same gene (as illustrated in Fig. 1) has been the overall similarity in phenotypes that has been observed when the mutant *Il1rn* alleles are brought onto the same genetic backgrounds, despite the detailed differences between the individual null alleles and the resulting positions of the selectable marker. Also, rigorous experiments have now been reported describing the complementation of the phenotype of the C57BL/6 $Il1rn^{-/-}$ mouse by overexpression of IL-1Ra from a transgene *(20)*. However, this strain does not normally develop any of the reported tissue-specific inflammatory pathologies that we describe below, so, strictly, some of the more interesting features of the knockout phenotype have not been tested for their dependence on IL-1Ra deficiency.

To avoid confusion, we have taken the liberty of naming the three "null" alleles after their cities of origin, to facilitate the discussion.

2.1. $Il1rn^{ny}$

The first report of disruption of *Il1rn* was from the Columbia College of Physicians and Surgeons in New York *(54)*, so we name this $Il1rn^{ny}$. Hirsch and colleagues used DNA from a 129λ library and an ES cell line, CCE, derived from a 129/Sv mouse. The gene disruption was achieved by homologous replacement with insertion of a short cytomegalovirus (CMV) promoter-driven *aph* cassette into an engineered site close to the beginning of exon a3/b4. Homologous arms were 2.0 kb at the 5'-flank and 8.9 kb at the 3'-flank (Fig. 1). No deletion was made, but the insertion of the CMV-*Neo* cassette disrupts the open reading frame of exon a3/b4. In theory, loss of the insertion could occur through deletion, which might restore gene activity. Alternatively, the function of the gene could be retained if transcripts could be produced that spliced around the mutation. However, there is no evidence of either problem. Exon a3/b4 is the second exon of the core of *Il1rn*, so transcription of the *ny* allele might result in the synthesis of a stub of protein, whether the gene is expressed from the s or the ic promoters. However, given the complex single fold of the mature IL-1Ra protein, it is extremely unlikely that the remaining peptide would have any IL-1-related activity. In fact, no mRNA was detected from the *ny* allele, in accordance with the current understanding of nonsense-mediated mRNA decay *(56)*.

The $Il1rn^{ny}$ allele was first studied in a cross, produced between the original chimera and C57BL/6J, generating a genetically heterogeneous population of mice. The allele was also backcrossed onto DBA/1, for use in studies of collagen-induced arthritis *(57)* and extensively onto C57BL/6J, on which background studies on atherogenesis have been made *(58)*, as well as an elegant genetic study of the basal and induced phenotypes *(20)*. Hirsch and colleagues have carried the $Il1rn^{ny}$ allele in heterozygous $Il1rn^{+/ny}$ breeding animals, because of breeding difficulties (as discussed later).

2.2. Il1rn^{t}

The second report of a null mutation in the IL-1Ra gene came from the University of Tokyo, and we have dubbed the allele $Il1rn^{t}$ *(17)*. Homologous DNA was prepared from a 129/SvJ λ library, and ES cells were the 129-derived R1 line *(59)*. In contrast to Hirsch et al., Horai et al. deleted almost all of the open reading frame of both forms of IL-1Ra. They used homologous arms of 2.1 and 4.5 kb (Fig. 1) that flanked a 5.3-kb deletion. The 5' start of the deletion is within the 5' untranslated region of exon a1. Consequently no sIL-1Ra-derived peptide could be produced from the $Il1rn^{t}$ allele. Since exon b2 was deleted, icIL-1Ra-derived peptides would terminate after the first 3–4 amino acids. No corresponding mRNA or protein could be detected from the mutant allele *(17)*. Horai and her colleagues also did initial studies on outcrossed 129 × C57BL/6J populations but then backcrossed the null allele onto C57BL/6J *(17)* and Balb/cA lines (CLEA-Japan) *(60)*. The latter strain was found to be susceptible to arthritis.

2.3. Il1rn^{s}

In collaboration with the Centre for Genome Research, Edinburgh, we generated a "null" allele, which we call $Il1rn^{s}$ (for the Sheffield allele) in the 129/Ola-derived ES cell-line E14 TG2A *(55)*. Our initial attempts to create a purebred 129 $Il1rn^{s}$ line were not successful because of the poor performance of the 129/Ola mice as breeders. Work instead began on an outcross onto a vigorous, outbred albino Swiss-derived population, MF1. Coinciding with the publication of the first results from Hirsch et al. *(54)*, which seemed to show no spontaneously inflammatory phenotype, the mice were inbred and retained in order to identify late-onset disease. Once interesting pathology had been observed and a second derivation of the knockout (twice backcrossed onto 129/Ola and then bred with another MF1) had yielded similar findings of vascular pathology *(55)*, we began to line breed and rederive the original group of $Il1rn^{+/s}$ animals. Two lines, Sf1 and Sf3, have been successfully developed and have been rederived into specific pathogen-free (SPF) conditions. At the time of writing, Sf3 is approaching its 20th sib-sib mated generation, which traditionally will entitle it to be regarded as an inbred line. Both *Il1rn*^{s} and wild-type alleles have been retained during the inbreeding, in order to provide *Il1rn*$^{-/-}$ and wild-type animals from the same stock. Backcrosses of *Il1rn*^{s} onto Balb/c, C57BL/6, and DBA/1 are now in their tenth or higher generations and so can also be regarded as genetically homogeneous.

3. The Basal Il1rn Phenotype

After the excitement about the likely roles of IL-1 in hematopoiesis, development, and reproduction, the observation of the great abundance of both IL-1 and IL-1Ra in epithelia and particularly the skin, and the general observation that almost everywhere that IL-1 is found, IL-1Ra is also present, the most startling feature of the first report of the *Il1rn*$^{-/-}$ phenotype *(54)* was its moderation. *Il1rn*$^{ny/ny}$ mice, on mixed 129 × C57BL/6 or purebred C57BL/6J backgrounds, were similar in weight to their wild-type littermates at the time they were weaned, but they failed to grow as fast as their wild-type littermates thereafter. This finding has been confirmed with C57BL/6J *Il1rn*$^{t/t}$ in Tokyo *(17)*. Irikura et al. *(20)* have extended the previous work from New York *(54)* and have recently published a thorough description of the phenotype of the C57BL/6 *Il1rn*$^{ny/ny}$ mouse. The authors remark that the primary difference between the wild-type and IL-1Ra-deficient animals is the sparseness of body fat in the latter. The age at which the difference in body mass becomes significant is between 6 and 8 wk, as has been reported by both the New York *(20,54)* and Tokyo groups *(17)*. The latter authors reported a shortfall of mass of 20% in males and 13% in females at 12 wk of age in *Il1rn*$^{t/t}$ mice, whereas the former *(20)* report that *Il1rn*$^{ny/ny}$ C57BL/6 mice show a 30% shortfall in mass by 14 wk.

In this respect, it is interesting to note that *Il1rn*$^{ny/ny}$ mice on a C57BL/6 × 129 background have also been reported to have constitutively elevated IL-6 levels *(61)*, which is consistent with the finding that IL-6 and IL-6 receptor-deficient mice become obese *(62)*. Irikura et al. also report that *Il1rn*$^{ny/ny}$ animals generally fail to breed, a point that is discussed later. Interestingly, however, although prone to malaise, the *Il1rn*$^{ny/ny}$ C57BL/6 mice do not show an identifiable, localized, spontaneous inflammatory disease. Irikura et al. also report high mortality in *Il1rn*$^{ny/ny}$ C57BL/6, with only 40% of *Il1rn*$^{ny/ny}$ mice surviving for 1 yr, compared with no losses among wild-type controls *(20)*. Among these mice, in the New York facility, the onset of malaise seemed to be predictable, and by 14 or 17 wk, 50% of males or females, respectively, were suffering piloerection and mild weight loss or other signs of illness. We also showed an effect of *Il1rn*$^{s/s}$ on weight gain during the first few generations that we inbred the 129/Ola x MF1 stock. At this stage, mice were not reared behind a barrier *(55)*.

We must conclude, though, that strain differences or environmental influences must be important in the development of this rather nonspecific phenotype, as we have not observed systematic illness in C57BL/6 *Il1rn*$^{s/s}$ mice in our own facility. However, we have not studied weight gain in this strain. Devlin et al. *(58)* mention that the survivors of their atherogenic regimen (discussed later), which were *Il1rn*$^{ny/ny}$ C57BL/6 or wild-type control animals, showed no difference in body weight, and only 2/19 of the knockout mice were suffering from piloerection and hunching at 16 wk, even though they were of the same strain as those studied by Irikura et al. *(20)*.

Because IL-1Ra-deficient mice in the four growth studies *(17,20,54,55)* subsequently became overtly ill, it is questionable at present whether the growth deficiency in these animals reflects a primary function of IL-1 in normal growth control or whether it is a sign of incipient illness.

Irikura et al. *(20)* were also the first to report substantial differences in the blood leukocyte content between wild-type and *Il1rn*$^{ny/ny}$ C57BL/6 mice. In 8–10-wk-old mice, the authors found small but significant increases in the numbers of circulating γδ+ T-cells and CD11b+ (Mac-1+) cells, which are mainly granulocytes, and a doubling of the proportion of neutrophils among the circulating leukocytes. A 50% expansion is also seen in the proportion of CD11b+ progenitors in bone marrow. Again, it is not clear whether these differences reflect the early stages of pathology, caused by the onset of chronic inflammation, or whether they might represent a difference in hematopoiesis that might be a factor in causing subsequent immune dysregulation and hence lead to disease. Further studies in other strains will be required to resolve this question.

4. The Induced Phenotype of *Il1rn*$^{-/-}$ Mice

Acute challenges with agents that elicit IL-1-dependent responses are likely to produce different results in wild-type mice from those that lack IL-1Ra. The functional overlap between the proinflammatory cytokines tends to obscure significant, measurable cytokine-specific effects unless protocols are first fine-tuned.

4.1. Endotoxin

Injection of endotoxin from Gram-negative bacteria results in the activation of monocytes and macrophages, which then release cytokines, including IL-1 and IL-1Ra *(46)*. The endpoint of the experiment is hemodynamic shock. There is considerable redundancy in the acute effects of inflammatory mediators, and injection of IL-1 or tumor necrosis factor (TNF), individually, can cause shock. The response to endotoxin is subject to a great deal of biologic variability, and before the most recent study by Irikura et al. *(20)* the literature includes not only a clear demonstration of the importance of the IL-1Ra gene *(54)*, which implies a significant role for IL-1 in the response, but also evidence that IL-1RI is not required *(63)*, suggesting either that there is no significant role for IL-1 or that the shock response is mediated by a different and unrecognized receptor from IL-1RI. Obviously, these findings are either inconsistent for technical reasons or imply that we need to reconsider the molecular biology of IL-1 signaling. Irikura et al. *(20)* argue the former case and point out that the response to endotoxin is protocol-dependent and that the conflict in the literature is most likely the result of different experimental methods. They therefore performed a parallel set of experiments on a number of different genotypes and established that the IL-1 receptor is required for the full response to endotoxin (under their chosen conditions) and that the response is inhibited by overexpression of IL-1Ra. They confirmed their previous findings *(54)* that *Il1rn*$^{ny/ny}$ mice are more sensitive to endotoxin than are wild-type animals and that this can be reversed and made subnormal by IL-1Ra overexpression or by complete deficiency of the IL-1RI gene.

Circulating IL-1β was measured in the *Il1rn*$^{ny/ny}$ mice *(20,54)* after they had been challenged with endotoxin. In previous studies, on isolated human peripheral blood mononuclear cells and transfected monocyte-like cell lines, it had been shown in vivo and in vitro that IL-1β is engaged in an autocrine activation loop *(64,65)*. It was therefore expected that the IL-1 system would be highly susceptible to autoactivation in the absence of IL-1Ra. The opposite appears to be the case in two studies of endotoxin challenge of *Il1rn*$^{ny/ny}$ 129 xC57BL/6 *(54)* and C57BL/6J *(20)*. Circulating IL-1β in IL-1Ra-deficient mice, after endotoxin challenge, was approximately one-half of that seen in the wild type, despite a more sensitive physiologic response in the mutant animals: an increased physiologic response with less IL-1 present is not self-contradictory because the effective activity of a given quantity of IL-1 is expected to be much greater in the absence of abundant competitor IL-1Ra.

Interestingly, inactivation of the IL-1Ra and IL-1RI genes together caused substantial elevation of IL-1β, after endotoxin challenge, compared with wild-type animals. The level of circulating IL-1β in challenged mice that lacked only IL-1RI was not distinguishable from the level in double knockouts *(20)*. Irikura et al. argue for the simplest explanation for their findings, based on the availability of receptors to adsorb free IL-1β. Thus, when IL-1Ra is not present, more IL-1β can be adsorbed by an unchanged number of receptors, but when the receptor is absent, the free concentration of IL-1β increases. It is also worth noting, though, that a generalized mechanism, whereby IL-1β expression is diminished in response to the amount of signal detected through the IL-1 receptor, would equally well explain these data. One experiment that would distinguish these two hypotheses would be the overexpression of a signaling-deficient IL-1 receptor or of IL-1RII on an $Il1r1^{-/-}$ background. The binding model would predict a reduction in circulating IL-β, compared with wild-type mice, whereas the signaling model would predict an increase.

4.2. Turpentine

Turpentine, injected subcutaneously, creates a sterile abscess and a sustained fever over several days that resolves over about a week. IL-1RI was shown to be necessary for a full response *(61,66)*. Horai et al. *(17)* showed that wild-type and IL-1α-deficient C57BL/6 mice develop a similar fever in response to turpentine injection. IL-1β-deficient mice responded much more weakly, allowing the authors to assign a specific role to IL-1β. As expected for an IL-1-mediated response, $Il1rn^{t/t}$ mice were more severely affected by the injection of turpentine than were the wild-type animals. The knockouts suffered a significantly higher immediate fever and a more sustained reaction. Turpentine injection causes a rapid increase in circulating glucocorticoid. Even though the late phase of the glucocorticoid response seems to be IL-1-mediated, the absence of IL-1Ra had no significant effect, suggesting that the response was already maximal. Working with $Il1rn^{ny/ny}$ on a mixed C57BL/6 × 129 background, Josephs et al. *(61)* have also looked at the effects of defects in the IL-1 system upon the response to turpentine injection. They report that 3/6 of the IL-1Ra-deficient mice died during the protocol, compared with none from any other group, suggesting that the IL-1Ra deficiency increases the reaction to turpentine injection.

4.3. Resistance to Listeria *monocytogenes*

Listeria is an opportunistic intracytoplasmic bacterial parasite that primarily infects monocytes and macrophages but can induce its own phagocytosis by normally nonphagocytic cells. The mechanism by which *Listeria* is controlled and eliminated from circulation by naive mice is not well understood, but presumably T-helper function is not required in the reponses that are monitored shortly after infection. In experimental primary listeriosis, a bolus of *Listeria* is injected intravenously and the bacteria multiply within cells and can be titred from extracts of the organs at the endpoint (7 d) or at the point of death through infection. Strain differences are crucial in this biologic assay, and Irikura et al. *(20)* used only extensively backcrossed C57BL/6, deriving both wild-type and $Il1rn^{ny/ny}$ mice from the same litters. There seems to be a specific role for IL-1, since IL-1RI-deficient mice do not clear *Listeria* efficiently, succumb to a smaller inoculum of bacteria than wild-type animals, and show a higher blood titer of the bacteria *(20)*, although these results conflict with those reported previously *(63)*. The difference between these two experiments is presumably the result of differences between the protocols used. As expected, overexpression of IL-1Ra has an effect similar to that IL-1RI-deficiency *(54,20)*. On the other hand, *Il1rn*$^{ny/ny}$ C57BL/6 mice clear *Listeria* over 10-fold more efficiently than do wild-type animals, and all of the group survived the treatment, which killed 20% of the wild-type animals.

These results are particularly revealing when placed alongside the data relating to spontaneous inflammatory diseases. Evolution of the innate immune response has apparently overlaid extremely potent cytokines with inhibitors and other regulatory mechanisms and has achieved a balance between insipidity, which results in a harmonious lack of self-reactivity, but at the same time causes susceptibility to infectious bacteria, and excessive force, which is highly effective against intracytoplasmic parasites, but which causes susceptibility to chronic inflammatory diseases.

4.4. Atherogenic Diet

The role of inflammation in atherosclerosis has been increasingly emphasized recently, both because of its systemic effects on lipid metabolism and because of the involvement of macrophages that secrete proinflammatory cytokines in atherosclerotic plaque (reviewed in ref. *67*). IL-1 is secreted by vascular endothelial cells, by smooth muscle cells, and by macrophages that become incorporated into atherosclerotic plaques. Some recent evidence has suggested that there is a correlation between human *IL1RN* genotype and susceptibility to a subtype of human coronary disease *(68)*. Devlin et al. *(58)* subjected *Il1rn*$^{ny/ny}$ C57BL/6 and control wild-type mice and heterozygotes to 12 wk of a highly atherogenic cholesterol/cholate diet, beginning at 4 wk. Mortality was high but not significantly associated with the genotype of the mice. Interestingly, no significant weight difference was found among the 16-wk-old survivors, and malaise was only reported in 2/19 of the IL-1Ra-deficient mice. Of the parameters tested, there was a significant threefold increase in the level of non-high-density cholesterol cholesterol in the serum of the *Il1rn*$^{ny/ny}$ compared with the wild-type C57BL/6 animals. More research will be needed to link this work to the known functions of IL-1 and IL-1Ra.

4.5. Collagen-Induced Arthritis

Subcutaneous injection of heterologous type II collagen (CII) into genetically susceptible mice causes an immune response to the collagen, which then develops into an autoimmune response, initially to type II collagen in the animals' own joints, which then progresses to include other antigens. The humoral and cell-mediated immune responses result in an arthritis that is among the best mouse models for rheumatoid arthritis. The process depends on the presentation of peptides from type II collagen and is consequently dependent on mouse MHC haplotype. Mouse strains used in collagen-induced arthritis (CIA) are generally *H-2*^{r} or *H-2*^{q}, and the most commonly used *H-2*^{q} strain is DBA/1. CIA is highly protocol-dependent. Ma et al. *(57)* used *Il1rn*$^{ny/ny}$ DBA/1 and DBA/1 control mice, in a mild CIA protocol, giving a single injection of bovine type II collagen . Under this protocol, fewer than half of the wild-type animals became affected by 50 d, with the affected animals developing arthritis between 30 and 40 d. By contrast, the *Il1rn*$^{ny/ny}$ mice developed arthritis between 20 and 35 d, and all were affected. The pathology resembled that normally seen in CIA, with formation of pannus and erosion of the cartilage and bone but was more severe than was observed with this protocol in the wild-type animals. Parallel experiments were done with transgenic IL-1Ra overexpressors, so that a full range of levels of IL-1Ra expression was studied. IL-1 is probably involved at a number of stages in the immune and subsequenct inflammatory responses, but Ma et al. *(57)* show that the humoral immune response to type II collagen is not significantly altered when IL-1Ra is overexpressed, suggesting that the major effect of IL-1Ra is on the subsequent inflammatory response.

4.6. Reproduction and IL-1Ra Deficiency

Important roles have been proposed for IL-1 in reproduction, ovulation, and implantation. All these suggestions have been put into doubt, in mice at least, by the observation that animals lacking IL-1 and IL-1RI seem to be fertile *(17,63)*. It remains possible that excessive IL-1 activity, caused by an absence of IL-1Ra, might have a detrimental effect on reproduction. In their recent characterization of the IL-1Ra phenotype of $Il1rn^{ny/ny}$ mice, Irikura et al. *(20)* have reported that C57BL/6 $Il1rn^{ny/ny}$ mice are relatively infertile, with a reproductive success rate of only 30% in female and 50% in male $Il1rn^{ny/ny}$ mice. The authors point out that mice who develop malaise become completely infertile, which suggests that the effect of genotype on fertility is likely to be secondary even in the New York colony. Moreover, Horai et al. *(17)* have reported that their IL-1Ra-deficient C57BL/6 ($Il1rn^{t/t}$) mice are fertile. We have not tested $Il1rn^{s/s}$ C57BL/6 mice, but we have bred Sf $Il1rn^{s/s}$ mice of both sexes either with $Il1rn^{+/s}$ or with $Il1rn^{s/s}$ partners, and we routinely breed from $Il1rn^{s/s}$ males. Balb/c $Il1rn^{s/s}$ males and females have also been successfully bred here with $Il1rn^{+/s}$ mates. We have generally refrained from mating $Il1rn^{s/s}$ mice together in the Sf1 subline, because the short life span of the females (around 100 d) and their tendency to develop arteritis early has often appeared to cause breeding or rearing to fail.

We also recently inbred F1 $Il1rn^{s/s}$ mice from a cross between Balb/c and C57BL/6 to create an F2. The study was not set up to measure fecundity, so no $Il1rn^{+/s}$ littermates were bred as controls. However, 11 homozygous F1 females were mated with four homozygous males. All animals bred successfully. The males each sired as many litters as they were allowed (4–6), with a mean litter size between 7.4 and 9.2 for each male. The females were allowed to breed twice, yielding 22 litters in total. The mean litter size at weaning was 8.4, with a mode of 12 and a range of 2–12. Time between litters was unremarkable, and the larger of the two litters produced by each female was between 7 and 12, with 5/11 females producing at least one litter of 12. Although in the absence of the control, we cannot assert that there is no diminution in fertility compared with a cross between wild-type Balb/c and C57BL/6, we have shown that these $Il1rn^{-/-}$ are very fertile. It is also possible that the hybrid vigor obtained from the interstrain cross might disguise low fertility, which might otherwise be apparent in a more delicate inbred strain. However, we can conclude that IL-1Ra is not required in a substantial way in reproduction.

5. Chronic Inflammatory Diseases in IL-1Ra-Deficient Mice

As discussed above, IL-1Ra is strongly inducible, except in epithelia, where it is constitutive, but low levels of the protein circulate in the plasma. This may have some role in limiting the extent of inflammation that is generated by release of a small bolus of IL-1. Given the general well-being of most young IL-1Ra-deficient mice, it seems a plausible hypothesis that IL-1Ra might only be required sporadically, in response to a proinflammatory insult. However, their primary immune systems could be regarded as insufficiently damped (against the effects of IL-1) and thus unstable. Consequently a large enough stimulus, or a spatial coincidence of smaller ones, might be sufficient to cause the accumulation of enough IL-1-secreting leukocytes to establish chronic inflammation.

5.1. Arterial Inflammation: A Model for Giant Cell Arteritis?

We detected excess mortality in mice that had been inbred from the original 129/Ola chimera and a single female from an outbred albino Swiss population carried by Harlan U.K. as the MF1. Although it was a genetically heterogeneous population, we soon discovered a 10-fold excess mortality in $Il1rn^{s/s}$ mice compared with their $Il1rn^{+/s}$ littermates, and we extended this study to include all available complete litters for up to 550 d of age. Included in the mortality statistics *(55)* were animals that were culled because they were showing signs of disease, occasionally with hunching and malaise, as has now been described by Irikura et al. *(20)*.

In contrast to their findings, we have not found malaise to be a constitutive phenotype in our $Il1rn^{s/s}$ colony in any strain. Signs of illness have been highly variable, generally very sudden in their onset, and have featured (in some cases) sudden death, rear limb paralysis, spinning, diabetes, cyanosis, audible breathing, and the sudden appearance of swellings, particularly in the popliteal region and on the neck and shoulders. We demonstrated *(55)* vasculitic lesions in the major arteries of more than 90% of $Il1rn^{s/s}$ animals that had become ill or had died. In many cases it was possible to associate a lesion with the infarction of a specific organ or stenosis of a particular artery and the signs exhibited by the mouse. With a single exception in a pulmonary artery, lesions were found in the high-pressure arterial system. The affected vessels were always the aorta or its large primary or secondary branches, and the sites of inflammation were focused on the junction between two vessels or a strong flexure (such as in the popliteal artery). These, interestingly, are the sites of low, chaotic shear stress caused by turbulence that also serve as foci for the development of atherosclerosis in humans.

The increased tendency for inflammation to develop at these sites has been explained in two ways. Gimbrone and colleagues *(69)* favor a direct affect of low shear stress on the arterial endothelium, which causes a failure of the activation of a shear-stress-induced anti-inflammatory gene program. Other workers have focused on the tendency for various types of proinflammatory debris to dither or even become deposited at sites of relatively low, inconsistent blood flow.

Our recent studies have not shown any constitutive activation of inflammatory markers such as E-selectin or intercellular adhesion molecule-1 (ICAM-1) at the aortic root of young, preaffected Sf3 mice. Indeed, the initial signs of infiltration of the arterial wall tend to include the full complement of inflammatory leukocytes, including activated CD4+ T-cells that contain interferon-γ (IFN-γ). Lesions progressively affect the entire thickness of the vessel wall. Leukocytes, including IL-1β-secreting macrophages, neutrophils, and activated CD4+ T-cells, seem to arrive from the vasa vasorum, which becomes expanded, causing massive swelling of the collagen-rich adventitia. The infiltrate penetrates toward the intima, destroying the elastic laminae. Smooth muscle takes on a noncontractile appearance and proliferates in the intima *(55)*. It is clear that despite the absence of IL-1Ra some of the lesions are self-limiting, and it is possible to section along an older lesion (Fig. 2)

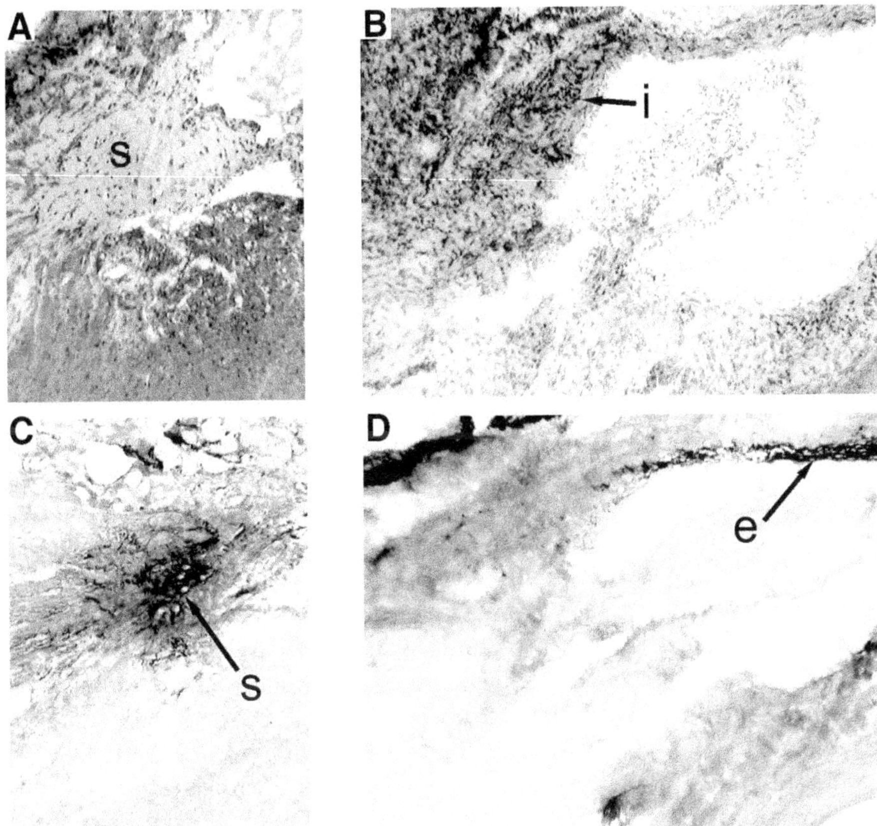

Fig. 2. Simultaneous scarring adjacent to an active lesion, seen in low-power images of frozen sections of arteritic lesions found at the aortic root of a 165-d-old Sf3 female. A glancing section has cut partly through the wall of a coronary artery as it enters the myocardium. (**A**) and (**B**) are stained with hematoxylin and eosin, and the picture has been adjusted to show the blue of the hematoxylin as black. (**C**) and (**D**) are stained with elastin and van Gieson stain, and the green channel from the image is shown. (**A**) and (**C**) are centered on the scar tissue, and (**B**) and (**D**) show the active area of the lesion. S, scar tissue; i, a heavily inflamed site; e, a surviving elastic lamina. The lighter areas in (**B**) and (**D**) are the lumen of the vessel.

from an actively inflamed portion to one that is apparently resolving and leaving disorganized elastin and scar tissue within the vessel wall *(55)* (J. S. and M. N., manuscript in preparation).

In many respects, the disease that we see resembles two human pathologies, "pulseless disease" or Takayasu arteritis (TA) and giant cell arteritis (GCA). Both diseases resemble one another but have different epidemiologies, GCA tending to affect both sexes from late middle age, and TA being reported predominantly in young Oriental women. In both diseases, highly destructive transmural inflammatory lesions are found to be highly localized in the high-pressure arterial system. The primary lesion is usually not noticed, but malaise may occur. Destruction of the elastic laminae causes aneurysms, particularly of the aorta, and vascular collapse and stenosis, which can cause ischemia. In the human diseases, pain through ischemia of the limbs and blindness through infarction of the retina are common problems. Remodeling and scarring are seen. Many features are shared with the mouse model disease; the one that is obviously missing is the presence of giant macrophages (the "giant cells") in the granulomas of GCA. However, it is not clear that these cells have a specific pathogenic role.

Even in the mouse model, the initiation of the inflammatory response is currently not observable, although it represents the most interesting phase of the immunology of the disease. The central arterial system is not easy to observe, and we have so far only been able to make postmortem studies. Longitudinal studies will be necessary, and the ability to monitor disease development by high-resolution magnetic resonance imaging scanning will be enormously beneficial. Also, a much more consistent genetic background, the fully inbred Sf3 strain, will be vital to eliminate all but stochastic effects and reveal the progress of the disease.

Because of the unconventional background of our *Il1rn*$^{s/s}$ mice, we set up backcrosses onto Balb/c (Harlan) mice. On screening six *Il1rn*$^{s/s}$ F2, we found that three had aortic root vasculitis. We also examined six formaldehyde-fixed cadavers of *Il1rn*$^{t/t}$ Balb/cA mice raised in Tokyo (J. S., M. N., and Y. Iwakura, unpublished observations), of which four showed aortic root arteritic lesions, confirming that the specific null allele of *Il1rn*, the precise strain background, and the details of the environment are not important in the development of arterial inflammation. Deeply backcrossed *Il1rn*$^{s/s}$ Balb/c (Harlan) mice are susceptible to the disease, as would be expected, but are generally not ideal animals for studying arteritis because they also develop arthritis and psoriasis over the same timescale.

C57BL/6 *Il1rn*$^{ny/ny}$ developed hunching, piloerection, and malaise *(20)*, but pathologic investigation of eight *Il1rn*$^{ny/ny}$ cadavers by ourselves did not reveal arterial inflammation, even after a thorough examination of all major arteries *(55)*. Irikura et al. *(20)* have also made an extensive pathologic investigation that has not yet revealed any specific cause of premature death of aged C57BL/6 *Il1rn*$^{ny/ny}$ mice. Faced with these results, we have questioned whether our Sf3 *Il1rn*$^{s/s}$ mice generally die or become ill as a result of arteritis, or whether they are dying of other causes while suffering from a nonlethal arteritis. We have certainly found many cases indicating that the signs of illness in an individual animal are correlated with the site of an aneurysm or collapsed vessel, but we have also observed cases of elderly, ostensibly healthy *Il1rn*$^{s/s}$ mice in our outbred population that were found, post mortem, to have extensive aortic lesions and scarring, indicating a long history of the disease.

5.2. Spontaneous Arthritis: A Model for Rheumatoid Arthritis?

Horai et al. *(60)* demonstrated that *Il1rn*$^{t/t}$ mice on the Balb/cA strain, a substrain of Balb/c (obtained from CLEA, Japan), were fully susceptible to spontaneous inflammatory arthritis, the pathology of which has many parallels with human rheumatoid arthritis. The authors established a severity scale in which reddening of the footpad or slight swelling resulted in a score of 1 per affected limb, graduating to 2 for obvious swelling and 3 for joint fixation. The disease was first detected at 5 wk of age, although at this stage the average score is less than 1, indicating less than one reddened footpad per animal. At 8 wk, 80% of the animals were affected, and a mean severity score of approx. 2.5 per animal was seen, indicating that most animals probably had one swollen hind ankle. Severity seemed to plateau around 12 wk, and at 14 wk, all animals were affected. Unlike human rheumatoid arthritis, there was no significant difference between males and females, and the severity score per animal of around 6 indicates at least two swollen limbs. The inflammation affected the hind ankle joints most obviously and was generally symmetric.

Histologic analysis revealed the formation of granulation tissue resembling the pannus of rheumatoid arthritis in the joint space. The tissue seemed to derive from proliferation of the synovial lining and showed extensive infiltration by neutrophils and lymphocytes. Fibrin clots were found in the joint space, and the pannus was associated with erosion of the synovial cartilage and bone. Inflammation was associated with slight splenomegaly and enlargement of the draining lymph nodes, but there was no evidence for a significant skewing of the ratios of either B- to T-cells or CD4+ to CD8+ T-cells. At a late stage in the disease (16 wk), the authors also investigated the potential humoral contribution to autoimmunity. The prominent rheumatoid factor of humans, an IgM anti-Ig, was *not* found to be elevated, nor was IgM generally, but there was strong elevation of both IgG1 and IgE and a significantly increased titer of self-reactive antiimmunoglobulin IgG levels. Serum from affected Balb/cA $Il1rn^{t/t}$ mice was found to have significantly elevated reactivity to double-stranded DNA and type II collagen compared with age-matched (unaffected) wild-type animals. Unaffected, age-matched C57BL/6 $Il1rn^{t/t}$ mice also showed no significant increase in autoreactive antibodies. The authors point out that there was no correlation between antibody titer and disease severity for any of these autoantigens, unlike in the human disease. It is likely, therefore, that if there is an important humoral component in this mouse model of rheumatoid arthritis, then the spectrum of pathogenic autoantigens is likely to be different from those seen in rheumatoid arthritis.

Horai et al. *(60)* also analyzed RNA expression in extracts from whole joints by nuclease protection assay. Increased expression of the inflammation-dependent markers IL-1β, IL-6, IL-1RII, and cyclooxygenase 2 were observed, but IL-1α was rather surprisingly suppressed and TNF-α expression was only slightly altered. The authors point out that there is a small increase in the levels of IL-1β mRNA even before onset of disease signs, but the differences are small. By contrast, $Il1rn^{t/t}$ C57BL/6 were only susceptible to spontaneous arthritis at much greater ages, and only 2 mice from a group of 19 became affected, the first case being seen at 24 wk. The report does not indicate how severe the arthritis was. We also set up a backcross with Balb/c mice from Harlan soon after establishing our own $Il1rn^{s/s}$ line.

We have not yet performed a detailed time-course study, but we found only 2/22 cases of swollen joints before 14 wk of age in Balb/c (Harlan) $Il1rn^{s/s}$ mice, but by 18 wk, 10/22 were affected. The oldest unaffected animals that we have seen were 26 wk old. The onset of florid arthritis is obviously slower, and the disease is less penetrant than was reported by Horai et al. in Balb/c $Il1rn^{t/t}$ mice, but nevertheless the onset is much more rapid and has much higher penetrance than in C57BL/6 $Il1rn^{t/t}$ or in our Sf3 $Il1rn^{s/s}$ line, where we have not seen a single case in several hundred animals. Sections of decalcified joints (Fig. 3A) reveal similar histopathology to that reported by Horai et al. *(60)*, with prominent formation of pannus (marked P in Fig. 3A) in some joints and dense infiltrate into the ankle joints of the hindlimbs in particular. Deep erosions of cartilage and bone are also clearly evident (indicated by arrows in Fig. 3A). We have also begun immunohistologic studies on frozen sections cut from whole affected joints (J. S. and M. N., unpublished results). We have shown that T-cells are present and IFN-γ+ cells (Fig. 3C) are as frequent as CD4+ cells (Fig. 3D), whereas IL-4+ cells seem to be absent (not shown), suggesting a predominance of Th1 cells, as we have also seen in aortic root arteritic lesions in the same animals. This

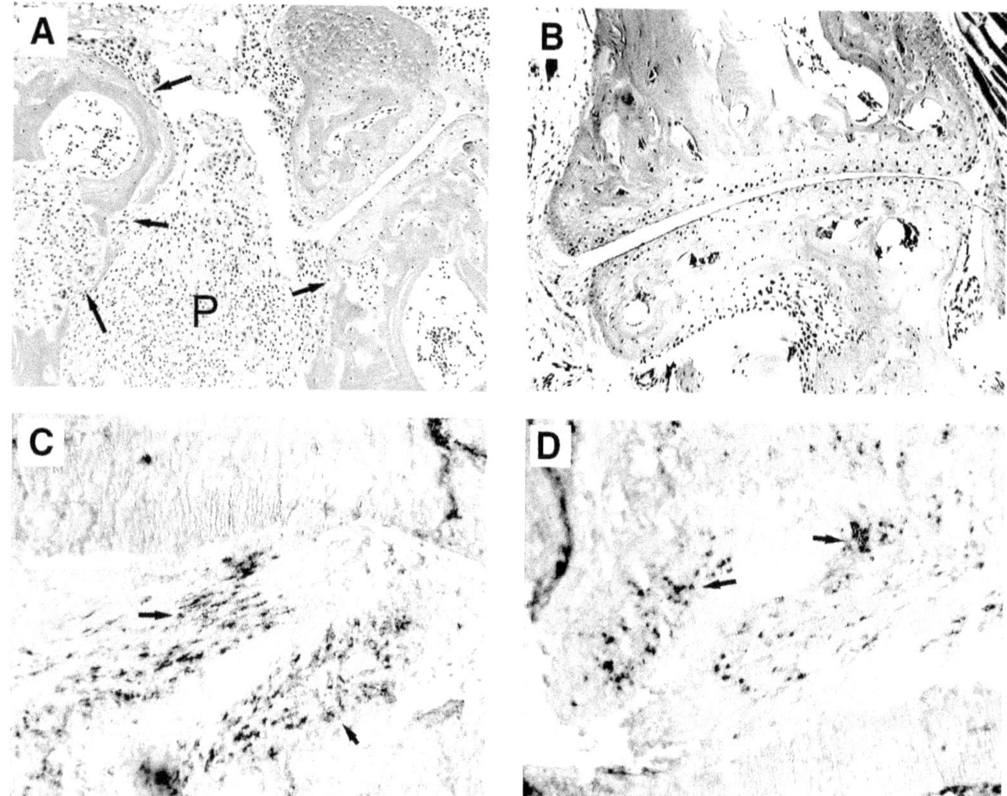

Fig. 3. Arthritis in a 132-d-old female *Il1rn*$^{s/s}$ Balb/c mouse compared with a similar joint from a 155-d-old female wild-type Balb/c. (**A**) and (**B**) are decalcified formaldehyde-fixed sections. (**A**) P indicates tissue resembling pannus of human rheumatoid arthritis. Arrows indicate sites of cartilage and bone erosion. The marrow space on the left appears to be filled with pannus. (**B**) A normal joint from the wild-type mouse. (**C**) and (**D**) Higher power immunohistologic images of fresh-frozen sections of whole bone, stained for IFN-γ (**C**), and CD4 (**D**). The pannus is seen in the center of the images, flanked by bone. Arrows indicate the areas of activated T-cells. The blue channel of the image only is shown, so that the yellow-brown of the peroxidase staining appears black.

contrasts sharply with our observations in the psoriasis-like disease seen in the same animals, in which considerable intracellular IL-4 was detected in dermal infiltrate cells.

The importance of lymphocytes and an acquired immune response in this model of arthritis has recently been confirmed *(70)* by Iwakura, who demonstrated that *Rag*$^-$ mutations (which prevent B- and T-cell development) when homozygous completely suppress the effect of IL-1Ra deficiency.

Clearly, there must be an allelic, background or environmental difference between the *Il1rn*$^{s/s}$ Balb/c (Harlan) mice held in our laboratory and the *Il1rn*$^{t/t}$ Balb/cA mice held in Tokyo. Despite their physical differences, it is very likely that both the *s* and *t* alleles of *Il1rn* are functionally null and therefore functionally equivalent, and the disease that we do see is essentially the same. Given the strong evidence for genetic modifiers from our own studies, we favor the hypothesis that the chief reason for difference in detail between our findings and those of Horai et al. lies in the genetic background of the two Balb/c substrains.

The tendency for Balb/c rather than C57BL/6 to develop rheumatoid-like arthritis has been regarded as surprising, since it has been asserted that rheumatoid arthritis is predominantly Th1-mediated *(71)* and that Balb/c mice is deficient in Th1 responses *(72)*. It is also noteworthy that the standard CIA-induced arthritis strain DBA/1, which carries the CIA-susceptible $H\text{-}2^q$ MHC haplotype, does not develop arthritis spontaneously when deficient in IL-1Ra *(57)*.

5.3. Spontaneous Inflammatory Dermatosis: A Model for Psoriasis?

In our SPF facility, we have found that IL-1Ra-deficient Balb/c (Harlan) mice have a tendency to develop redness and scaling of their ears. Recent detailed examination (Shepherd et al., submitted) has revealed a close resemblance between the histopathology of the mouse skin and that of human psoriasis. We have observed extensive thickening of the cornified and subcorneal layers of the epidermis and dermis. The overall thickness of the pinna increases at least fourfold. The disease incidence was found to be at least 59% in $Il1rn^{s/s}$ Balb/c mice. The earliest cases appear at around 54 d of age, but some animals seem never to become affected. Thickening of the skin of the ears has also been observed frequently in Balb/cA $Il1rn^{t/t}$ mice by Iwakura and colleagues (Y. Iwakura, personal communication). Figure 4 illustrates the thickening of the skin of the pinna of the ear. In Fig. 4A and B, we compare wild-type skin with affected skin from an $Il1rn^{s/s}$ Balb/c mouse with $Il1rn^{+/+}$ of a comparable age.

The following features all resemble human psoriasis. The epidermis and the dermis are massively thickened, and the epidermis has become highly convoluted, as is also seen in human psoriasis. Staining for keratin 6 (Fig. 4E and F) reveals that this marker of undifferentiated cells is expressed widely in the epidermis, whereas it is restricted to the cells of the sheath of the hair follicle in normal skin, except occasionally and at sites of damage, where it tends also to be expressed in the basal layer of the epidermis. The nuclei of kera-tinocytes appear to be retained, even in the outer cornified cellular layer, and there is a neutrophilic infiltrate beneath it, forming sterile microabscesses. The dermis is heavily infiltrated with leukocytes and also becomes hypervascular. There is also a high density of mast cells in the dermis. Immunohistology reveals the presence of large numbers of MHC class II+ dendritic cells within the epidermis and the dermis (Fig. 4C and D), and those in the epidermis have the characteristic appearance of Langerhans cells. CD4+ cells are also abundant in the infiltrates found in the dermis and epidermis, and recent work (J. Shepherd, unpublished data) has shown convincingly that these cells are also CD3+ and are therefore not dendritic cells. Macrophages, or perhaps dermal dendritic cells, are indicated by the F4/80 marker on cells of the dermis (not shown).

Cytokine expression is interesting in that it appears to differ from that seen in floridly inflamed aortic tissue, even from the same mouse. We expect and find IL-1 expression, and a Th1 response, as has been implicated in psoriasis, would be expected to show an abundance of IFN-γ+ T-cells. These are observed in both the psoriasis-like inflammation and the arteritis. IL-5 has previously been reported in psoriasis *(73)*; we observe it here, but it is conspicuously absent in aortitis from the same animal. IL-4 is also abundant in the psoriasis-like disease but is absent from the aortic lesion. The presence of IL-4 in psoriasis is rather controversial, and investigators have disagreed over its presence at the mRNA level *(73–75)*. In $Il1rn^{-/-}$ mice at least, there appears to be more of a Th2 response in inflamed ear skin than in arterial inflammation.

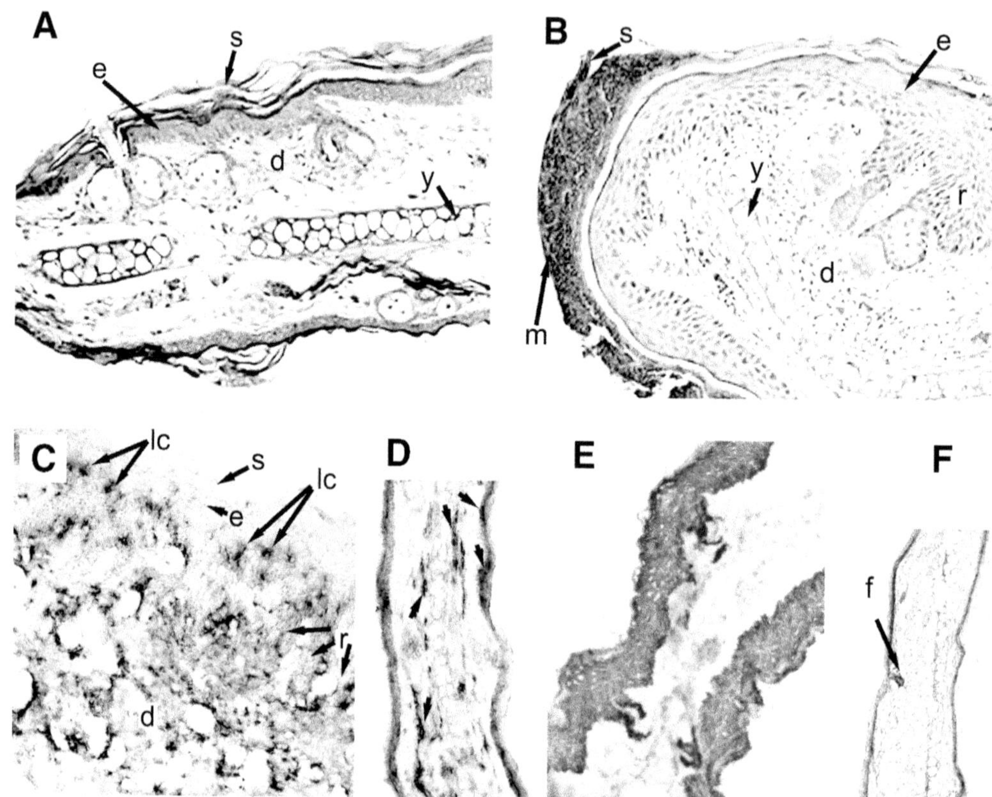

Fig. 4. Normal and psoriasiform lesional ear skin in a Balb/c wild-type and $Il1rn^{s/s}$ mice. (**A**) and (**B**) Low-power view of a formaldehyde-fixed section, stained with hematoxylin and eosin. (**A**) Ear of a wild-type animal. s, the stratum corneum, which tends to become detached in preparation from the subcorneal epidermis (e) The epidermis is smooth and the dermis (d), is thin. y, the yellow elastic tissue at the core of the ear flap. (**B**) Psoriasiform skin. A neutrophil-rich microabscess, (m) has appeared beneath the stratum corneum (s). The subcorneal epidermis is grossly thickened, forming rete ridges (r) that penetrate into the dermis (d), which is also grossly thickened. (**C**) Higher power image of a frozen section of the epidermis and dermis of an affected mouse that has been stained for the presence of class II MHC (Ia^d antigen), revealing abundant dermal and epidermal dendritic cells. The latter [Langerhans cells (lc)] have obviously branched morphology. (**D**) Occasional Ia^{d+} cells (some indicated by arrows) in the epidermis and dermis of a wild-type Balb/c mouse. (**E**) A frozen section of an affected mouse ear that has been stained for the presence of keratin 6, showing extensive expression in the thickened epidermis. (**F**) Image from the ear of a wild-type animal, stained similarly for keratin 6. The only stong staining is seen at the hair follicle (f). As in Fig. 3, only the blue channel from the color images is shown in (**C**)–(**F**).

5.4. Unpicking the Mechanism of Chronic Inflammation

Mice that are deficient in IL-1Ra tend to develop chronic inflammatory diseases at specific sites, and a study of the development of each mouse model disease is likely to illuminate the mechanisms of the corresponding human disorder. Deficiency of IL-1Ra is expected only to increase the effective activity of IL-1, and the well-established role of IL-1 is to trigger local acute inflammation. At present we are still at the stage of observing the development of the three diseases. We need to develop methods to study the development of the three diseases longitudinally, so that animals can be investigated post mortem at different stages in the development of the disease. The age of onset is too broad to be used to identify the beginning of the phenotype. Thus we have so far observed early, mild lesions, but even they are all associated with most of the cell types and activation markers that are seen in later, severe lesions. We are thus missing the causative events of the diseases. When it comes to investigating the progress of the disease, the psoriasiform dermatosis is continuously visible and so may be more suitable for a continuous study. The arthritis is manifested externally, but only by swellings when well advanced. The arteritis, though, is usually only detected post mortem.

If chronic inflammation requires an adaptive immune response and thus the chronic presentation of an antigen, then we would expect mutations or treatments that suppress T-cell activation to suppress development of the disease phenotype as well. If the triggering antigen in a chronic inflammatory disease is initially exogenous, then we would expect that antibiotics or germ-free conditions would suppress the appearance of the disease. Genetic analysis is likely to reveal whether MHC haplotype is a significant factor in disease susceptibility, which would most easily be interpreted, as it has in human diseases, as evidence that the dominant presentation of a certain antigen or class of antigens by antigen-presenting cells is required to drive the disease. Studies on the reactivity and clonality of T-cell receptors might reveal evidence that specific autoantigens predominate in each of the three chronic diseases, and eventually it will be possible to isolate specific autoantigens.

In general, the steps that lead from acute to chronic inflammation are of great medical significance, and yet they are poorly delineated. Studies of IL-1Ra-deficient mice might reveal some possible routes. We need to discover how excessive IL-1 activity leads to autoantigen presentation. With the current intense interest in dendritic cells, we have begun to focus on their possible role in the three inflammatory diseases. Dendritic cells potentially bridge the gap between a response to IL-1 and autoantigen presentation. IL-1, like TNF or the microbial agonists of the Toll-like receptors, has the capacity to activate the maturation of dendritic cells in the presence of CD40 *(76,77)*. All the inflammatory diseases that we observe involve connective tissues, which probably contain antigenic epitopes that are generally cryptic and can only be presented after tissue has been destroyed by macrophages or neutrophils in response to inflammation. Immature dendritic cells would collect debris from inflammatory sites, and their oversensitivity to IL-1, in the absence of IL-1Ra, would tend to increase their rate of maturation and trafficking to draining lymph nodes. Once in the lymph nodes, dendritic cells could efficiently present material, including cryptic antigens, captured at the acutely inflamed site, resulting in the development of autoimmunity.

5.5 Suppression of the IL-1Ra-Deficient Phenotype by Epistatic Genetic Changes

It is fairly obvious that overexpression of IL-1Ra from a transgene should suppress any phenotype of IL-1Ra deficiency, as long as the domain of the trangene's expression includes that of the endogenous gene. This test, and a study in epistasis with IL-1RI have recently been reported by Irikura et al. *(20)*. Since IL-1Ra is believed to act solely as an inhibitor of the binding of IL-1 (IL-1α and IL-1β) to IL-1RI, and only IL-1 is believed to activate IL-1RI, then in the absence of IL-1RI, all biologic activity of IL-1 would be lost.

Consequently mice that lacked both IL-1Ra and IL-1RI should have no inflammatory phenotype and in fact should have no phenotype other than that ascribed to IL-1RI deficiency.

If the above statements are true, then it should also be true that mice deficient in both IL-1α and IL-1β should be identical to IL-1RI knockouts. Moreover, IL-1Ra deficiency should have no phenotype in the absence of either IL-1RI or of both forms of IL-1. Irikura et al. *(20)* showed that the growth deficiency of the $Il1rn^{ny/ny}$ mouse is significantly improved and delayed by a heterozygous null mutation in IL-1RI, but is completely corrected in homozygous nulls at this locus. Overexpression of the sIL-1Ra transcript has an indistinguishable suppressive effect. The early mortality of the $Il1rn^{ny/ny}$ C57BL/6 is also rescued either by deficiency of IL-1RI or by overexpression of sIL-1Ra. In the same way, hypersensitivity to toxic shock in $Il1rn^{ny/ny}$ mice is converted to hyposensitivity. The one apparently beneficial effect of IL-1Ra deficiency, the highly effective clearing of intracellular *L. monocytogenes*, was also abrogated and made subnormal (compared with wild-type mice) by deficiency of IL-1RI or IL-1Ra overexpression *(20)*.

All of these findings were completely in agreement with the expectations of the conservative model of IL-1Ra and IL-1 function described above in that there is no independent effect of *Il1rn* deficiency in the absence of the IL-1 receptor. Strictly speaking, there is one detail yet to be confirmed: that *Il1a/Il1b* double mutants *(17)* on the correct strain background are equivalent to *Il1r1*-deficient mice, which will establish that only IL-1 signals through the type I IL-1 receptor. Thus *Il1a/Il1b* double deficiency should, if this is true, completely suppress *Il1rn* deficiency.

We have also studied the ability of *Il1r1* deficiency to suppress the development of arterial inflammation in *Il1rn*-deficient Sf3 mice (J. S., M. N., unpublished data). We inbred $Il1rn^{s/s}/Il1r1^{+/-}$ parents and retained $Il1r1^{+/+}$ and $Il1r1^{-/-}$ littermates, which were necessarily completely deficient in IL-1Ra. At 200 d, 11/16 of the $Il1r1^{+/+}$ animals had clear arteritic lesions at the first site that we investigated, the aortic root, whereas 0/19 $Il1r1^{-/-}$ mice were affected. We conclude that one of the chronic inflammatory phenotypes, arteritis, is mediated through the IL-1 receptor and therefore probably involves IL-1. Further experiments with knockouts of the IL-1 genes will be needed to identify their roles in the development of the disease.

An extra interesting detail of the study by Irikura et al. *(20)* is their demonstration that sIL-1Ra overexpression is sufficient to suppress all of the phenotype of IL-1Ra deficiency. The authors interpret these results as demonstrating that icIL-1Ra is dispensable. Because the reverse experiment has not been done, though, an alternative interpretation might be that either form of IL-1Ra may be sufficient to suppress the phenotype caused by the absence of the other. It will be particularly interesting to know whether icIL-1Ra is required to suppress the psoriasiform phenotype, given the predominance of this form in the epidermis.

Conclusions

Three laboratories have developed their own null alleles of the mouse IL-1Ra gene. It is apparent that many of the inflammatory pathways mediated by IL-1 are redundantly served by other cytokines. Thus, in severe induced responses, the effect of IL-1Ra deficiency can be subtle and difficult to detect. It has taken several years to discover the potential of the IL-1Ra-deficient mouse to provide models for human diseases, specifically giant cell arteritis, rheumatoid arthritis, and psoriasis. The mouse diseases are sporadic although common, possibly influenced by environment, and more or less dependent on the genetic background of the mutant mouse. With the aid of further genetics and more sophisticated, longitudinal studies, the IL-1Ra-deficient mouse will at least illustrate how acute and chronic inflammation become linked.

Acknowledgments

J. S. is supported by a grant from the British Heart Foundation, which has also funded some of our work, described here. Other funding has been provided by a cooperative project under the European Union Framework V Quality of Life Programme.

References

1. Eisenberg, S. P., Evans, R. J., Arend, W. P., et al. (1990) Primary structure and functional expression from complementary-DNA of a human interleukin-1 receptor antagonist. *Nature* **343,** 341–346.
2. Hannum, C. H., Wilcox, C. J., Arend, W. P., et al. (1990) cDNA cloning of an intracellular form of the human interleukin-1 receptor antagonist associated with epithelium. *Nature* **343,** 336–340.
3. Dripps, D. J., Verderber, E., Ng, R. K., Thompson, R. C., and Eisenberg, S. P. (1991) Interleukin-1 receptor antagonist binds to the type-II interleukin-1 receptor on B-cells and neutrophils. *J. Biol. Chem.* **266,** 20311–20315.
4. Kassiotis, G. and Kollias, G. (2001) TNF and receptors in organ-specific autoimmune disease: multi-layered functioning mirrored in animal models. *J. Clin. Invest.* **107,** 1507–1508.
5. Niki, Y., Yamada, H., Seki, S., et al. (2001) Macrophage- and neutrophil-dominant arthritis in human IL-1 alpha transgenic mice. *J. Clin. Invest.* **107,** 1127–1135.
6. Nicklin, M. J. H., Barton, J. L., Nguyen, M., FitzGerald, M. G., Duff, G. W., and Kornman, K. (2002) A sequence-based map of the nine genes of the human interleukin-1 cluster. *Genomics* **79,** 718–725.
7. Taylor, S. L., Renshaw, B. R., Garka, K. E., Smith, D. E., and Sims, J. E. (2002) Genomic organization of the interleukin-1 locus. *Genomics* **79,** 726–733.
8. Graves, B. J., Hatada, M. H., Hendrickson, W. A., Miller, J. K., Madison, V. S., and Satow, Y. (1990) Structure of interleukin 1-alpha at 2.7-a resolution. *Biochemistry* **29,** 2679–2684.
9. Priestle, J. P., Schar, H. P., and Grutter, M. G. (1989) Crystallographic refinement of interleukin-1-beta at 2.0 Å resolution. *Proc. Natl. Acad. Sci. USA* **86,** 9667–9671.
10. Vigers, G. P. K., Caffes, P., Evans, R. J., Thompson, R. C., Eisenberg, S. P., and Brandhuber, B. J. (1994) X-ray structure of interleukin-1 receptor antagonist at 2.0-Ångstrom resolution. *J. Biol. Chem.* **269,** 12874–12879.
11. Sims, J. E., Nicklin, M. J. H., Bazan, J. F., et al. (2001) A new nomenclature for IL-1-family genes. *Trends Immunol.* **22,** 536–537.
12. Dunn, E., Sims, J. E., Nicklin, M. J. H., and O'Neill, L. A. J. (2001) Annotating genes with potential roles in the immune system: six new members of the IL-1 family. *Trends Immunol.* **22,** 533–536.
13. Barton, J. L., Herbst, R., Bosisio, D., Higgins, L., and Nicklin, M. J. H. (2000) A tissue specific IL-1 receptor antagonist homolog from the IL-1 cluster lacks IL-1, IL-1ra, IL-18 and IL-18 antagonist activities. *Eur. J. Immunol.* **30,** 3299–3308.
14. Lin, H. S., Ho, A. S., Haley-Vicente, D., et al. (2001) Cloning and characterization of IL-1HY2, a novel interleukin-1 family member. *J Biol. Chem.* **276,** 20597–20602.
15. Silver, A. R. J., Masson, W. K., George, A. M., Adam, J., and Cox, R. (1990) The IL-1-alpha-gene and IL-1-beta-gene are closely linked (less-than 70 kb) on mouse chromosome-2. *Somat. Cell Mol. Genet.* **16,** 549–556.
16. Zahedi, K., Seldin, M. F., Rits, M., Ezekowitz, R. A. B., and Whitehead, A. S. (1991) Mouse IL-1 receptor antagonist protein—molecular characterization, gene-mapping, and expression of messenger-RNA in vitro and in vivo. *J. Immunol.* **146,** 4228–4233.
17. Horai, R., Asano, M., Sudo, K., et al. (1998) Production of mice deficient in genes for interleukin (IL)-1 alpha, IL-1 beta, IL-1 alpha/beta, and IL-1 receptor antagonist shows that IL-1 beta is crucial in turpentine-induced fever development and glucocorticoid secretion. *J. Exp. Med.* **187,** 1463–1475.
18. Zahedi, K. A., Uhlar, C. M., Rits, M., Prada, A. E., and Whitehead, A. S. (1994) The mouse interleukin-1 receptor antagonist protein—gene structure and regulation in-vitro. *Cytokine* **6,** 1–9.

19. Gabay, C., Porter, B., Fantuzzi, G., and Arend, W. P. (1997) Mouse IL-1 receptor antagonist isoforms: complementary DNA cloning and protein expression of intracellular isoform and tissue distribution of secreted and intracellular IL-1 receptor antagonist in vivo. *J. Immunol.* **159,** 5905–5913.
20. Irikura, V. M., Lagraoui, M., and Hirsh, D. (2002) The epistatic relationships between IL-1, IL-1 receptor antagonist, and the type I IL-1 receptor. *J. Immunol.* **169,** 393–398.
21. Malyak, M., Guthridge, J. M., Hance, K. R., Dower, S. K., Freed, J. H., and Arend, W. P. (1998a) Characterization of a low molecular weight isoform of IL-1 receptor antagonist. *J Immunol.* **161,** 1997–2003.
22. Haskill, S., Martin, G., Van Le, L., et al. (1991) cDNA cloning of an intracellular form of the human interleukin-1 receptor antagonist assocviated with epithelium. *Proc. Natl. Acad. Sci. USA* **88,** 3681–3685.
23. Muzio, M., Polentarutti, N., Facchetti, F., et al. (1999) Characterization of type II intracellular IL-1 receptor antagonist (IL-1ra3): a depot IL-1ra. *Eur. J. Immunol.* **29,** 781–788.
24. Seckinger, P., Williamson, K., Balavoine, J. F., et al. (1987) A urine inhibitor of interleukin-1 activity affects both interleukin 1α and 1β but not tumor necrosis factor α. *J. Immunol.* **139,** 1541–1545.
25. Seckinger, P., Lowenthal, J. W., Williamson, K., Dayer, J. M., and MacDonald, H. R. (1987) A urine inhibitor of interleukin 1 activity that blocks ligand binding. *J. Immunol.* **139,** 1546–1549.
26. Greenfeder, S. A., Nunes, P., Kwee, L., Labow, M., Chizzonite, R. A., and Ju, G. (1995) Molecular cloning and characterization of a second subunit of the interleukin 1 receptor complex. *J. Biol. Chem.* **270,** 13757–13765.
27. Korherr, C., Hofmeister, R., Wesche, H., and Falk, W. (1997) A critical role for interleukin-1 receptor accessory protein in interleukin-1 signaling. *Eur. J. Immunol.* **27,** 262–267.
28. Schreuder, H., Tardif, C., Trump-Kallmeyer, S., et al. A new cytokine-receptor binding mode revealed by the crystal structure of the IL-1 receptor with an antagonist. *Nature* **386,** 194–200.
29. Vigers, G. P. A., Anderson, L. J., Caffes, P., and Brandhuber, B. J. (1997) Crystal structure of the type-I interleukin-1 receptor complexed with interleukin-1 beta. *Nature* **386,** 190–194.
30. Colotta, F., Re, F., Muzio, M., et al. (1993) Interleukin-1 type II receptor—a decoy target for IL-1 that is regulated by IL-4. *Science* **261,** 472–475.
31. Malinowsky, D., Lundkvist, J., Laye, S., and Bartfai, T. (1998) Interleukin-1 receptor accessory protein interacts with the type II interleukin-1 receptor. *FEBS Lett.* **429,** 299–302.
32. McMahan, C. J., Slack, J. L., Mosley, B., et al. (1991) A novel IL-1 receptor, cloned from B cells by mammalian expression, is expressed in many cell-types. *EMBO J.* **10,** 2821–2832.
33. Watson, J. M., Lofquist, A. K., Rinehart, C. A., et al. (1995) The intracellular IL-1 receptor antagonist alters IL-1-inducible gene-expression without blocking exogenous signaling by IL-1β. *J. Immunol.* **155,** 4467–4475.
34. Janson, R. W., Hance, K. R., and Arend, W. P. (1991) Production of IL-1-receptor antagonist by human *in vitro*-derived macrophages—effects of lipopolysaccharide and granulocyte-macrophage colony-stimulating factor. *J. Immunol.* **147,** 4218–4223.
35. Lore, K., Sonnerborg, A., Spetz, A. L., Andersson, U., and Andersson, J. (1998) Immunocytochemical detection of cytokines and chemokines in Langerhans cells and in vitro derived dendritic cells. *J. Immunol. Methods* **214,** 97–111.
36. McColl, S. R., Paquin, R., Menard, C., and Beaulieu, A. D. (1992) Human neutrophils produce high-levels of the interleukin-1 receptor antagonist in response to granulocyte macrophage colony-stimulating factor and tumor necrosis factor α. *J. Exp. Med.* **179,** 593–598.
37. Malyak, M., Smith, M. F., Abel, A. A., and Arend, W. P. (1994) Peripheral-blood neutrophil production of interleukin-1 receptor antagonist and interleukin-1β. *J. Clin. Immunol.* **14,** 20–30.
38. Dewberry, R. M., Holden, H., Crossman, D. C., and Francis, S. E. (2000) Interleukin-1 receptor antagonist expression in human endothelial cells and atherosclerosis. *Arterioscler. Thromb. Vasc. Biol.* **20,** 2394–2400.
39. Hagaman, D. D., Okayama, Y., D'Ambrosio, C., Prussin, C., Gilfillan, A. M., and Metcalfe, D. D. (2001) Secretion of interleukin-1 receptor antagonist from human mast cells after immunoglobulin E-mediated activation and after segmental antigen challenge. *Am. J. Respir. Cell Mol. Biol.* **25,** 685–691.
40. Chan, L. S., Hammerberg, C., Kang, K., Sabb, P., Tavakkol, A., and Cooper, K. D. (1992) Human dermal fibroblast interleukin-1 receptor antagonist (IL-1Ra) and interleukin-1-beta (IL-1β) mes-

senger-RNA and protein are co-stimulated by phorbol ester—implication for a homeostatic mechanism. *J. Invest. Derm.* **99,** 315–322.

41. Silvera, M. R. and Phipps, R. P. (1995) Synthesis of interleukin-1 receptor antagonist by Thy-1(+) and Thy-1(-) murine lung fibroblast subsets. *J. Interferon Cytokine Res.* **15,** 63–70.
42. Steinkasserer, A., Estaller, C., Weiss, E. H., and Sim, R. B. (1992) Human interleukin-1 receptor antagonist is expressed in liver. *FEBS Lett.* **310,** 60–62.
43. Gabay, C., Porter, B., Guenette, D., Billir, B., and Arend, W. P. (1999) Interleukin-4 (IL-4) and IL-13 enhance the effect of IL-1 beta on production of IL-1 receptor antagonist by human primary hepatocytes and hepatoma HepG2 cells: differential effect on C-reactive protein production. *Blood* **93,** 1299–1307.
44. Cerretti, D. P., Kozlosky, C. J., Mosley, B., et al. (1992) Molecular-cloning of the interleukin-1-beta converting enzyme. *Science* **256,** 97–100.
45. MacKenzie, A., Wilson, H. L., Kiss-Toth, E., Dower, S. K., North, R. A., and Surprenant, A. (2001) Rapid secretion of interleukin-1 beta by microvesicle shedding. *Immunity* **15,** 825–835.
46. Arend, W. P. and Leung, D. Y. M. (1994) IgG induction of IL-1 receptor antagonist production by human monocytes. *Immunol. Rev.* **139,** 71–78.
47. Arend, W. P., Smith, M. F. Jr., Janson, R., and Joslin, F. G. (1991) IL-1 receptor antagonist and IL-1-beta production in human monocytes are regulated differently. *J. Immunol.* **147,** 1530–1536.
48. Fenton, M. J., Buras, J. A., and Donnelly, R. P. (1992) IL-4 reciprocally regulates IL-1 and IL-1 receptor antagonist expression in human monocytes. *J. Immunol.* **149,** 1283–1288.
49. Vannier, E., Miller, L. C., and Dinarello, C. (1992) Co-ordinated anti-inflammatory effects of interleukin-4. Interleukin-4 suppresses interleukin-1 production but up-regiulates gene-expression and synthesis of interleukin-1 receptor antagonist. *Proc. Natl. Acad. Sci. USA* **89,** 4076–4080.
50. Beasley, D., McGuiggin, M. E., and Dinarello, C. A. (1995) Human vascular smooth-muscle cells produce an intracellular form of interleukin-1 receptor antagonist. *Am. J. Physiol.* **38,** C961–C968.
51. Bigler, C. F., Norris, D. A., Weston, W. L., and Arend, W. P. (1992) Interleukin-1 receptor antagonist production by human keratinocytes. *J. Invest. Dermatol.* **98,** 38–44.
52. Levine, S. J., Wu, T., and Shelhamer, J. H. (1997) Extracellular release of the type I intracellular IL-1 receptor antagonist from human airway epithelial cells—differential effects of IL-4, IL-13, IFN-gamma, and corticosteroids. *J. Immunol.* **158,** 5949–5957.
53. Merot, Y., Didienean, L., Dayer, J. M., Fournier, C., Carraux, P., and Saurat, J. H. (1987) Immunoreactive interleukin-1 (IL-1) alpha and beta in normal human-skin. *J. Invest. Dermatol.* **89,** 327.
54. Hirsch, E., Irikura, V. M., Paul, S. M., and Hirsh, D. (1996) Functions of interleukin 1 receptor antagonist in gene knockout and overproducing mice. *Proc. Natl. Acad. Sci. USA* **93,** 11008–11013.
55. Nicklin, M. J. H., Hughes, D. E., Barton, J. L., Ure, J. M., and Duff, G. W. (2000) Arterial inflammation in mice lacking the interleukin 1 receptor antagonist gene. *J. Exp. Med.* **191,** 303–311.
56. Hentze, M. W. and Kulozik, A. E. (1999) A perfect message: RNA surveillance and nonsense-mediated decay. *Cell* **96,** 307–310.
57. Ma, Y. H., Thornton, S., Boivin, G. P., Hirsh, D., Hirsch, R., and Hirsch, E. (1998) Altered susceptibility to collagen-induced arthritis in transgenic mice with aberrant expression of interleukin-1 receptor antagonist. *Arthritis Rheum.* **41,** 1798–1805.
58. Devlin, C. M., Kuriakose, G., Hirsch, E., and Tabas, I. (2002) Genetic alterations of IL-1 receptor antagonist in mice affect plasma cholesterol level and foam cell lesion size. *Proc. Natl. Acad. Sci. USA* **99,** 6281–6285.
59. Nagy, A., Rossant, J., Nagy, R., Abramow-Newerly, W., and Roder, J. C. (1990) Derivation of completely cell culture-derived mice from early-passage embryonic stem-cells. *Proc. Natl. Acad. Sci USA* **90,** 8424–8428.
60. Horai, R., Saijo, S., Tanika, M., et al. (2000) Development of chronic inflammatory arthropathy resembling rheumatoid arthritis in interleukin 1 receptor antagonist-deficient mice. *J. Exp. Med.* **191,** 313–320.
61. Josephs, M. D., Solorzano, C. C., Taylor, M., et al. (2000) Modulation of the acute phase response by altered expression of the IL-1 type 1 receptor or IL-1ra. *Am. J. Physiol.* **278,** R824–R830.
62. Wallenius, V., Wallenius, K., Ahren, B., et al. (2002) Interleukin-6-deficient mice develop mature onset obesity. *Nature Med.* **8,** 75–79.

63. Glaccum, M. B., Stocking, K. L., Charrier, K., et al. (1997) Phenotypic and functional characterization of mice that lack the type I receptor for IL-1. *J. Immunol.* **159,** 3364–3371.
64. Dinarello, C. A., Ikejima, T., Warner, S. J. C., et al. (1987) Interleukin-1 induces interleukin-1. 1. Induction of circulating interleukin-1 in rabbits in vivo and in human mononuclear cells in vitro. *J. Immunol.* **139,** 1902–1910.
65. Warner, S. J. C., Auger, K. R., and Libby, P. (1987) Human interleukin-1 induces interleukin-1 gene-expression in human vascular smooth-muscle cells. *J. Exp. Med.* **165,** 1316–1331.
66. Leon, L. R., Conn, C. A., Glaccum, M., and Kluger, M. J. (1996) IL-1 type I receptor mediates acute phase response to turpentine, but not lipopolysaccharide, in mice. *Am. J. Physiol.* **271,** R1668–R1675.
67. Ross, R. (1995) Cell biology of atherosclerosis. *Annu. Rev. Physiol.* **57,** 791–804.
68. Francis, S. E., Camp, N. J., Dewberry, R. M., et al. (1999) Interleukin-1 receptor antagonist gene polymorphism and coronary artery disease. *Circulation* **99,** 861–866.
69. Garcia-Cardena, G., Comander, J., Anderson, K. R., Blackman, B. R., and Gimbrone, M. A. (2001) Biomechanical activation of vascular endothelium as a determinant of its functional phenotype. *Proc. Natl. Acad. Sci. USA* **98,** 4478–4485.
70. Iwakura, Y. (2002) Roles of IL-1 in the development of rheumatoid arthritis: consideration from mouse models. *Cytokine Growth Factor Rev.* **13,** 341–355.
71. Simon, A. K., Seipelt, E., and Seiper, J. (1994) Divergent T cell cytokine patterns in inflammatory arthritis. *Proc. Natl. Acad. Sci USA* **91,** 8562–8566.
72. Chatelain, R., Varkila, K., and Cofman, R. L. (1992) IL-4 induces a TH2 response in *Leishmania major*-infected mice. *J. Immunol.* **148,** 1182–1187.
73. Vollmer, S., Menssen, A., and Prinz, J. C. (1994) T lymphocytes derived from skin lesions of patients with psoriasis vulgaris express a novel cytokine pattern that is distinct from that of T helper type 1 and type 2 cells. *Eur. J. Immunol.* **24,** 3277–3282.
74. Schlaak, J. F., Buslau, M., Jochum, W., et al. (1994) T-cells involved in psoriasis vulgaris belong to the TH1 subset. *J. Invest. Dermatol.* **102,** 145–149.
75. Uyemura, K., Yamamura, M., Fivenson, D. F., Modlin, R. L., and Nickoloff, B. J. (1993) The cytokine network in lesional and lesion-free psoriatic skin is characterized by T-helper type–1 cell-mediated response. *J. Invest. Dermatol.* **101,** 701–705.
76. Sallusto, F., Cella, M., Danieli, C., and Lanzavecchia, A. (1995) Dendritic cells use macropinocytosis and the mannose receptor to concentrate macromolecules in the major histocompatability complex class II compartment: downregulation by cytokines and bacterial products. *J. Exp. Med.* **182,** 389–400.
77. Roake, J. A., Rao, A. S., Morris, P. J., Larsen, C. P., Hankins, D. F., and Austyn, J. M. (1995) Dendritic cell loss from nonlymphoid tissue after systematic administration of lipopolysaccharide, tumor necrosis factor, and interleukin 1. *J. Exp. Med.* **181,** 2237–2247.

8

A Unique Role for IL-2 in Self-Tolerance

Thomas Hünig and Anneliese Schimpl

Summary

A decade ago, it was discovered unexpectedly that mice defective in IL-2 signalling do not suffer from impaired T-cell development or immune responsiveness, but rather from hyperactivation of the immune system leading to the autoimmune-inflammatory "IL-2 deficiency syndrome." Here we discuss the mechanisms unravelled so far which are likely to contribute to this immunopathological disorder. Definite evidence has been obtained for a defect in the generation and/or the maintenance of "regulatory" suppressor T-cells, and for a cell autonomous defect in the susceptibility of activated CD4 T-cells to apoptosis, which normally serves to terminate immune responses by clonal contraction. In addition, an as-yet unconfirmed defect in the negative selection of autoreactive CD4 T-cells is being discussed. In conclusion, it has become clear that while redundant as a T-cell growth factor, IL-2 serves a unique role as a negative regulator of the immune system with an essential task in maintaining self tolerance.

Key words

IL-2, apoptosis, autoimmunity, tolerance, regulatory T-cells, suppressor T-cells

1. Introduction

Interleukin-2 (IL-2), a prototypic member of the hematopoietins, has pleiotropic effects on cells of the immune system, some of which are shared with other cytokines of the 4 α-helical bundle family such as IL-4, IL-7, and IL-15. This partial overlap in function is explained by the modular structure of the corresponding cytokine receptors: They signal through a common γ-chain supplemented by one or two additional subunits that convey cytokine specificity and that again can be shared between distinct cytokine receptors of the family (reviewed in ref. *1*). With regard to IL-2, the "common" γ-chain (γc) is supplemented by a β-chain [IL-2 receptor β (IL-2Rβ), CD122] also used by IL-15. IL-2 specificity is conveyed by a third receptor chain, IL-2Rα (CD25) required for high-affinity binding but not for signal transduction.

Beyond the T-cell growth factor activity originally described as the function of IL-2, additional effects on the generation, proliferation, and differentiation of T- and B-cells, as well as natural killer (NK) cells, were discovered *(2)*, suggesting a central function of IL-2 in the development and response of the immune system. With the advent of knockout technology, these proposed "positive" functions of IL-2 were put to the test in vivo. Surprisingly, mice deficient in IL-2 *(3)* or in the α- *(4)* or β- *(5)* subunits of its receptor developed

From: *Contemporary Immunology: Cytokine Knockouts, 2nd Edition*
Edited by: Giamila Fantuzzi © Humana Press Inc., Totowa, NJ

an apparently complete immune system, which, rather than being sluggish, overreacts against both self and non-self, leading to multiorgan autoimmunity and inflammation *(3–5)*. The massive defect in clonal control observed in the absence of IL-2 suggested that the only unique function of IL-2 is a negative, rather than a positive one. In the meantime, however, IL-2 is back as a factor required for differentiation and survival of T-cells—this time for a subset suppressing pathologic immune responses, the currently much discussed regulatory T-cells (T*reg* cells) *(6,7)*.

In the present chapter, we first review the generation and function of the immune system in mice lacking IL-2 or components of IL-2R and then discuss how defective IL-2R signaling may affect lymphopoiesis and peripheral immune regulation, leading to the complex immunopathology we have previously called the *IL-2 deficiency syndrome (8)*.

2. Cellular Immunology of Mice Defective in IL-2 Signaling

2.1. Lymphopoiesis in the Absence of IL-2R Signals

2.1.1. Expression of IL-2R Subunits

The three subunits of IL-2R are differentially expressed on developing lymphocytes: as part of the IL-7 receptor, the common γ-chain is found in early stages of B- and T-cell development, allowing stromal cell-derived IL-7 to promote the expansion of B-cell precursors *(9)* and early thymocytes *(10)*. Curiously, the IL-2Rα chain (CD25) is transiently expressed on pro B-cells *(11)* and on a subset of $CD3^-/4^-/8^-$ immature thymocytes *(12–14)* in mice. The absence of IL-2Rβ (CD122) on these early B- and T-cell precursors, however, puts the physiologic significance of CD25 expression at that stage into question, rather, IL-2Rβ expression in primary lymphoid organs of mice is restricted to γ/δ thymocytes including the precursors of dendritic epidermal γ/δ T-cells *(15)*, and to a small subset of phenotypically mature α/β T-cells in the postnatal thymus *(16)*, where it is apparently induced by self-antigen recognition *(17)*.

2.1.2. Effects of IL-2 and IL-2R Deficiency on Lymphopoiesis

2.1.1.1. Generation of Lymphocyte Subsets

Inactivation of the γc gene results in a complete lack of γ/δ T-cells and NK cells *(18)* and greatly impairs mainstream T- and B-cell development *(18,19)* primarily as a result of defective IL-7 signaling. This mutation is thus the least informative with regard to the requirement for IL-2 in lymphopoiesis.

In peripheral lymphoid organs of IL-2-deficient mice, the representation of B-cells, CD4, and CD8 T-cell subsets and of T-cell receptor $(TCR)^-$ NK1.1 (NK) cells is initially normal *(20)*. In IL-2Rα- *(4)* and IL-2Rβ-deficient mice *(5)*, T- and B-cells also seed the periphery in normal numbers, confirming that IL-2 is not required for their development or export and extending this finding to IL-15.

With regard to minor T-cell subsets, earlier work reported on IL-2-deficient mice has demonstrated that γ/δ T-cells *(21)* as well as the progeny of the earliest wave of thymic γ/δ T-cell development, the dendritic epidermal T-cells in the skin *(22)*, are also normally represented in IL-2-deficient mice; these IL-2Rβ/γ-expressing cells may, however, utilize IL-15 for their development and/or survival. Importantly, however, recent work has suggested that another T-cell subset generated in the thymus, the T*reg* cells, are lacking in the absence of IL-2R signaling.

2.1.1.2. Defective *Treg* Generation?

Treg cells are CD45R^{low}, CD62L+ CD4 T-cells that make IL-10 and transforming growth factor-β (TGF-β) but not IL-2 and that suppress inflammation and autoimmunity in a broad spectrum of experimental systems (reviewed in refs. *6* and *7*). Of particular importance for the present discussion, *Treg* cells express CD25 *(23)* and are completely dependent on exogenous IL-2 for growth or survival *(24,25)*. Evidence for a *Treg* defect as a causative factor of the immunopathology of IL-2-deficient mice will be discussed below. With regard to a defect in their thymic generation in the absence of IL-2R signaling, the following findings can be summarized:

1. *Treg* cells are produced in the thymus (*26*; reviewed in ref. *27*) but can also develop in the periphery (*28*; reviewed in ref. *7*).
2. CD4+/CD25+ thymocytes and peripheral T-cells are lacking in IL-2-deficient mice *(24)*. The caveat with this result is that IL-2 is required for phenotypic upregulation of CD25, but additional data on cytokine production and *Treg* function support the notion of defective *Treg* production in the absence of IL-2 signaling (see below).
3. Among the minute subset of IL-2Rα^{-}/β^{+} TCR-α/β^{+} thymocytes, IL-2 deficiency leads to a shift from the major CD4^{-}/8^{-} to a CD4^{-}/8^{+} phenotype *(17)*. Conceivably, these are end products of a dysregulated differentiation pathway from which *Treg* cells normally branch off if IL-2 is provided and the IL-2R α-chain is transiently coexpressed. In line with this hypothetical scheme, studies with TCR transgenic mice have shown that self-antigen recognition during T-cell development can induce IL-2Rβ expression *(17)*, indicating that IL-2Rβ-expressing thymocytes may be on their way to enter the pool of *Treg* cells with autoreactive receptors but suppressive function.
4. Immunopathology of IL-2Rβ-deficient mice is abolished by transient IL-2Rβ expression in the thymus *(29)*. This supports the concept that signals through the IL-2 (or IL-15) receptor during T-cell development are required for the generation of functional *Treg* cells.

2.1.1.3. Thymic Repertoire Selection

In IL-2 knockout mice, negative selection of CD4 and CD8 T-cells expressing TCR Vβ segments reactive with endogenous superantigens proceeds normally *(30)*, and deletion of thymocytes bearing an MHC class I restricted transgenic TCR by confrontation with cognate peptide is comparable between wild-type and IL-2-deficient cells both in vitro and in vivo *(31)*. However, deletion of CD4+/8+ thymocytes expressing the MHC class II restricted OVA-specific DO11.10 receptor is impaired in IL-2 knockout mice and can be restored by application of IL-2 *(32)*. Taken together, evidence for defective negative selection in the absence of IL-2 is so far restricted to the CD4 lineage, in which dependence of apoptosis induction on the Fas/CD95 pathway at high- but not at low-antigen doses was recently reported *(33)*. Since IL-2-deficient mice display a defect in CD95-mediated apoptosis (see below), CD95-dependent deletion of maturing CD4 T-cells, as postulated for high antigen doses, may be partially defective in IL-2 knockout mice. Thus, endogenous superantigen stimulation, which deletes developing CD4 T-cells also in the absence of IL-2, may represent a low-antigen dose scenario not requiring CD95 signaling for deletion. If, indeed, CD4 T-cell deletion by high antigen doses is defective, mature T-cells from IL-2 knockout mice may have a more autoimmune-prone T-cell repertoire.

2.2. Humoral Immune Responses

Even without intentional immunization, serum immunoglobulin levels in IL-2-deficient mice are strongly elevated up to the time point when B-cell destruction sets in *(3,34)*.

Although the most dramatic effects were observed in the "TH2-dependent" isotypes IgG1 and IgE, no selective cytokine skewing but rather an overall increase in prototypic Th1 and Th2 cytokines is detected (I. Berberich, A. Schimpl, unpublished data). In mice lacking the IL-2Rα- or β-chains, IgG1 and IgE levels were similarly increased *(4,5)* whereas, not unexpectedly, all "switched" isotypes were diminished in γc knockout mice, which are both B- and T-lymphopenic *(18)*.

After immunization with T-dependent antigens *(21)* or after virus infection *(35)*, IL-2-deficient mice mount close to normal antibody responses including the production of neutralizing antibodies. This is in contrast to the lack of neutralizing IgG or IgM in vesicular stomatitis virus (VSV) infected IL-2Rβ-deficient mice *(5)*, suggesting a role for IL-15 in the response to infectious virus.

2.3. CD4 T-Cell Responses

2.3.1. In Vivo Responses

2.3.1.1. Model Protein Antigens

In vivo priming for proliferative in vitro responses with protein antigens is unaffected by IL-2 deficiency, and T-helper function for B-cell isotype switching in these responses is even elevated *(20)*, indicating efficient Th2 function. On the other hand, the Th1-skewed response and inflammatory bowel disease (IBD) observed after immunization of gnotobiotic IL-2-deficient mice with trinitrophenyl/keyhole limpet hemocyanin (TNP/KLH) in the adjuvant was interpreted as a defect in Th2 development *(36)*; in light of more recent findings, however, the IL-2 dependence of antiinflammatory regulatory T-cells seems a more likely explanation. In fact, our own analysis showed that, with the exception of IL-5, most prototypic Th1 and Th2 cytokines are overproduced by the activated CD4 T-cells accumulating in IL-2 knockout mice (unpublished data).

To follow the clonal dynamics of stimulated CD4 T-cells in vivo more closely, responses to superantigens and, in the case of TCR transgenic IL-$2^{-/-}$ mice, to MHC class II presented peptides were studied.

2.3.1.2. Superantigens

In response to staphylococcal enterotoxin A or B (SEA or SEB), IL-2-deficient C57BL/6 and C3H mice, respectively, showed both the early deletion and subsequent expansion phases known from wild-type animals. The late deletion of CD4 cells was, however, reduced in IL-2 knockout mice *(37)*. Similar observations were also made in mice lacking IL-2Rα *(4)*. Importantly, IL-2-deficient CD4 T-cells isolated from superantigen-stimulated animals at this late phase of the response proliferated vigorously in vitro when restimulated with the same superantigen *(37)*. This is in marked contrast to CD4 T-cells from wild-type mice, which had become anergic or died when restimulated in cell culture.

2.3.1.3. Peptide Response of TCR Transgenic Cells

To avoid crowding effects in vivo, the corresponding experiments with TCR transgenic CD4 T-cells were done by adoptive transfer of small T-cell numbers into athymic mice. Similarly to the observations with superantigens, the classical dynamics of such a response originally observed by Jenkins and colleagues *(38)*, i.e., an initial expansion followed by a "crash," was altered in the absence of IL-2: IL-$2^{-/-}$ TCR transgenic DO.11.10 CD4 T-cells increased in number throughout the 3 wk of the observation period, whereas control cells declined after d 7 *(39)*.

Together, these observations indicate that antigen-driven clonal expansion of CD4 T-cells does not require IL-2 in vivo, whereas clonal contraction is defective in the absence of IL-2. This phenotype is the key feature of the dysregulated immune response in mice defective in IL-2 signaling and provides an explanation for the attenuating effects of a germ-free environment and TCR repertoire restriction on the development of the IL-2 deficiency syndrome (see below).

2.3.2. In Vitro Responses

2.3.2.1. POLYCLONAL ACTIVATION

In vitro, proliferation of unseparated lymph node T-cells upon polyclonal stimulation with concanavalin A, anti-CD3, or allogeneic spleen cells is only two to threefold lower than that of wild-type controls. Furthermore, purified IL-2-deficient CD4 T-cells activated with plate-bound anti-CD3 monoclonal antibody (MAb) are readily costimulated by anti-CD28, even if, in the responder cells, the IL-4 gene was additionally inactivated (unpublished). Incidentally, this also holds true for thymocytes from $\gamma c^{-/-}$ mice *(18)*, confirming our conclusion that CD28-mediated costimulation does not depend on IL-2 or IL-4 in driving T-cell proliferation.

2.3.2.2. SUPERANTIGENS AND PEPTIDE ANTIGENS

Using more physiologic stimuli, IL-2-deficient CD4 T-cells were also found to proliferate in response to bacterial superantigens *(37)* or, when carrying a transgenic TCR, to the relevant MHC class II peptide presented *(40)*. We also used the TCR-transgenic DO.11.10 system to test directly the claim that IL-2 is required for the generation of IL-4-producing cells in vitro *(41)*, and we found no evidence for such a requirement *(40)*.

2.4. CD8 T-Cell Responses

2.4.1. In Vivo Responses

2.4.1.1. RESPONSE TO VIRUS INFECTION

IL-2 deficiency has only a small impact on primary cytotoxic T-lymphocyte (CTL) responses against vaccinia virus and lymphocytic choriomeningitis virus (LCMV) *(35)*. Furthermore, virus clearance and early delayed-type hypersensitivity (DTH) reactions were normal. This is in contrast to IL-2Rβ-deficient mice, in which virus-specific CD8 T-cell responses were absent *(5)*, suggesting a role of IL-15. Indeed, there is increasing evidence for the importance of this cytokine for the maintenance of CD8 T-cell responses in vivo *(42)*.

2.4.1.2. ALLOREACTIVE CTL RESPONSES

Islet allografts are rejected by IL-2-deficient mice with a delay of about 10 d *(43)*. The potential participation of CTL in this response is illustrated by generation of CTL activity in injected allogeneic tumor cells, albeit with greatly reduced efficiency compared with IL-2 wild-type mice *(44)*. Conceivably, a contribution of IL-15 to this system is much less pronounced than in the antiviral response.

2.4.1.3. PEPTIDE-DRIVEN CTL RESPONSES

IL-2-deficient mice expressing a transgenic TCR specific for $H2D^b$ plus influenza nucleoprotein show normal T-cell proliferation in response to peptide injection in short-term assays *(31)*. However, CTLs thus activated only displayed CTL activity when isolated from

IL-2 wild-type mice, again suggesting the participation of additional cytokines in the CTL responses to infectious viruses described above, which may not be recruited by antigenic peptides given in isolation.

2.4.1.4. Superantigen Responses

Injection of bacterial superantigens led to a transient expansion of the Vβ-defined superantigen-reactive CD8 and CD4 T-cells in both IL-2 wild-type and IL-2-deficient mice *(37)*. However, CTL activity was only observed in the former, paralleling the results obtained with peptide-driven activation of a transgenic TCR. Importantly and in contrast to CD4 T-cells (see above), superantigen-expanded CD8 T-cells were strongly depleted from peripheral lymphoid organs during the further time-course and accumulated in the liver *(37)*.

Taken together, initial induction of proliferation of CD8 T-cells seems to be independent of IL-2 in vivo. Differences between IL-2 and IL-2Rβ knockout mice with regard to the antiviral CTL response suggest, furthermore, that for the functional differentiation of CTL, IL-2Rβ-mediated signals are required, allowing IL-15 to substitute partially for IL-2. Finally, the availability of IL-15 for CTL differentiation seems to depend on the mode of immunization, i.e., it supports responses to infectious viruses but not to peptides or allogeneic cells.

2.4.2. CD8 Responses Depend on IL-2 In Vitro

In agreement with the original definition of IL-2 as an important growth and differentiation factor for CD8 T-cells, a strict dependence on exogenous IL-2 was observed for the induction of primary and secondary antiviral responses from IL-2-deficient mice in vitro *(35)*. Similarly, peptide stimulation of IL-2-deficient TCR transgenic CD8 cells, although inducing transient DNA synthesis, failed to yield cytotoxic activity *(31)*. Since even polyclonal activation with anti-CD3 antibodies or in mixed lymphocyte reactions did not yield cytotoxic activity unless IL-2 was added *(45)*, the results in all systems studied lead to the conclusion that in vitro activation of CD8 T-cells is strongly IL-2-dependent. As mentioned above, this discrepancy between results obtained in cell culture and in some in vivo systems may be explained by the availability of IL-15 in the latter but not the former situation.

3. Cellular and Molecular Basis of the IL-2 Deficiency Sydrome

3.1. Immunopathology of Mice Defective in IL-2 Signaling

IL-2 knockout mice suffer from autoimmunity and inflammation affecting multiple organs *(34,46,47)*. Although strain-specific background genes modify the kinetics of disease development, all mice with an intact T-cell compartment but lacking IL-2 invariably succumb to lethal immunopatholoy.

Initially, an increase in CD4 T-cells expressing activation markers is observed at the expense of CD4 cells of the naive phenotype, followed by massive activation of B-cells and, to a lesser extent, CD8 T-cells *(20,34)*. Spleens and lymph nodes become dramatically hyperplastic and lose their normal architecture. The hyperactivated immune system then attacks multiple organs and cell types with both its cell-mediated and humoral arms. In strains rapidly succumbing to the IL-2 deficiency syndrome, anemia resulting from autoantibody production and/or destruction of bone marrow cells by infiltrating T-cells as well as IBD are prime causes of death *(34,46,47)*. The general breakdown of self-tolerance is, however, illustrated by the mononuclear infiltrations and lesions observed in the pancreas, lung, heart, blood vessels, and liver, as well as the production of autoantibodies with multiple organ specifities *(47)*.

Among mice targeted for the three chains of the IL-2R, those lacking the α-chain develop an autoimmune-inflammatory syndrome most similar to that found in IL-2-deficient mice, including the accumulation of activated lymphocytes, anemia, and IBD *(4)*. Since the murine IL-2Rβ/γ fails to bind IL-2 but contributes to the receptor for IL-15 *(48)*, the role of IL-2 in maintaining self-tolerance seems to be unique within this closely related cytokine subfamily. With the exception of massive lymphocytic infiltration in the gut, the pathologic features of the IL-2 deficiency syndrome observed in IL-$2^{-/-}$ and IL-2R$\alpha^{-/-}$ lines are also found in IL-2Rβ-deficient animals *(5)*. Although at face value, this would point to a protective role of IL-15 in gut inflammation, the strong influence of antigenic load and genetic background on the onset of IBD severity in IL-2 knockout mice makes such conclusions uncertain.

Deletion of the third chain of IL-2R, the "common" γ-chain (γc), abolishes reactivity not only to IL-2 and IL-15 but also to IL-4, IL-7, IL-9, and the recently discovered IL-21 *(1)*. In view of the strongly impaired T-cell development *(18,19)*, it is not surprising that the generalized T-cell-mediated inflammation characteristic of the IL-2 deficiency syndrome is not observed in these animals. Nevertheless, in spite of the absence of gut-associated lymphoid tissue and intestinal intraepithelial lymphocytes, mononuclear infiltrates of the lamina propria resulting in a distinct form of IBD was reported *(18,49)*. Furthermore, activated CD4 T-cells also accumulate in the spleens of $\gamma c^{-/-}$ mice *(18)*, lending further support to the concept of a role of IL-2R in the containment of T-cell expansion.

3.2. Importance of Thymus-Derived CD4 T-Cells and Antigen

The central role of pathogenic CD4 T-cells for the development of the IL-2 deficiency syndrome is indicated by the following findings:

1. The absence of T- and B-lymphocytes induced by inactivation of the RAG-2 gene prevents the development of immunopathology *(50)*. Since transfer of IL-2-deficient, but not of wild-type bone marrow results in disease development *(51)*, cells responsible for the IL-2 deficiency syndrome map to the hematopoietic system.
2. IL-2-deficient athymic mice do not develop disease, indicating that thymus-derived T-cells initiate immune pathology and secondarily destroy the B-cell compartment *(51)*.
3. B-cell-deficient IL-2 knockout mice develop IBD but not hemolytic anemia, indicating that an intact T-cell compartment suffices for inflammation and that autoantibody production by B-cells, helped by abnormally activated T-cells, is the primary cause of anemia *(50)*.
4. Treatment of IL-2-deficient mice with CD40 ligand-specific MAb inhibits activation of B- and CD4 T-cells and delays disease development *(46)*. Similarly, IL-2Rβ-deficient mice are protected from immunopathology by treatment with depleting CD4-specific antibodies *(5)*.

The importance of antigen in the abnormal CD4 T-cell activation with ensuing immune pathology is indicated by the absence of IBD in germ-free IL-2-deficient mice *(34)* and by the marked delay in the onset of disease in mice with a restricted TCR repertoire achieved by the introduction of a transgenic TCR *(39)*.

Taken together, these findings have established that peripheral activation of thymus-derived CD4 T-cells is essential for the development of the IL-2 deficiency syndrome. Since responding to antigens is what CD4 T-cells are normally supposed to do, their aggressive behavior must be explained by defects in regulation and, possibly, a partial lack of central tolerance (see above).

3.3. Evidence for Dysregulation in *cis* and *trans*

The accumulation of T-cells with an activated phenotype in untreated IL-2-deficient mice as well as the impaired clonal contraction in response to superantigens or a peptide recognized by a transgenic TCR suggested a defect in peripheral T-cell death following activation and/or in indirect regulatory effects such as the deactivation of antigen-presenting cells and proliferating T-cells by counterregulatory cells. At present, there is experimental evidence for both proposed mechanisms.

3.3.1. Defective CD95-Mediated Apoptosis in the Absence of IL-2 Signals

Lenardo *(52)* first showed that Vβ-specific T-cell deletion induced in vivo by the injection of bacterial superantigens is incomplete when IL-2 signaling is blocked by the injection of IL-2Rα-specific antibodies. These findings are in full agreement with the later observations made by us and by Willerford et al. using mice deficient in IL-2 *(37)* or the IL-2Rα chain *(4)*, respectively (see above). Furthermore, we could show in vitro that activated CD4 T-cells from IL-2-deficient mice are relatively resistant to the induction of apoptosis by superantigen restimulation *(37)*.

Since activation-induced cell death (AICD) following religation of the antigen receptor depends on the expression of the death receptor CD95 and the induction of its ligand, CD95L *(53)*, defects in the expression of this receptor/ligand pair as well as modifications of downstream signaling events were investigated. Activated IL-2-deficient CD4 T-cells express normal levels of CD95, but CD95L induction is partially impaired *(4,37,54)*. This reduced CD95L expression, however, is insufficient to explain the defect in AICD since activated, CD95 expressing IL-2-deficient CD4 T-cells are also resistant to the induction of apoptosis by artificially crosslinking CD95 with MAb *(37,54)*. Thus, the downstream signaling machinery of CD95 must also be affected.

Analysis of stimulatory and inhibitory components of the death-inducing signaling complex (DISC) revealed the following differences between activated CD4 T-cells from IL-2-deficient versus wild-type mice: Refaeli et al. *(54)* reported that although activated IL-2-sufficient T-cells downregulate the antiapoptotic DISC component c-Flip, c-Flip expression remained high in the absence of IL-2. In our own experiments with IL-2-deficient CD4 T-cells expressing the Ova-specific DO11.10 TCR *(30)*, we only observed a twofold difference in c-Flip expression compared with wild-type TCR transgenic cells. In addition, however, we also found that caspase 8, which competes with c-Flip for its place in the DISC, was downregulated in the absence of IL-2, again by about a factor of 2. Thus, an overall fourfold difference in caspase 8/c-Flip ratios could affect the sensitivity to CD95-mediated cell death. As a caveat, it should be mentioned that increased resistance to CD95-mediated cell death in the absence of IL-2 is not observed in all experimental settings: Thus, when we hypercrosslinked CD95 with biotinylated antibodies and streptavidin, activated CD4 cells from IL-2 knockout mice died with even faster kinetics than wild-type cells *(30)*. Clearly, the relevance of these findings for the in vivo situation needs to be clarified by further experiments.

Signaling through death receptors initiates the activation of a cascade of caspases culminating in the activation of effector caspases that cleave the relevant death substrates. In addition to this so-called type I pathway, a type II pathway exists that depends on a mitochondrial amplification loop of caspase activation that is negatively regulated by antiapoptotic molecules of the bcl-2 family *(55)*. Among those, we observed a clear-cut overexpression of the A1 protein in IL-2-deficient compared with IL-2-sufficient CD4 T-cells analyzed ex vivo *(30)*. Further activation of IL-2-deficient cells led to further upregulation of A1, which was maintained throughout the in vitro observation period. In CD4 T-cells with an intact IL-2 gene, in contrast, A1 expression induced by in vitro activation is only transient. Again, however, there seem to be no simple answers: We consistently failed to detect the prototypic member of this antiapoptotic family of proteins, bcl-2 itself, in activated CD4+/IL-$2^{-/-}$ cells *(30)*. This possibly explains the increased apoptosis of these cells following the hyper-crosslinking of CD95 described above; additionally, lack of bcl-2 could even contribute to the relative apoptosis resistance at low levels of CD95 crosslinking, because bcl-2 can be converted by cleavage from an antiapoptotic to a proapoptotic molecule. We are currently trying to understand the complex regulation of apoptotic pathways by bcl-2 family members using retroviral complementation assays.

In summary, the following differences in the CD95-dependent apoptotic machinery between wild-type and IL-2-deficient CD4 T-cells have so far been discovered and may contribute to the enhanced survival of activated cells in vivo: lower levels of CD95L, an increased c-Flip/caspase 8 ratio, and upregulation of the antiapoptotic A1 protein.

3.3.2. Evidence for Defects in trans-*Regulation*

The earliest experiments indicating that in vivo, accumulation of pathogenic IL-2-deficient CD4 T-cells can be suppressed by wild-type cells were studies in which IL-2-sufficient and IL-2-deficient bone marrow were cotransplanted into $RAG^{-/-}$ mice *(51)*. They showed that the progeny of cells with an intact IL-2 gene completely suppressed the dysregulated T-cell activation and immunopathology observed with IL-2-deficient bone marrow alone. An important extension of this approach was the analysis of mixed bone marrow chimeras in which the wild-type component suppressed the abnormal activation of IL-2Rβ-deficient cells (which cannot receive an IL-2 signal), demonstrating regulation in *trans* by a mechanism distinct from paracrine IL-2 delivery *(56)*.

Finally, Freitas and colleagues recently provided further strong evidence for the importance of the IL-2/IL-2R system in the establishment of negative regulation in *trans (56a)*. Using homeostasis of peripheral CD4 T-cells as a readout for the presence or absence of regulatory cells in IL-2- or IL-2Rα-deficient mice (which both develop the disease), they found that cotransfer of IL-2-deficient with IL-2Rα-deficient bone marrow reconstitutes a normal phenotype, whereas with either bone marrow source used in isolation, immunopathology develops. In the framework of the regulatory T-cell hypothesis, these results are explained in the following way: IL-2Rα-deficient T-cells initially produce IL-2 used by IL-2-deficient T-cell precursors to generate regulatory CD4+/CD25+ T-cells, allowing their survival and function in the periphery. This population of T*reg* cells would then mediate homeostatic control of CD4 T-cells derived from both the IL-2- and the IL-2Rα-deficient bone marrow.

3.3.3. Suppression of the IL-2 Deficiency Syndrome by Transfer of Treg *Cells*

The first experiments that aimed at identifying means to suppress the immunopathology associated with defective IL-2R signaling by interfering with immunoregulation simply involved postnatal treatment with IL-2. Not unexpectedly, injection of IL-2 into IL-2-deficient mice for a defined time-window suppressed disease development—unless treatment was initiated later than 4 d after birth *(57)*. In an extension of these experiments, Klebb et al. *(57)* provided the first direct evidence for the ability of an IL-2-dependent regulatory T-cell subset to contain the abnormal T-cell activation of IL-2-deficient mice: they showed that transfer of spleen cells or thymocytes from IL-2-deficient mice treated from birth with IL-2 conferred disease resistance in a fraction of IL-2-deficient recipients and suggested that IL-2 is required for the postnatal differentiation or maturation of regulatory cells required for self/non-self discrimination. However, protection conferred by the transferred cells was never indefinite, pointing to a role of IL-2 in the maintenance of T*reg* function or survival. The apparent contradiction of these findings to the results obtained by Malek et al., in which thymus-specific expression of an IL-2Rβ transgene fully prevented the development of immune pathology in IL-2Rβ-deficient mice *(29)*, may be explained by the fact that the IL-2Rβ transgene introduced was not completely absent on peripheral T-cells, thus allowing the peripheral survival of T*reg* cells generated in the thymus.

We have recently obtained direct evidence for the ability of CD4+/CD25+ T*reg* cells to control the abnormal activation of IL-2-deficient CD4 T-cells *(39)*. Using the cell transfer system described above, in which IL-2-deficient T-cells expressing the Ova-specific DO11.10 TCR were injected into athymic mice and challenged with antigen, we found that the abnormal expansion observed in the absence of IL-2 was efficiently suppressed by both CD25+ and $CD25^-$ subsets of wild-type CD4 T-cells. Importantly, the T*reg* cells transferred do not produce IL-2, excluding paracrine IL-2 delivery in this system. On the other hand, the mechanism by which the $CD25^-$/CD4+ T-cells conveyed protection could either have been paracrine IL-2 delivery, or alternatively, suppression by a CD25- T*reg* subset, as had been described in other systems (reviewed in ref. *7*).

3.3.4. Importance of CD25-Treg Cells?

Phenotypic definition of T*reg* cells by expression of CD25 is complicated not only by the fact that IL-2 is required for the full upregulation of the IL-2Rα chain (the CD25 marker) *(58)* but also by the description in multiple systems of T-cells with regulatory function that do not express CD25 (reviewed in ref. *7*). The lineage relationships between these various phenotypically defined T*reg* cells are not fully understood. Of interest, thymic T*reg* cells in the rat are exclusively CD25+, whereas in the periphery, T*reg* function is also expressed by other CD4 cells within the $CD45R^{low}$ subset *(59)*, suggesting that either thymic CD25+ T*reg* cells further differentiate into CD25+ and CD25– cells in the periphery, or that additional T*reg* cells lacking CD25 are generated outside the thymus. A candidate for such a population has been defined in mice based on the expression of CD38 *(60)*. CD38+ T*reg* cells overlap only partially with the CD25+ subset. Such CD4+/CD38+ T-cells are present in IL-2-deficient mice and at least in vitro, they exhibit the functional features of T*reg* cells *(60)*. Their effectiveness as T*reg* cells in vivo is not yet known, however.

Although expression of CD25 is certainly an incomplete and sometimes misleading way to identify T*reg* cells, when we look at the data together, the correlation of immunopathology with defective IL-2 signaling and the expression of CD25 on at least one important subset of T*reg* cells (together with the ability of this subset to suppress uncontrolled T-cell activation) suggest that a defect in T*reg* generation or survival is a central event in the development of the IL-2 deficiency syndrome.

3.4. Newly Discovered Functions of IL-2: Do They Relate to the IL-2 Deficiency Syndrome?

Until recently, it was believed that IL-2 is only produced by activated T-cells. This has recently been challenged by Ricciardi-Castagnoli and colleagues *(61)*, who showed that transient production of IL-2 by dendritic cells (DCs) may be important for their function.

Since, again contrary to a prevailing dogma, it was recently shown that DCs not only potently induce T-cell activation but also that a DC subset can actually tolerize *(62)*, modifications in DC function by endogenously produced IL-2 could contribute to the autoimmune phenotype of IL-2- and IL-2R-deficient mice. Further experimentation will be needed to clarify this point.

One paradoxic finding relating to the autoimmune-prone phenotype of IL-2-deficient mice is their increased resistance to experimental autoimmune encephalomyelitis (EAE) induction, which is overcome by injection of IL-2 *(63)*. Since there is no *a priori* reason why T-cell activation by myelin oligodendrocyte glycoprotein (MOG) could be less efficient than priming with the other protein antigens so far studied in IL-2-deficient mice, pathomechanisms downstream of T-cell activation could be affected by the absence of IL-2. Indeed, the absence of perivascular inflammatory infiltrates in MOG-immunized IL-2-deficient mice suggested that migration and homing to the central nervous system might be defective *(63)*. This has become a likely possibility with the recent description of IL-2-dependent induction of homing receptors on activated T-cells *(64)*. Thus, in CD8 T-cells, induction of a glycosyltransferase required for the generation of the core structures of the P-selectin ligands is primarily controlled by IL-2 in CD8 T-cells. It is speculated that CD4 T-cells are similarly affected. Accordingly, in a special setting of an organ-specific (auto-) immune response, defective IL-2 signaling may alter cell migration, resulting in an abnormal balance of lymphocyte subsets at certain sites. Although in the setting of EAE, this may actually be protective to the host, in other situations this could also contribute to the harmful dysregulated immune response of IL-2-deficient mice.

4. Concluding Remarks

A decade after the surprising phenotype of mice defective in IL-2 signaling was reported, several mechanisms have been identified that may contribute to the immunopathology of the IL-2 deficiency syndrome. As summarized in Fig. 1, these are a defective generation of regulatory T-cells and a cell-autonomous defect in the susceptibility to AICD. In addition, an as yet unconfirmed defect in the negative selection of autoreactive CD4 T-cells seems possible. It will be the task of the next years to evaluate the relative contributions of these defects to the overall phenotype—unless, again, an unexpected new function of IL-2 will add further complexity to its role in controlling homeostasis of the immune system.

Acknowledgments

We thank A. Freitas and colleagues for communicating their unpublished results and all our colleagues at the Institute for Virology and Immunology who have coauthored the original literature on IL2-deficient mice from our group referenced here.

Note Added in Proof

The dependence of regulatory T-cells protecting from EAE on IL-2 was shown by Lafaille and colleagues *(65)*.

References

1. Ozaki, K. and Leonard, W. J. (2002) Cytokine and cytokine receptor pleiotropy and redundancy. *J. Biol. Chem.* **277,** 29355–29358.
2. Smith, K. A. (1988) Interleukin-2: inception, impact and implications. *Science* **240,** 1169–1176.

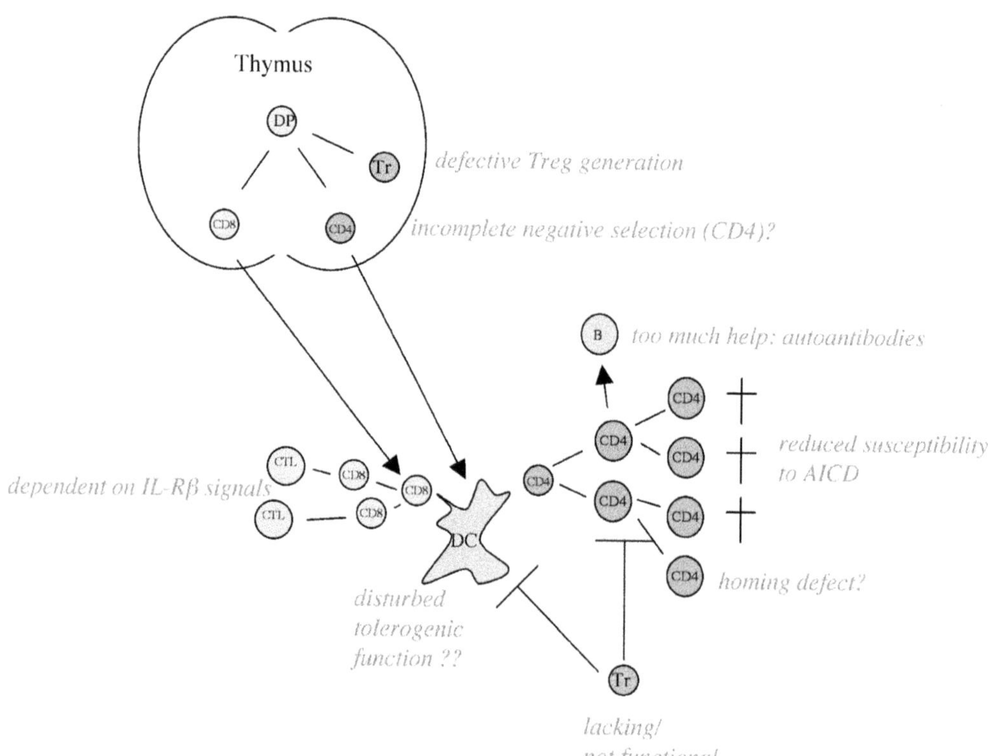

Fig. 1. Known and possible defects of the immune system in mice deficient in IL-2 signaling. In the thymus, defective generation of T*reg* cells appears to be of prime importance for the development of immunopathology. In addition, negative selection of CD4 cells may be incomplete at high antigen doses. Although a contribution of a defect in dendritic cell (DC) function is still hypothetical, both increased resistance to apoptosis and impaired T*reg* activity contribute to the hyperactivation and accumulation of CD4 T-cells, including autoreactive cells, which in turn provide help to B-cells making autoantibodies. The partial defect in the activation and maturation of CD8 T-cells can be overcome in interleukin (IL)-2 and IL-2Rα-deficient (but not IL-2Rβ-deficient) mice by endogenous IL-15 if infectious virus is used for immunization. AICD, activation-induced cell death.

3. Schorle, H., Holtschke, T., Hünig, T., Schimpl, A., and Horak, I. (1991) Development and function of T-cells in mice rendered interleukin-2 deficient by gene targeting. *Nature* **352,** 621–624.
4. Willerford, D. M., Chen, J., Ferry, J. A., Davidson, L., Ma, A., and Alt, F. W. (1995) Interleukin-2 receptor α chain regulates the size and content of the peripheral lymphoid compartment. *Immunity* **3,** 521–530.
5. Suzuki, H., Kündig, T. M., Furlonger, C., et al. (1995) Deregulated T cell activation and autoimmunity in mice lacking interleukin-2 receptor beta. *Science* **268,** 1472–1476.
6. Shevach, E. M. (2002) CD4+ CD25+ suppressor T cells: more questions than answers. *Nat. Rev. Immunol.* **2,** 389–400.
7. Maloy, K. J. and Powrie, F. (2001) Regulatory T cells in the control of immune pathology. *Nat. Immunol.* **2,** 816–822.
8. Hünig, T. and Schimpl, A. (1997) The IL-2 deficiency syndrome: a lethal disease caused by abnormal lymphocyte survival. In: Durum, S. and Muegge, K., eds. *Cytokine Knockouts*. Humana Press, Totowa, pp. 1–19.
9. Namen, A., Lupton, S., Hjerrild, K., et al. (1988) Stimulation of B-cell progenitors by cloned murine interleukin-7. *Nature* **333,** 571–573.

10. Watson, J. D., Morrissey, P. J., Namen, A. E., Conlon, P. J., and Widmer, M. B. (1989) Effect of IL-7 on the growth of fetal thymocytes in culture. *J. Immunol.* **143,** 1215–1222.
11. Rolink, A., Grawunder, U., Winler, T. H., Karasuyama, H., and Melchers, F. (1994) IL-2 receptor α chain expression defines a crucial stage in pre-B cell devlopment. *Int. Immunol.* **6,** 1257–1268.
12. Takacs, L., Osawa, H., and Diamantstein, T. (1984) Detection and localization by the monoclonal anti-interleukin 2 receptor antibody AMT-13 of IL-2 receptor-bearing cells in the developing thymus of the mouse embryo and in the thymus of cortisone treated mice. *Eur. J. Immunol.* **14,** 1152–1156.
13. Raulet, D. H. (1985) Expression and function of interleukin-2 receptors in immature thymocytes. *Nature (Lond.)* **314,** 101–103.
14. Ceredic, R., Lowenthal, J. W., Nabholtz, M., and MacDonald, H. R. (1985) Expression of Interleukin-2 receptors as a differentiation marker on intrathymic stem cells. *Nature* **314,** 98–100.
15. Tanaka, T., Takeuchi, Y., Shiohara, T., et al. (1992) In utero treatment with monoclonal antibody to IL-2 receptor beta-chain completely abrogates development of Thy-1+ dendritic epidermal cells. *Int. Immunol.* **4,** 487–491.
16. Takeuchi, Y., Tanaka, T., Hamamura, K., et al. (1992) Expression and role of interleukin-2 receptor β chain on CD4-8- T-cell receptor α/β + cells. *Eur. J. Immunol.* **22,** 2929–2935.
17. Hanke, T., Mitnacht, R., Boyd, R., and Hünig, T. (1994) Induction of interleukin-2 receptor β chain expression by self-recognition in the thymus. *J. Exp. Med.* **180,** 1629–1636.
18. Cao, X., Shores, W., Hu-Li, J., et al. (1995) Defective lympoid development in mice lacking expression of the common cytokine receptor γ chain. *Immunity* **2,** 223–238.
19. Di Santo, J. P., Müller, W., Guy-Grand, D., Fischer, A., and Rajewsky, K. (1995) Lymphoid development in mice with a targeted deletion of the interleukin-2 receptor γ chain. *Proc. Natl. Acad. Sci. USA* **92,** 377–381.
20. Schimpl, A., Hünig, T., Berberich, I., et al. (1992) Lymphocyte development and immunoreactivity in IL-2 deficient mice. In: Gergely, J., Benczur, M., and Erdei, A., eds. *Progress in Immunology VIII.* Springer-Verlag, Hungary, pp. 305–311.
21. Schimpl, A., Schorle, H., Hünig, T., Berberich, I., and Horak, I. (1992) Lymphocyte subsets and immunoreactivity in IL-2 deficient mice. In: Romangnani, S., Mosmann, T. R., and Abbas, A. K. eds. *New Advances on Cytokines.* Raven Press, New York, pp. 87–95.
22. Schimpl, A., Hünig, T., Elbe, A., et al. (1994) Development and function of the immune system in mice with targeted disruption of the interleukin 2 gene. In: Bluethmann, H. and Ohashi, P., eds. *Transgenesis and Targeted Mutagenesis in Immunology.* Academic, San Diego, pp. 191–201.
23. Sakaguchi, S., Sakaguchi, N., Asano, M., Itoh, M., and Toda, M. (1995) Immunologic self-tolerance maintained by activated T cells expressing IL-2 receptor alpha-chains (CD25). Breakdown of a single mechanism of self-tolerance causes various autoimmune diseases. *J. Immunol.* **155,** 1151–1164.
24. Papiernik, M., de Moraes, M. L., Pontoux, C., Vasseur, F., and Penit, C. (1998) Regulatory CD4 T cells: expression of IL-2R alpha chain, resistance to clonal deletion and IL-2 dependency. *Int. Immunol.* **10,** 371–378.
25. Thornton, A. M. and Shevach, E. M. (1998) CD4+CD25+ immunoregulatory T cells suppress polyclonal T cell activation in vitro by inhibiting interleukin 2 production. *J. Exp. Med.* **188,** 287–296.
26. Asano, M., Toda, M., Sakaguchi, N., and Sakaguchi, S. (1996) Autoimmune disease as a consequence of developmental abnormality of a T-cell subpopulation. *J. Exp. Med.* **184,** 387–396.
27. Seddon, B. and Mason, D. (2000) The third function of the thymus. *Immunol. Today* **21,** 95–99.
28. Taguchi, O., Kontani, K., Ikeda, H., Kezuka, T., Takeuchi, M., and Takahashi, T. (1994) Tissue-specific suppressor T-cells involved in self-tolerance are activated extrathymically by self-antigens. *Immunology* **82,** 365–369.
29. Malek, T. R., Porter, B. O., Codias, E. K., Scibelli, P., and Yu, A. (2000) Normal lymphoid homeostasis and lack of lethal autoimmunity in mice containing mature T cells with severely impaired IL-2 receptors. *J. Immunol.* **164,** 2905–2914.
30. Schimpl, A., Berberich, I., Kneitz, B., et al. (2002) IL-2 and autoimmune disease. *Cytokine Growth Factor Rev.* **13,** 369–378.
31. Krämer, S., Mamalaki, C., Schimpl, A., Horak, I., Kioussis, D., and Hünig, T. (1994) Thymic selection and peripheral activation of TCR-transgenic CD8 T-cells in IL-2 deficient mice: requirement for IL-2 is restricted to the induction of cytotoxic effector function. *Eur. J. Immunol.* **24,** 2317–2322.

32. Bassiri, H. and Carding, S. R. (2001) A requirement for IL-2/IL-2 receptor signaling in intrathymic negative selection. *J. Immunol.* **166,** 5945–5954.
33. Kishimoto, H., Surh, C. D., and Sprent, J. (1998) A role for Fas in negative selection of thymocytes in vivo. *J. Exp. Med.* **187,** 1427–1438.
34. Sadlack, B., Merz, H., Schorle, H., Schimpl, A., Feller, A. C., and Horak, I. (1993) Ulcerative colitis-like disease in mice with a disrupted interleukin-2 gene. *Cell* **75,** 253–261.
35. Kündig, T. M., Schorle, H., Bachmann, M. F., Hengartner, H., Zinkernagel, R. M., and Horak, I. (1993) Immune responses in interleukin-2 deficient mice. *Science* **262,** 1059–1061.
36. Ehrhardt, R. O., Ludviksson, B. R., Gray, B., Neurath, M., and Strober, W. (1997) Induction and prevention of colonic inflammation in IL-2-deficient mice. *J. Immunol.* **158,** 566–573.
37. Kneitz, B., Herrmann, T., Yonehara, S., and Schimpl, A. (1995) Normal clonal expansion but impaired Fas-mediated cell death and anergy induction in IL-2 deficient mice. *Eur. J. Immunol.* **25,** 2572–2577.
38. Kearney, E. R., Pape, K. A., Loh, D. Y., and Jenkins, M. K. (1994) Visualization of peptide-specific T cell immunity and peripheral tolerance induction in vivo. *Immunity* **1,** 327–339.
39. Wolf, M., Schimpl, A., and Hunig, T. (2001) Control of T cell hyperactivation in IL-2-deficient mice by CD4(+)CD25(–) and CD4(+)CD25(+) T cells: evidence for two distinct regulatory mechanisms. *Eur. J. Immunol.* **31,** 1637–1645.
40. Santner, B., Wagner, S., Wolf, M., Kneitz, B., Hünig, T., and Schimpl, A. (1998) In vitro skewing of TCR-transgenic T-cells from IL-2 dficient mice towards TH1 and TH2 in the absence of exogenous IL-2. *Eur. Cytok. Network* **9,** 17–25.
41. Le Gros, G., Ben-Sasson, S. Z., Seder, R., Finkelman, F. D., and Paul, W. E. (1990) Generation of interleukin 4 (IL-4)-producing cells in vivo and in vitro: IL-2 and IL-4 are required for in vitro generation of IL-4-producing cells. *J. Exp. Med.* **172,** 921–929.
42. Sprent, J. and Surh, C. D. (2001) Generation and maintenance of memory T cells. *Curr. Opin. Immunol.* **13,** 248–254.
43. Steiger, J., Nickerson, P. W., Steurer, W., Moscovitch-Lopatin, M., and Strom, T. B. (1995) IL-2 knockout recipient mice refect islet cell allografts. *J. Immunol.* **155,** 489–498.
44. Steiger, J., Nickerson, P. W., Steurer, W., Moscovitch Lopatin, M., and Strom, T. B. (1995) IL-2 knockout recipient mice reject islet cell allografts. *J. Immunol.* **155,** 489–498.
45. Schimpl, A. and Hünig, T. (1994) *Overexpression and Knockout of Cytokines in Transgenic Mice.* Academic, San Diego, pp. 31–45.
46. Sadlack, B., Löhler, J., Schorle, H., et al. (1995) Generalized autoimmune disease in interleukin-2 deficient mice is triggered by an uncontrolled activation and proliferation of CD4+ T cells. *Eur. J. Immunol.* **25,** 3053–3059.
47. Horak, I., Löhler, J., Ma, A., and Smith, K. A. (1995) Interleukin-2 deficient mice: a new model to study autoimmunity and self-tolerance. *Immunol. Rev.* **148,** 35–44.
48. Nemoto, T., Takeshita, T., Ishii, N., et al. (1995) Differences in the interleukin-2 (IL-2) receptor system in human and mouse: α chain is required for formation of the functional mouse IL-2 receptor. *Eur. J. Immunol.* **25,** 3001–3005.
49. Leonard, W., Shores, E. W., and Love, P. E. (1995) Role of the common cytokine receptor γ chain in cytokine signaling and lymphoid development. *Immunol. Rev.* **148,** 97–114.
50. Ma, A., Datta, M., Margosian, E., and Horak, I. (1995) T cells, but not B cells, are required for bowel inflammation in IL-2 deficient mice. *J. Exp. Med.* **182,** 1567–1572.
51. Krämer, S., Schimpl, A., and Hünig, T. (1995) Immunopathology of Interleukin (IL) 2-deficient mice: thymus dependence and suppression by thymus-dependent cells with an intact IL-2 gene. *J. Exp. Med.* **182,** 1769–1776.
52. Lenardo, M. J. (1991) Interleukin-2 programs mouse α/β T-lymphocytes for apoptosis. *Nature* **353,** 858–861.
53. Krammer, P. H. (2000) CD95's deadly mission in the immune system. *Nature* **407,** 789–795.
54. Refaeli, Y., Van Parijs, L., London, C. A., Tschopp, J., and Abbas, A. K. (1998) Biochemical mechanisms of IL-2-regulated Fas-mediated T cell apoptosis. *Immunity* **8,** 615–623.
55. Scaffidi, C., Fulda, S., Srinivasan, A., et al. (1998) Two CD95 (APO-1/Fas) signaling pathways. *EMBO J.* **17,** 1675–1687.

56. Suzuki, H., Zhou, Y. W., Kato, M., Mak, T. W., and Nakashima, I. (1999) Normal regulatory alpha/beta T cells effectively eliminate abnormally activated T cells lacking the interleukin 2 receptor beta in vivo. *J. Exp. Med.* **90,** 1561–1572.
56a. Almeida, A. R., Legrand, N., Papiernik, M., and Freitas, A. A. (2002) Homeostasis of peripheral CD4+ T cells: IL-2R alpha and IL-2 shape a population of regulatory cells that controls CD4+ T cell numbers. *J. Immunol.* **169,** 4850–4860.
57. Klebb, G., Autenrieth, I. B., Haber, H., et al. (1996) Interleukin-2 is indispensable for development of immunological self-tolerance. *Clin. Immunol. Immunopathol.* **81,** 282–286.
58. Plaetinck, G., Combe, M. C., Corthesy, P., et al. (1990) Control of IL-2 receptor-alpha expression by IL-1, tumor necrosis factor, and IL-2. Complex regulation via elements in the 5' flanking region. *J. Immunol.* **145,** 3340–3347.
59. Stephens, L. and Mason, D. (2000) CD25 is a marker for CD4+ thymocytes that prevent autoimmune diabetes in rats, but peripheral T cells with this function are found in both CD25+ and CD25- subpopulations. *J. Immunol.* **165,** 3105–3110.
60. Singh, B., Read, S., Asseman, C., et al. (2001) Control of intestinal inflammation by regulatory T cells. *Immunol. Rev.* **182,** 190–200.
61. Granucci, F., Vizzardelli, C., Pavelka, N., et al. (2001) Inducible IL-2 production by dendritic cells revealed by global gene expression analysis. *Nat. Immunol.* **2,** 882–888.
62. Lutz, M. B., Suri, R. M., Niimi, M., et al. (2000) Immature dendritic cells generated with low doses of GM-CSF in the absence of IL-4 are maturation resistant and prolong allograft survival in vivo. *Eur. J. Immunol.* **30,** 1813–1822.
63. Petitto, J. M., Streit, W. J., Huang, Z., Butfiloski, E., and Schiffenbauer, J. (2000) Interleukin-2 gene deletion produces a robust reduction in susceptibility to experimental autoimmune encephalomyelitis in C57BL/6 mice. *Neurosci. Lett.* **285,** 66–70.
64. Carlow, D. A., Corbel, S. Y., Williams, M. J., and Ziltener, H. J. (2001) IL-2, -4, and -15 differentially regulate O-glycan branching and P-selectin ligand formation in activated CD8 T cells. *J. Immunol.* **167,** 6841–6848.
65. Furtado, G. C., Curotto de Lafaille, M. A., Kutchukhidze, N., and Lafaille, J. J. (2002) Interleukin 2 signaling is required for CD4(+) regulatory T cell function. *J. Exp. Med.* **196,** 851–857.

9

Molecular Basis for Binding Multiple Cytokines by γc

Implications for X-SCID and Impaired γc-Dependent Cytokine Receptor Function

Ferenc Olosz and Thomas R. Malek

Summary

Mutations in γc, a shared receptor subunit for interleukin (IL)-2, IL-4, IL-7, IL-9, IL-15, and IL-21, lead to profound impairment in T-cell and natural killer (NK) cell development and are responsible for X-linked severe combined immunodeficiency disease (X-SCID). Considerable attention has been paid to how the lack of γc expression and signaling results in failed lymphocyte development. However, γc is also an essential ligand binding subunit for γc-dependent cytokine receptors. Molecular modeling in conjunction with site-directed mutagenesis of γc indicates that a common mechanism is responsible for the ability of γc to bind multiple cytokines. This notion is related to instances in which mutations in the extracytoplasmic region of γc resulted in X-SCID.

Key words

IL-2 receptor, IL-4 receptor, IL-7 receptor, IL-15 receptor, molecular modeling, common gamma chain, X-linked severe combined immunodeficiency disease, site-directed mutagenesis, lymphocyte development

1. Introduction

The common cytokine receptor γ-chain (γc) is a well-known example of a shared receptor subunit. First identified as a membrane glycoprotein necessary for high-affinity interleukin-2 (IL-2) binding *(1)*, γc is now known to be part of the oligomeric receptors (R) for IL-2, IL-4, IL-7, IL-9, IL-15, and IL-21*(2–9)*. This group of four helix-bundled cytokines has been extensively studied for their critical involvement in the regulation of the immune system, especially in the development and function of T-cells, B-cells, and natural killer (NK) cells.

γc is absolutely required for mediating the activities of these cytokines. If γc is absent or functionally impaired, T-lymphocyte development is blocked at an early stage, NK cells are missing, and B-cells are either blocked in development in γc-deficient mice or nonfunctional in humans with an inherited γc defect. Genetic mutations of the human γc gene on chromosome Xq13 have been identified as the leading cause of a lethal syndrome known as X-linked severe combined immunodeficiency disease (X-SCID) *(10,11)*.

From: *Contemporary Immunology: Cytokine Knockouts, 2nd Edition*
Edited by: Giamila Fantuzzi © Humana Press Inc., Totowa, NJ

The biologic function of γc is mainly dependent on its cytoplasmic tail, which participates directly in the initiation of signaling *(12,13)*. However, no signaling can occur without extracellular events, i.e., capture of the cytokines by interleukin-specific subunits and subsequent ligand-induced recruitment of γc into the oligomeric receptor complex. γc recruitment often leads to enhanced ligand binding affinity by the receptor and involves direct molecular interactions between the extracellular domain of γc with both cytokines and other receptor subunits.Therefore, this review focuses primarily on the molecular basis by which γc contributes to ligand binding and how such defects might relate to X-SCID.

2. The Role of γc in Ligand Binding

2.1. Structure of γc

γc was initially discovered as a subunit of IL-2R (reviewed in refs. *14* and *15*). Its existence was first postulated because co-expression of IL-2Rα and -β in fibroblasts was insufficient to reconstitute a functional complex with full binding and signaling capability. In 1992, the human IL-2R γ-chain was co-immunoprecipitated with IL-2Rβ from extracts of a lymphoid cell line expressing intermediate-affinity IL-2R *(1)*. The new protein, about 64 kDa in size, was isolated by two-dimensional polyacrylamide gel electrophoresis. Based on its N-terminal amino acid sequence, primers were designed for the subsequent cloning of the γc cDNA. Mouse γc was cloned 1 year later, using the human sequence as a probe *(16)*. Canine *(17)* and bovine *(18)* are two additional mammalian γc genes that have been cloned (Fig. 1). A putative γc sequence from rainbow trout has also been reported *(19)*, exhibiting striking similarities to its mammalian counterparts (Fig. 1). Interestingly, two translated expressed sequence tag (EST) sequences from chicken (Genbank accessions BG713313 and BG713418) also show high similarity to the extracellular region of γc (Fig. 1). These conserved regions are probably important for the structural features of γc and, as discussed below, include amino acids important for ligand binding.

The human γc cDNA encodes 369 amino acids, including a signal peptide (22 amino acids), followed by the mature γc sequence (347 amino acids). Mature γc is a type I membrane glycoprotein that has a 232-amino acid extracellular region, a 29-amino acid single transmembrane domain, and an 86-amino acid cytoplasmic tail (Fig. 2). The calculated molecular weight of this protein is about 40,000, which is increased to 64 kDa owing to glycosylation. The extracellular domain of human γc contains six predicted sites for N-glycosylation. The mouse γc amino acid sequence is approximately 70% identical to human γc (Fig. 1). Characterization of mouse γc indicates that its mature protein has a higher molecular weight (75–80 kDa) owing to heavy N-linked glycosylation *(20)*.

The primary structure of γc shows significant homology to other receptors involved in the binding of four-helix bundled cytokines. The γc extracellular region contains typical sequence elements of the type I cytokine receptor superfamily, including four highly conserved Cys residues in the N-terminal domain and a membrane-proximal WSXWS motif (Fig. 2). The human γc gene spans about 4.2 kb on the X chromosome (region Xq13) and is composed of eight exons and seven introns *(21)*. The 5'-untranslated region (UTR) and the signal peptide are encoded by exon 1, the extracellular domain by exons 1–5, the transmembrane domain by exon 6, and the cytoplasmic tail by exons 7 and 8. Exon 8 also contains sequences of the 3'-UTR.

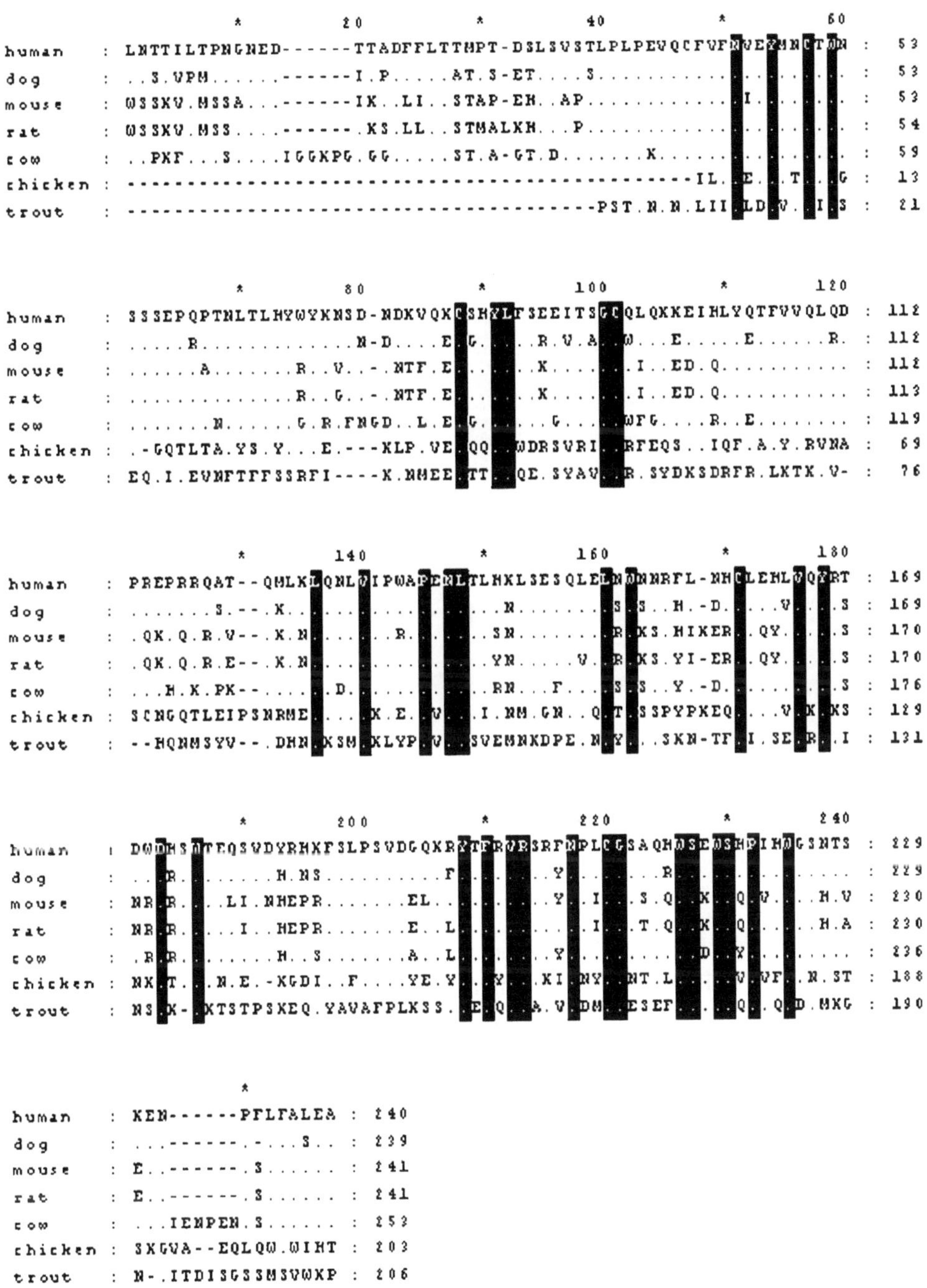

Fig. 1. Protein sequence alignment of known γc extracellular sequences. Residues conserved in all sequences are highlighted.

2.2. γc-Dependent Cytokine Interactions

Although γc does not appreciably bind cytokines by itself, kinetic studies have shown that the recruitment of γc to receptor complexes contributes to augmented ligand binding affinity *(22)*. For example, upon addition of γc to IL-2Rαβ, the IL-2 binding affinity increases

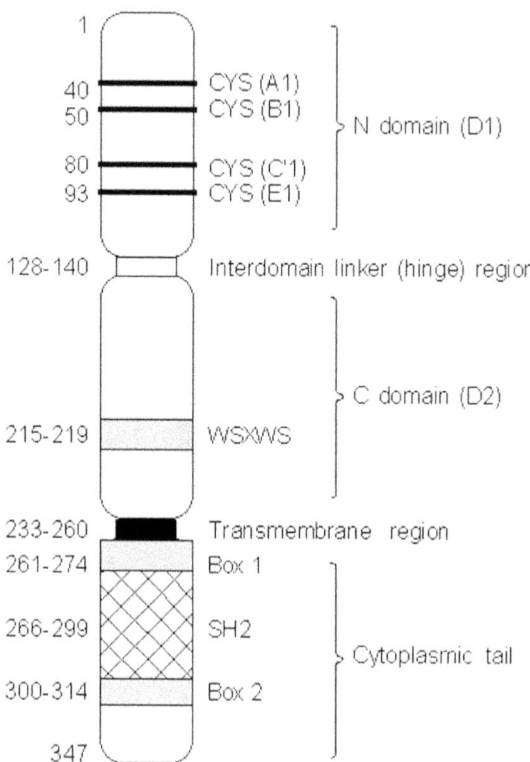

Fig. 2. Conserved structural properties of γc. Sequence features characteristic of the type I cytokine receptor superfamily are highlighted. Residue numbers are based on the mature γc sequence.

at least 10-fold (K_d-10^{-11} M), owing to both faster association and decreased dissociation rates of the cytokine. Dimerization of human IL-2Rβ/γc results in an even higher increase, from barely detectable IL-2 or IL-15 binding by individual IL-2Rβ and γc subunits to intermediate-affinity binding (K_d-10^{-9} M) by the dimeric complex. Similar, but more modest effects, have also been observed with IL-4 and IL-7 (threefold and fivefold increase, respectively) *(2–5)*. In contrast, γc does not appear to enhance the binding of IL-9 significantly *(6)*.

Based on the distinct binding properties of individual receptor subunits and the inability of γc to bind cytokines directly, it has been hypothesized that ligand binding involves a sequential mechanism *(23,24)*. In this model, the cytokine is first captured by private subunits with some intrinsic binding affinity (e.g., IL-2Rα, IL-15Rα, IL-2Rβ, IL-4Rα, or IL-7Rα), concentrating the ligand on the cell surface. The cytokine is then delivered to other subunits that are recruited into the receptor complex in a ligand-dependent fashion.

The recruitment of γc into the cytokine receptors and its effects on ligand binding are thought to involve direct physical interactions of γc with the ligands and/or the other receptor subunits. Such interactions have been strongly suggested by biochemical studies in which γc was co-immunoprecipitated with either the cytokines or other receptor subunits using anti-cytokine or anti-receptor antibodies. For example, human γc was first isolated by co-precipitation with IL-2Rβ using anti-IL-2Rβ monoclonal antibody (MAb), without the need for chemical crosslinking agents *(1)*. A direct interaction between IL-2 and γc

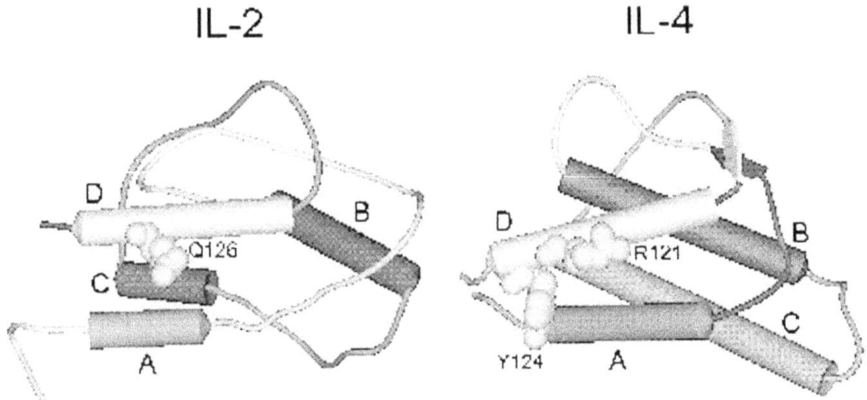

Fig. 3. Schematic diagram of interleukin (IL)-2 and IL-4 showing α-helices and potential γc-contacting residues.

and formation of a stable IL-2/IL-2Rβ/γc complex has also been demonstrated by co-immunoprecipitation experiments *(25)*. All three subunits of the mouse IL-2R have been crosslinked to radiolabeled IL-2 that was co-precipitated by the anti-IL-2Rα MAb 7D4 *(26)*. Radiolabeled IL-4, IL-7, IL-9, IL-15, and IL-21 have been co-immunoprecipitated with γc from cells expressing γc and IL-4Rα, IL-7Rα, IL-9Rα, IL-2Rβ, or IL-21Rα, respectively *(2–6,9,27,28)*.

The interactions of IL-2 and IL-4 with their receptors have been studied extensively by mutagenesis. A model of IL-2 and IL-4 highlighting γc contact residues is shown in Fig. 3. A comprehensive survey of 1090 mutations of mouse IL-2 has revealed several potential contact residues involved in binding to the IL-2Rα, β, and γc subunits *(29)*. Although several residues in the AB overhand loop were required for binding to the IL-2Rα chain, only three residues in the A and C helices were necessary for binding to IL-2Rβ, and only one residue in the D helix (Q141) was critical for interaction of mouse IL-2 with γc. A critical role of residues 119–141 of the D helix of mouse IL-2 has also been demonstrated by deletion analysis *(30)*. The D helix of human IL-2 has also been mutated, and the equivalent Q126D mutation was shown to inhibit specifically high-affinity binding and growth signaling mediated by γc, whereas interactions with IL-2Rα and -β remained unaffected *(31)*. A similar mutation, Q108S, was also identified in the putative D helix of IL-15 *(32)*.

In the IL-4 molecule, three residues of the D helix, R121, Y124, and S125 have been found to be important for interactions of this cytokine with γc and/or the IL-13Rα chain (Fig. 3) *(33–35)*. Substitution of Y124 to aspartate, but not to Phe or His, strongly inhibited IL-4 bioactivity and reduced the affinity of ligand binding to the IL-4Rα/γc complex *(34)*. However, in contrast to the weak antagonistic properties of mutant Q126D of IL-2, the Y124D mutant of IL-4 strongly inhibited IL-4 bioactivity in competitive proliferation assays *(34)*. A recent mutagenesis study of human IL-4 suggested that residues of the A helix (I11, N15) may also contribute to IL-4 interactions with γc *(23)*. It has been proposed that the γc binding site of IL-4 is largely hydrophobic, since substitution of R121, Y124, or S125 with large hydrophobic amino acids had minimal effect on IL-4 function *(23)*. In contrast, the IL-4:IL-4Rα interface involves mostly polar interactions surrounding residues E9 of the A helix, and R88 of the C helix of IL-4 *(36,37)*.

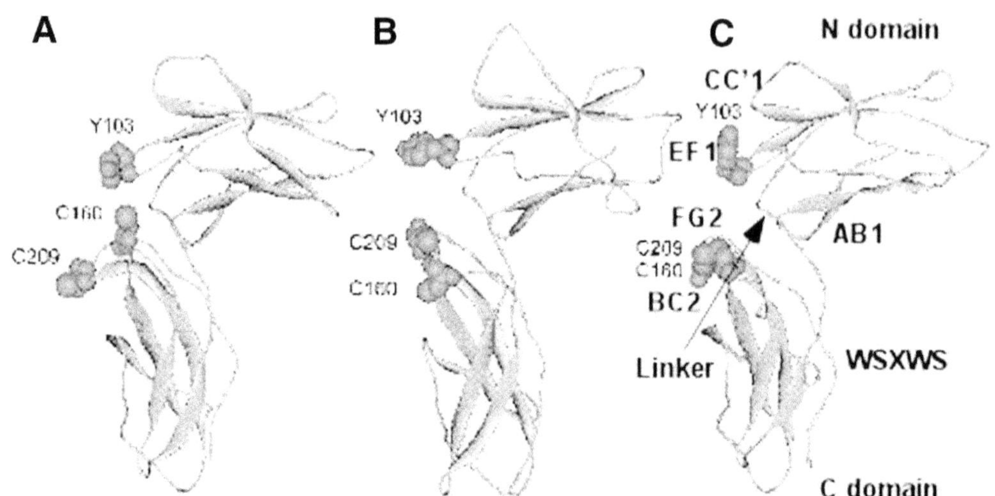

Fig. 4. Comparison between theoretical models of the human γc. Shown are models of γc by Bamborough et al. *(56)* (**A**), Gustchina et al. *(53)* (**B**), and Kroemer and Richards *(57)* (**C**). Highlighted residues in all models illustrate similar predictions for Tyr103 in the N domain, and distinct predictions for Cys160 and Cys209 in the C domain. Ligand binding loops, the linker region, and the WSXWS motif are depicted in (**C**).

Recently, the D helix of IL-7 has also been implicated in γc-dependent signaling. A homology model-based mutagenesis study of IL-7 demonstrated that the mutation W143D strongly inhibited IL-7 bioactivity, and this mutant acted as an antagonist of the wild-type cytokine in competition assays *(38)*. Other D-helix mutations that partially inhibited IL-7 function included K121A, L136A, and K140A.

2.3. Properties of Antagonistic MAbs to γc

The development of antagonistic MAbs that specifically inhibit γc-dependent activities of various cytokines and mapping their epitopes has also provided valuable insights into the structure and function of γc. Two rat anti-mouse γc MAbs, TUGm2 and TUGm3, have been extensively used in the study of γc-containing receptors *(2,6,39)*. TUGm2 has strong antagonistic properties on IL-4 and IL-7 bioactivity and inhibits the binding of all known γc-dependent cytokines. Cytokines bound to γc cannot be co-precipitated by TUGm2. In contrast, TUGm3 does not appear to interfere with receptor-ligand interactions and was used to precipitate radiolabeled cytokines crosslinked to γc. Alanine scanning mutagenesis of the γc ectodomain resulted in identification of a discontinuous TUGm2 epitope involving residues 158–162 of the BC2 loop and 210–211 of the FG2 loop *(40)*. The location of these loops in a structural model of γc is shown in Fig. 4C. Within this epitope, K158, E159, and R160 are the likely antigenic determinants, as these residues are not conserved, and their mutations strongly and selectively inhibited the binding of TUGm2 to the γc. As discussed below, it is likely that the TUGm2 site partially overlaps the cytokine binding region of γc. Thus, this MAb directly blocks the access of cytokines to the surface of γc.

A novel anti-human γc MAb (PC.B8) has been described that inhibits IL-2, IL-4, and IL-15 bioactivity *(41)*. Using alanine scanning mutagenesis of the human γc, the epitope of PC.B8 has been mapped to five discontinuous segments of the γc: the AB1, EF1, BC2,

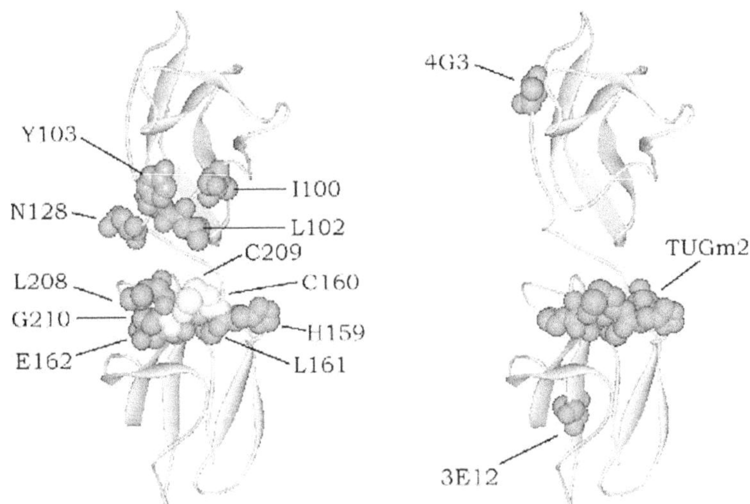

Fig. 5. Model of γc highlighting amino acid side chains important for ligand binding (left) or contributing to MAb epitopes (right).

and FG2 loops, and the linker region *(41)*. These data indirectly suggest that one or more of these regions may be involved in γc-cytokine interactions. The PC.B8 antibody was also used in combination with surface plasmon resonance (SPR) analysis of ligand binding to study the mechanism of intermediate-affinity IL-2 binding *(24)*. The results of this study provided evidence that ligand binding to the IL-2Rβγc dimer occurs as a two-step process involving capture of the cytokine by IL-2Rβ, followed by association of γc with the IL-2Rβ:IL-2 complex. PC.B8 interferes with the latter step of the oligomerization process by preventing recruitment of γc.

4G3 and 3E12 are two rat MAbs prepared in our laboratory that recognize separate epitopes of the mouse γc extracellular domain and have distinct properties *(42)*. 4G3 strongly inhibits the bioactivities of IL-7, IL-9, and IL-15, with weaker effects on IL-2 and IL-4 function *(43)*. Nevertheless, the binding of IL-2 and IL-4 is inhibited by 4G3 in radioligand binding assays *(42)*. Importantly, 4G3 cannot precipitate receptor-ligand complexes containing IL-2 or IL-7, suggesting that recognition of γc by 4G3 is blocked by the presence of these cytokines. In contrast, 4G3 is able to bind γc in the presence of IL-4 and can be used to precipitate IL-4:γc complexes. The 4G3 epitope was localized to the vicinity of residue V121 in the E1 strand of the N domain because the V121E mutation abrogated 4G3 binding *(44)*.

The 3E12 antibody selectively inhibits the bioactivity of IL-4, IL-9, and IL-15 and interferes with the binding of IL-4 and IL-7 but not IL-2 *(42,43)*. 3E12 co-precipitates IL-2, IL-4, and IL-7 crosslinked to the γc, and therefore it does not appear to block directly the interactions of the cytokines with the γc. Epitope mapping studies indicated that the 3E12 epitope of γc is located near R197 within the membrane proximal region of the C domain *(44)*. Therefore, 3E12 most probably inhibits cytokine bioactivity by interfering with receptor-receptor interactions. The location of the TUGm2, 4G3, and 3E12 epitopes in the context of a structural model of mouse γc is shown in Fig. 5.

2.4. Participation of γc in Receptor-Receptor Interactions

Owing to the complex nature of the cytokine receptors, very little is known about the interactions between receptor subunits. Crystal structures of the growth hormone (GH), erythropoietin (EPO), and prolactin (PRL) receptors *(45–47)* suggested that such interactions are established through membrane-proximal regions of the C domain. In at least two reports, kinetic measurements of ligand binding were used to estimate indirectly the strength of intersubunit interactions within the IL-4R complex *(23,48)*. These studies suggested that interactions between the IL-4Rα and γc chains are weak and do not contribute significantly to overall binding. Attempts have also been made to establish whether cytokine receptor subunits can preassociate on the cell surface in the absence of ligand binding. One study using fluorescence resonance energy transfer (FRET) measurements suggested that the IL-2Rα, -β, and γc subunits are not randomly distributed on the cell surface but are clustered in close proximity to each other *(49)*. However, the issue of receptor preassembly remains controversial and has not been clearly confirmed by other means.

Nevertheless, at least some receptors in this superfamily may preassociate in the absence of cytokines. It has been shown that unliganded EPO receptors can be crystallized as dimers, associated in a nonsignaling orientation *(50)*. An activation mechanism has been proposed in which the binding of the cytokine induces conformational changes in the preassociated receptor subunits that subsequently allow the dimerization of the cytoplasmic signaling domains *(51)*. Whether such a mechanism plays any role in the function of γc-containing receptors remains to be determined.

3. Molecular Basis for Cytokine Binding by γc

3.1. Homology Modeling of γc-Dependent Cytokine Receptors

Although the exact three-dimensional organization of γc is not known, many of its molecular features can be deduced from its sequence, based on homology to other members of the type I cytokine receptor superfamily. For example, analysis of the γc sequence allows predictions of the general folding pattern of γc, its domain organization, potential glycosylation sites, secondary structure, and even solvent accessibility of its residues. Although such predictions are useful, they are insufficient to explain adequately the molecular interactions of γc within heteromeric cytokine receptor complexes. However, a major turning point was reached when the first crystal structure of a type I cytokine receptor was published *(46)*. This structure showed the extracellular portions of a 2:1 GHR:GH complex, in which two identical GHR subunits contacted opposite surfaces of the same GH molecule and also interacted with each other through their membrane-proximal domains. This molecular organization was subsequently used as a paradigm for the homology modeling of a number of type I cytokine receptors that were either homodimers (EPOR) *(52)* or hetero-oligomers (receptors for granulocyte/macrophage colony-stimulating factor (GM-CSF), IL-2, IL-3, IL-4, and IL-7) *(53–57)*. Homology modeling followed by site-directed mutagenesis has been successfully used to identify potential ligand binding regions of GM-CSF *(54,58)* and gp130 *(59)*, confirming the credibility of this approach for the study of type I cytokine receptors.

Several attempts have been made to predict the structure of γc-containing complexes, including the high-affinity IL-2R *(56)*, IL-4R *(53,56)*, and IL-7R *(57)*. These studies used GHR as a template for the folding of IL-2Rβ, IL-4Rα, and IL-7Rα extracellular domains and incorporated known crystal structures of the helical cytokines IL-2 *(60)* and IL-4 *(61,62)*. For IL-7, a previously published theoretical structure was used *(63)*, whereas IL-2Rα was modeled from complement factor H *(64,65)*. The receptor subunits and the cytokines were assembled using the GHR:GH complex as the template *(46)*, and the models were optimized using energy minimization procedures. All models were refined to fit general structural quality criteria for proteins, such as correct bond lengths and angles, compactness, lack of large holes, no collisions between atoms, and few unfavorable side-chain interactions.

As expected, the models of γc, IL-2Rβ, IL-4Rα, and IL-7Rα share numerous features with the GHR structure. A model for γc is shown in Fig. 4C. Each receptor extracellular region is predicted to contain two domains that are similar in size, shape, and folding topology. These domains form an angle of approximately 90° with each other, exposing six loops (AB1, CC'1, EF1, BC2, FG2, and C'E2) and part of the interdomain linker toward the predicted ligand binding interface. Other loops point away from the ligand (BC1, C'E1, FG1) or are directed towards the plasma membrane (AB2, CC'2, EF2). Receptor-receptor contacts are predicted to involve most likely the AB2 and C'E2 loops, and the E2 strand. The highly conserved Cys residues in the N domains of γc, IL-2Rβ, and IL-4Rα occupy positions equivalent to similar cysteines in the GHR and are predicted to form disulfide bonds between the A1 and B1, and the C'1 and E1 strands, respectively. A slightly different pattern has been proposed for the N domain of IL-7Rα, in which only the A1-B1 disulfide bridge is conserved, but the C'1-E1 connection is replaced by another cysteine bond between strands C1 and C'1 *(57)*. The predicted C domains of γc, IL-2Rβ, IL-4Rα, and IL-7Rα also show similarities to each other and to the GHR, especially in their core structure and regions surrounding the WSXWS motif. This motif corresponds to a YGEFS sequence in the membrane-proximal domain of GHR, which does not participate directly in ligand binding but may be important for maintaining the structure of the FG2 loop and/or the rigidity of the whole receptor through highly conserved interactions with charged residues of the F2 strand.

The models have been used to predict a number of potential contact residues involved in receptor-ligand or receptor-receptor interactions. A view of three models of γc is shown in Fig. 4. Whereas IL-2Rβ, IL-4Rα, and IL-7Rα are thought to interact with the A and C helices of the cytokines, the γc chain is proposed to bind primarily to residues in the cytokine D helix (Fig. 3). At least five regions of the γc ectodomain have been implicated in these interactions: the AB1, EF1, BC2, and FG2 loops and the linker segment (Fig. 4C).

Although different predictions have been made regarding the sets of contact residues involved in the binding of IL-2, IL-4, and IL-7, respectively, the models suggest that all three cytokines interact with the same general region of γc. This putative ligand binding interface is located at neighboring regions of both the N and C domains that surround Y103 of the EF1 loop. All available γc models predicted that Y103 functions as a contact residue for IL-2, IL-4, and IL-7 *(53,56,57)* (Fig. 4).

The BC2 and FG2 loops in the membrane-proximal domain of γc are also likely to participate in cytokine binding. However, the modeling predictions in this region diverge significantly, owing to the usage of different γc-GHR sequence alignments for the construction of various models. These differences are most apparent when the predicted positions of Cys160 (BC2 loop) and C209 (FG2 loop) of the human γc are compared (Fig. 4). In the models of Bamborough et al. *(56)* (Fig. 4A) and Gustchina et al. *(53)* (Fig. 4B), the

BC2 and FG2 loops point in opposite directions, separating the two cysteines from each other. In contrast, in the model of Kroemer et al. *(57)* (Fig. 4C), the conformation of the BC2 and FG2 loops brings C160 and C209 in close proximity to each other, allowing formation of a putative disulfide bond between them.

The theoretical structures are consistent with the notion that potential N-glycosylation of either the receptors or the cytokines does not interfere with receptor assembly *(56)*. Also, several predictions of the IL-2R model are in good agreement with mutagenesis data regarding the interactions of IL-2 with IL-2Rα and IL-2Rβ *(29,56,66)*. The models are also consistent with the role of the cytokine D helix in interactions with the γc chain, and with epitope-mapping studies suggesting the involvement of the AB1, EF1, linker, BC2, and FG2 regions in ligand binding to the γc *(40,41)*. Several contacts at the IL-4Rα:IL-4 interface have also been correctly predicted by modeling of the IL-4R *(36,37,53,56)*. However, comparison of the IL-4R models with a recently determined crystal structure of the IL-4Rα:IL-4 complex *(36)* also highlights the limitations of modeling. Whereas the theoretical models were reasonably accurate in the core structure of IL-4Rα, errors in the loop regions were much higher. In the case of cytokine receptors, for which the ligand binding interface is formed by a combination of several loops, such errors may have a particularly strong influence on the accuracy of predictions.

3.2. Site-Directed Mutagenesis of γc to Identify Potential Ligand Contact Site

We *(40,44)* and Zhang et al. *(67)* have experimentally tested the importance of individual residues of γc for cytokine binding by site-directed mutagenesis of mouse and human γc, respectively. Our work *(40,44)* investigated γc-dependent binding using transfected cells that expressed heterodimeric cytokine receptors to IL-2, IL-4, IL-7, and IL-15. Zhang et al. *(67)* directly examined the binding of IL-4 to purified wild-type and mutant γc by BIAcore analysis. Generally similar results were obtained from both type of analysis.

A model of key ligand binding sites and antagonistic MAb epitopes of γc in the context of a heterodimeric IL-7/IL-7R complex is shown in Fig. 5. As predicted by the structural models, the first 34 residues of γc are not required for cytokine binding. This region shows no homology to other members of the type I cytokine receptor superfamily and has the least similarity in amino acid sequences when the extracellular domains of γc are compared between mammalian species (Fig. 1). Also, as predicted by the models, Y103 is necessary for the binding of IL-2, IL-4, IL-7, and IL-15. Our cell-based binding assays revealed that mutation of Y103 to alanine or arginine resulted in a partial inhibition of binding by all four cytokines. Although we did not detect a role for neighboring I100 or L102 in binding IL-2 or IL-7, mutation of these residues to alanine in human γc resulted in impaired binding of IL-4 by BIAcore analysis. We believe that these difference simply reflect that the BIAcore assay is more sensitive, although we can not rule out that I100 and L102 might uniquely contribute to IL-4 binding. Substitutions of Y103 did not impair the binding of MAbs to mouse γc, indicating that mutation of Y103 did not obviously affect the folding of γc. Based on these results and the fact that Y103 of γc is homologous to known receptor-ligand contact sites in the GHR *(68)* and EPOR *(69)*, it is highly likely that this residue of mouse and human γc is directly involved in receptor-ligand interactions with IL-2, IL-4, IL-7, and IL-15.

A second region of γc that appears to function directly is the γc-dependent cytokine binding that surrounds amino acid N128 in the linker region *(44,67)*. This area of γc seems to display more variability in its specific contribution in binding individual γc-dependent cytokines, presumably to accommodate distinctive features of each cytokine. Our work established the importance of this area based on its proximity to the 4G3 anti-γc epitope. We found that the N128A mutation of mouse γc partially reduced IL-7 binding while minimally affecting IL-2 or IL-15 binding. Importantly, γc containing a double mutation at Y103 and N128 substantially inhibited γc-dependent IL-2, IL-7, and IL-15 binding, implicating N128 in binding these three cytokines. N128A did not obviously affect the binding of IL-4 when it was directly examined for cell surface IL-4R. However, a modest decrease in binding was observed for IL-4 binding to the N128A mutant of human γc by BIAcore analysis *(67)*. Therefore, this or surrounding residues may also provide a contribution to IL-4/γc interaction.

A third region of γc that contributes to binding IL-2, IL-4, IL-7, and IL-15 encompasses amino acids C161, C210, and G211 of mouse γc or C160, C209, or G210 of human γc *(40,44,67)*. (The numbering of amino acids for mature human and mouse γc differs by one after position 158 owing to a single amino acid insertion, i.e., lysine, into mouse γc.) When mouse C161 and C210 were mutated to serine, these γc molecules were unable to support IL-2 or IL-7 γc-dependent cytokine binding *(40)*. This result suggests that C161 and C210 may form a disulfide bond connecting the BC2 and FG2 loops of the C domain. When L208, which neighbors C209 of human γc, was mutated to alanine, direct binding of IL-4 to γc was greatly impaired *(67)*. These data, in conjunction with the mutagenesis of IL-4 *(33–35,67)*, support a model in which L209 in conjunction with I100, L102, and Y103 of γc forms a hydrophobic interface to interact with the Y124 of IL-4.

With respect to anti-γc epitoping mapping, comparison of the rat and mouse γc sequences confirmed the location of the TUGm2 epitope identified earlier, which is centered around a unique lysine residue of the mouse γc sequence at position 158. The predicted positions of the putative 4G3, 3E12, and TUGm2 epitopes are in distinct regions of the mouse γc ectodomain (Fig. 5), consistent with biochemical data that these MAbs do not block each other's binding. The 4G3 site is proximal to Y103 and N128, and the TUGm2 epitope is likely to overlap partially the ligand binding site of γc at residues C161, C210, and G211. Epitope mapping studies of the antagonistic PC.B8 MAb that reacts with a discontinuous site on human γc are also consistent with a role for this region of γc in cytokine binding *(41)*. Based on the locations of the epitopes and the inhibitory properties of the MAbs *(2,5, 6,42,70)*, it is highly likely that 4G3, TUG2, and PC.B8 antagonize γc-dependent cytokines by directly interfering with their access to the ligand binding region of γc.

3.3. *Implications for γc Structural Models*

The data presented here partially confirm the predictions of several homology modeling studies of the human γc *(53,56,63,71)*. All models predicted that Y103 may function as a contact residue and that the ligand binding region of γc includes amino acids contributed by the EF1, BC2, and FG2 loops, as well as the linker region. Overall, the theoretical model of γc proposed by Kroemer et al. *(63)* appears to be best supported by the mutagenesis and epitope mapping data, as it has predicted the participation of Y103 and the involvement of linker residues in IL-7 binding, as well as the possibility of disulfide bond formation in the C domain of γc. Additionally, all seven residues found to be critical for the binding of TUGm2 were confined to a small area on the surface of γc, constituting a putative epitope. In contrast, in other models *(53,56)* the TUGm2 epitope is divided into two different surface regions on γc, separated by residues whose mutations did not affect TUGm2 binding. Interestingly, the IL-4R model proposed by Gustchina et al. *(53)* also had some predictions confirmed regarding the contributions of Y103, N128, and backbone atoms of C160 to the putative ligand binding interface. However, this model does not readily explain the inhibitory effects of mouse γc mutations at C210 and G211 on either cytokine binding or the TUGm2 epitope. The same is true for models proposed by Bamborough et al. *(56)*, which seem to be least confirmed by site-directed mutagenesis of γc.

4. X-SCID and Extracytoplasmic Mutations in γc

4.1. X-Linked SCID and the Role of γc in T, B, and NK Cell Development

Severe combined immunodeficiency (SCID) is the most severe form of primary immune diseases in humans, characterized by profound defects in T- and B-cell-mediated immunity. The consequences of SCID are lethal if not reversed by successful bone marrow transplantation. In the future, gene therapy may also serve as a viable treatment for this disease *(72)*. Affected children appear initially healthy owing to the protective effect of maternal antibodies, but within 6 months of age they become ill with severe recurring bacterial or viral infections and die within their first year of life *(14)*.

Human SCID occurs in approximately 1/80,000 live births and can be caused by numerous genetic mutations (reviewed in ref. *73*). X-linked severe combined immunodeficiency (X-SCID) is the most common form of SCID, accounting for approximately 50% of SCID cases. The genetic defect causing X-SCID was initially mapped to the SCIDX1 locus on the X chromosome, between the regions Xq11 and Xq13. Subsequently, the human γc (IL2RG) gene was cloned and localized to the Xq13 region, and mutations of the γc gene have been established as the primary cause of X-SCID *(10,11)*. A large number of such mutations have been identified and will be discussed in more detail below.

SCID patients are characterized by a block in T-cell development, whereas the B-cell and NK cell compartments are variably affected. Accordingly, the SCID phenotypes can be divided into four groups: T–B–NK–, T–B–NK+, T–B+NK–, and T–B+NK+ *(74)*. Typical human X-SCID is T–B+NK–, characterized by greatly reduced T-cell numbers, absence of NK cells, and normal or even increased number of B-cells. However, B-cell function is defective, partly because of the absence of T-cell help and partly because of intrinsic defects caused by the mutation of the γc gene. The latter notion is supported by nonrandom X chromosome inactivation in surface IgM– mature B-cells, but not in immature B-cells of X-SCID carrier females, indicating a possible requirement for γc during terminal B-cell differentiation *(75)*.

Typical T–B+NK–X-SCID results from severe dysfunction of γc-mediated ligand binding and/or signal transduction. However, atypical cases of X-SCID have also been reported, in which patients exhibited normal numbers of nonfunctional peripheral T-cells *(76,77)* or had reduced numbers of T-lymphocytes but normal numbers of NK cells *(78)*. It is likely that in such cases the mutant γc chains have retained some of their signaling function.

Symptoms similar to those of X-SCID can arise not only from mutations of the γc gene but also from genetic defects of downstream signaling molecules associated with γc. One molecule that is critical for γc-dependent signal transduction is the JAK3 tyrosine kinase. JAK3 physically associates with the cytoplasmic tail of γc and is activated upon γc stimulation by cytokines. Mutations of the human JAK3 gene has been shown to cause an autosomal form of T–B+NK–SCID that is clinically and immunologically indistinguishable from X-SCID *(79)*. Animal studies have also confirmed the close similarity between γc-deficient *(80,81)* and JAK3-deficient mice *(82–84)*.

Mice with targeted disruption of cytokine or cytokine receptor genes have also been useful for establishing the in vivo contributions of different γc-dependent cytokines to lymphoid development and their role in the etiology of X-SCID. As in humans, γc deficiency in mice results in impaired T-cell and NK cell development *(80,81,84)*. However, the T-cell defect is less severe in mice, and both CD4+ and CD8+ T-cells can be readily detected in the periphery. T-cell numbers and splenic cellularity tend to increase with age, and many of the peripheral CD4+ cells have a characteristic activated or memory cell phenotype. T-cell receptor (TCR)γδ T-cells and intraepithelial lymphocytes are not detected in γc-deficient mice. However, in contrast, human X-SCID in which normal B-cell production is observed, γc-deficient mice have significantly reduced numbers of conventional B-cells owing to a developmental block at the pre-B-cell stage in the bone marrow. Similar observations were made in mouse models of X-SCID in which irradiated bone marrow chimeric animals were treated in vivo with antagonistic anti-γc MAbs *(85)*.

It is thought that many of the symptoms observed in γc-deficient mice and in X-SCID patients are caused by the lack of IL-7 signaling. Mice deficient in IL-7 or IL-7Rα *(86,87)* show similar reductions in T- and B-cell numbers as γc knockout animals. Recently, a number of mutations of the IL-7Rα gene have been identified in human SCID patients with a T–B+NK+ phenotype *(74,88)*. Mice deficient in IL-2, IL-4, IL-2Rα, or IL-4Rα are not defective in T-cell, B-cell, or NK cell development. However, targeted disruption of the IL-2Rβ, IL-15, or IL-15Rα genes inhibits the production of NK cells, suggesting an important role of IL-15 in the development of this lineage of cells. Thus, IL-7 and IL-15 appear to be primarily responsible for the observed T-cell, B-cell, and NK cell defects caused by γc deficiency *(70)*. This notion is also supported by the finding that IL-7Rα/IL-2Rβ double knockout animals recapitulate most of the phenotypic effects observed in γc-deficient mice *(89)*.

4.2. Human γc Mutations That Cause X-SCID

A large number of human γc mutations have been described *(90–99)* that cause both typical and atypical *(76–78,100,101)* forms of X-SCID. A comprehensive database of these mutations (IL2RGbase) has been created and is publicly available via the Internet (http://www.nhgri.nih.gov/DIR/GMBB/SCID) *(91)*. X-SCID mutations have been found in all exons of the γc gene, encoding both extracellular and cytoplasmic regions of the receptor. Additional mutations affect intronic sequences that interfer with splicing γc mRNA. Analysis of the γc genes from 220 X-SCID patients revealed 147 unique genetic defects, including 51 missense and 27 nonsense mutations, 37 insertions or deletions causing frame shifts, 3 in-frame deletions or insertions, 27 splicing mutations, and 2 complex mutations (IL2RGbase; *see* ref. *91*). Although the effects of most nonsense, deletion, or splice mutations can be readily explained by premature termination of the protein and/or loss of critical functional domains of γc, missense mutations are more difficult to interpret. In the context of this review, those amino acid substitutions that affect the extracellular region of γc are of particular interest, as they may provide important clues about ectodomain residues required for γc structure and/or ligand binding.

Currently, at least 45 extracellular missense mutations of γc are known (Table 1), only part of which have been characterized in terms of γc mRNA and surface protein expression *(90)*. In a number of cases, the mutations have been shown to interfere with the folding of γc, resulting in undetectable or trace expression of γc protein on the cell surface (mutants E46K, Y65C, Y69C, G92D, C93F, H101P, V130A, L150Q, C160R, R202W, R204C, R204H, F205C, L208P, G210R, W218C). Several mutations affect highly conserved structural motifs in the N domain (C80Y, C93R), or the C domain of γc (W215R, W218C, S219I) and presumably also disrupt the folding of the receptor. Importantly, the most frequent types of missense mutations found in X-SCID patients were amino acid substitutions to or from Pro, Cys, or Gly, all of which may alter protein structure. Thus, it is likely that a substantial fraction of the known X-SCID mutations causes severe conformational changes in γc. However, for some extracellular missense mutations (N68K, Y103N, I131N, A134V, H163R), the available data are insufficient to explain the molecular mechanisms contributing to the X-SCID phenotype. It is especially interesting that for three of these mutations, Y103N, I131N, and A134V, detectable γc surface expression has been reported, yet patients with these mutations developed X-SCID *(78,90)*.

4.3. Relationship Between X-SCID Mutation and Site-Directed Mutagenesis of γc

Human Y103, C160, L208, C209, and G210 and their mouse counterparts have not only been implicated in cytokine binding by site-directed mutagenesis but also in X-SCID. Therefore, some instances of X-SCID may be the direct result of missense mutations that impair γc-dependent cytokine binding without drastic alteration of the structure of γc. Site-directed mutagenesis of γc indicates that the BC2 and FG2 loops participate in cytokine binding, and several other X-SCID mutations (C160R, L161R, F205C, L209P, C209Y, G210Y) are found in these two loops, consistent with the functional importance of these regions of γc. The linker region is highly conserved in mammalian γc and also appears to be important in cytokine binding *(40,44,67)*. Four X-SCID mutations in the linker region (V130A, I131N, A134V, and P135S) neighbor N128, which has been directly implicated in γc-dependent cytokine binding by site-directed mutagenesis. These X-SCID mutations are candidates for additional ligand contact sites of γc. The X-SCID A134V mutation of γc may be of particular interest as this mutant γc was expressed on the cell surface but exhibited a selective defect in γc-dependent IL-4 and IL-7, but not IL-2 and IL-15 signaling *(78)*. Two other X-SCID mutations (I131N and L150P) are possible candidates to represent ligand binding amino acids, as these γc molecules were also expressed *(90)*.

5. Concluding Remarks

Current data support a model in which IL-2, IL-4, IL-7, and IL-15 use a common mechanism for their interactions with γc. So far three sites have been identified for γc-dependent binding of IL-2, IL-4, IL-7, and IL-15. Two of these sites are necessary for binding all four of these cytokines. The region surrounding Y103 may function as a structurally conserved residue for ligand binding, whereas the region surrounding C161, C210, and G211 may be required to maintain the local structure of the receptor-ligand interface. The region surrounding N128 may provide a topography that controls specificity for binding distinct ligands. Some patients with X-SCID have missense mutations within these regions strongly suggesting that these individuals have this disease because of impaired cytokine binding

Table 1
Extracellular Missense Mutations of γc in X-SCID

Mutation	mRNA	γc protein	Comments
C40G			Conserved Cys
E46K	+	–	
E46G			
Y52G			
Y52C			Mutation to Cys
N62K			Potential N-glycosylation site
T64P			Mutation to Pro
Y65C	+	Trace	Mutation to Cys
Y69C		–	Mutation to Cys
K76E			
C80Y			Conserved Cys
Y83C			Mutation to Cys
S86P			Mutation to Pro
G92D	+	Trace	
C93R			Conserved Cys
C93F	+	Trace	Conserved Cys
H101P	+	–	Mutation to Pro
Y103N	+	+	Protein expression detected
Q109P			Mutation to Pro
L110F			
Q122P	+	–	Mutation to Pro
L124P			Mutation to Pro
V130A		–	
I131N	+	+	Protein expression detected
A134V		+	Selective IL-4/IL-7 defect
P135S			Conserved Pro
L140H			
L140R			
L150Q	+	–	
L150P		+	Mutation to Pro; protein expression detected
C160R		–	Cys
L161S			
H163R			
R200C			F2 strand
R202W	+	–	F2 strand
R204C	+	Trace	F2 strand
R204H	+	Trace	F2 strand
F205C	+	Trace	Mutation to Cys
L208P	+	–	Mutation to Pro
C209R			Cys
C209Y			Cys
G210R	+	Trace	
W215R			WSXWS motif
W218C	+	Trace	WSXWS motif
S219I			WSXWS motif

Information compiled from IL2RGbase *(91)* and Kumaki et al. *(93)*.

by γc. The validity of structural models and a more precise definition of ligand binding properties of γc await the solving of the crystal structure of this protein complexed with ligand as a heterodimer receptor.

Acknowledgments

Our research is supported by NIH grants AI40114 and CA45957.

References

1. Takeshita, T., Asao, H., Ohtani, K., et al. (1992) Cloning of the γ-chain of the human IL-2 receptor. *Science* **257,** 379–382.
2. Kondo, M., Takeshita, T., Ishii, N., et al. (1993) Sharing of the interleukin-2 (IL-2) receptor γ-chain between receptors for IL-2 and IL-4 [see comments]. *Science* **262,** 1874–1877.
3. Russell, S. M., Keegan, A. D., Harada, N., et al. (1993) Interleukin-2 receptor γ-chain: a functional component of the interleukin-4 receptor [see comments]. *Science* **262,** 1880–1883.
4. Noguchi, M., Nakamura, Y., Russell, S. M., et al. (1993) Interleukin-2 receptor γ-chain: a functional component of the interleukin-7 receptor. *Science* **262,** 1877–1880.
5. Kondo, M., Takeshita, T., Higuchi, M., et al. (1994) Functional participation of the IL-2 receptor γ-chain in IL-7 receptor complexes. *Science* **263,** 1453–1454.
6. Kimura, Y., Takeshita, T., Kondo, M., et al. (1995) Sharing of the IL-2 receptor γ-chain with the functional IL-9 receptor complex. *Int. Immunol.* **7,** 115–120.
7. Giri, J. G., Anderson, D. M., Kumaki, S., Park, L. S., Grabstein, K. H., and Cosman, D. (1995) IL-15, a novel T cell growth factor that shares activities and receptor components with IL-2. *J. Leukoc. Biol.* **57,** 763–766.
8. Parrish-Novak, J., Dillon, S. R., Nelson, A., et al. (2000) Interleukin 21 and its receptor are involved in NK cell expansion and regulation of lymphocyte function. *Nature* **408,** 57–63.
9. Asao, H., Okuyama, C., Kumaki, S., et al. (2001) The common γ-chain is an indispensable subunit of the IL-21 receptor complex. *J. Immunol.* **167,** 1–5.
10. Noguchi, M., Yi, H., Rosenblatt, H. M., et al. (1993) Interleukin-2 receptor γ-chain mutation results in X-linked severe combined immunodeficiency in humans. *Cell* **73,** 147–157.
11. Puck, J. M., Deschenes, S. M., Porter, J. C., et al. (1993) The interleukin-2 receptor γ-chain maps to Xq13.1 and is mutated in X-linked severe combined immunodeficiency, SCIDX1. *Hum. Mol. Genet.* **2,** 1099–1104.
12. Nakamura, Y., Russell, S. M., Mess, S. A., et al. (1994) Heterodimerization of the IL-2 receptor β- and γ-chain cytoplasmic domains is required for signalling. *Nature* **369,** 330–333.
13. Nelson, B. H., Lord, J. D., and Greenberg, P. D. (1994) Cytoplasmic domains of the interleukin-2 receptor β and γ chains mediate the signal for T-cell proliferation. *Nature* **369,** 333–336.
14. He, Y. W. and Malek, T. R. (1998) The structure and function of γc-dependent cytokines and receptors: regulation of T lymphocyte development and homeostasis. *Crit. Rev. Immunol.* **18,** 503–524.
15. Nelson, B. H. and Willerford, D. M. (1998) Biology of the interleukin-2 receptor. *Adv. Immunol.* **70,** 1–81.
16. DiSanto, J. P., Certain, S., Wilson, A., et al. (1994) The murine interleukin-2 receptor γ chain gene: organization, chromosomal localization and expression in the adult thymus. *Eur. J. Immunol.* **24,** 3014–3018.
17. Henthorn, P. S., Somberg, R. L., Fimiani, V. M., Puck, J. M., Patterson, D. F., and Felsburg, P. J. (1994) IL-2R γ-gene microdeletion demonstrates that canine X-linked severe combined immunodeficiency is a homologue of the human disease. *Genomics* **23,** 69–74.
18. Yoo, J., Stone, R. T., Solinas-Toldo, S., Fries, R., and Beattie, C. W. (1996) Cloning and chromosomal mapping of bovine interleukin-2 receptor γ gene. *DNA Cell Biol.* **15,** 453–459.
19. Wang, T. and Secombes, C. J. (2001) Cloning and expression of a putative common cytokine receptor γ-chain (γc) gene in rainbow trout (*Oncorhynchus mykiss*). *Fish Shellfish Immunol.* **11,** 233–244.

20. Malek, T. R., Furse, R. K., Fleming, M. L., Fadell, A. J., and He, Y. W. (1995) Biochemical identity and characterization of the mouse interleukin-2 receptor β and γc subunits. *J. Interferon Cytokine Res.* **15,** 447–454.
21. Noguchi, M., Adelstein, S., Cao, X., and Leonard, W. J. (1993) Characterization of the human interleukin-2 receptor γ-chain gene. *J Biol Chem.* **268,** 13601–13608.
22. Balasubramanian, S., Chernov-Rogan, T., Davis, A. M., et al. (1995) Ligand binding kinetics of IL-2 and IL-15 to heteromers formed by extracellular domains of the three IL-2 receptor subunits. *Int. Immunol.* **7,** 1839–1849.
23. Letzelter, F., Wang, Y., and Sebald, W. (1998) The interleukin-4 site-2 epitope determining binding of the common receptor γ-chain. *Eur. J. Biochem.* **257,** 11–20.
24. Baker, D. P., Whitty, A., Zafari, M. R., et al. (1998) The murine anti-human common γ-chain monoclonal antibody PC.B8 blocks the second step in the formation of the intermediate affinity IL-2 receptor. *Biochemistry* **37,** 14337–14349.
25. Voss, S. D., Leary, T. P., Sondel, P. M., and Robb, R. J. (1993) Identification of a direct interaction between interleukin 2 and the p64 interleukin 2 receptor γ-chain. *Proc. Natl. Acad. Sci. USA* **90,** 2428–2432.
26. Saragovi, H. and Malek, T. R. (1987) The murine interleukin 2 receptor. Irreversible cross-linking of radiolabeled interleukin 2 to high affinity interleukin 2 receptors reveals a noncovalently associated subunit. *J. Immunol.* **139,** 1918–1926.
27. Giri, J. G., Ahdieh, M., Eisenman, J., et al. (1994) Utilization of the β and γ chains of the IL-2 receptor by the novel cytokine IL-15. *EMBO J.* **13,** 2822–2830.
28. de Jong, J. L., Farner, N. L., Widmer, M. B., Giri, J. G., and Sondel, P. M. (1996) Interaction of IL-15 with the shared IL-2 receptor β and γc subunits. The IL-15/β/γc receptor-ligand complex is less stable than the IL-2/β/γc receptor-ligand complex. *J. Immunol.* **156,** 1339–1348.
29. Zurawski, S. M., Vega, F. Jr., Doyle, E. L., et al. (1993) Definition and spatial location of mouse interleukin-2 residues that interact with its heterotrimeric receptor. *EMBO J.* **12,** 5113–5119.
30. Zurawski, S. M. and Zurawski, G. (1988) Identification of three critical regions within mouse interleukin 2 by fine structural deletion analysis. *EMBO J.* **7,** 1061–1069.
31. Buchli, P. and Ciardelli, T. (1993) Structural and biologic properties of a human aspartic acid-126 interleukin-2 analog. *Arch. Biochem. Biophys.* **307,** 411–415.
32. Pettit, D. K., Bonnert, T. P., Eisenman, J., et al. (1997) Structure-function studies of interleukin 15 using site-specific mutagenesis, polyethylene glycol conjugation, and homology modeling. *J. Biol. Chem.* **272,** 2312–2318.
33. Kruse, N., Tony, H. P., and Sebald, W. (1992) Conversion of human interleukin-4 into a high affinity antagonist by a single amino acid replacement. *EMBO J.* **11,** 3237–3244.
34. Kruse, N., Shen, B. J., Arnold, S., Tony, H. P., Muller, T., and Sebald, W. (1993) Two distinct functional sites of human interleukin 4 are identified by variants impaired in either receptor binding or receptor activation. *EMBO J.* **12,** 5121–5129.
35. Schnarr, B., Ezernieks, J., Sebald, W., and Duschl, A. (1997) IL-4 receptor complexes containing or lacking the γc chain are inhibited by an overlapping set of antagonistic IL-4 mutant proteins. *Int. Immunol.* **9,** 861–868.
36. Hage, T., Sebald, W., and Reinemer, P. (1999) Crystal structure of the interleukin-4/receptor α-chain complex reveals a mosaic binding interface. *Cell* **97,** 271–281.
37. Wang, Y., Shen, B. J., and Sebald, W. (1997) A mixed-charge pair in human interleukin 4 dominates high-affinity interaction with the receptor α-chain. *Proc. Natl. Acad. Sci. USA* **94,** 1657–1662.
38. Cosenza, L., Rosenbach, A., White, J. V., Murphy, J. R., and Smith, T. (2000) Comparative model building of interleukin-7 using interleukin-4 as a template: a structural hypothesis that displays atypical surface chemistry in helix D important for receptor activation. *Protein Sci.* **9,** 916–926.
39. Sugamura, K., Asao, H., Kondo, M., et al. (1995) The common γ-chain for multiple cytokine receptors. *Adv. Immunol.* **59,** 225–277.
40. Olosz, F. and Malek, T. R. (2000) Three loops of the common γ-chain ectodomain required for the binding of interleukin-2 and interleukin-7. *J. Biol. Chem.* **275,** 30100–30105.
41. Raskin, N., Jakubowski, A., Sizing, I. D., et al. (1998) Molecular mapping with functional antibodies localizes critical sites on the human IL receptor common gamma (γc) chain. *J. Immunol.* **161,** 3474–3483.

42. He, Y. W., Adkins, B., Furse, R. K., and Malek, T. R. (1995) Expression and function of the gamma c subunit of the IL-2, IL-4, and IL-7 receptors. Distinct interaction of γc in the IL-4 receptor. *J. Immunol.* **154,** 1596–1605.
43. Malek, T. R., Levy, R. B., Adkins, B., and He, Y. W. (1998) Monoclonal antibodies to the common gamma-chain as cytokine receptor antagonists in vivo: effect on intrathymic and intestinal intraepithelial T lymphocyte development. *J. Leukoc. Biol.* **63,** 643–649.
44. Olosz, F. and Malek, T. R. (2002) Structural basis for binding multiple ligands by the common cytokine receptor γ-chain. *J. Biol. Chem.* **277,** 12047–12052.
45. Elkins, P. A., Christinger, H. W., Sandowski, Y., et al. (2000) Ternary complex between placental lactogen and the extracellular domain of the prolactin receptor. *Nat. Struct. Biol.* **7,** 808–815.
46. de Vos, A. M., Ultsch, M., and Kossiakoff, A. A. (1992) Human growth hormone and extracellular domain of its receptor: crystal structure of the complex. *Science* **255,** 306–312.
47. Syed, R. S., Reid, S. W., Li, C., et al. (1998) Efficiency of signalling through cytokine receptors depends critically on receptor orientation. *Nature* **395,** 511–516.
48. Whitty, A., Raskin, N., Olson, D. L., et al. (1998) Interaction affinity between cytokine receptor components on the cell surface. *Proc. Natl. Acad. Sci. USA* **95,** 13165–13170.
49. Damjanovich, S., Bene, L., Matko, J., et al. (1997) Preassembly of interleukin 2 (IL-2) receptor subunits on resting Kit 225 K6 T cells and their modulation by IL-2, IL-7, and IL-15: a fluorescence resonance energy transfer study. *Proc. Natl. Acad. Sci. USA* **94,** 13134–13139.
50. Livnah, O., Stura, E. A., Middleton, S. A., Johnson, D. L., Jolliffe, L. K., and Wilson, I. A. (1999) Crystallographic evidence for preformed dimers of erythropoietin receptor before ligand activation. *Science* **283,** 987–990.
51. Remy, I., Wilson, I. A., and Michnick, S. W. (1999) Erythropoietin receptor activation by a ligand-induced conformation change. *Science* **283,** 990–993.
52. Caravella, J. A., Lyne, P. D., and Richards, W. G. (1996) A partial model of the erythropoietin receptor complex. *Proteins* **24,** 394–401.
53. Gustchina, A., Zdanov, A., Schalk-Hihi, C., and Wlodawer, A. (1995) A model of the complex between interleukin-4 and its receptors. *Proteins* **21,** 140–148.
54. Rajotte, D., Cadieux, C., Haman, A., et al. (1997) Crucial role of the residue R280 at the F'-G' loop of the human granulocyte/macrophage colony-stimulating factor receptor α-chain for ligand recognition. *J. Exp. Med* **185,** 1939–1950.
55. Layton, J. E., Iaria, J., Smith, D. K., and Treutlein, H. R. (1997) Identification of a ligand-binding site on the granulocyte colony-stimulating factor receptor by molecular modeling and mutagenesis. *J. Biol. Chem* **272,** 29735–29741.
56. Bamborough, P., Hedgecock, C. J., and Richards, W. G. (1994) The interleukin-2 and interleukin-4 receptors studied by molecular modeling. *Structure* **2,** 839–851.
57. Kroemer, R. T. and Richards, W. G. (1996) Homology modeling study of the human interleukin-7 receptor complex. *Protein Eng.* **9,** 1135–1142.
58. Layton, J. E., Iaria, J., and Nicholson, S. E. (1997) Neutralising antibodies to the granulocyte colony-stimulating factor receptor recognise both the immunoglobulin-like domain and the cytokine receptor homologous domain. *Growth Factors* **14,** 117–130.
59. Horsten, U., Muller-Newen, G., Gerhartz, C., et al. (1997) Molecular modeling-guided mutagenesis of the extracellular part of gp130 leads to the identification of contact sites in the interleukin-6 (IL-6).IL-6 receptor.gp130 complex. *J. Biol. Chem.* **272,** 23748–23757.
60. Brandhuber, B. J., Boone, T., Kenney, W. C., and McKay, D. B. (1987) Three-dimensional structure of interleukin-2. *Science* **238,** 1707–1709.
61. Wlodaver, A., Pavlovsky, A., and Gustchina, A. (1992) Crystal structure of human recombinant interleukin-4 at 2.25 A resolution. *FEBS Lett.* **309,** 59–64.
62. Smith, L. J., Redfield, C., Boyd, J., et al. (1992) Human interleukin 4. The solution structure of a four-helix bundle protein. *J. Mol. Biol.* **224,** 899–904.
63. Kroemer, R. T., Doughty, S. W., Robinson, A. J., and Richards, W. G. (1996) Prediction of the three-dimensional structure of human interleukin-7 by homology modeling. *Protein Eng.* **9,** 493–498.
64. Barlow, P. N., Norman, D. G., Steinkasserer, A., et al. (1992) Solution structure of the fifth repeat of factor H: a second example of the complement control protein module. *Biochemistry* **31,** 3626–3634.

65. Barlow, P. N., Steinkasserer, A., Norman, D. G., et al. (1993) Solution structure of a pair of complement modules by nuclear magnetic resonance. *J. Mol. Biol.* **232,** 268–284.
66. Imler, J. L., Miyajima, A., and Zurawski, G. (1992) Identification of three adjacent amino acids of interleukin-2 receptor beta chain which control the affinity and the specificity of the interaction with interleukin-2. *EMBO J.* **11,** 2047–2053.
67. Zhang, J. L., Buehner, M., and Sebald, W. (2002) Functional epitope of common γ chain for interleukin-4 binding. *Eur. J. Biochem.* **269,** 1490–1499.
68. Clackson, T., Ultsch, M. H., Wells, J. A., and de Vos, A. M. (1998) Structural and functional analysis of the 1:1 growth hormone:receptor complex reveals the molecular basis for receptor affinity. *J. Mol. Biol.* **277,** 1111–1128.
69. Middleton, S. A., Johnson, D. L., Jin, R., et al. (1996) Identification of a critical ligand binding determinant of the human erythropoietin receptor. Evidence for common ligand binding motifs in the cytokine receptor family. *J. Biol. Chem.* **271,** 14045–14054.
70. Malek, T. R., Porter, B. O., and He, Y. W. (1999) Multiple γc-dependent cytokines regulate T-cell development. *Immunol. Today* **20,** 71–76.
71. Bamborough, P., Grant, G. H., Hedgecock, C. J., West, S. P., and Richards, W. G. (1993) A computer model of the interleukin-4/receptor complex. *Proteins* **17,** 11–19.
72. Cavazzana-Calvo, M., Hacein-Bey, S., de Saint Basile, G., et al. (2000) Gene therapy of human severe combined immunodeficiency (SCID)-X1 disease. *Science* **288,** 669–672.
73. Leonard, W. J. (2000) X-linked severe combined immunodeficiency: from molecular cause to gene therapy within seven years. *Mol. Med. Today* **6,** 403–407.
74. Puel, A. and Leonard, W. J. (2000) Mutations in the gene for the IL-7 receptor result in T(−)B(+) NK(+) severe combined immunodeficiency disease. *Curr. Opin. Immunol.* **12,** 468-473.
75. Conley, M. E., Lavoie, A., Briggs, C., Brown, P., Guerra, C., and Puck, J. M. (1988) Nonrandom X chromosome inactivation in B cells from carriers of X chromosome-linked severe combined immunodeficiency. *Proc. Natl. Acad. Sci. USA* **85,** 3090–3094.
76. DiSanto, J. P., Rieux-Laucat, F., Dautry-Varsat, A., Fischer, A., and de Saint Basile, G. (1994) Defective human interleukin 2 receptor γ chain in an atypical X chromosome-linked severe combined immunodeficiency with peripheral T cells. *Proc. Natl. Acad. Sci. USA* **91,** 9466–9470.
77. Sharfe, N., Shahar, M., and Roifman, C. M. (1997) An interleukin-2 receptor γ chain mutation with normal thymus morphology. *J. Clin. Invest.* **100,** 3036–3043.
78. Kumaki, S., Ishii, N., Minegishi, M., et al. (1999) Functional role of interleukin-4 (IL-4) and IL-7 in the development of X-linked severe combined immunodeficiency. *Blood* **93,** 607–612.
79. Russell, S. M., Tayebi, N., Nakajima, H., et al. (1995) Mutation of Jak3 in a patient with SCID: essential role of Jak3 in lymphoid development. *Science* **270,** 797–800.
80. Cao, X., Shores, E. W., Hu-Li, J., et al. (1995) Defective lymphoid development in mice lacking expression of the common cytokine receptor γ chain. *Immunity* **2,** 223–238.
81. DiSanto, J. P., Muller, W., Guy-Grand, D., Fischer, A., and Rajewsky, K. (1995) Lymphoid development in mice with a targeted deletion of the interleukin 2 receptor γ chain. *Proc. Natl. Acad. Sci. USA* **92,** 377–381.
82. Nosaka, T., van Deursen, J. M., Tripp, R. A., et al. (1995) Defective lymphoid development in mice lacking Jak3. *Science* **270,** 800–802.
83. Park, S. Y., Saijo, K., Takahashi, T., et al. (1995) Developmental defects of lymphoid cells in Jak3 kinase-deficient mice. *Immunity* **3,** 771–782.
84. Suzuki, K., Nakajima, H., Saito, Y., Saito, T., Leonard, W. J., and Iwamoto, I. (2000) Janus kinase 3 (Jak3) is essential for common cytokine receptor γ chain (γc)-dependent signaling: comparative analysis of γc, Jak3, and γc and Jak3 double-deficient mice. *Int. Immunol.* **12,** 123–132.
85. He, Y. W., Levy, R. B., and Malek, T. R. (1995) Blockade of T- and B-lymphocyte development by antibody to the γc subunit of the receptors for interleukins 2, 4, and 7. *Proc. Natl. Acad. Sci. USA* **92,** 5689–5693.
86. von Freeden-Jeffry, U., Vieira, P., Lucian, L. A., McNeil, T., Burdach, S. E., and Murray, R. (1995) Lymphopenia in interleukin (IL)-7 gene-deleted mice identifies IL-7 as a nonredundant cytokine. *J. Exp. Med.* **181,** 1519–1526.
87. Peschon, J. J., Morrissey, P. J., Grabstein, K. H., et al. (1994) Early lymphocyte expansion is severely impaired in interleukin 7 receptor-deficient mice. *J. Exp. Med.* **180,** 1955–1960.

88. Puel, A., Ziegler, S. F., Buckley, R. H., and Leonard, W. J. (1998) Defective IL7R expression in T(–)B(+)NK(+) severe combined immunodeficiency. *Nat. Genet.* **20,** 394–397.
89. Porter, B. O. and Malek, T. R. (1999) IL-2Rbeta/IL-7Ralpha doubly deficient mice recapitulate the thymic and intraepithelial lymphocyte (IEL) developmental defects of γc–/– mice: roles for both IL-2 and IL-15 in CD8αα IEL development. *J. Immunol.* **163,** 5906–5912.
90. Puck, J. M., Pepper, A. E., Henthorn, P. S., et al. (1997) Mutation analysis of IL2RG in human X-linked severe combined immunodeficiency. *Blood* **89,** 1968–1977.
91. Puck, J. M. (1996) IL2RGbase: a database of γc-chain defects causing human X-SCID. *Immunol. Today* **17,** 507–511.
92. Niemela, J. E., Puck, J. M., Fischer, R. E., Fleisher, T. A., and Hsu, A. P. (2000) Efficient detection of thirty-seven new IL2RG mutations in human X-linked severe combined immunodeficiency. *Clin. Immunol.* **95,** 33–38.
93. Kumaki, S., Ishii, N., Minegishi, M., et al. (2000) Characterization of the gamma c chain among 27 unrelated Japanese patients with X-linked severe combined immunodeficiency (X-SCID). *Hum. Genet.* **107,** 406–408.
94. Fugmann, S. D., Muller, S., Friedrich, W., Bartram, C. R., and Schwarz, K. (1998) Mutations in the gene for the common γ chain (γc) in X-linked severe combined immunodeficiency. *Hum. Genet.* **103,** 730–731.
95. Clark, P. A., Lester, T., Genet, S., et al. (1995) Screening for mutations causing X-linked severe combined immunodeficiency in the IL-2R γ chain gene by single-strand conformation polymorphism analysis. *Hum. Genet.* **96,** 427–432.
96. Markiewicz, S., Subtil, A., Dautry-Varsat, A., Fischer, A., and de Saint Basile, G. (1994) Detection of three nonsense mutations and one missense mutation in the interleukin-2 receptor γ chain gene in SCIDX1 that differently affect the mRNA processing. *Genomics* **21,** 291–293.
97. DiSanto, J. P., Dautry-Varsat, A., Certain, S., Fischer, A., and de Saint Basile, G. (1994) Interleukin-2 (IL-2) receptor γ chain mutations in X-linked severe combined immunodeficiency disease result in the loss of high-affinity IL-2 receptor binding. *Eur. J. Immunol.* **24,** 475–479.
98. Ishii, N., Asao, H., Kimura, Y., et al. (1994) Impairment of ligand binding and growth signaling of mutant IL-2 receptor γ-chains in patients with X-linked severe combined immunodeficiency. *J. Immunol.* **153,** 1310–1317.
99. Kanai, N., Yanai, F., Hirose, S., et al. (1999) A G to A transition at the last nucleotide of exon 6 of the γc gene (868G-->A) may result in either a splice or missense mutation in patients with X-linked severe combined immunodeficiency. *Hum. Genet.* **104,** 36–42.
100. Kumaki, S., Ochs, H. D., Kuropatwinski, K. K., et al. (1999) A novel mutant γc chain from a patient with typical phenotype of X-linked severe combined immunodeficiency (SCID) has partial signalling function for mediating IL-2 and IL-4 receptor action. *Clin. Exp. Immunol.* **115,** 356–361.
101. Schmalstieg, F. C., Leonard, W. J., Noguchi, M., et al. (1995) Missense mutation in exon 7 of the common γ chain gene causes a moderate form of X-linked combined immunodeficiency. *J. Clin. Invest.* **95,** 1169–1173.

10

G-CSF, GM-CSF, and IL-3 Knockout Mice

Thomas Enzler and Glenn Dranoff

Summary

Granulocyte colony stimulating factor (G-CSF), granulocyte-macrophage colony stimulating factor (GM-CSF), and interleukin-3 (IL-3) stimulate the proliferation, differentiation, and activation of multiple hematopoietic cells. G-CSF acts primarily on mature neutrophils and their precursors, and the ability of this cytokine to promote granulopoiesis in vivo underlies its clinical application in the setting of neutropenia. GM-CSF influences a broader range of cells, including neutrophils, eosinophils, macrophages, erythroid progenitors, megakaryocyte progenitors, and dendritic cells. These properties result in marked immunostimulation, and have led to clinical testing of the cytokine as a vaccine adjuvant. IL-3 augments the numbers and functions of hematopoietic progenitors, mast cells, basophils, neutrophils, macrophages, eosinophils, erythrocytes, megakaryocytes, and dendritic cells.

In this chapter we review the generation and characterization of mice deficient in each of these cytokines. These studies have delineated essential roles for the molecules in hematopoiesis, immunity, and pulmonary homeostasis.

Key words

G-CSF, GM-CSF, IL-3, hematopoiesis, immunity, pulmonary homeostasis

1. Introduction

Granulocyte colony-stimulating factor (G-CSF), granulocyte-macrophage colony stimulating factor (GM-CSF), and interleukin-3 (IL-3) stimulate the proliferation, differentiation, and activation of blood cells in many similar ways *(1)*. Nonetheless, the generation of mice singly and multiply deficient in these cytokines has established unique roles for these molecules in hematopoiesis, immunity, and pulmonary homeostasis.

G-CSF is a glycoprotein of 208 amino acids (mouse) that enhances the survival, proliferation, differentiation, and function of mature neutrophils and their precursors *(2)*. The ability of the cytokine to promote granulopoiesis in vivo was revealed by injecting mice with pharmacologic doses of recombinant protein *(3–5)* and by reconstituting lethally irradiated animals with bone marrow transduced with a retroviral vector expressing the gene product *(6)*. Consistent with these findings, low numbers of circulating neutrophils in humans were associated with high serum G-CSF levels in some clinical situations *(7,8)*.

GM-CSF is a glycoprotein of 124 amino acids (mouse) that has a broad range of actions on neutrophils, eosinophils, macrophages, erythroid progenitors, megakaryocyte progenitors,

From: *Contemporary Immunology: Cytokine Knockouts, 2nd Edition*
Edited by: Giamila Fantuzzi © Humana Press Inc., Totowa, NJ

and dendritic cells *(9–13)*. The effects of GM-CSF overproduction *in vivo* were examined by generating GM-CSF transgenic mice *(14)* and by reconstituting animals with bone marrow transduced with a retrovirus expressing GM-CSF *(15)*. In these cases, marked increases in granulocytes, macrophages, and committed precursors were observed, although this myeloproliferative syndrome did not progress to frank leukemia *(15)*. GM-CSF also has marked immunostimulatory capabilities, and vaccination with irradiated tumor cells engineered to secrete GM-CSF generated potent, specific, and long-lasting antitumor immunity in multiple murine models *(16)*.

IL-3 is a glycoprotein of 166 amino acids (mouse) that promotes the differentiation and proliferation of hematopoietic progenitors, mast cells, basophils, neutrophils, macrophages, eosinophils, erythrocytes, megakaryocytes, and dendritic cells *(17–23)*. IL-3 also stimulates antigen presentation for T-cell-dependent responses, augments macrophage cytotoxicity and adhesion, and enhances the activities of eosinophils, basophils, and mast cells *(24–28)*.

2. G-CSF-Deficient Mice

2.1. The Disrupted G-CSF Allele

The murine G-CSF gene resides on chromosome 11 *(29)*, separated from the GM-CSF/IL-3 locus by 28 c*M (30,31)*. G-CSF-deficient mice were generated by the deletion of three exons and the insertion of a *lac*-Z cassette under the control of the G-CSF promoter. The disrupted G-CSF allele was confirmed by polymerase chain reaction (PCR) analysis of genomic DNA *(32)*.

2.2. Survival and Fertility

G-CSF-deficient mice were viable, fertile, and clinically healthy. Homozygous deficient males and females could be interbred efficiently and produced normal-sized litters.

2.3. Hemopoiesis

G-CSF-deficient mice manifested a chronic neutropenia *(32)*. Peripheral blood neutrophil levels were 20–30% of wild-type values, and heterozygous deficient mice showed intermediate levels, suggesting a possible gene-dosage effect (Fig. 1). Although there were no alterations in the femoral cellularity of 6–8-wk-old G-CSF-deficient mice, mutant marrows contained reduced numbers of early and late granulocyte precursors *(32)*. No compensatory splenic granulopoiesis was detected under steady-state conditions. As granulocytes in the marrow and spleen together constitute approximately 90% of total body neutrophils *(33)*, G-CSF-deficient mice displayed a major reduction in total neutrophil mass.

To determine the number of neutrophils available for immediate mobilization from noncirculating reserves, Lieschke and colleagues *(32)* injected recombinant G-CSF into mutant animals and wild-type controls. The increase in peripheral neutrophils in G-CSF-deficient mice was only 21% of that achieved in wild-type animals 3 h after injection, revealing a substantial reduction in the neutrophil reserve.

2.4. Rescue of Granulopoiesis

To determine whether therapeutic G-CSF administration could correct the effects of chronic G-CSF deficiency, Lieschke and associates *(32)* administered recombinant G-CSF (250 µg/kg) subcutaneously for several days. This regimen promptly "rescued" G-CSF-deficient

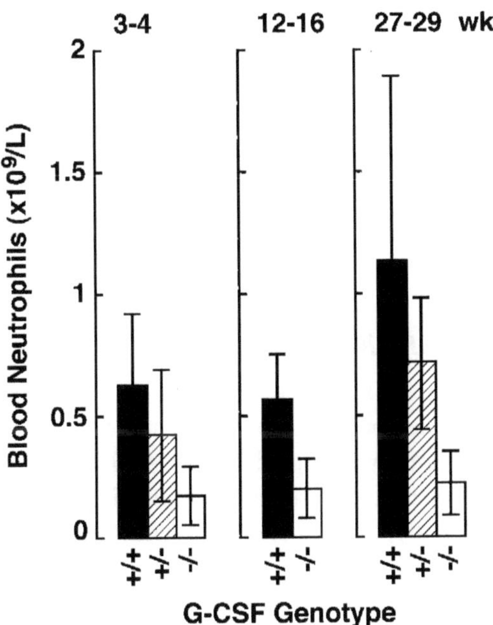

Fig. 1. Chronic neutropenia in granulocyte colony-stimulating factor (G-CSF)-deficient mice, as reported in Lieschke et al. *(32)*. Data shown are the mean ± SD for mice of three different ages. G-CSF genotypes are as follows: +/+, homozygous wild-type; +/–, heterozygous; –/–, homozygous null. Reprinted with permission.

granulopoiesis. After only 1 d of G-CSF therapy, mutant mice attained blood neutrophil numbers that were equivalent to basal levels in wild-type mice, although marrow granulopoiesis was still reduced. However, after 4 d of therapy, marrow granulopoiesis exceeded the basal levels found in wild-type animals.

2.5. Infection

The response of G-CSF-deficient mice to infection with *Listeria monocytogenes* was investigated *(32)*. Five days after inoculation, the liver and spleen of G-CSF$^{-/-}$ mice showed significantly higher levels of *L. monocytogenes* compared with wild-type animals, indicating an impaired response to infectious challenge. The mortality in G-CSF$^{-/-}$ mice by d 5 was 50%, whereas no deaths occurred in G-CSF$^{+/+}$ mice over the same time. The G-CSF$^{-/-}$ mice that succumbed to infection harbored high bacterial burdens. The granulopoietic response to infection was markedly diminished in the mutant mice. One day after inoculation, the increase in peripheral blood neutrophils was only 15% of that of wild-type mice. Whereas a neutrophilia was maintained in infected wild-type mice, neutrophil numbers gradually decreased to baseline levels in surviving G-CSF-deficient mice, although circulating immature forms were increased. Interestingly, G-CSF-deficient mice also showed a delay in the characteristic monocytosis induced in wild-type mice as a consequence of *L. monocytogenes* inoculation.

2.6. The Physiologic Role of G-CSF

Steady-state granulopoiesis maintains circulating neutrophil levels within a narrow range, probably through both positive and negative regulators *(1,2,34,35)*. The finding that some cases of neutropenia in humans are associated with high levels of G-CSF provides indirect evidence that this cytokine may contribute to homeostatic regulation *(7)*. Nonetheless, the defects delineated in G-CSF$^{-/-}$ mice established a critical role for the cytokine in maintaining normal steady-state granulopoiesis, the size of the reserve pool, and circulating neutrophil numbers. Moreover, G-CSF was also required for "emergency" granulopoiesis in response to acute infection *(2,34)*. Recent studies revealed that whereas G-CSF is dispensable for neutrophil trafficking, the primary function of the cytokine is to promote the survival of myeloid precursors and cells of the neutrophil lineage *(36)*.

3. GM-CSF-Deficient Mice

3.1. The Disrupted GM-CSF Allele

The murine GM-CSF gene is located on chromosome 11 and is within 14 kb of the IL-3 locus *(31)*. The GM-CSF gene contains four exons and encodes a major transcript of 780 nucleotides *(37,38)*. Our laboratory disrupted the GM-CSF locus in embryonic stem cells by deleting exons 3 and 4. Homozygous deficient mutant animals were confirmed by Southern analysis *(39)*. In a parallel study, Stanley and colleagues *(40)* generated GM-CSF deficient mice by deleting exons 1 and 2.

3.2. Phenotype

The phenotypes of the GM-CSF-deficient mice produced by the two groups were virtually identical. GM-CSF-deficient mice developed normally and appeared healthy at birth. Adult mutant animals showed a partial impairment in fertility. The mean number of resorbed and malformed fetuses was increased, and the mean litter sizes were slightly reduced compared with controls *(41)*.

3.3. Hemopoiesis

Surprisingly, despite the ability of GM-CSF to stimulate hematopoiesis, homozygous inactivation of the GM-CSF gene did not alter steady-state blood cell production *(39,40)*. Normal numbers of peripheral blood cells, bone marrow progenitors, and tissue hematopoietic populations, including splenic dendritic cells, were maintained throughout the life span of the animals *(42,43)*. Lethally irradiated mutant recipients were also efficiently reconstituted with mutant bone marrow *(42)*. However, in response to infection with *L. monocytogenes*, GM-CSF-deficient mice showed a modest impairment in granulocyte and macrophage responses *(44)*.

3.4. Pulmonary Homeostasis

Pathologic analysis of GM-CSF-deficient mice unexpectedly revealed abnormalities in the lungs. By the age of 2 mo, amorphous, eosinophilic material was present in the alveolar spaces of all mutant mice, but not in heterozygotes or wild-type controls (Fig. 2) *(39)*. Electron microscopy and immunohistochemistry demonstrated that the material was surfactant *(39)*. Pulmonary surfactant is a complex mixture of phospholipid and protein that functions primarily to reduce surfactant tension at the air-liquid interface, although it may also contribute to lung defense *(45)*. Surfactant proteins and lipids are synthesized by type II pneumocytes and cleared from the alveolar space through both recycling and degradation by type II cells and, to a lesser extent, alveolar macrophages *(46)*. Bronchoalveolar lavage obtained from the mutant animals was highly enriched in pulmonary surfactant lipid and

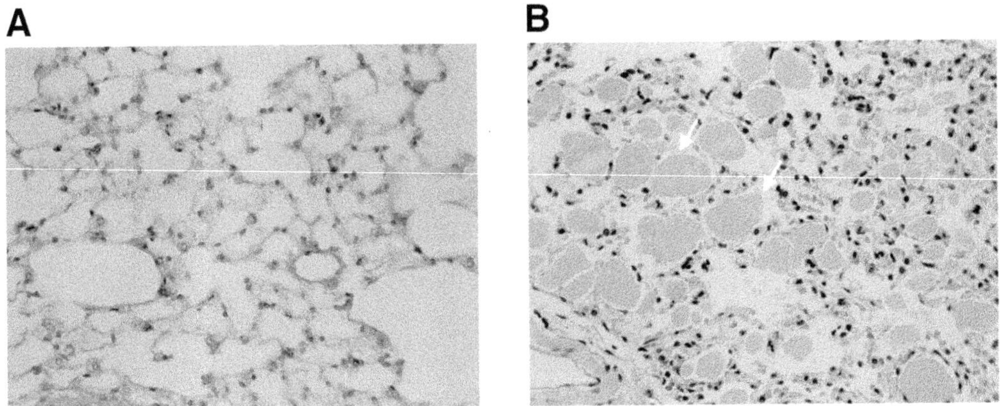

Fig. 2. Pulmonary alveolar proteinosis in GM-CSF-deficient mice. (**A**) Normal lung from a wild-type animal. (**B**) Extensive proteinosis with aggregates of eosinophilic lipoproteinaceous material (arrows) within the alveoli. Reprinted with permission from ref. *39*.

proteins. Western analysis demonstrated a marked increase in the amount of surfactant proteins SP-A, -B, -C, and -D, as well as an increased abundance of nonreducing oligomers of SP-A *(39,47)*. Collectively, these morphologic and biochemical findings were reminiscent of an idiopathic human disorder, pulmonary alveolar proteinosis (PAP) *(48)*. The mechanisms underlying the surfactant accumulation in GM-CSF-deficient mice primarily reflected the decreased clearance and catabolism by mutant alveolar macrophages *(47,49, 50)*. Lastly, the pulmonary-specific expression of GM-CSF corrected the lung pathology, revealing a crucial role for the cytokine in the pulmonary microenvironment *(51–53)*.

3.5. Pulmonary Alveolar Proteinosis

Human PAP is a heterogenous group of congenital and acquired lung disorders characterized by the accumulation of surfactant protein and lipid within alveoli *(48)*. Patients with PAP manifest a restrictive lung defect and show increased susceptibility to pulmonary infection. Based on the findings in the GM-CSF-deficient mice, studies were undertaken to examine the possible involvement of GM-CSF dysfunction in human PAP. Kitamura and colleagues *(54)* demonstrated that 11 individuals with idiopathic PAP, but not healthy controls or patients with other lung disease, showed high titers of neutralizing IgG antibodies against GM-CSF. This work suggests that some cases of PAP may involve an autoimmune response to GM-GSF. Other patients with PAP were found to harbor mutations in the β_c-subunit of the GM-CSF receptor *(55)* or manifest an aberrant alveolar macrophage response in which excessive IL-10 production suppressed GM-CSF function *(56,57)*. Consistent with these findings, the therapeutic administration of GM-CSF resulted in symptomatic, physiologic, and radiographic improvements in some affected patients *(58–60)*.

3.6. Macrophage Function

Macrophages in GM-CSF-deficient mice showed multiple abnormalities. These included decreased catabolism of surfactant lipids and proteins *(49,50)*, defective phagocytosis of microbes *(61)*, decreased oxygen radical production *(62)*, and compromised tumor necrosis factor-α (TNF-α) and leukotriene secretion *(63)*. GM-CSF-deficient mice displayed impaired pulmonary clearance of bacterial and fungal pathogens with abnormal cytokine responses *(61,62)*. These defects could be corrected by the intratracheal administration of GM-CSF or by the pulmonary expression of a GM-CSF transgene *(51–53)*. Recently, the transcription factor PU.1 was shown to be a critical mediator of GM-CSF signaling *(64)*. The ectopic expression of PU.1 in alveolar macrophages from GM-CSF-deficient mice reversed most of the defects examined *(64)*. Mutant mice also showed increased susceptibility to systemic challenge with *L. monocytogenes*, probably because of peritoneal macrophage and granulocyte abnormalities *(44,65)*.

3.7. Inflammation

GM-CSF$^{-/-}$ mice demonstrated an extensive pulmonary lymphoid hyperplasia around both airways and pulmonary veins *(39)*. Additionally, aggregates of mononuclear cells were sometimes found around intralobular vessels. Immunohistochemistry revealed the presence of mostly B220-positive cells, with smaller numbers of CD4- or CD8-positive T-cells *(39,40)*. The cause of the lymphoid hyperplasia remains unclear. Since infectious agents typically were not detected in the lungs of mice reared under specific-pathogen free conditions, the absence of GM-CSF may lead to an exaggerated response against innocuous inhaled antigens *(39)*. Indeed, normal alveolar macrophages inhibit mitogen-induced lymphocyte proliferation *(66)*, suggesting that abnormalities in immunoregulation might be involved.

Several defects in the immune response of GM-CSF-deficient mice were delineated. Reduced antigen-specific T-cell interferon-γ (IFN-γ) production and cytotoxicity and decreased antibody titers were found following immunization *(67,68)*. These defects rendered GM-CSF-deficient mice relatively resistant to the toxicities of lipopolysaccharide (LPS) and to the development of collagen-induced arthritis and experimental autoimmune encephalomyelitis *(69–71)*.

4. IL-3-Deficient Mice

4.1. The Disrupted IL-3 Allele

To generate a null allele of the IL-3 gene, our group introduced a neomycin-resistance cassette into the third exon of the IL-3 locus by homologous recombination in embryonic stem cells *(72)*. Homozygous deficient mice were identified by Southern analysis.

4.2. Phenotype

IL-3-deficient mice developed normally and appeared clinically healthy. Adult animals were fertile and produced normal-sized litters. Pathologic examination of IL-3-deficient mice revealed no abnormalities.

4.3. Hemopoiesis

Surprisingly, IL-3-deficient mice demonstrated no alterations in steady-state hematopoiesis and maintained normal numbers of mast cells *(72)*. Bone marrow cultures from IL-3-deficient mice did, however, yield fewer mast cells in response to stem cell factor (SCF) than controls *(73,74)*. Nonetheless, the daily subcutaneous injection of recombinant SCF elicited clear increases in mast cell numbers *in vivo*; in some tissues mast cell expansion was significantly greater (up to 140%) after treatment in IL-3-deficient mice than in controls *(74)*.

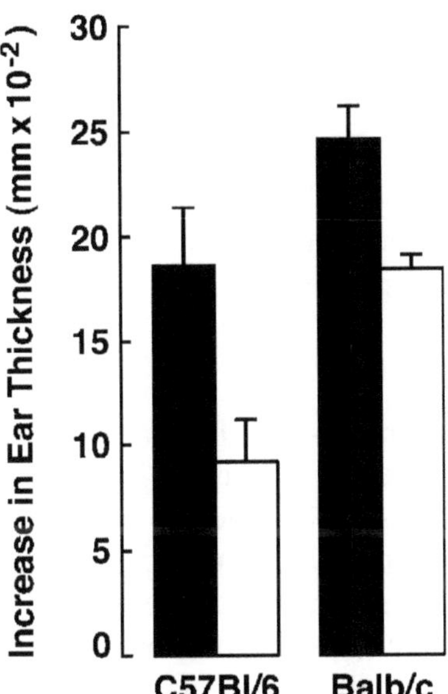

Fig. 3. Delayed-type hypersensitivity reactions, reprinted with permission from ref. *72*. Contact hypersensitivity reactions to oxazolone in wild-type (■) and IL-3-deficient (□) littermates.

4.4. Parasite Infection

IL-$3^{-/-}$ mice showed two striking abnormalities in response to infection with the intestinal nematode *Strongyloides venezuelensis*, a naturally occurring parasite of rodents. First, although baseline percentages of bone marrow basophils were comparable in IL-$3^{-/-}$ and wild-type mice, *S. venezuelensis* infection induced a significant increase in basophil levels in wild-type, but not IL-$3^{-/-}$ animals *(74)*. These findings revealed a requirement for IL-3 in the infection-induced expansion of basophils. Second, IL-3 contributed to a substantial proportion (about 76%) of the mast cell hyperplasia in the jejunum of infected mice *(74)*. Moreover, mice deficient in both IL-3 and c-kit signaling displayed more severe defects in mast cell expansion and worm expulsion following *S. venezuelensis* infection than mice lacking either cytokine alone *(74)*.

4.5. Delayed-Type Hypersensitivity

To evaluate the potential role of IL-3 in T-cell-dependent immunity, we compared the abilities of wild-type and mutant animals to develop contact hypersensitivity to epicutaneously applied oxazolone *(72)*. Contact hypersensitivity is a form of delayed-type hypersensitivity in which hapten-protein conjugates formed in the skin are presented by epidermal Langerhans cells, following their migration to regional lymph nodes, to hapten-specific CD4-positive and CD8-positive T-lymphocytes *(75–77)*. Sensitized T-cells initiate a local inflammatory response in the skin upon secondary hapten challenge. Although IL-3-deficient mice were indistinguishable from wild-type littermates in the magnitude of their immunologically nonspecific response to initial hapten challenge, they exhibited significantly compromised reactivity upon secondary hapten challenge, as measured by ear swelling (Fig. 3). In wild-type animals, the inflammatory response was characterized by an intense cellular infiltrate consisting predominantly of neutrophils, lymphocytes, and eosinophils, as well as substantial dermal edema, hyperkeratosis, and focal intraepidermal abscesses. IL-3-deficient animals, in contrast, developed a dramatically less intense cellular infiltrate, although the cellular composition was similar to that of wild-type animals. IL-3-deficient mice also demonstrated less edema, fewer and smaller intraepidermal abscesses, and little keratinocyte activation. The number of Langerhans cells in the skin of untreated IL-3-deficient mice, as determined by immunofluorescence staining of MHC class II positive cells in epidermal ear sheets, was comparable, however, to that of wild-type controls.

5. β_c-Deficient Mice

The cloning of the receptors for GM-CSF, IL-3, and IL-5 revealed a common signaling chain (β_c) coupled with cytokine-specific α-subunits *(78,79)*. Murine IL-3 also signals through a second chain, β_{IL3}, which shows 91% homology to β_c *(80,81)*. β_c-deficient mice were thus unresponsive to GM-CSF and IL-5, whereas the retention of β_{IL3} preserved IL-3 function *(82,83)*. β_c-deficient mice manifested defects that were similar to those revealed in GM-CSF- or IL-5-deficient mice *(84)*. β_c knockout animals developed pulmonary alveolar proteinosis *(82,83)*, although subtle differences in surfactant homeostasis were noted compared with GM-CSF mutant mice *(82,85)*. Interestingly, the transplantation of wild-type bone marrow into β_c-deficient mice corrected the alveolar proteinosis, establishing a critical role for alveolar macrophages in the surfactant accumulation *(86)*. Indeed, abnormalities in β_c-deficient peritoneal cells were also delineated *(87)*. β_c knockout mice showed reduced numbers of eosinophils, consistent with a crucial role for IL-5 in stimulating eosinophil production *(88)*. The animals also failed to mount an eosinophil response following infection with the nematode *Nippostrongylus brasiliensis (82)*. In contrast to these findings, mice deficient in β_{IL3} did not manifest significant abnormalities, consistent with the preservation of IL-3 function through β_c signaling *(82,89)*.

6. Compound Deficiencies of Colony Stimulating Factors

6.1. Mice Deficient in G-CSF and GM-CSF

G-CSF-deficient mice were interbred with GM-CSF-deficient mice to generate double knockouts *(90)*. Newborn animals manifested a greater degree of neutropenia compared with single G-CSF knockouts, and this was associated with increased mortality. In contrast, adult doubly deficient mice showed similar neutrophil numbers as G-CSF-deficient animals *(90)*. These findings revealed a selective role for GM-CSF in maintaining neutrophil numbers in young G-CSF-deficient mice.

6.2. Mice Deficient in GM-CSF and IL-3

To study the impact of dual GM-CSF and IL-3 ablation, without a concurrent loss in IL-5 signaling (which was the case in IL-3/β_c knockouts; see below), our group generated mice lacking both GM-CSF and IL-3 *(91)*. Because these genes are separated by only 14 kb on chromosome 11 *(92)*, doubly deficient mice could not be obtained by interbreeding single knockout animals. Thus, mice lacking both cytokines were generated through sequential gene targeting in embryonic stem cells. A hygromycin cassette replacing exons 3 and 4 of the GM-CSF locus was introduced by homologous recombination into IL-3 heterozygous deficient embryonic stem cells *(91)*.

Homozygous GM-CSF/IL-3-deficient mice were obtained at the expected frequencies and were clinically healthy. Pathologic examination of 2–4-mo-old mutant mice revealed abnormalities restricted to the lungs that were similar to those found in the GM-CSF-deficient animals *(42,91)*. Hematocrits, total circulating white blood cells, and platelets were normal in GM-CSF/IL-3-deficient mice. Surprisingly, examination of stained blood smears revealed that circulating eosinophils were increased (about four times) in doubly deficient mice, com-pared with single knockouts and wild-type controls *(91)*. The eosinophilia required IL-5 function, as mice lacking GM-CSF, IL-3, and β_c showed reduced numbers of eosinophils comparable to IL-5-deficient mice *(91)*. Although GM-CSF/IL-3-deficient mice were indistinguishable from wild-type littermates in the initial reaction to oxazolone challenge, they exhibited a strongly reduced response on secondary challenge, as measured by ear swelling. The degree of compromise was significantly greater than that for IL-3-deficient mice *(72,91)*.

6.3. Mice Deficient in GM-CSF and M-CSF

To delineate possible overlapping roles for GM-CSF and M-CSF in regulating the proliferation and function of monocyte/macrophages, Lieschke and colleagues *(93)* crossed GM-CSF knockout mice with *op/op* mice. These latter animals have a naturally occurring point mutation in the M-CSF gene that results in a truncated, biologically crippled protein *(94,95)*. *op/op* mice manifested a severe deficiency of macrophages and osteoclasts, resulting in excessive bone formation, occlusion of the marrow cavity, and reduced marrow hemopoietic activity *(96,97)*. Interestingly, the osteopetrosis and hemopoietic defects of *op/op* mice attenuated with age *(98–100)*. Mice doubly deficient in GM-CSF and M-CSF showed a significantly higher mortality than either single knockout. Severe bacterial pneumonia commonly resulted in death, and the alveolar proteinosis appeared worse than in GM-CSF single knockouts *(93)*. Despite the severe pulmonary pathology, however, doubly deficient mice produced circulating monocytes and tissue macrophages, demonstrating that additional factors regulate the formation of this lineage.

6.4. Mice Deficient in GM-CSF or IL-3 and the Erythropoietin Receptor

Erythropoietin (EPO) and its receptor (EpoR) are critical for definitive erythropoiesis, as mice lacking either gene product died during embryogenesis with severe anemia *(101–103)*. Mice retaining one functional allele of the EpoR also manifested lower hematocrits and increased mortality in response to phenylhydrazine-induced anemia *(104)*. $EpoR^{+/-}$ erythroid colony-forming units (CFU-E) demonstrated attenuated responses to EPO. To evaluate a potential interaction between EPO and GM-CSF or IL-3, $EpoR^{+/-}$ mice were interbred with $GM\text{-}CSF^{-/-}$ and $IL\text{-}3^{-/-}$ animals *(104)*. The compound knockouts displayed a further reduction in CFU-E, indicating that GM-CSF and IL-3 cooperate with EPO to promote erythropoiesis *(104)*.

6.5. Mice Deficient in IL-3 and β_c

Since β_c-deficient mice retain the β_{IL3} subunit, IL-3 function is preserved. To clarify the role of the entire IL-3/GM-CSF/IL-5 system in hematopoiesis in vivo, the β_c mutant mice were crossed with IL-3-deficient mice *(105)*. The compound knockout mice were clinically healthy and fertile. They showed comparable lung pathology to $GM\text{-}CSF^{-/-}$ mice and similar defects in steady-state and parasite-induced eosinophil production as IL-5 deficient mice *(105)*. The kinetics of bone marrow recovery after 5-fluorouracil administration was also similar to that of wild-type controls, indicating that the IL-3/GM-CSF/IL-5 axis is dispensable for hematopoiesis *(105)*.

6.6. Mice Deficient in IL-3 and c-Mpl

Mice deficient in thrombopoietin (TPO) or its receptor c-Mpl display impaired platelet development and reduced hematopoitic progenitors *(106–108)*. Although administration of IL-3 stimulates megakaryocytopoiesis *(20)*, IL-3/c-Mpl compound knockout mice displayed no greater deficiencies in megakaryocytes or platelets than c-Mpl-mutant animals *(109)*. These findings indicate that IL-3 does not contribute to the residual megakaryocytopoiesis in the absence of c-Mpl *(109)*.

Conclusions

The generation of mice singly and multiply deficient in G-CSF, GM-CSF, and IL-3 revealed unique physiologic roles for each cytokine. G-CSF-deficient mice manifested a chronic neutropenia, establishing this CSF as a critical regulator of granulopoiesis in vivo. Whereas GM-CSF-deficient mice maintained normal hematopoiesis, they developed a lung disorder resembling human PAP. Clinical investigations revealed defects in the GM-CSF pathway in many patients with the disorder, and the administration of recombinant protein has induced substantial clinical benefits. IL-3-deficient mice mounted impaired basophil and mast cell responses to parasite infection and displayed compromised contact hypersensitivity. Compound cytokine knockouts have provided evidence for redundancy and complementarity of cytokine function. As CSF knockout mice are interbred with other growth factor-deficient animals, a more detailed understanding of the cytokine network will emerge.

Acknowledgments

We thank the Medical Arts Department of the Dana-Farber Cancer Institute and Ashley Dunn (Ludwig Institute for Cancer Research, Melbourne) for permission to reprint Fig. 1. We also thank the staff of the Redstone Animal Facility for maintenance of the mouse colony. This work was supported by the Hanne Liebermann Foundation, Zurich, Switzerland (T.E.) and the Cancer Research Institute/Partridge Foundation, grants CA74886 and CA39542 (G.D.). G.D. is a Clinical Scholar of the Leukemia and Lymphoma Society.

References

1. Metcalf, D. (1993) Hematopoietic regulators: redundancy or subtlety? *Blood* **82,** 3515–3523.
2. Demetri, G. D. and Griffin, J. D. (1991) Granulocyte colony-stimulating factor and its receptor. *Blood* **78,** 2791–808.
3. Moore, M. A., Welte, K., Gabrilove, J., and Souza, L. M. (1987) Biological activities of recombinant human granulocyte colony stimulating factor (rhG-CSF) and tumor necrosis factor: in vivo and in vitro analysis. In: Neth, R., et al., eds. *Haematology and Blood Transfusion.* Springer-Verlag, Berlin.
4. Tamura, M., Hattori, K., Namura, H., et al. (1987) Induction of neutrophilic granulocytosis in mice by administration of purified human native granulocyte colony-stimulating factor (G-CSF). *Biochem. Biophys. Res. Commun.* **142,** 454–660.
5. Pojda, Z., Molineux, G., and Dexter, T. M. (1990) Hemopoietic effects of short-term in vivo treatment of mice with various doses of rhG-CSF. *Exp. Hematol.* **18,** 27–31.

6. Chang, J. M., Metcalf, D., Gonda, T. J., and Johnson, G. R. (1989) Long-term exposure to retrovirally expressed granulocyte-colony-stimulating factor induces a nonneoplastic granulocytic and progenitor cell hyperplasia without tissue damage in mice. *J. Clin. Invest.* **84,** 1488–1496.
7. Watari, K., Asano, S., Shirafuji, N., et al. (1989) Serum granulocyte colony-stimulating factor levels in healthy volunteers and patients with various disorders as estimated by enzyme immunoassay. *Blood* **73,** 117–122.
8. Mempel, K., Pietsch, T., Menzel, T., Seidler, C., and Welte, K. (1991) Increased serum levels of granulocyte colony-stimulating factor in patients with severe congenital neutropenia. *Blood* **77,** 1919–1922.
9. Gasson, J. C., Weisbart, R. H., Kaufman, S. E., et al. (1984) Purified human granulocyte-macrophage colony-stimulating factor: direct action on neutrophils. *Science* **226,** 1339–1342.
10. Cannistra, S. A. and Griffin, J. D. (1988) Regulation of the production and function of granulocytes and monocytes. *Semin. Hematol.* **25,** 173–188.
11. Caux, C., Massacrier, C., Vanbervliet, B., et al. (1996) CD34+ hematopoietic progenitors from human cord blood differentiate along two independent dendritic cell pathways in response to GM-CSF+TNF alpha. *J. Exp. Med.* **184,** 695–706.
12. Lopez, A. F., Williamson, D. J., Gamble, J. R., et al. (1986) Recombinant human granulocyte-macrophage colony-stimulating factor stimulates in vitro mature human neutrophil and eosinophil function, surface receptor expression, and survival. *J. Clin. Invest.* **78,** 1220–1228.
13. Ferrero, D., Tarella, C., Badoni, R., et al. (1989) Granulocyte-macrophage colony-stimulating factor requires interaction with accessory cells or granulocyte-colony stimulating factor for full stimulation of human myeloid progenitors. *Blood* **73,** 402–405.
14. Lang, R. A., Metcalf, D., Cuthbertson, R. A., et al. (1987) Transgenic mice expressing a hemopoietic growth factor gene (GM-CSF) develop accumulations of macrophages, blindness, and a fatal syndrome of tissue damage. *Cell* **51,** 675–686.
15. Johnson, G. R., Gonda, T. J., Metcalf, D., Hariharan, I. K., and Cory, S. (1989) A lethal myeloproliferative syndrome in mice transplanted with bone marrow cells infected with a retrovirus expressing granulocyte-macrophage colony stimulating factor. *EMBO J.* **8,** 441–448.
16. Dranoff, G., Jaffee, E., Lazenby, A., et al. (1993) Vaccination with irradiated tumor cells engineered to secrete murine granulocyte-macrophage colony-stimulating factor stimulates potent, specific, and long-lasting anti-tumor immunity. *Proc. Natl. Acad. Sci. USA* **90,** 3539–3543.
17. Rennick, D. M., Lee, F. D., Yokota, T., Arai, K. I., Cantor, H., and Nobel, G. J. (1985) A cloned MCGF cDNA encodes a multilineage hematopoietic growth factor: multiple activities of interleukin 3. *J. Immunol.* **134,** 910–914.
18. Suda, T., Suda, T., Ogawa, M., and Ihle, J. N. (1985) Permissive role of interleukin 3 (IL-3) in proliferation and differentiation of multipotential hemopoietic progenitors in culture. *J. Cell. Physiol.* **124,** 182–190.
19. Caux, C., Vanberbliet, B., Massacrier, C., Durand, I., and Banchereau, J. (1996) Interleukin-3 cooperates with tumor necrosis factor alpha for the development of human dendritic/Langerhans cells from cord blood CD34+ hematopoietic progenitor cells. *Blood* **87,** 2376–2385.
20. Metcalf, D., Beley, C. G., Johnson, G. R., Nicola, N. A., Lopez, A. F., and Williamson, D. J.. (1986) Effects of purified bacterially synthesized murine multi-CSF (IL-3) on hematopoiesis in normal adult mice. *Blood* **68,** 46–57.
21. Kindler, V., Thorens, B., de Kossodo, S., et al. (1986) Stimulation of hematopoiesis in vivo by recombinant bacterial murine interleukin 3. *Proc. Natl. Acad. Sci. USA* **83,** 1001–1005.
22. Donahue, R. E., Seehra, J., Metzger, M., et al. (1988) Human IL-3 and GM-CSF act synergistically in stimulating hematopoiesis in primates. *Science* **241,** 1820–1823.
23. Gianella-Borradori, A. (1994) Present and future clinical relevance of interleukin 3. *Stem Cells* **12(Suppl. 1),** 241–248.
24. Rothenberg, M. E., Owen, W. F. Jr., Silberstein, D. S., et al. (1988) Human eosinophils have prolonged survival, enhanced functional properties, and become hypodense when exposed to human interleukin 3. *J. Clin. Invest.* **81,** 1986–1992.
25. Kimoto, M., Kinder, V., Higaki, M., Ody, C., Izui, S., and Vassalli, P. (1988) Recombinant murine IL-3 fails to stimulate T or B lymphopoiesis in vivo, but enhances immune responses to T cell-dependent antigens. *J. Immunol.* **140,** 1889–1894.

26. Cannistra, S. A., Vellenga, E., Groshek, P., Rambaldi, A., and Griffin, J. D. (1988) Human granulocyte-monocyte colony-stimulating factor and interleukin 3 stimulate monocyte cytotoxicity through a tumor necrosis factor-dependent mechanism. *Blood* **71,** 672–676.
27. Madden, K. B., Urban, J. F. Jr., Ziltener, H. J., Shcrader, J. W., Finkelman, F. D., and Katona, I. M. (1991) Antibodies to IL-3 and IL-4 suppress helminth-induced intestinal mastocytosis. *J. Immunol.* **147,** 1387–1391.
28. Pulaski, B. A., Yeh, K. Y., Shastri, N., et al. (1996) Interleukin 3 enhances cytotoxic T lymphocyte development and class I major histocompatibility complex "re-presentation" of exogenous antigen by tumor-infiltrating antigen-presenting cells. *Proc. Natl. Acad. Sci. USA* **93,** 3669–3674.
29. Buchberg, A. M., Bedigian, H. G., Taylor, B. A., et al. (1988) Localization of Evi-2 to chromosome 11: linkage to other protooncogene and growth factor loci using interspecific backcross mice. *Oncogene Res.* **2,** 149–165.
30. Buchberg, A. M., Brownell, E., Nagata, S. Jenkins, N. A., and Copeland, N. G. (1989) A comprehensive genetic map of murine chromosome 11 reveals extensive linkage conservation between mouse and human. *Genetics* **122,** 153–161.
31. Barlow, D. P., Bucan, M., Lehrach, H., Hogan, B. L, and Gough, N. M. (1987) Close genetic and physical linkage between the murine haemopoietic growth factor genes GM-CSF and Multi-CSF (IL3). *EMBO J.* **6,** 617–623.
32. Lieschke, G. J., Grail, D., Hodgson, G., et al. (1994) Mice lacking granulocyte colony-stimulating factor have chronic neutropenia, granulocyte and macrophage progenitor cell deficiency, and impaired neutrophil mobilization. *Blood* **84,** 1737–1746.
33. Metcalf, D., Lindeman, G. J., and Nicola, N. A. (1995) Analysis of hematopoiesis in max 41 transgenic mice that exhibit sustained elevations of blood granulocytes and monocytes. *Blood* **85,** 2364–2370.
34. Lieschke, G. J. and Dunn, A. R. (1992) Physiologic role of granulocyte colony stimulating factor: insights from in vivo studies. In: Abraham, N. G., et al., ed. *Molecular Biology of Haematopoiesis.* Andover, Hants, UK, p. 201.
35. Layton, J. E., Hockman, H., Sheridan, W. P., and Morstyn, G. (1989) Evidence for a novel in vivo control mechanism of granulopoiesis: mature cell-related control of a regulatory growth factor. *Blood* **74,** 1303–1307.
36. Basu, S., Hodgson, G., Katz, M., and Dunn, A. R. (2002) Evaluation of role of G-CSF in the production, survival, and release of neutrophils from bone marrow into circulation. *Blood* **100,** 854–861.
37. Stanley, E., Metcalf, D., Sobieszczuk, P., Gough, N. M., and Dunn, A. R. (1985) The structure and expression of the murine gene encoding granulocyte-macrophage colony stimulating factor: evidence for utilisation of alternative promoters. *EMBO J.* **4,** 2569–2573.
38. Miyatake, S., Otsuka, T., Yokota, T., Lee, F., and Arai, K. (1985) Structure of the chromosomal gene for granulocyte-macrophage colony stimulating factor: comparison of the mouse and human genes. *EMBO J.* **4,** 2561–2568.
39. Dranoff, G., Crawford, A. D., Sadelain, M., et al. (1994) Involvement of granulocyte-macrophage colony-stimulating factor in pulmonary homeostasis. *Science* **264,** 713–716.
40. Stanley, E., Lieschke, G. J., Grail, D., et al. (1994) Granulocyte/macrophage colony-stimulating factor-deficient mice show no major perturbation of hematopoiesis but develop a characteristic pulmonary pathology. *Proc. Natl. Acad. Sci. USA* **91,** 5592–5596.
41. Robertson, S. A., Roberts, C. T., Farr, K. L., Dunn, A. R., and Seamark, R. F. (1999) Fertility impairment in granulocyte-macrophage colony-stimulating factor-deficient mice. *Biol. Reprod.* **60,** 251–261.
42. Dranoff, G. and Mulligan, R. C. (1994) Activities of granulocyte-macrophage colony-stimulating factor revealed by gene transfer and gene knockout studies. *Stem Cells* **12(Suppl. 1),** 173–182; discussion 182–184.
43. Vremec, D., Lieschke, G. J., Dunn, A. R., Robb, L., Metcalf, D., and Shortman, K. (1997) The influence of granulocyte/macrophage colony-stimulating factor on dendritic cell levels in mouse lymphoid organs. *Eur. J. Immunol.* **27,** 40–44.

44. Zhan, Y., Lieschke, G. J., Grail, D., Dunn, A. R., and Cheers, C. (1998) Essential roles for granulocyte-macrophage colony-stimulating factor (GM-CSF) and G-CSF in the sustained hematopoietic response of *Listeria monocytogenes*-infected mice. *Blood* **91,** 863–869.
45. Wright, J. R. and Clements, J. A. (1987) Metabolism and turnover of lung surfactant. *Am. Rev. Respir. Dis.* **136,** 426–444.
46. Wright, J. R. and Dobbs, L. G. (1991) Regulation of pulmonary surfactant secretion and clearance. *Annu. Rev. Physiol.* **53,** 395–414.
47. Ikegami, M., Hull, W. M., Yoshida, M., Wert, S. E., and Whitsett, J. A. (2001) SP-D and GM-CSF regulate surfactant homeostasis via distinct mechanisms. *Am. J. Physiol. Lung Cell. Mol. Physiol.* **281,** L697–L703.
48. Rosen, S. H., Castleman, B., and Liebow, A. A. (1958) Pulmonary alveolar proteinosis. *N. Engl. J. Med.* **258,** 1123–1142.
49. Yoshida, M., Ikegami, M., Reed, J. A., Chroneos, Z. C., and Whitsett, J. A. (2001) GM-CSF regulates protein and lipid catabolism by alveolar macrophages. *Am. J. Physiol. Lung Cell. Mol. Physiol.* **280,** L379–L386.
50. Ikegami, M., Veda, T., Hull, W., et al. (1996) Surfactant metabolism in transgenic mice after granulocyte macrophage-colony stimulating factor ablation. *Am. J. Physiol.* **270,** L650–L658.
51. Huffman, J. A., Hull, W. M., Dranoff, G., Mulligan, R. C., and Whitsett, J. A. (1996) Pulmonary epithelial cell expression of GM-CSF corrects the alveolar proteinosis in GM-CSF-deficient mice. *J. Clin. Invest.* **97,** 649–655.
52. Zsengeller, Z. K., Reed, J. A., Bachurski, C. J. et al. (1998) Adenovirus-mediated granulocyte-macrophage colony-stimulating factor improves lung pathology of pulmonary alveolar proteinosis in granulocyte-macrophage colony-stimulating factor-deficient mice. *Hum. Gene Ther.* **9,** 2101–2109.
53. Reed, J. A., Ikegami, M., Cianciolo, E. R., et al. (1999) Aerosolized GM-CSF ameliorates pulmonary alveolar proteinosis in GM-CSF-deficient mice. *Am. J. Physiol.* **276(4 Pt 1),** L556–L563.
54. Kitamura, T., Tanaka, N., Watanabe, J., et al. (1999) Idiopathic pulmonary alveolar proteinosis as an autoimmune disease with neutralizing antibody against granulocyte/macrophage colony-stimulating factor. *J. Exp. Med.* **190,** 875–880.
55. Dirksen, U., Nishinakamura, R., Groneck, P., et al. (1997) Human pulmonary alveolar proteinosis associated with a defect in GM-CSF/IL-3/IL-5 receptor common beta chain expression. *J. Clin. Invest.* **100,** 2211–2217.
56. Tchou-Wong, K. M., Harkin, T. J., Chi, C., Bodkin, M., and Rom, W. N. (1997) GM-CSF gene expression is normal but protein release is absent in a patient with pulmonary alveolar proteinosis. *Am. J. Respir. Crit. Care Med.* **156,** 1999–2002.
57. Thomassen, M. J., Yi, T., Raychaudhuri, B., Malur, A., and Kavuru, M. S. (2000) Pulmonary alveolar proteinosis is a disease of decreased availability of GM-CSF rather than an intrinsic cellular defect. *Clin. Immunol.* **95,** 85–92.
58. Barraclough, R. M. and Gillies, A. J. (2001) Pulmonary alveolar proteinosis: a complete response to GM-CSF therapy. *Thorax* **56,** 664–665.
59. Kavuru, M. S., Sullivan, E. J., Piccin, R., Thomassen, M. J., and Stoller, J. K. (2000) Exogenous granulocyte-macrophage colony-stimulating factor administration for pulmonary alveolar proteinosis. *Am. J. Respir. Crit. Care Med.* **161,** 1143–1148.
60. Seymour, J. F., Dunn, A. R., Vincetn, J. M., Presneill, J. J., and Pain, M. C. (1996) Efficacy of granulocyte-macrophage colony-stimulating factor in acquired alveolar proteinosis. *N. Engl. J. Med.* **335,** 1924–1925.
61. Paine, R. 3rd, Preston, A. M., Wilcoxen, S., et al. (2000) Granulocyte-macrophage colony-stimulating factor in the innate immune response to *Pneumocystis carinii* pneumonia in mice. *J. Immunol.* **164,** 2602–2609.
62. LeVine, A. M., Reed, J. A., Kurak, K. E., Cianciolo, E., and Whitsett, J. A. (1999) GM-CSF-deficient mice are susceptible to pulmonary group B streptococcal infection. *J. Clin. Invest.* **103,** 563–569.
63. Paine, R. 3rd, Morris, S. B., Jin, H., et al. (2001) Impaired functional activity of alveolar macrophages from GM-CSF-deficient mice. *Am. J. Physiol. Lung Cell. Mol. Physiol.* **281,** L1210–L1218.

64. Shibata, Y., Berclaz, P. Y., Chroneos, Z. C., Yoshida, M., Whitsett, J. A., and Trapnell, B. C. (2001) GM-CSF regulates alveolar macrophage differentiation and innate immunity in the lung through PU.1. *Immunity* **15,** 557–567.
65. Zhan, Y., Basu, S., Lieschke, G. J., Grail, D., Dunn, A. R., and Cheers, C. (1999) Functional deficiencies of peritoneal cells from gene-targeted mice lacking G-CSF or GM-CSF. *J. Leukoc. Biol.* **65,** 256–264.
66. Bilyk, N. and Holt, P. G. (1993) Inhibition of the immunosuppressive activity of resident pulmonary alveolar macrophages by granulocyte/macrophage colony-stimulating factor. *J. Exp. Med.* **177,** 1773–1777.
67. Wada, H., Noguchi, Y., Marino, M. W., Dnn, A. R., and Old, L. J. (1997) T cell functions in granulocyte/macrophage colony-stimulating factor deficient mice. *Proc. Natl. Acad. Sci. USA* **94,** 12557–12561.
68. Noguchi, Y., Wada, H., Marino, M. W., and Old, L. J. (1998) Regulation of IFN-gamma production in granulocyte-macrophage colony-stimulating factor-deficient mice. *Eur. J. Immunol.* **28,** 3980–3988.
69. Campbell, I. K., Rich, M. J., Bischof, R. J., Dunn, A. R., Grail, D., and Hamilton, J. A. (1998) Protection from collagen-induced arthritis in granulocyte-macrophage colony-stimulating factor-deficient mice. *J. Immunol.* **161,** 3639–3644.
70. McQualter, J. L., Darwiche, R., Ewing, C., et al. (2001) Granulocyte macrophage colony-stimulating factor: a new putative therapeutic target in multiple sclerosis. *J. Exp. Med.* **194,** 873–882.
71. Basu, S., Dunn, A. R., Marino, M. W., et al. (1997) Increased tolerance to endotoxin by granulocyte-macrophage colony-stimulating factor-deficient mice. *J. Immunol.* **159,** 1412–1417.
72. Mach, N., Lantz, C. S., Galli, S. J., et al. (1998) Involvement of interleukin-3 in delayed-type hypersensitivity. *Blood* **91,** 778–783.
73. Galli, S. J., Zsebo, K. M., and Geissler, E. N. (1994) The kit ligand, stem cell factor. *Adv. Immunol.* **55,** 1–96.
74. Lantz, C. S., Boesiger, J., Song, C. H., et al. (1998) Role for interleukin-3 in mast-cell and basophil development and in immunity to parasites. *Nature* **392,** 90–93.
75. Eisen, H. N., Orris, L., and Belman, S. (1952) Elicitation of delayed allergic skin reactions with haptens: the dependence of elicitation on hapten combination with protein. *J. Exp. Med.* **95,** 473–475.
76. Silberberg, I., Baer, R. L., and Rosenthal, S. A. (1976) The role of Langerhans cells in allergic contact hypersensitivity. A review of findings in man and guinea pigs. *J. Invest. Dermatol.* **66,** 210–217.
77. Gocinski, B. L. and Tigelaar, R. E. (1990) Roles of CD4+ and CD8+ T cells in murine contact sensitivity revealed by in vivo monoclonal antibody depletion. *J. Immunol.* **144,** 4121–4128.
78. Kitamura, T., Onishi, M., Kinoshita, S., Shibuya, A., Miyajima, A., and Nolan G. P. (1991) Expression cloning of the human IL-3 receptor cDNA reveals a shared beta subunit for the human IL-3 and GM-CSF receptors. *Cell* **66,** 1165–1174.
79. Tavernier, J., Devos, R., Cornelis, S., et al. (1991) A human high affinity interleukin-5 receptor (IL5R) is composed of an IL5-specific alpha chain and a beta chain shared with the receptor for GM-CSF. *Cell* **66,** 1175–1184.
80. Itoh, N., Yonehara, S., Schreurs, J., et al. (1990) Cloning of an interleukin-3 receptor gene: a member of a distinct receptor gene family. *Science* **247,** 324–327.
81. Gorman, D. M., Itoh, N., Kitamura, T., et al. (1990) Cloning and expression of a gene encoding an interleukin 3 receptor-like protein: identification of another member of the cytokine receptor gene family. *Proc. Natl. Acad. Sci. USA* **87,** 5459–5463.
82. Nishinakamura, R., Nakayama, N., Hirabayashi, Y., et al. (1995) Mice deficient for the IL-3/GM-CSF/IL-5 beta c receptor exhibit lung pathology and impaired immune response, while beta IL3 receptor-deficient mice are normal. *Immunity* **2,** 211–222.
83. Robb, L., Drinkwater, C. C., Metcalf, D., et al. (1995) Hematopoietic and lung abnormalities in mice with a null mutation of the common beta subunit of the receptors for granulocyte-macrophage colony-stimulating factor and interleukins 3 and 5. *Proc. Natl. Acad. Sci. USA* **92,** 9565–9569.
84. Kopf, M., Brombacher, F., Hodgkin, P. D., et al. (1996) IL-5-deficient mice have a developmental defect in CD5+ B-1 cells and lack eosinophilia but have normal antibody and cytotoxic T cell responses. *Immunity* **4,** 15–24.

85. Reed, J. A., Ikegami, M., Robb, L., Begley, C. G., Ross, G., and Whitsett, J. A. (2000) Distinct changes in pulmonary surfactant homeostasis in common beta- chain- and GM-CSF-deficient mice. *Am. J. Physiol. Lung Cell. Mol. Physiol.* **278,** L1164–L1171.
86. Nishinakamura, R., Wiler, R., Dirksen, U., et al. (1996) The pulmonary alveolar proteinosis in granulocyte macrophage colony-stimulating factor/interleukins 3/5 beta c receptor-deficient mice is reversed by bone marrow transplantation. *J. Exp. Med.* **183,** 2657–2662.
87. Scott, C. L., Hughes, D. A., Cary, D., Nicola, N. A., Begley, C. G., and Robb, L. (1998) Functional analysis of mature hematopoietic cells from mice lacking the betac chain of the granulocyte-macrophage colony-stimulating factor receptor. *Blood* **92,** 4119–4127.
88. Yamaguchi, Y., Hayashi, Y., Sughama, Y., et al. (1988) Highly purified murine interleukin 5 (IL-5) stimulates eosinophil function and prolongs in vitro survival. IL-5 as an eosinophil chemotactic factor. *J. Exp. Med.* **167,** 1737–1742.
89. Nicola, N. A., Robb, L., Metcalf, D., Cary, D., Drinkwater, C. G., and Begley, C. G. (1996) Functional inactivation in mice of the gene for the interleukin-3 (IL-3)-specific receptor beta-chain: implications for IL-3 function and the mechanism of receptor transmodulation in hematopoietic cells. *Blood* **87,** 2665–2674.
90. Seymour, J. F., Lieschke, G. J., Grail, D., Quilici, C., Hodgson, G., and Dunn, A. R. (1997) Mice lacking both granulocyte colony-stimulating factor (CSF) and granulocyte-macrophage CSF have impaired reproductive capacity, perturbed neonatal granulopoiesis, lung disease, amyloidosis, and reduced long-term survival. *Blood* **90,** 3037–3049.
91. Gillessen, S., Mach, N., Small, C., Mihm, M., and Dranoff, G. (2001) Overlapping roles for granulocyte-macrophage colony-stimulating factor and interleukin-3 in eosinophil homeostasis and contact hypersensitivity. *Blood* **97,** 922–9928.
92. Lee, J. S. and Young, I. G. (1989) Fine-structure mapping of the murine IL-3 and GM-CSF genes by pulsed-field gel electrophoresis and molecular cloning. *Genomics* **5,** 359–362.
93. Lieschke, G. J., Stanley, E., Grail, D., et al. (1994) Mice lacking both macrophage- and granulocyte-macrophage colony-stimulating factor have macrophages and coexistent osteopetrosis and severe lung disease. *Blood* **84,** 27–35.
94. Wiktor-Jedrzejczak, W., Bartocci, A., Ferrante, A. W. Jr., et al. (1990) Total absence of colony-stimulating factor 1 in the macrophage-deficient osteopetrotic (op/op) mouse. *Proc. Natl. Acad. Sci. USA* **87,** 4828–4832.
95. Yoshida, H., Hayashi, S., Kunisada, T., et al. (1990) The murine mutation osteopetrosis is in the coding region of the macrophage colony stimulating factor gene. *Nature* **345,** 442–444.
96. Marks, S. C. Jr. and Lane, P. W. (1976) Osteopetrosis, a new recessive skeletal mutation on chromosome 12 of the mouse. *J. Hered.* **67,** 11–18.
97. Wiktor-Jedrzejczak, W. W., Ahmed, A., Szczylik, C., and Skelly, R. R. (1982) Hematological characterization of congenital osteopetrosis in op/op mouse. Possible mechanism for abnormal macrophage differentiation. *J. Exp. Med.* **156,** 1516–1527.
98. Begg, S. K., Radley, J. M., Pllard, J. W., Chisholm, O. T., Stanley, E. R., and Bertoncello, I. (1993) Delayed hematopoietic development in osteopetrotic (op/op) mice. *J. Exp. Med.* **177,** 237–242.
99. Begg, S. K. and Bertoncello, I. (1993) The hematopoietic deficiencies in osteopetrotic (op/op) mice are not permanent, but progressively correct with age. *Exp. Hematol.* **21,** 493–495.
100. Nilsson, S. K. and Bertoncello, I. (1994) Age-related changes in extramedullary hematopoiesis in the spleen of normal and perturbed osteopetrotic (op/op) mice. *Exp. Hematol.* **22,** 377–383.
101. Wu, H., Liu, X., Jaenisch, R., and Lodish, H. F. (1995) Generation of committed erythroid BFU-E and CFU-E progenitors does not require erythropoietin or the erythropoietin receptor. *Cell* **83,** 59–67.
102. Lin, C. S., Lim, S. K., D'Agati, V., and Constantini, F. (1996) Differential effects of an erythropoietin receptor gene disruption on primitive and definitive erythropoiesis. *Genes Dev.* **10,** 154–164.
103. Wu, H., Lee, S. H., Gao, J., Liu, X., and Iruela-Arispe, M. L. (1999) Inactivation of erythropoietin leads to defects in cardiac morphogenesis. *Development* **126,** 3597–3605.
104. Jegalian, A. G., Acurio, A., Dranoff, G., and Wu, H. (2002) Erythropoietin receptor haploinsufficiency and in vivo interplay with granulocyte-macrophage colony-stimulating factor and interleukin 3. *Blood* **99,** 2603–2605.

105. Nishinakamura, R., Miyajima, A., Mee, P. J., Tybulewicz, V. L., and Murray, R. (1996) Hematopoiesis in mice lacking the entire granulocyte-macrophage colony-stimulating factor/interleukin-3/interleukin-5 functions. *Blood* **88,** 2458–2464.
106. Gurney, A. L., Carver-Moore, K., de Sauvage, F. J., and Moore, M. W. (1994) Thrombocytopenia in c-mpl-deficient mice. *Science* **265,** 1445–1447.
107. Alexander, W. S., Roberts, A. W., Nicola, N. A., Li, R., and Metcalf, D. (1996) Deficiencies in progenitor cells of multiple hematopoietic lineages and defective megakaryocytopoiesis in mice lacking the thrombopoietic receptor c-Mpl. *Blood* **87,** 2162–2170.
108. de Sauvage, F. J., Carver-Moore, K., Luoh, S. M., et al. (1996) Physiological regulation of early and late stages of megakaryocytopoiesis by thrombopoietin. *J. Exp. Med.* **183,** 651–656.
109. Gainsford, T., Roberts, A. W., Kimura, S., et al. (1998) Cytokine production and function in c-mpl-deficient mice: no physiologic role for interleukin-3 in residual megakaryocyte and platelet production. *Blood* **91,** 2745–2752.

11

IL-4 Knockout Mice

Pascale Kropf and Ingrid Müller

Summary

The pleiotropic cytokine interleukin-4 is a major regulator of the immune system. It has a multitude of biological effects, and participates in protective as well as in pathological responses. IL-4 can affect a variety of cells in multiple ways by regulating antibody production, hematopoiesis, the development of effector T-helper cell responses, and inflammatory responses. Therefore, IL-4-deficient mice are a powerful tool to assess the role of IL-4 in vivo in different experimental animal models. Here we review studies using genetically different strains of IL-4-deficient mice infected with a variety of parasites and assess the importance of the genetic background of the mice. In addition, we discuss the biological importance of IL-4 in targeting class switching to particular classes in B-cells and in different models of allergic asthma. Finally, a possible role of IL-4 as an immunoregulatory cytokine is discussed.

Key words

IL-4, immune response, Th1/Th2, parasites, protection/pathology; immunoregulation

1. Introduction

Interleukin 4 (IL-4) is a pleiotropic cytokine that plays a critical role in the regulation of the immune system; it exerts its biologic activities on B- and T-cells, as well as many nonlymphoid cells including monocytes, endothelial cells, and fibroblasts. IL-4 is mainly derived from a subset of activated CD4+ T-helper (Th) 2 cells *(1)* and is also produced by basophils *(2)*, mast cells *(3)*, eosinophils *(4)*, NK1.1$^-$/CD4+ T-cells *(5)*, NK1.1+/CD4+ T-cells *(4)*, and γδ T-cells *(6)*. IL-4 was first described as a cofactor in the proliferation of resting B-cells *(7)* and exerts different effects on B-cells at distinct stages in the cell cycle. It has been shown to increase the expression of MHC class II on resting B-cells *(8)* and to drive their clonal expansion selectively *(9)*. In addition, IL-4 preferentially induces immunoglobulin isotype switching to IgG1 and IgE *(10)*.

IL-4 is the hallmark cytokine secreted by polarized CD4+ Th2 cells. Antigen recognition in the presence of appropriate costimulatory signals can induce naive CD4+ Th cells to differentiate into functionally distinct subsets, Th1 and Th2 *(11,12)*. These two Th cell subsets can be classified by the cytokine pattern they secrete; Th1 cells produce IL-2, interferon-γ (IFN-γ), and tumor necrosis factor-β (TNF-β), and Th2 cells produce IL-4, IL-5, IL-6, IL-10, and IL-13. Th2 cells favor humoral immune responses, contributing to the resolution of a variety of helminth infections, but also to atopy in susceptible individuals and to the severe, nonhealing forms of leishmaniasis *(1,13)*.

From: *Contemporary Immunology: Cytokine Knockouts, 2nd Edition*
Edited by: Giamila Fantuzzi © Humana Press Inc., Totowa, NJ

One of the important influences on the differentiation of mature uncommitted cells into Th2 cells is thought to be exerted by the cytokine environment itself. IL-4 has been demonstrated to have the greatest influence in driving Th2 differentiation *(14)*, and IL-4-secreting Th2 cells suppress the expansion of Th1 cells *(15)*. The ability of CD4+ T-cells to produce IL-4 upon restimulation correlates directly with the concentration of exogenous IL-4 added to primary cultures, IFN-γ-producing Th cells being suppressed at the higher doses of IL-4 *(14)*. To assess the biologic functions of IL-4 in vivo, a widely used strategy is to inject anticytokine and/or anticytokine receptor monoclonal antibodies (MAbs) into experimental animals *(16–20)*. For example, in the experimental model of cutaneous leishmaniasis, the crucial role of IL-4 during progressive, nonhealing disease was demonstrated by injections of neutralizing anticytokine MAb in vivo: a nonhealing strain of mice treated with anti-IL-4 MAb could control the replication of *Leishmania* parasites, resolve the cutaneous lesions, and switch from a detrimental Th2 response to a protective Th1 response *(20)*.

2. IL-4-Deficient Mice

The major disadvantage to injecting neutralizing MAb in vivo is that one cannot be absolutely sure that the MAb completely blocks the action of the cytokine. Indeed, a study by Finkelman et al. *(21)* showed that anticytokine antibodies can act as carrier proteins in vivo and can prolong the half-life of the cytokine. The alteration of genes in embryonic stem (ES) cell lines represents an alternative strategy for analyzing gene functions *in vivo*. The manipulated ES cells can be reintroduced into blastocysts and can repopulate mouse tissue, including the germline. IL-4-deficient (IL-4$^{-/-}$) mice were generated by targeting the IL-4 gene in murine ES cells *(22)*. These mice provide a powerful tool for assessing the role of IL-4 in vivo in a multitude of experimental animal models. The first IL-4$^{-/-}$ mice were generated by targeting the IL-4 gene in ES cells derived from the mouse strain 129/Sv: ES cell clones carrying the mutation were injected into blastocysts from C57BL/6 mice, and the resulting chimeras were mated to C57BL/6 mice. The hybrids (129/Sv × C57BL/6) were interbred to obtain mice homozygous for the disrupted IL-4 (gene) *(22,23)*.

Although effective, targeting of the IL-4 gene in ES cells from 129/Sv mice has its disadvantages since mice from this strain are genetically resistant to a wide variety of infectious diseases including leishmaniasis *(24)*, schistosomiasis *(25)* and murine (M)AIDS *(26)*. In contrast, BALB/c mice are susceptible to a number of diseases such as leishmaniasis *(13,27)* and intestinal nematodes *(28)*. Thus, in order to analyze the influence of IL-4 on a background that is susceptible to the disease of interest, it is necessary to backcross the mice. To avoid the use of mice with mixed susceptible and resistant genetic backgrounds and time-consuming backcrossing of 129/Sv × C57BL/6 mice onto the BALB/c background, Noben-Trauth and colleagues *(29)* generated genetically pure IL-4-deficient mice by using ES cells derived from BALB/c mice. Similarly, genetically pure C57BL/6 mice were generated by disrupting the IL-4 gene in ES cells derived from C57BL/6 mice *(29)*.

2.1. Phenotype of IL-4-Deficient Mice

All the strains of IL-4-deficient mice reported on here *(22,23,29)* display a normal phenotype, and IL-4 was shown not to be required for a normal lymphocyte composition in the

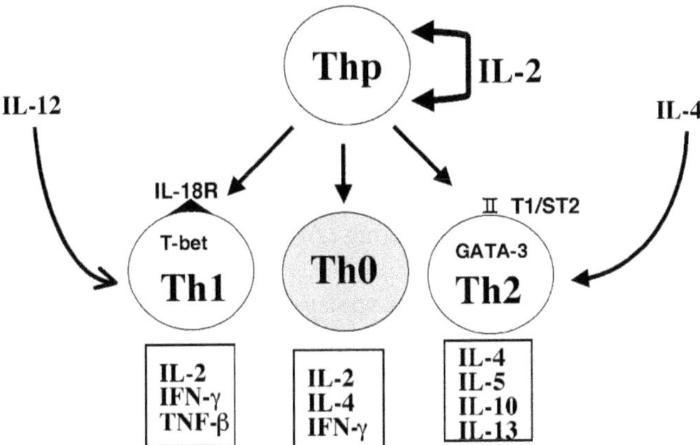

Fig. 1. Differentiation of naïve T helper precursor cells into distinct T helper effector cells.

thymus, spleen, and lymph nodes *(22,23,30)*. However, the levels of IgG1 and IgE were strongly reduced in the serum of IL-4-deficient mice compared with their littermate controls, whereas IgM, IgG2a, IgG2b, and IgA were normal *(22)*.

IL-4 has been shown to have the greatest influence in driving Th2 differentiation and the production of Th2 cytokines like IL-5 and IL-10 by polarized Th2 cells in response to polyclonal stimulation *(14,31)*. It was therefore expected that the lymphoid cells from IL-$4^{-/-}$ mice would mount impaired Th2 responses and have reduced production of Th2 cytokines compared with wild-type mice. However, contradictory results have been obtained by different groups: Kühn et al. *(32)* showed that the levels of IL-5 and IL-10 produced by CD4+ T-cells upon anti-CD3 stimulation were similar in the wild-type and the IL-4-deficient mice derived from targeted ES cells from 129/Sv mice. Similar results were obtained by Noben-Trauth et al. *(30)* with genetically pure IL-$4^{-/-}$ BALB/c mice. In contrast, in a study by Kopf et al. *(23)*, the Th2 response and the production of IL-5 and IL-10 was impaired in response to polyclonal activation. Although difficult to reconcile, these differences may be caused by the different protocols used to stimulate the cells.

3. Animal Models

The balance between cell-mediated and humoral immune responses is critical in determining the outcome of infection by various pathogens. The selection of immune effector functions is largely controlled by antigen-specific Th cells *(33,34)*. Naive T-helper cells can differentiate from a common precursor cell into functionally distinct effector cells that mediate different functions in protection and pathology (Fig. 1). Cytokines released by one T-helper cell subset can crossregulate the development of the other subset: Th2 cells suppress Th1 cells by secreting IL-4, whereas IFN-γ, the key cytokine released by Th1 cells, inhibits Th2 cell expansion *(15,35)*. In a range of infectious diseases, IL-4 has been shown either to protect against or to exacerbate diseases caused by a variety of pathogens, and the generation of IL-$4^{-/-}$ mice provided a powerful tool to assess the role of IL-4 in these infections (Table 1).

Table 1
Outcome of Parasitic Infections in IL-4-Deficient Mice

Pathogen	$IL\text{-}4^{+/+}$ T-helper response	$IL\text{-}4^{-/-}$ Predicted result	$IL\text{-}4^{-/-}$ Unexpected result
O. volvulis	Th2 *(36)* Keratitis	Healing *(18)*	Nonhealing *(37)*
N. brasiliensis	Th2 *(38)* Expulsion of worms	No expulsion (NR)	Expulsion of worms *(28)*
T. muris	Th2 *(38)* Expulsion of worms	No expulsion *(41)*	Expulsion of worms *(42)*
S. mansoni	Th2 *(43)* Granulomas	No granulomas *(45,46)*	Granulomas *(46)*
L. major	Th2 *(13,27)* Uncontrolled parasite replication	Clearance of parasites *(65)*	Uncontrolled parasite replication *(30,62,69)*

NR, not reported.

3.1. Filarial Nematodes

In experimental onchocercal keratitis, a filarial disease caused by *Onchocerca volvulis*, the immune response is predominantly Th2-like, with elevated levels of IL-4 and IL-5 and low levels of IFN-γ *(36)*; this Th2-mediated inflammation is thought to be responsible for keratitis. The use of IL-4-deficient mice confirmed the importance of IL-4 in the development of the disease, as in the absence of IL-4, mice failed to develop or had a diminished corneal disease *(36)*. A later study by Pearlman et al. *(37)* showed that in the IL-4-deficient mice, the Th2 cytokines IL-5, IL-10, and IL-13 were present in the cornea, demonstrating that Th2 differentiation can occur in an IL-4-independent manner. The authors suggested that the reduced severity of onchocercal keratitis in $IL\text{-}4^{-/-}$ mice was not owing to the failure to mount a Th2 response, but rather to a failure to recruit inflammatory cells into the corneal stroma *(37)*. In this case, $IL\text{-}4^{-/-}$ mice were not only a useful tool in confirming the importance of IL-4 in the inflammatory reaction but also in demonstrating that IL-4 is not a prerequisite for Th2 differentiation. The capacity of IL-4 to suppress the differentiation of Th1 cells *(13,15)* was also confirmed *in vivo*, as the production of IFN-γ was clearly increased in the $IL\text{-}4^{-/-}$ mice immunized with soluble *O. volvulis* antigen, compared with IL-4-competent mice *(37)*.

Infection of mice with *Nippostrongylus brasiliensis* is characterized by a strong Th2 response, and IL-4 was thought to be a prerequisite for the expulsion of *N. brasiliensis* and the development of immunity *(38)*. However, $IL\text{-}4^{-/-}$ mice were able to expel adult worms as effectively as fully immunocompetent animals *(28)*, demonstrating that IL-4 was not essential for the control of *N. brasiliensis*. In addition, infection of IL-4-deficient mice with *N. brasiliensis* resulted in an impaired, but still detectable, production of IL-5, IL-9, and IL-10 *(23)*, suggesting that, similarly to the experimental model of *O. volvulis*, Th2 cytokines can be produced in an IL-4-independent manner. Another study has revealed that IL-13, a Th2 cytokine sharing the IL-4 receptor α (IL-4Rα) chain among many other features with IL-4 *(39)*, can regulate Th2 responses to nematode infection *(40)*.

In contrast to infection with *N. brasiliensis*, IL-4-deficient mice infected with the nematode *Trichuris muris* displayed a severely impaired capacity to expel the worms *(41)*. They displayed an impaired production of Th2 cytokines and a stronger production of IFN-γ in response to polyclonal activation *(41)*. Interestingly, only IL-4$^{-/-}$ mice on the C57BL/6 background were susceptible to *T. muris* infection, whereas IL-4$^{-/-}$ mice on the BALB/c background could resist infection *(42)*. The latter mice produced similar levels of Th2 and Th1 cytokines in response to antigenic stimulation as wild-type BALB/c mice *(42)*. In addition, gender plays an important role as, in contrast to female IL-4$^{-/-}$ BALB/c mice, male IL-4$^{-/-}$ BALB/c mice were susceptible to *T. muris* infection *(42)*. In this model, expulsion of the worms was shown to be IL-13-dependent, as in vivo neutralization of IL-13 in female IL-4$^{-/-}$ BALB/c mice prevented *T. muris* expulsion *(42)*.

3.2. Helminths

Like the experimental model of infection with *N. brasiliensis*, IL-4-deficient mice have also revealed an important role for IL-13 in schistosomiasis. In this model, the immune response to the egg antigen (SEA) has been shown to be of a Th2 nature *(43)*, and this Th2 response has been proposed to be responsible for granuloma formation around tissue-trapped parasite eggs. However, following percutaneous infection of mice with *Schistoma mansoni* cercariae, IL-4$^{-/-}$ mice developed hepatic granulomas similar to those observed in IL-4$^{+/+}$ wild-type BALB/c mice, even though the deficient mice displayed a Th1-type response and an impaired Th2-type response *(44)*. In contrast, other studies showed that IL-4$^{-/-}$ mice did not switch to a type 1 response, in spite of a lower production of Th2 cytokines, and developed smaller hepatic granulomas *(45,46)*.

The divergent results obtained in the studies outlined above *(44–46)* may be caused by the different lines of IL-4-deficient mice used or by differences in the methods used to determined the levels of cytokines produced. Interestingly, however, the use of IL-4-deficient mice in experimental schistosomiasis revealed a key role for IL-13 in the formation of granulomas during *S. mansoni* infection. Indeed, IL-13 blockade in IL-4-deficient mice almost completely abrogated granuloma development *(47)*. In addition, these experiments demonstrate that IL-13 can be produced in an IL-4-independent manner and that IL-4 was not responsible for the granuloma formation in the liver. Moreover, a recent study by Brunet et al. *(48)* suggested that IL-4 prevents severe disease during schistosomiasis by regulating macrophage activation: it was shown that in the absence of IL-4, C57BL/6 mice displayed enhanced morbidity and mortality, owing to an uncontrolled production of proinflammatory cytokines. Therefore, it was concluded that IL-4 has a protective role in *S. mansoni* infection *(48,49)*.

3.3. Allergic Asthma

The evidence for the importance of IL-4 in the development of allergic asthma has been compelling *(50–52)*. In a model of allergen-induced airway inflammation, blockade of IL-4 abrogated the development of asthma *(53)*, and IL-4-deficient mice develop substantially less peribronchial inflammation and have fewer eosinophils in bronchoalveolar lavage compared with IL-4 competent mice *(52,54,55)*. The production of IL-5 in the lung tissue and the levels of antigen-specific IgE were both impaired in the IL-4$^{-/-}$ mice *(54,55)*, suggesting that IL-4 is a central mediator of allergic asthma. However, blockade of IL-4 before or during antigen challenge did not inhibit allergic inflammation *(56)*, indicating that

IL-4 is not necessary for the expression of allergic asthma. Indeed, IL-13 was found to be necessary and sufficient for the expression of allergen-induced inflammation, as blockade of IL-13 resulted in a complete reversal of the pathophysiologic features of asthma *(56)*. Also, exposure of the skin to soluble protein and subsequent airway challenge demonstrated a marked difference in the IL-4 dependence of Th2 responses: IL-4$^{-/-}$ mice epicutaneously exposed to soluble protein develop an similar inflammatory response and IL-5 and IL-13 production similar to that of wild-type mice *(55)*. In contrast, depletion of IL-13 in epicutaneously sensitized mice resulted in a loss of Th2 activation, indicating that IL-13 could effectively induce a Th2 response after epicutaneous protein exposure *(55)*. Furthermore, these results demonstrate that an IL-4-independent Th2 response to a protein antigen can also occur in mice.

In summary, these results demonstrate a critical role for IL-13 in the expression of murine asthma and suggest that, although IL-4 may be of immunoregulatory importance, IL-4 is not a prime effector molecule. IL-4-deficient mice in the model of allergen-induced airway inflammation were proved to be a useful tool in the analysis of the Th2 response; they revealed the importance of IL-13 in the development of allergic asthma and confirmed the existence of an IL-4-independent pathway of Th2 differentiation.

3.4. Leishmaniasis

Infection of mice with the protozoan parasite *Leishmania major* is one of the best characterized models of Th1 and Th2 differentiation. When they are infected subcutaneously in the footpads, most inbred strains of mice like B10.D2, C57BL/6 and CBA develop small lesions that heal spontaneously after a few weeks; these mice can mount a strong delayed-type hypersensitivity (DTH) response and can acquire immunity to subsequent challenge *(27)*. On the other hand, a few strains of mice such as BALB/c cannot control the replication of the parasites and will develop nonhealing ulcerating lesions. It has been extensively documented that nonhealing is associated with a strong Th2 and a downregulated Th1 response *(13,57–59)*. Indeed, the production of IFN-γ by lymphoid cells of *L. major*-infected BALB/c mice has been shown to be low or undetectable, whereas high and sustained levels of IL-4 are produced during the entire course of infection *(13,57,60,61)*. The detrimental role of IL-4 during the course of infection with *L. major* has been confirmed by the fact that treatment of BALB/c mice with neutralizing anti-IL-4 MAb enables them to switch to a Th1 phenotype, to control the replication of the parasites and to resolve the cutaneous lesions *(61)*.

However, the outcome of *L. major* infection in IL-4-deficient BALB/c mice has been a controversial subject. We and others have shown that IL-4-deficient BALB/c mice infected with *L. major* developed progressive lesions and could not contain the replication of the parasites *(30,62,63)*, whereas other studies have reported that IL-4-deficient mice infected with *L. major* displayed an intermediate phenotype *(64)* or were able to control the disease *(65,66)*. In the study in which control of experimental leishmaniasis was observed *(65)*, a different line of IL-4$^{-/-}$ BALB/c mice was used: the IL-4 gene was inactivated in an ES cell line derived from the 129Sv mouse strain, and these IL-4-deficient mice (F2:129Sv × C57BL/6) were backcrossed for six generations onto the BALB/c background (IL-4$^{-/-}$ ES:129Sv). Since the 129Sv mice have been reported to heal infection with *L. major (67)*, the possibility cannot be excluded that resistance genes closely linked to the mutated IL-4 gene were carried over during the backcrossing from a healer (129Sv mice) to a nonhealer

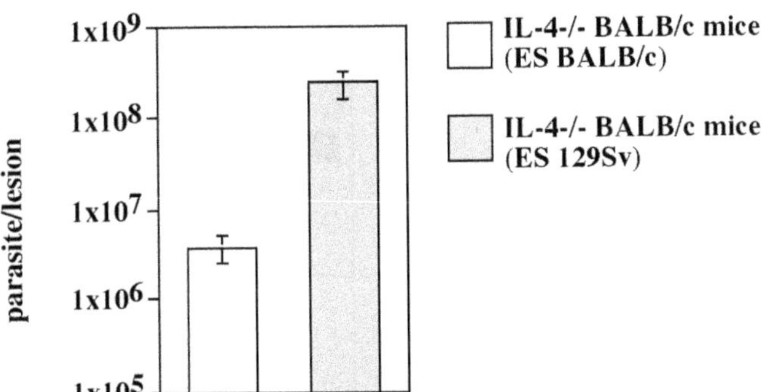

Fig. 2. Groups of interleukin (IL)-4$^{-/-}$ BALB/c mice generated from different embryonic stem (ES) cells (BALB/c, open bar; 129Sv mice, gray bar) were infected with *L. major* LV39 promastigotes. The progression of the infection was monitored by measuring the footpad thickness. Two months post infection, the numbers of viable parasites were determined in the infected footpads. Values are the average ± SEM. Data show the results of one representative experiment out of two.

background (BALB/c mice). Indeed, the loci for susceptibility to leishmaniasis (*Scl1*), for IL-12p40 (*Il12b*), and for inducible nitric oxide synthase (*Nos2*) are linked to the IL-4 structural gene (*Il4*) on chromosome 11 *(68)*.

To test the hypothesis that a carryover of resistance genes is responsible for the reported differences in the outcome of *L. major* infection, we infected the backcrossed IL-4$^{-/-}$ BALB/c mice of mixed susceptible and resistant backgrounds (ES:129Sv x C57BL/6) with *L. major* parasites and compared their lesion development with that of genetically pure IL-4$^{-/-}$ BALB/c mice (ES:BALB/c). Both groups of IL-4$^{-/-}$ BALB/c mice developed progressive lesions (data not shown) and could not control the parasite replication in their lesions (Fig. 2). Thus, these experiments show that the conflicting results are not owing to a carryover of resistance genes.

Another major difference that could be responsible for the conflicting outcomes of *L. major* infection in IL-4-deficient BALB/c mice *(30,65)* is the isolate of *L. major* parasites used: resistance was observed after infection with *L. major* MHOM/IL/81/FEBNI (*L. major* FEBNI), whereas while nonhealing occurred after infection with the *L. major* LV39 MRHO/SU/59/P-strain *(30)*. It has been shown that different isolates of *L. major* parasites can induce different disease outcomes in IL-4R$\alpha^{-/-}$ BALB/c mice *(62)*. Therefore, IL-4$^{-/-}$ BALB/c mice were infected with *L. major* FEBNI, and lesion development was compared with that of IL-4$^{-/-}$ mice infected with *L. major* LV39. The onset of lesion development was similar in both groups; however, 4 weeks post infection, 75% of BALB/c mice infected with *L. major* LV39 had developed ulcerating lesions, whereas 12.5% of IL-4$^{-/-}$ BALB/c mice infected with *L. major* FEBNI had an ulcer (data not shown). The lesions from the latter group did not resolve; they remained stationary, and some animals developed open ulcers at later time points. Thus, the onset of pathology was delayed after infection with *L. major* FEBNI. The determination of the number of viable parasites per lesion showed that even though a smaller number of parasites was detected in the footpads of IL-4$^{-/-}$ BALB/c mice infected with *L. major* FEBNI 4 weeks post infection, the parasites kept on multiplying in the footpad and a higher parasite load was present 8 wk after parasite inoc-

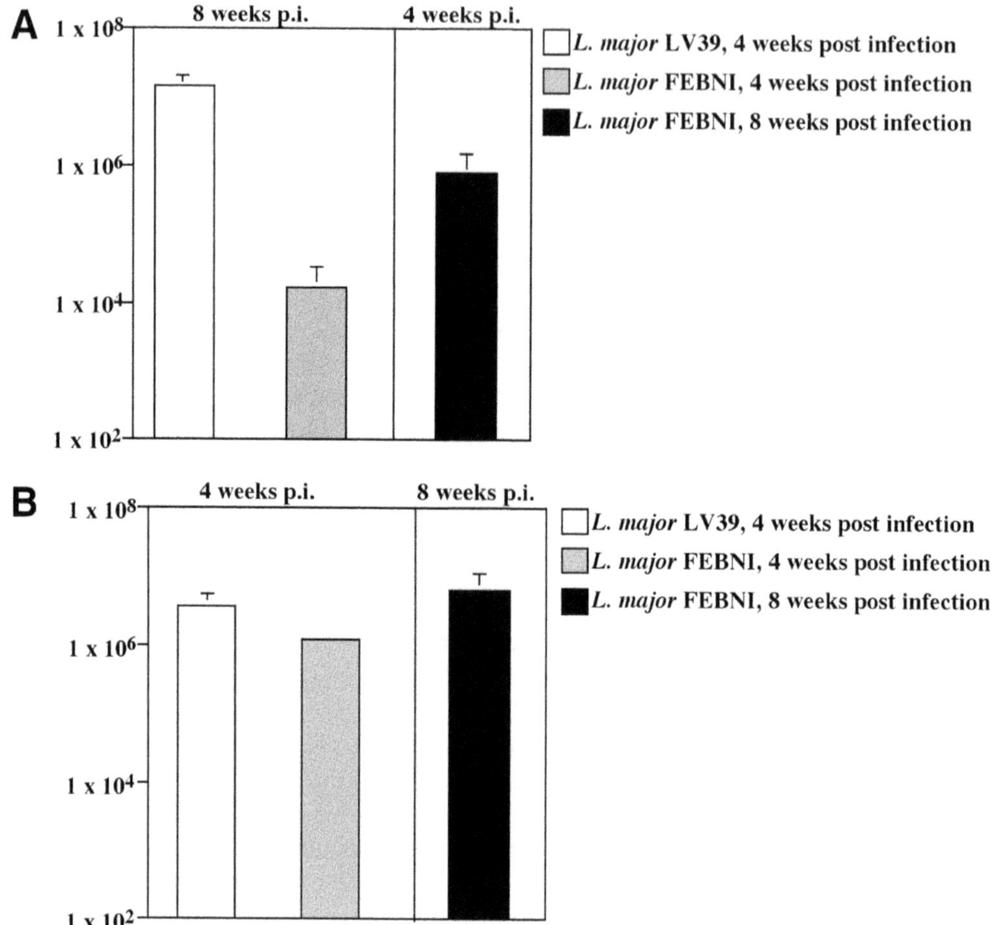

Fig. 3. Parasite load in the organs of IL-$4^{-/-}$ BALB/c mice infected with different strains of *L. major*. Groups of IL-$4^{-/-}$ BALB/c were infected with *L. major* LV39 or *L. major* FEBNI. The progression of the infection was monitored by measuring the footpad thickness. At the indicated time points post infection (p. i.), the numbers of viable parasites were determined in the infected footpad (**A**) or in the popliteal lymph node (**B**). Values are the average ± SEM. Data show the results of one representative experiment out of two. LN, lympth node.

ulation (Fig. 3), whereas no parasites were detectable in a healer strain of mice, C57BL/6 at this time (data not shown). In addition, the parasite loads were similar in both groups in the lymph nodes draining the lesions (Fig. 3). Thus, despite reduced pathology and delayed parasite growth in the footpads, these results demonstrate that IL-$4^{-/-}$ BALB/c mice can by no means "resist" infection with *L. major* FEBNI. Moreover, IL-$4^{-/-}$ BALB/c mice were also shown to be susceptible to infection with *L. major* Seidman [WHOM/SN/74 Seidman *(69)*] and *L. major* IR173 WHOM/IR/-173 *(62)*.

Factors such as the environment in which animals are bred *(70)* or the maintenance of parasites *(71)* are of crucial importance and can influence the outcome of the disease. In addition, age is another factor influencing the onset of lesion development in *L. major*-

infected IL-4-deficient BALB/c mice; indeed, the lesions of 6-wk-old IL-4$^{-/-}$ BALB/c mice were larger and contained significantly more viable parasites compared with 6-mo-old mice. The older mice developed progressive lesions with time, and after 4 mo of infection, 75% of them had developed open ulcers (P. Kropf, S.I. Herath, and I. Müller, submitted). Therefore, if the mice are not kept long enough, the initially smaller lesions in these mice could be misinterpreted as a healer phenotype. Indeed, in a study by Mohrs et al. *(64)*, IL-4$^{-/-}$ BALB/c mice had relatively small lesions at 80 d post infection; however, after 20 wk they started to ulcerate, and 23 wk post infection, the mice had to be killed because of the extent of the ulceration.

The role of IL-13, a cytokine sharing a receptor chain and many biologic activities with IL-4 *(39,72)*, in the susceptibility of IL-4$^{-/-}$ BALB/c mice to *L. major* infection is subject to controversy: Matthews et al. *(66)* have shown that *L. major*-infected IL-13-deficient mice can control their lesion development. However, a study by Kropf et al. *(69)* showed that after neutralization of IL-13 in vivo, IL-4$^{-/-}$ BALB/c mice developed similar lesions as the wild-type mice after *L. major* infection. The IL-13-deficient BALB/c mice used *(66)* were derived from C57BL/6 ES cells and backcrossed for four generations on the BALB/c background. Since C57BL/6 mice are genetically resistant and able to heal infection with *L. major*, the possibility cannot be excluded that resistance genes closely linked to the mutated IL-13 gene were carried over during the backcrosses. Indeed, the IL-13 gene is in a genomic region associated with susceptibility to leishmaniasis *(66)*.

Previous studies have already suggested that the use of different strains of IL-4$^{-/-}$ mice may account for the different outcome observed in experimental models in which susceptibility or resistance is associated to the genetic background: for example, *S. mansoni*-infected IL-4$^{-/-}$ mice on a mixed genetic background (C57BL/6x129Sv) developed liver granulomas and a Th2 response similar to those of the wild-type mice *(44)*, whereas genetically pure C57BL/6 IL-4$^{-/-}$ mice developed smaller granulomas and a lower Th2 response *(45)*. Similarly, IL-4-deficient mice (C57BL/6 × 129Sv) were resistant to MAIDS *(73)*, whereas IL-4-deficient mice derived from a different ES cell line (C57BL/6 × 129Ola) were as susceptible as the wild-type mice *(74)*.

These results suggest that other genetic factors, independent of IL-4, are responsible for these discrepant results. In addition, these experiments indicate that results obtained with cytokine gene-deficient mice on mixed resistant and genetic backgrounds might be difficult to interpret since the possibility of a carryover of small numbers of genes in close proximity to the targeted region is hard to exclude. These experiments further strengthen the importance of using genetically pure IL-4$^{-/-}$ mice to test the role of IL-4.

The work outlined above suggests that IL-4 alone is not responsible for the nonhealing phenotype of *L. major*-infected BALB/c mice. Indeed, in a study presented by Kane et al. *(75)*, IL-10$^{-/-}$ BALB/c mice infected with *L. major* controlled the disease progression, suggesting that IL-10 is crucial for the disease progression and that IL-4 alone cannot be responsible for the nonhealing phenotype of BALB/c mice.

Infection of BALB/c mice with *L. major* parasites is widely used as model to study the differential development of CD4+ T-cells into polarized Th1 or Th2 cells *(13,27)*. IL-4 is thought to be responsible for the induction and maintenance of the detrimental Th2 response during the course of infection and for the downregulation of the beneficial Th1 response *(13,27)*. However, the antigen-specific production of Th2 cytokines was shown to be similar during the course of *L. major* infection in IL-4$^{-/-}$ and IL-4-competent BALB/c mice *(30,69)*; thus, it can be concluded that IL-4 is not required for the development of a Th2 response and the secretion of Th2 cytokines in this experimental system. This conclusion is further supported by results showing that a stable cell surface marker for Th2 cells, T1/ST2 *(76)*, was expressed at similar levels after *L. major* infection in the presence or absence of IL-4 *(69,77)*.

These results clearly demonstrate that IL-4 is not necessary for the induction of *L. major*-specific Th2 responses and confirm our previous work showing that genetically pure IL-4-deficient BALB/c mice develop nonhealing *L. major* infections *(30)*. Indeed, our findings were confirmed by a study from another group showing that IL-$4^{-/-}$ BALB/c mice remained susceptible to *L. major* infection and produced lower, but still clearly detectable, levels of IL-10 and IL-13 *(62)*. In the studies outlined above, the levels of IFN-γ were similar in the IL-4-deficient BALB/c mice and the wild-type BALB/c controls *(30,62,69)*. In the study in which the IL-$4^{-/-}$ mice were shown to resist *L. major* infection, the levels of Th2 cytokines were reduced or not detectable in the absence of IL-4, and the production of IFN-γ was similar in the IL-$4^{-/-}$ and the IL-$4^{+/+}$ BALB/c mice 3 wk post infection and reduced 9 wk post infection (65). Importantly, the in vitro stimulation conditions were different in the studies summarized above *(30,65,69)*: the number of cells, the type of cells (total lymphoid cells versus purified CD4+ T-cells), the stimuli (live parasite, soluble fraction or polyclonal), and the time of stimulation before the supernatants were harvested for the determination of the cytokine content by enzyme-linked immunosorbent assay (ELISA) all varied.

The results presented here show that the role of IL-4 in the nonhealing phenotype of *L. major*-infected BALB/c mice and the generation of Th2 responses are disputed. IL-4 is clearly not the only determining factor for the nonhealing disease and the induction of Th2 responses; in contrast, this cytokine might be required for the development of efficient Th1 response and healing. Indeed, a possible role for IL-4 in protective responses has already been described: it has been shown recently that IL-4 may have a role in the differentiation of Th1 cells *(78,79)*. Several studies have shown that IL-4 can indeed induce a Th1 response. Lingnau et al. *(78)* have shown that IL-4, in combination with transforming growth factor-β (TGF-β), can induce naive CD4+ T-cells to differentiate into Th1 cells in response to polyclonal activation. IL-4 was shown to be indispensable for the induction of protective immunity mediated by Th1 cells in a model of infection with *Candida albicans, (79)*. IL-$4^{-/-}$ BALB/c mice were highly resistant to *C. albicans* during the primary infection, but died after secondary challenge. This susceptibility is thought to be owing to an impaired Th1 response: in the absence of IL-4, neutrophils could not be primed to produce the IL-12 necessary for the maintenance of the protective Th1 response.

Recently, a study established a crucial role for IL-4 in the generation of a protective Th1 response in experimental leishmaniasis *(80)*: it was shown that during the early phase of activation, IL-4 was inducing dendritic cells to differentiate and to produce IL-12 and thereby promoting the development of a protective Th1 response. This elegant work demonstrated that IL-4 was contributing to the ability of BALB/c mice to develop a Th1 response and to heal *L. major* infection. These results confirm the results we obtained with the IL-$4^{-/-}$ BALB/c mice: in the absence of IL-4, IL-$4^{-/-}$ BALB/c mice were not able to mount a protective Th1 response *(30,63,69)* and remain susceptible to *L. major* infection.

The studies outlined above show that IL-4 can contribute to the induction of Th1 differentiation. Moreover, these results could also explain why IL-$4^{-/-}$ BALB/c mice cannot control *L. major* infection: in the absence of IL-4, IL-$4^{-/-}$ BALB/c mice may not be able to mount and/or maintain an appropriate Th1 response.

4. Immunoglobulin Isotype Switching

B-cells can alter the class of antibody they produce by immunoglobulin class switch recombination. During this process, B-cells exchange the gene segments encoding the constant regions of the Ig heavy chain and thereby alter the class and the effector function of the antibody. Cytokines target the recombination to particular switch regions, and this targeting is accompanied by the induction of transcription through the targeted switch region. The role of cytokines in targeting class switching to particular classes lies in the induction of these switch transcripts.

Various cytokines secreted by activated T-helper cells have been shown to induce B-cells to switch to a particular isotype. IL-4 has been shown to induce Ig class switching to IgE and IgG1 *(10)*; indeed, blockade of IL-4 with anti-IL-4 MAb or anti-IL-4 receptor MAb abrogated the polyclonal induction of IgE in vivo *(81)*. In addition, after *N. brasiliensis* or *Heligmosomoides polygyrus* infection, the serum levels of IgE were clearly reduced in anti-IL-4-treated mice *(81)*, confirming the relevance of IL-4 for IgE production. In naive IL-4-deficient mice, the levels of IgG1 were reduced compared with their wild-type littermates *(22)*. Infection of IL-4-deficient mice with a variety of pathogens [*N. brasiliensis (82)*, *Plasmodium chabaudi (83)*, *S. mansoni (44)*, and *L. major (30)*] further confirmed the importance of IL-4 in the induction of class switching, as IgE and/or IgG1 responses were reduced. The residual production of IgE and/or IgG1 is likely to be caused by IL-13: simultaneous disruption of IL-4 and IL-13 revealed that these two cytokines cooperate to initiate isotype switching. Indeed, in a model of pulmonary granuloma induced by *S. mansoni*, the antigen-specific levels of IgE and IgG1 were below the detection limit in IL-4- and IL-13-double deficient mice, whereas they were only partially reduced in IL-13- and IL-4-deficient mice *(84)*.

5. Immunoregulation

CD8+ T-cells, like CD4+ T-cells, can also develop into functionally distinct type 1 and type 2 subsets *(85,86)*. The role of IL-4 in the regulation of CD8+ T cell responses is, however, poorly understood. IL-4 has been shown to augment the growth of CD8+ T-cells but also to act as a negative regulator of effector functions in CD8+ T-cells. IL-4-deficient mice have been used to investigate the disparate roles of IL-4 in the regulation of CD8 responses. The absence of IL-4 during viral infections was associated with enhanced cytolytic activity of CD8+ effector T-cells *(87)*. CD8+ splenocytes from IL-4-deficient mice were more responsive to antigenic stimulation than those of IL-4 competent wild-type mice *(87)*.

This enhanced responsiveness of CD8+ T-cells was not owing to differences in the precursor frequency or in the viral load. In contrast, tumor immunity requires IL-4 for the priming of cytotoxic T-lymphocytes (CTLs), since IL-4-deficient mice exhibited severely impaired antitumor responses associated with undetectable CTL activity and reduced IFN-γ production *(88)*. It is likely that the defective CTL response in IL-4-deficient mice was the result of defective help by Th1 cells. T-cell help for CTL activation is provided as a result of a crosstalk between T-helper cells and antigen-presenting cells. Differences in the dependence of CTL responses on help provided by CD4+ T-cells could account for the discrepancies (enhanced versus lacking CTL activity) in the results outlined above. Indeed, IL-4 secreted by CD4+ T-cells has been shown to mediate the crosstalk between CD4 and CD8 cells and to be crucial for the development of the CD8+ T-cell responses that can inhibit the development of the liver stages in malaria infections *(89)*.

6. Conclusions

The use of IL-4-deficient mice has proved to be a valuable tool for the analysis of Th responses and for the role of Th cell subsets in many diseases, ranging from helminth and protozoan infections to autoimmunity and to sensitization with protein antigen. These mice have been useful in demonstrating that the generally accepted notion that IL-4 alone is responsible for the generation of detrimental or beneficial Th2 responses is an oversimplification and that the immune system frequently does not rely on only one mechanism: it can use alternative pathways. Also importantly, the use of IL-4-deficient BALB/ mice has revealed the existence of an IL-4-independent pathway of Th2 differentiation: it is now obvious that other cytokines like IL-13 and IL-10 play a large role in the generation of Th2 responses. In addition, from the studies presented in this chapter, it is clear that Th1 responses can be downregulated independently of IL-4. They have also highlighted the importance of the genetic background of the cytokine-deficient mice and showed that the use of mixed susceptible and resistant backgrounds can lead to results that are difficult to interpret. Although some of the findings obtained with IL-4-deficient mice were unexpected, and some are controversial, overall, studies with IL-4-deficient mice have contributed intriguing new aspects to our still incomplete understanding of immune responses.

Acknowledgments

The authors would like to thank Dr. Martin Goodier, Imperial College, London, for critical reading of the manuscript. Because of limited space, we could not cover all the fascinating aspects of this rapidly developing field, and we therefore apologize to all the researchers whose work has not been mentioned.

The preparation of this book chapter as well as some of the work summarized was made possible by financial support from The Wellcome Trust, London, UK.

References

1. Seder, P. and Paul, W. E. (1994) Acquisition of lymphokine-producing phenotype by CD4$^+$ T cells. *Annu. Rev. Immunol.* **12,** 635–673.
2. Seder, R. A., Plaut, M., Barbieri, S., Urban, J. D. F. F., and Paul, W. E. (1991) Mouse splenic and bone marrow cell population that express high affinity Fc epsilon receptors and produce interleukin 4 are highly enriched in basophils. *Proc. Natl. Acad. Sci. USA* **88,** 2835–2839.
3. Plaut, M., Pierce, J. H., Watson, C. J., Hanley, H. J., Nordan, R. P., and Paul, W. E. (1989) Mast cell lines produce lymphokines in response to cross-linkage of FcERI or to calcium ionophores. *Nature* **339,** 64–67.
4. Scott, D. E., Gause, W. C., Finkelman, F. D., and Steinberg, A. D. (1990) Anti-CD3 antibody induces rapid expression of cytokine genes *in vivo. J. Immunol.* **145,** 2183–2188.
5. Launois, P., Ohteki, T., Swihart, K., MacDonald, H. R., and Louis, J. (1995) In susceptible mice, *Leishmania major* induce very rapid interleukin-4 production by CD4+ T cells which are NK1.1-. *Eur. J. Immunol.* **25,** 3298–3307.
6. Ferrick, D. A., Schrenzel, M. D., Mulvania, T., Hsieh, B., GFerlin, W. G., and Lepper, H. (1995) Differential production of IFN-γ and IL-4 in response to Th1 and Th2-stimulating pathogens by γδ T cells *in vivo. Nature* **373,** 255–257.

7. Howard, M., Farrar, J., Hilfiker, M., et al. (1982) Identification of a T cell-derived factor distinct from interleukin 2. *J. Exp. Med.* **155,** 914–923.
8. Noelle, R., Krammer, R. P., Ohara, J., Uhr, J. W., and Vitetta, E. S. (1984) Increased expression of Ia antigens on resting B cells: an additional role for B cell growth factor. *Proc. Natl. Acad. Sci. USA* **81,** 6149–6153.
9. Coffman, R. L., Lebman, D. A., and Rothman, P. (1993) Mechanism and regulation of immunoglobulin isotype switching. *Adv. Immunol.* **54,** 229–270.
10. Stavnezer, J. (1996) Immunoglobulin class switching. *Curr. Opin. Immunol.* **8,** 199–205.
11. Mosmann, T. R., Cherwinski, H., Bond, M. W., Giedlin, M. A., and Coffman, R. L. (1986) Two types of murine helper T cell clone. I. Definition according to profiles of lymphokine activities and secreted proteins. *J. Immunol.* **136,** 2348–2357.
12. Mosmann, T. R., Schumacher, J. H., Street, N. F., et al. (1991) Diversity of cytokine synthesis and function of mouse $CD4^+$ T cells. *Immunol. Rev.* **123,** 209–229.
13. Reiner, S. L. and Locksley, R. M. (1995) The regulation of immunity to *Leishmania major*. *Annu. Rev. Immunol.* **13,** 151–177.
14. Constant, S. L. and Bottomly, K. (1997) Induction of Th1 and Th2 $CD4^+$ T cell responses: the alternative approaches. *Annu. Rev. Immunol.* **15,** 297–322.
15. Gajewski, T. F. and Fitch, F. W. (1988) Anti-proliferative effect of IFN-γ in immune regulation. I. IFN-γ inhibits the proliferation of Th2 but not Th1 murine T helper lymphocyte clones. *J. Immunol.* **140,** 4245–4252.
16. Haak-Frenscho, M., Brown, J. F., Iizawa, Y., Wagner, R. D., and Czuprynski, C. J. (1992) Administration of anti-IL-4 antibody 11b11 increases the resistance of mice to *Listeria monocytogenes* infection. *J. Immunol.* **148,** 3978–3985.
17. Yoshino, S. (1998) treatment of mice with an anti-IL-4 mAb blocks supression of collagen-induced arthritis in mice by oral administration of type II collagen. *J. Immunol.* **160,** 3067–3071.
18. Sher, A., Coffman, R. L., Hieny, S., and Cheever, A. W. (1990) Ablation of eosinophil and IgE responses with anti-IL-5 and anti-IL-4 antibodies fails to affect immunity against *Schistosoma mansoni* in the mouse. *J. Immunol.* **145,** 3911–3916.
19. Lukacs, N. W., Striter, R. M., Chensue, S. W., and Kunkel, S. L. (1994) Interleukin-4-dependent pulmonary eosinophil infiltration in a murine model of asthma. *Am. J. Respir. Cell. Mol. Biol.* **10,** 526–532.
20. Sadick, M. D., Heinzel, F. P., Holaday, B. J., Pu, R. T., Dawkins, R. S., and Locksley, R. M. (1990) Cure of murine leishmaniasis with anti-interleukin 4 monoclonal antibody. *J. Exp. Med.* **171,** 115–117.
21. Finkelman, F. D., Madden, K. B., Morris, S. C., et al. (1993) Anti-cytokine antibodies as carrier proteins. Prolongation of *in vivo* effects of exogenous cytokines by injection of cytokine-anti-cytokine antibody complexes. *J. Immunol.* **151,** 1235–1244.
22. Kühn, R., Rajewski, K., and Müller, W. (1991) Generation and analysis of interleukin-4 deficient mice. *Science* **254,** 707–710.
23. Kopf, M., Le Gros, G., Bachmann, M., Lamers, M. C., Bluethmann, H., and Koehler, G. (1993) Disruption of the murine IL-4 gene blocks Th2 cytokine response. *Nature* **362,** 245–248.
24. DeTolla, L. J., Scott, P. A., and Farrell, J. P. (1981) Single gene control of resistance to cutaneous leishmaniasis in mice. *Immunogenetics* **14,** 29–39.
25. Coulson, P. S. and Wilson, R. A. (1989) Portal shunting and resistance to *Schistosomiasis mansoni* in 129 strain mice. *Parasitology* **3,** 383–389.
26. Norse, H. C. 3rd, Chattopadhyay, S. K., Makino, M., Fredrickson, T. N., Hugin, A. W., and Hartley, J. W. (1992) Retrovirus-induced immunodeficiency in the mouse: MAIDS as a model for AIDS. *AIDS* **6,** 607–621.
27. Etges, B. and Müller, I. (1998) Progressive disease or protective immunity to *Leishmania major* infection: the result of a network of stimulatory and inhibitory interactions. *J. Mol. Med.* **76,** 372–390.
28. Lawrence, R. A., Gray, C. A., Osborne, J., and Maizels, R. M. (1996) *Nippostrongylus brasiliensis*: cytokine responses and nematode expulsion in normal and IL-4 deficient mice. *Exp. Parasitol.* **84,** 65–73.

29. Noben-Trauth, N., Köhler, G., Bürki, K., and Ledermann, B. (1996) Efficient targeting of the IL-4 gene in a BALB/c embryonic stem cell line. *Transgenic Res.* **5,** 487–491.
30. Noben-Trauth, N., Kropf, P., and Müller, I. (1996) Susceptibility to *Leishmania major* infection in interleukin-4-deficient mice. *Science* **271,** 987–990.
31. Ben-Sasson, S. Z., Makedonski, K., Li-Hu, J., and Paul, W. E. (2000) Survival and cytokine polarisation of naive T cells in vitro is largely dependent on exogenous cytokines. *Eur. J. Immunol.* **30,** 1308–1317.
32. Müller, W., Rajewsky, K., and Kühn, R. (1993) Interleukin-4-deficient mice. *Res. Immunol.* **144,** 637–638.
33. Murphy, K. M. (1998) T lymphocyte differentiation in the periphery. *Curr. Opin. Immunol.* **10,** 226–232.
34. O'Garra, A. (1998) Cytokines induce the development of functionally heterogeneous T helper cell subsets. *Immunity* **8,** 275–283.
35. Mosmann, T. R. and Coffman, R. L. (1989) Th1 and Th2 cells: different patterns of lymphokine seretion lead to different functional properties. *Annu. Rev. Immunol.* **7,** 145–173.
36. Pearlman, E., Lass, J. H., Bardenstein, D. S., et al. (1995) Interleukin 4 and T helper type 2 cells are required for the development of experimental onchocercal keratitis (river blindness). *J. Exp. Med.* **182,** 931–940.
37. Pearlman, E., Lass, J. H., Bardenstein, D. S., et al. (1996) *Onchocerca volvulus*-mediated keratitis: cytokine production by IL-4-deficient mice. *Exp. Parasitol.* **84,** 274–281.
38. Urban, J. F., Fayer, F., Sullivan, C., et al. (1996) Local Th1 and Th2 responses to parasitic infection in the intestine: regulation by IFN-γ and IL-4. *Vet. Immunol. Immunopathol.* **54,** 337–344.
39. Callard, R. E., Mathews, D. J., and Hibbert, L. (1996) IL-4 and IL-13 receptors: are they one or the same? *Immunol. Today* **17,** 108–110.
40. Barner, M., Mohrs, M., Brombacher, K. F., and Kopf, M. (1998) Differences between IL-4Rα-deficient and IL-4-deficient mice reveal a role for IL-13 in the regulation of Th2 responses. *Curr. Biol.* **8,** 667–672.
41. Bancroft, A. J., McKenzie, A. N. J., and Grencis, R. K. (1998) A critical role for IL-13 in resistance to intestinal nematode infection. *J. Immunol.* **160,** 3453–3461.
42. Bancroft, A., Artis, D., Donaldson, D. D., Sypek, J. P., and Grencis, R. K. (2000) Gastrointestinal nematode expulsion in IL-4 knockout mice is IL-13 dependent. *Eur. J. Immunol.* **30,** 2083–2091.
43. Pearce, E. J., Caspar, P., Grzych, J. M., Lewis, F. A., and Sher, A. (1991) Downregulation of the Th1 cytokine production accompanies induction of the Th2 responses by a parasitic helminth, *S. mansoni*. *J. Exp. Med.* **173,** 159–166.
44. Pearce, E. J., Cheever, A., Leonard, S., et al. (1996) *Schistosoma mansoni* in IL-4-deficient mice. *Int. Immunol.* **8,** 435–444.
45. Metwali, A., Elliott, D., Blum, A. M., et al. (1996) The granulomatous response in murine *Schistosoma mansoni* does not switch to a Th1 in IL-4-deficient C57BL/6 mice. *J. Immunol.* **157,** 4546–4553.
46. Wynn, T. A., Morawetz, R., Scharton-Kersten, T., et al. (1997) Analysis of granuloma formation in double cytokine-deficient mice reveals a central role for IL-10 in polarizing both T helper cell 1- and T helper cell 2-type cytokine responses in vivo. *J. Immunol.* **159,** 5014–5023.
47. Chiaramonte, M. G., Schopf, L., Neben, T. Y., Cheever, A. W., Donaldson, D. D., and Wynn, T. A. (1999) IL-13 is a key regulatory cytokine for Th2 cell-mediated pulmonary granuloma formation and IgE reponse induced in *Schistosoma mansoni* eggs. *J. Immunol.* **162,** 920–930.
48. Brunet, L. R., Finkelman, F. D., Cheever, A. W., Kopf, M. A., and Pearce, E. J. (1997) IL-4 protects against TNF-α-mediated cachexia and death during acute phase of schistosomiasis. *J. Immunol.* **159,** 777–785.
49. Hoffmann, K. F., Cheever, A. W., and Wynn, T. A. (2000) IL-10 and the danger of immune polarisation: excessive type1 and type 2 cytokines responses induce distinct forms of lethal immunopathology in murine schistosomiasis. *J. Immunol.* **164,** 6406–6416.
50. Finkelman, F. D., Katona, I. M., Urban, J. F., et al. (1988) IL-4 is required to generate and sustain in vivo IgE responses. *J. Immunol.* **141,** 2335–2341.
51. Rankin, J. A., Picarella, D. E., Geba, G. P., et al. (1996) Phenotypic and physiologic characterisation of transgenic mice expressing interleukin 4 in the lung: lymphocytic and eosinophilic inflammation without airway hyperreactivity. *Proc. Natl. Acad. Sci. USA* **93,** 7821–7825.

52. Brusselle, G. G., Kips, J. C., Tavernier, J. H., et al. (1994) Attenuation of allergic airway inflammation in IL-4 deficient mice. *Clin. Exp. Allergy* **24,** 73–80.
53. Coyle, A. J., Le Gros, G., Tsuyuki, S., Heusser, C. H., Kopf, M., and Anderson, G. P. (1995) Interleukin-4 is required for the induction of lung Th2 mucosal immunity. *Am. J. Respir. Cell. Mol. Biol.* **13,** 54–59.
54. Hamelmann, E., Takeda, K., Haczku, A., et al. (2000) Interleukin-5, but not immunoglobulin E reconstitutes airway inflammation and airway hyperresponsiveness in IL-4-deficient mice. *Am. J. Respir. Cell Mol. Biol.* **23,** 327–334.
55. Herrick, C. A., MacLeod, H., Glusa, C. E., Tigelaar, R. E., and Bottomly, K. (2000) Th2 responses induced by epicutaneous or inhalational protein exposure are differentially dependent on IL-4. *J. Clin. Invest.* **105,** 765–775.
56. Wills-Karp, M., Luyimabazi, J., Xu, X., et al. (1998) Interleukin-13: central mediator of allergic asthma. *Science* **282,** 2258–2261.
57. Locksley, R. M., Heinzel, F. P., Sadick, M. D., Holaday, B. J., and Gardner, K. D. (1987) Murine cutaneous leishmaniasis. Susceptibility correlates with differential expansion of helper T cell subsets. *Ann. Inst. Pasteur Immunol.* **138,** 744–749.
58. Heinzel, F. P., Sadick, M. D., Holaday, B. J., Coffman, R. L., and Locksley, R. M. (1989) reciprocal expression of interferon-γ or interleukin-4 during the resolution or progression of murine leishmaniasis. Evidence for expansion of distinct helper T cell subsets. *J. Exp. Med.* **169,** 59–72.
59. Reiner, S. L. and Seder, R. A. (1995) T helper cell differentiation in immune response. *Curr. Opin. Immunol.* **7,** 360–366.
60. Launois, P., Swihart, K. G., Milon, G., and Louis, J. A. (1997) Early production of IL-4 in susceptible mice infected with *Leishmania major* rapidly induces IL-12 unresponsiveness. *J. Immunol.* **158,** 3317–3324.
61. Sadick, M. D., Heinzel, F. P., Holaday, B. J., Pu, R. T., Dawkins, R. S., and Locksley, R. M. (1990) Cure of murine leishmaniasis with anti-interleukin-4 monoclonal antibody. Evidence for a T-cell-dependent, interferon-γ-independent mechanism. *J. Exp. Med.* **171,** 115–127.
62. Noben-Trauth, N., Paul, W. E., and Sacks, D. L. (1999) IL-4- and IL-4 Receptor-alpha deficient BALB/c mice reveal differences in susceptibility to *Leishmania major* parasite substrains. *J. Immunol.* **162,** 6132–6140.
63. Kropf, P., Etges, R., Schopf, L., Chang, C., Sypek, J., and Müller, I. (1997) Characterisation of T cell-mediated responses in nonhealing and healing *Leishmania major* infections in the absence of endogenous IL-4. *J. Immunol.* **159,** 3434–3443.
64. Mohrs, M., Ledermann, B., Köhler, G., Dorfmüller, A., Gessner, A., and Brombacher, F. (1999) Differences between IL-4- and IL-4 receptor a-deficient mice in chronic leishmaniasis reveal a protective role for IL-13 receptor signaling. *J. Immunol.* **162,** 7302–7308.
65. Kopf, M., Brombacher, F., Köhler, G., et al. (1996) IL-4-deficient BALB/c mice resist infection with *L. major*. *J. Exp. Med.* **184,** 1127–1136.
66. Matthews, D. J., Emson, C. L., McKenzie, G. J., Jolin, H. E., Blackwell, J. M., and McKenzie, A. N. J. (2000) IL-13 is a susceptibility factor for *L. major* infection. *J. Immunol.* **164,** 1458–1462.
67. Leal, L. M., Moss, D. W., Kuhn, R., Muller, W., and Liew, F. Y. (1993) IL-4 transgenic mice of resistant background are susceptible to *Leishmania major* infection. *Eur. J. Immunol.* **23,** 566–569.
68. Mock, B., Blackwell, J., Hilgers, J., Potter, M., and Nacy, C. (1994) The inducible form of nitric oxide synthase (NOS2) isolated from murine macrophages maps near the nude mutation on mouse chromosome 11. *Eur. J. Immunogenet.* **21,** 231–238.
69. Kropf, P., Schopf, R. L., Chung, C. L., et al. (1999) Expression of Th2 cytokines and the stable Th2 marker ST2L in the absence of IL-4 during *L. major* infection. *Eur. J. Immunol.* **29,** 3621–3628.
70. Julia, V., McSorley, S. S., Malherbe, L., et al. (2000) Priming by microbial antigens from the intestinal flora determines the ability of CD4+ T cells to rapidly secrete IL-4 in BALB/c mice infected with *L. major*. *J. Immunol.* **165,** 5637–5645.
71. Da Silva, R. and Sacks, D. L. (1987) Metacyclogenesis is a major determinant of *Leishmania* promastigotes virulence and attenuation. *Infect. Immun.* **55,** 2082–2086.
72. Zurawski, G. and de Vries, J. E. (1994) IL-13, an IL-4-like cytokine that acts on monocytes and B cells, but not on T cells. *Immunol. Today* **15,** 19–26.

73. Kanagawa, O., Vaupel, B. A., Gayama, S., Köhler, G., and Kopf, M. (1993) Resistance of mice deficient in IL-4 to retrovirus-induced immunodeficieny syndrome (MAIDS). *Science* **262,** 240–242.
74. Morawetz, R. A., Doherty, T. M., Giese, N. A., et al. (1994) Resistance to muring acquired immunodeficiency syndrome (MAIDS). *Science* **252,** 264–266.
75. Mentink Kane, M. and Mosser, D. M. (2001) The role of IL-10 in promoting disease progression in leishmaniasis. *J. Immunol.* **166,** 1141–1147.
76. Xu, D., Chan, W. L., Leung, B. P., et al. (1998) Selective expression of a stable cell surface molecule on type 2 but not type 1 helper T cells. *J. Exp. Med.* **187,** 787–794.
77. Kropf, P., Bickle, Q., Herath, S. H., Klemenz, R., and Müller, I. (2002) Organ-specific distribution of CD4+T1/ST2+ Th2 cells in *Leishmania major* infection. *Eur. J. Immunol.* **9,** 2450–2459.
78. Lingnau, K., Hoehn, P., Kerdine, S., et al. (1998) IL-4 in combination with TGF-β favors an alternative pathway of Th1 development independent of IL-12. *J. Immunol.* **161,** 4709–4718.
79. Mencacci, A., Del Sero, G., Cenci, E., et al. (1998) Endogenous IL-4 is required for the development of protective CD4+ T helper1 cells responses to *Candida albicans. J. Exp. Med.* **187,** 207–317.
80. Biedermann, T., Zimmermann, S., Himmelrich, H., et al. (2001) IL-4 instructs Th1 responses and resistance to *Leishmania major* in susceptible BALB/c mice. *Nat. Immunol.* **2,** 1054–1060.
81. Finkelman, F. D., Holmes, J., Katona, I. M., et al. (1990) Lymphokine control of in vivo immunoglobulin isoltype selection. *Annu. Rev. Immunol.* **8,** 303–333.
82. Morawetz, R. A., Gabriele, L., Rizzo, L. V., et al. (1996) Interleukin-4-independent immunoglobulin class switch to immunoglobulin (Ig)E in the mouse. *J. Exp. Med.* **184,** 1651–1661.
83. von der Weid, T., Kopf, M., and Langhorne, J. (1994) The immune response to *Plasmodium chabaudi* malaria in interleukin-4-deficient mice. *Eur. J. Immunol.* **24,** 2285–2293.
84. McKenzie, G. J., Fallon, G. P., Emson, C. L., Grencis, R. K., and McKenzie, A. N. J. (1999) Simultaneous disruption of IL-4 and IL-13 defines individual roles in T helper cell type 2-mediated responses. *J. Exp. Med.* **189,** 1565–1572.
85. Sad, S., Marcotte, R., and Mosmann, T. R. (1995) Cytokine-induced differentiation of precursor mouse $CD8^+$ T cells into cytotoxic $CD8^+$ T cells secreting Th1 or Th2 cytokines. *Immunity* **2,** 271–279.
86. Li, L., Sad, S., Kägi, D., and Mosmann, T. R. (1997) CD8Tc1 and Tc2 cells secrete distinct cytokine patterns in vitro and in vivo but induce similar inflammatory reactions. *J. Immunol.* **158,** 4152–4161.
87. Villacres, M. C. and Bergmann, C. C. (1999) Enhanced cytotoxic T cell activity in IL-4-deficient mice. *J. Immunol.* **162,** 2663–2770.
88. Schüler, T., Qin, Z., Ibe, S., Noben-Trauth, N., and Blankenstein, T. (1999) T helper cell type 1-associated and cytotoxic T lymphocyte-mediated tumor immunity is impaired in IL-4-deficient mice. *J. Exp. Med.* **189,** 803–810.
89. Carvalho, L. H., Sano, G.-I., Hafalla, J. C. R., et al. (2002) IL-4-secreting $CD4^+$ T cells are crucial to the development of $CD8^+$ T-cell responses against malaria liver stages. *Nat. Med.* **8,** 166–170.

12

Role of IL-5 in Immune and Pathological Responses in the Mouse

Paul S. Foster and Simon P. Hogan

Summary

Studies in interleukin (IL)-$5^{-/-}$ mice have shown that this cytokine plays a critical role in the regulation of eosinophil expansion in the bone marrow and blood in response to allergic and parasitic stimuli. IL-5 also plays a central role in regulating baseline blood and tissue eosinophil numbers but is not essential for eosinophil development or migration. Thus, eosinophil accumulation into allergic tissues should not be viewed as a process that is exclusively regulated by IL-5, but one that is greatly enhanced by this cytokine. Although IL-5 regulated eosinophilia plays an important role in the regulation of allergic inflammation and the subsequent development of disease, its role in the elimination of parasites and in nonallergic disease processes is less clear. This may stem from the observation that eosinophils can accumulate in tissues independently of IL-5 and that these alternative pathways coexist in many disease and immune responses. Importantly, studies in IL-$5^{-/-}$ mice are disclosing an important role for this cytokine in the regulation of immune responses by modulating lymphocyte function.

Key words

cytokines, interleukin 5, eotaxin, eosinophils, allergic disease

1. Introduction

The generation of mice deficient in interleukin- (IL)-5 (IL-$5^{-/-}$ mice) by Kopf and Matthaei, described in a landmark publication in 1996 *(1)*, has facilitated the dissection of the role of IL-5 and eosinophils in a range of immune and pathologic events. In this chapter we highlight investigations in IL-$5^{-/-}$ mice that have provided new information on the role of IL-5-regulated processes in allergic disease, parasite infection, reproduction, transplantation, viral infection and tumor clearance mechanisms.

2. IL-5 in Models of Allergic Disease

The infiltration of eosinophils into the airway wall is thought to play a major pathologic role in asthma *(2)*. Eosinophils have also been implicated in the development of allergic disease of the skin (dermatitis), upper respiratory tract (rhinitis), and gastrointestinal tract (food allergy) *(2–4)*. Migration of eosinophils to sites of allergic disease is thought to be primarily regulated by the secretion of IL-5 from activated CD4+ T-helper 2 (Th2) cells. Through the release of highly toxic granular proteins and a wide range of proinflammatory molecules, eosinophils are thought to induce tissue damage and promote inflammation.

From: *Contemporary Immunology: Cytokine Knockouts, 2nd Edition*
Edited by: Giamila Fantuzzi © Humana Press Inc., Totowa, NJ

Although IL-5-regulated eosinophilia has been implicated in the development of allergic disease, it was not until the generation of IL-$5^{-/-}$ mice that the role of this cytokine in disease induction and progression could be unequivocally identified *(1,5)*.

2.1. IL-5 and Mouse Models of Asthma and Allergy

IL-$5^{-/-}$ mice have been extensively employed to gain insights into the role of eosinophils in asthma and allergy by employing acute and chronic models of allergic airways disease (mouse asthma models) *(6,7)* and antigen-induced Th2 responses in the skin, gastrointestinal tract, and nasal mucosa.

2.1.1. Regulation of Eosinophilia in Asthma Models

Although the etiology and pathophysiology of asthma are complex, a central paradigm in pathogenesis has emerged whereby CD4+ Th-2 type lymphocytes (Th2 cells) regulate disease processes through the recruitment and activation of eosinophils in the allergic lung *(6)*. In this model, Th2 cells, through the secretion of IL-5, regulate eosinophil recruitment to the lung and thereby pathogenic processes that predispose to the development of airway obstruction and remodeling, as well as enhanced bronchial reactivity [airway hyperreactivity (AHR)] to nonspecific spasmogenic stimuli. The idea that IL-5-regulated eosinophilia plays a central role in the pathogenesis of asthma is based on extensive clinical and experimental investigations showing a strong correlation between IL-5 and eosinophils and their secreted products with severity and exacerbation of disease *(8)*.

We have extensively characterized IL-$5^{-/-}$ mice at baseline and during allergic inflammatory conditions *(1,5,9–15)*. At steady-state conditions, mature eosinophils are found in the bone marrow and in blood and tissues (albeit significantly reduced), indicating that IL-5 is not essential for eosinophil differentiation, maturation, survival, or subsequent migration from the bone marrow *(1,5)*. IL-3 and granulocyte/macrophage colony-stimulating factor (GM-CSF) are known to prime progenitor cells for IL-5 responsiveness, and all three cytokines employ the β-common chain to transduce signals *(16)*. However, although IL-5, IL-3, and GM-CSF all contribute to eosinopoiesis, mature eosinophils are found in the bone marrow of mice deficient in these factors or in common components of their receptor signaling systems (β-common chain) *(5,17)*. Thus, studies in these factor-deficient mice demonstrate the presence of alternative, as yet unidentified pathways, that regulate eosinophil differentiation and maturation. Furthermore, a rapid blood eosinophilia can also be induced in naive IL-$5^{-/-}$ mice by the intravenous instillation of the eosinophil-specific chemokine eotaxin, indicating that these eosinophils are functional and can migrate in response to specific chemotactic stimuli.

By contrast to wild-type mice, allergic IL-$5^{-/-}$ mice (systemically sensitized to antigen) do not generate eosinophilia in the blood or bone marrow compartments in response to antigen inhalation (aeroallergen challenge), and this greatly reduces the level of eosinophils that are available to be recruited to the airways. However, since basal levels of eosinophils are still produced in IL-$5^{-/-}$ mice, residual tissue eosinophilia persists in the allergic airways of these mice *(10,18)*. Interestingly, tissue eosinophilia (although reduced) is also a predominant feature of IL-$5^{-/-}$ mice with allergic inflammation of the gastrointestinal tract and in the pulmonary compartment after *Toxocara canis* infection *(12,19)*. Eosinophils also fluctuate normally (in reduced numbers) in the uterus of IL-$5^{-/-}$ mice during the estrus cycle *(20)*.

The production of IL-5 by recombinant vaccinia virus (rVV-IL-5) in the airways of allergic IL-$5^{-/-}$ mice restores eosinophilia in the bone marrow, blood, and lung to levels normally observed in allergic wild-type mice after antigen inhalation *(18)*. In contrast, expression of IL-5 in the airways of IL-$5^{-/-}$ mice at baseline by rVV-IL-5 infection (over days) does not induce eosinophilia in these compartments, indicating that other factors are required to promote eosinopoiesis and migration in conjunction with IL-5. Th2 cells play a central role in eliciting these additional signals that promote eosinophil expansion in association with IL-5. Adoptive transfer of antigen-responsive Th2 cells (IL-5-producing) from wild-type mice to naive or allergic IL-$5^{-/-}$ mice during antigen inhalation results in the induction of eosinophilia and allergic disease of the lung *(11)*. Thus, eosinopoiesis and migration is regulated by IL-5 and signals derived from Th2 cells.

The adoptive transfer of wild-type or IL-$5^{-/-}$ eosinophils to the blood of allergic IL-$5^{-/-}$ mice during antigen inhalation also increases the number of eosinophils recruited to the lung, indicating that the homing of this leukocyte is not solely regulated by IL-5 *(9)*. Notably, these homing mechanisms that operate independently of IL-5 may play an important role in eosinophil accumulation under some pathologic conditions.

Our results suggest that IL-5 is critical for expansion of the eosinophils in the bone marrow and blood in response to allergic stimulation. These data are supported by studies in IL-$5^{-/-}$ mice showing that IL-5 predominantly acts systemically and does not play a central role in the recruitment of this cell to the lung when expressed in the airways *(21)*. However, IL-5 does promote tissue recruitment of eosinophils in response to locally derived chemotactic signals, primarily by increasing the number of eosinophils in the circulation. This cytokine also participates in the maintenance of baseline levels of eosinophils in the blood and tissues. However, additional factors that are under the control of Th2 cells regulate eosinophil homing to sites of allergic disease and amplify eosinopoiesis.

2.1.2. Regulation of AHR in Experimental Models of Asthma

In experimental models of allergic lung disease, inhibition of the actions of IL-5 suppresses eosinophilia (blood and lung) in response to antigen inhalation; however, this effect does not always correlate with abolition of AHR *(9)*. For example, allergic IL-$5^{-/-}$ mice of the C57BL/6 strain do not develop antigen-induced AHR, whereas BALB/c mice develop enhanced reactivity independently of this factor *(10,18)*. AHR also persists in C57BL/6 IL-$5^{-/-}$ mice that have been infected with *Nippostrongylus brasiliensis (22)*. *N. brasiliensis* infection produces a pronounced pulmonary eosinophilia, AHR, and extensive morphologic changes to the lung. IL-5 also contributes to inflammatory and pathologic effects in response to primary *Trichinella spiralis* infection but is not essential for the development of the enhanced smooth muscle contractility that is associated with infection *(22)*. However, whether the mechanisms underlying the induction of enhanced smooth muscle responsiveness in the allergic lung are similar to those induced by parasites remains to be determined.

Although eosinophil recruitment to sites of allergic disease or parasite infection is markedly attenuated in IL-$5^{-/-}$ mice in comparison with wild-type responses, a marked residual tissue eosinophilia can persist in these mice at the site of inflammation *(9,13)*. Tissue levels of eosinophils in allergic mice are significantly greater than those observed in naive wild-type mice. In models of allergic airways disease, the degree of residual tissue eosinophilia in IL-$5^{-/-}$ mice directly correlates with the persistence of AHR *(13)*. In allergic C57BL/6

IL-5$^{-/-}$ mice in which AHR is abolished, tissue eosinophilia is significantly less than in BALB/c mice, in which hyperresponsiveness of smooth muscle persists. However, AHR does not develop in allergic BALB/c mice deficient in both IL-5 and eotaxin (IL-5/eotaxin$^{-/-}$ mice), in which tissue eosinophilia is abolished in response to antigen inhalation *(13)*. Notably, in IL-5/eotaxin$^{-/-}$ mice, Th2 cells are limited in their ability to produce IL-13, a cytokine that potently primes airways smooth muscle to cholinergic agonists. After transfer of wild-type eosinophils to IL-5/eotaxin$^{-/-}$ mice, T-cell production of IL-13 is reestablished to normal levels. These data suggest that eosinophils may directly or indirectly modulate Th2 immunity and, importantly IL-13 production, smooth muscle function, and mucus secretion.

We have also investigated the role of IL-5 in chronic models of asthma that more closely mimic human disease. After chronic administration of low doses of antigen, inflammation and eosinophilia are confined to the epithelium and lamina propria of the airways *(23)*. The airways also exhibit many morphologic features of chronic asthma (subepithelial fibrosis, epithelial hypertrophy, mucus cell metaplasia, and hyperplasia) *(23)*. In the chronic model, IL-5 regulates eosinophil migration, inflammation (numbers of infiltrating cells in the lamina propria), and AHR; however, this cytokine does not contribute to subepithelial collagenization or epithelial thickening *(24)*.

2.1.2. Allergic Models of Rhinitis, Dermatitis, and Gastrointestinal Disease

Employment of IL-5$^{-/-}$ mice in allergic models of the skin and the gastrointestinal tract and of rhinitis has further enhanced our understanding of eosinophils and IL-5 in the pathogenesis of these disorders *(12,25–33)*. In a model of experimental allergic rhinitis, the importance of IL-5 in the induction of eosinophilia and subsequent recruitment to the site of allergic disease (nasal mucosa) in response to allergen challenge was further highlighted *(25)*. However, in this model clinical symptoms of disease and nasal reactivity to histamine were not completely attenuated owing to the presence of additional pathways in IL-5$^{-/-}$ mice that maintained inflammation of the nasal mucosa *(25)*. By contrast, in a model of allergic dermatitis no eosinophils were recruited to sites if inflammation and epidermal and dermal thickening were significantly decreased in IL-5$^{-/-}$ mice, identifying an important role for IL-5 in inflammation and hypertrophy of the skin in this disorder *(26)*.

Eosinophil numbers are increased in the gastrointestinal tract in numerous clinical disorders; however, information on the role of this cell in disease and on the processes regulating recruitment to this mucosal surface is very limited *(4,34)*. In naive IL-5$^{-/-}$ mice, eosinophil numbers in the gastrointestinal mucosa are significantly decreased, but only in the eotaxin-deficient mice (eotaxin$^{-/-}$ mice) were they absent *(27,29)*. Both molecules appear to have similar roles in the recruitment of eosinophils to the gastrointestinal tract during allergic inflammation *(12,27)*. In a model of allergic inflammation of the gastrointestinal tract, characterized byTh2-regulated inflammation, the development of gastric dysmotility, gastromegaly, cachexia, and tissue eosinophilia (albeit reduced) was still a predominant feature of IL-5$^{-/-}$ mice *(12,27)*. By contrast, in eotaxin$^{-/-}$ mice, eosinophil recruitment and the development of pathophysiologic responses were almost abolished.

Eosinophil infiltration of the esophagus is also observed in a range of diseases (e.g., gastroesophageal reflux and allergic gastroenteritis) *(4)*. In a model of experimental esophagitis, eosinophil recruitment was impaired in eotaxin$^{-/-}$ mice, whereas in the absence of IL-5, eosinophil accumulation and epithelial hyperplasia were ablated *(31)*. Thus, anti-IL-5 treatment may be a rational approach to the treatment of eosinophilic esophageal disorders, whereas targeting eotaxin may be more beneficial for disorders of the gastrointestinal mucosa *(31)*. Collectively, these studies indicate that eosinophil accumulation in various tissues is differentially regulated and that targeting eosinophils in diseased states will require a firm understanding of the mechanisms of tissue-specific migration.

3. IL-5 and Parasitic Infection

Although eosinophils are a predominant feature of parasitic infections and are thought to play a central role in host defence, very few studies have employed IL-$5^{-/-}$ mice to examine the effect of eosinophilia on worm clearance and persistence during infection. IL-$5^{-/-}$ mice infected with the helminth *Mesocestoides cortido* did not develop blood or tissue eosinophilia *(1)*. Notably, the absence of IL-5 did not affect worm burden in these infected mice, suggesting that eosinophilia does not play a significant role in the host defence in this parasite model *(1)*. Comparison of schistosomiasis infection in wild-type and IL-$5^{-/-}$ mice also suggested that IL-5-regulated processes played only a small role in the development of Th2 responses, susceptibility to primary infections, and the ability to resist subsequent infections *(35)*. Hepatic pathology was also similar in both the presence and absence of IL-5, although eosinophil numbers were markedly decreased in liver tissue of IL-$5^{-/-}$ mice after infection *(35)*. Interestingly, during chronic schistosomiasis infection, mast cell numbers increased and were observed in the granulomas of IL-$5^{-/-}$ mice, and IL-4 production from non-T- and non-B-cells was reduced *(35)*. Studies in IL-$5^{-/-}$ mice have also shown an important role for IL-5 and eosinophils in the *Schistosoma mansoni* egg-induced early production of IL-4 and potentially in the development of egg-specific Th2 cells *(36)*.

Peripheral and tissue eosinophilia is a prominent feature of enteric nematode infections, such as *T. spiralis (37,38)*. Infection of wild-type or IL-$5^{-/-}$ mice with *T. spiralis* resulted in expulsion of the parasite by d 21 *(38)*. In response to secondary infection, IL-$5^{-/-}$ mice had little increase in eosinophil numbers within the intestine in comparison with wild-type mice. However, during the course of the infection, IL-$5^{-/-}$ mice developed larger worm burdens, and the kinetics of elimination of the parasite were significantly slower than those observed in wild-type mice. Thus, in response to secondary infection of *T. spiralis*, IL-5 plays a key role in regulating eosinophilia and contributes to parasite elimination, demonstrating an important role for IL-5 in host defence against this parasite *(38)*. Although in the nematode-infected mice IL-5 appears essential for intestinal eosinophilia, it only partially contributes to development of enhanced smooth muscle reactivity in response to infection *(37)*. IL-5 and eosinophils have also been shown to have a protective role in response to primary *Strongyloides ratti* infection *(39)*.

By contrast, a detrimental role for IL-5 has been suggested in the early phases of infection with *Toxoplasma gondii (40)*. After oral administration of this parasite, IL-$5^{-/-}$ mice are less susceptible to infection. IL-$5^{-/-}$ mice had reduced mortality rates and less severe morphologic changes in the small intestine 8 d after infection. Reduction in disease progression correlated with increased serum levels of IL-12 and interferon-γ and an absence of eosinophils in the blood of IL-$5^{-/-}$ mice. Interestingly, no differences in mortality or pathophysiologic features were observed between wild-type and IL-$5^{-/-}$ mice infected intraperitoneally with *T. gondii (40)*. Zhang and Denkers *(41)*, in a chronic model of *T. gondii* infection, found that IL-$5^{-/-}$ mice had increased mortality and weight loss in comparison with wild-type mice, suggesting different roles for IL-5 in regulating the immune response and disease progression during acute and chronic infection *(41)*. These studies with *T. gondii* further suggest that IL-5, by regulating eosinophilia, can alter the Th1/Th2 balance in response to infectious agents.

Eosinophilia in the peripheral blood and bone marrow compartments is a prominent feature of C57Bl/6 wild-type but not IL-5$^{-/-}$ mice infected with embryonated eggs of *T. canis* *(19)*. Although the number of eosinophils recruited to tissues decreased during the acute phase of infection in IL-5$^{-/-}$ mice, this granulocyte was still present in significant numbers. Eosinophils were detected in reduced numbers in the lung, liver, heart, and skeletal muscle of infected IL-5$^{-/-}$ mice in comparison with wild-type mice. Notably, IL-5 had no effect on the number and location of *Toxocara canis* larvae. However, tissue damage to the infected lung in IL-5$^{-/-}$ mice was less extensive than that observed in wild-type mice. These results suggest that eosinophils regulate pathologic responses in mice infected with *T. canis.*

4. IL-5-Regulated Eosinophilia in Immune and Physiologic Responses and Nonallergic Disorders

Although eosinophils are predominating features of allergic diseases and parasitic infections, this leukocyte also participates in immune responses associated with many disorders (cancer, transplantation, idiopathic bowel disease, and other forms of colonic inflammation). However, the role of this cell in disease processes remains largely unknown *(2)*. Although IL-5 and eosinophils have been linked to tissue rejection during transplantation, employment of IL-5$^{-/-}$ mice failed to demonstrate a role for this granulocyte in the rejection of neovascularized pig proislet xenografts in mice *(42)*. CD4 T-cells and eosinophils are features of the inflammatory response associated with the rejection of neovascularized pig proislet (islet precursor) xenografts in mice. Eosinophil accumulation at the transplant site was ablated in IL-5$^{-/-}$ mice, but the kinetics of xenograft rejection were unaltered. Prolonged xenograft survival was only achieved in anti-CD4 monoclonal antibody (mAb)-treated mice, suggesting that CD4+ T-cells and not eosinophils play a central role in the rejection process *(42)*. However, the role of IL-5-regulated eosinophilia in the survival of skin grafts within species remains controversial *(43)*.

Eosinophils have also been observed infiltrating disease tissues of the bowel, suggesting a pathogenic role for this cell. In a dextran sulphate sodium (DSS)-induced colitis model of inflammatory bowel disease, tissue eosinophilia was reduced significantly in IL-5$^{-/-}$ mice, but this effect did not correlate with differences in disease severity or extent of tissue damage to the colon *(44)*.

Although IL-5 has been primarily thought of as a key regulator of eosinophil function, it was first identified as a terminal differentiation factor for B-lymphocytes *(45)*. Indeed, studies with IL-5$^{-/-}$ mice are disclosing important roles for this cytokine in the regulation of immune responses by modulating lymphocyte function. Initial studies in IL-5$^{-/-}$ mice showed that the number of CD5+ (B-1) cells was reduced in 2 wk-old mice but returned to normal by 6–8 wk *(1)*. In recent studies a more sustained effect on B-1 lymphocytes and mucosal IgA levels has been proposed in the absence of IL-5 *(46)*. In limited in vitro studies, IL-5 has also been implicated in regulating cytotoxic lymphocyte (CTL) development *(47)*. These studies have been extended in IL-5$^{-/-}$ mice, in which a role for this cytokine in the generation of CTL responses to modified tumor antigens was as identified *(48)*. IL-5 was as effective as IL-2 for the induction of CTL responses from spleen cells, and CTL precursor frequency was greatly diminished in IL-$5^{-/-}$ mice, which correlated with an inability to reject antigen-specific tumors *(48)*.

Evidence is also emerging that IL-5 may modulate Th2 cell function. However, whether IL-5 directly modulates T-cell function or exerts its effects through eosinophils or other mechanisms is not yet established *(13,36,49,50)*. Although eosinophil trafficking is profoundly impaired in the allergic lung of IL-$5^{-/-}$ mice, the recruitment of lymphocytes to the lung compartment is also significantly attenuated *(10,18)*. Recently, we have also shown that IL-5 deficiency results in lower levels of IL-13 production in the allergic lung, owing to impaired secretion of this cytokine from Th2 cells *(13)*. Analysis of CD4+ T-cells from naive IL-$5^{-/-}$ mice shows that they have an intrinsic defect in their ability to produce IL-13 after polarization to the Th2 phenotype. Notably, normal production of IL-13 was restored in Th2 cells after transfer of eosinophils to mice deficient in this cytokine. Importantly, these data show that IL-5 and/or eosinophils play a fundamental role in regulating Th2 immunity by influencing T-lymphocyte function.

Thus, the proinflammatory actions of IL-5 may stem from the fact that it regulates not only eosinophilia but also T-cell function. IL- 5 may directly influence the lymphocyte pool or may regulate T-cell responses through eosinophils. In this regard, we and others have recently shown that eosinophils can modulate CD4+ T-cell function *(49,50)*. Eosinophils in the allergic lung can present antigen and traffic to local lymph nodes, where they colocalize with T-cells, and this granulocyte can induce proliferation and cytokine secretion from Th2 cells. Eosinophils are also known to secrete a wide range of T-cell growth and chemotactic factors. Thus, evidence is emerging that eosinophils may not only act as terminal effector cells but also actively modulate allergic inflammation by amplifying the type 2 cytokine response. IL-5 plays an important role in these processes by regulating eosinophil accumulation at sites of allergic disease.

References

1. Kopf, M., Brombacher, F., Hodgkin, P. D., et al. (1996) IL-5-deficient mice have a developmental defect in $CD5^+$ B-1 cells and lack eosinophilia but have normal antibody and cytotoxic T cell responses. *Immunity* **4,** 15–24.
2. Rothenberg, M. (1998) Eosinophilia. *N. Engl. J. Med.* **338,** 1592–1600.
3. Weller, P. F. (1994) Eosinophils: structure and functions. *Curr. Opin. Immunol.* **6,** 85–90.
4. Rothenberg, M. E., Mishra, A., Brandt, E. B., and Hogan, S. P. (2001) Gastrointestinal eosinophils in health and disease. *Adv. Immunol.* **78,** 291–328.
5. Foster, P. S., Hogan, S. P., Ramsay A. J., Matthaei, K. I., and Young, I. G. (1996) Interleukin 5 deficiency abolishes eosinophilia, airways hyperreactivity, and lung damage in a mouse asthma model [see comments]. *J. Exp. Med.* **183,** 195–201.
6. Wills-Karp, M. (1999) Immunologic basis of antigen-induced airway hyperresponsiveness. *Annu. Rev. Immunol.* **17,** 255–281.
7. Wills-Karp, M. (2000) Murine models of asthma in understanding immune dysregulation in human asthma. *Immunopharmacology* **48,** 263–268.
8. Robinson, D. S., Durham, S. R., and Kay, A. B. (1993) Cytokines in asthma. *Thorax* **48,** 845–853.
9. Foster, P., Mould, A., Yang, M., et al. (2001) Elemental signals regulating eosinophil accumulation in the lung. *Immunol. Rev.* **179,** 173–181.
10. Hogan, S. P., Matthaei, K. I., Young, J. M., Koskinen, A., Young, I. G., and Foster, P. S. (1998) A novel T cell-regulated mechanism modulating allergen-induced airways hyperreactivity in BALB/c mice independently of IL-4 and IL-5. *J. Immunol.* **161,** 1501–1509.

11. Hogan, S. P., Koskinen, A., Matthaei, K. I., Young, I. G., and Foster, P. S. (1998) Interleukin-5-producing CD4+ T cells play a pivotal role in aeroallergen-induced eosinophilia, bronchial hyperreactivity, and lung damage in mice. *Am. J. Respir. Crit. Care Med.* **157,** 210–218.
12. Hogan, S., Mishra, E., Brandt, E., Foster, P., and Rothenberg, M. (2000) A critical role for eotaxin in experimental aral antigen-indcued eosinophilic gastrointestinal allergy. *Proc. Natl. Acad. Sci.* **97,** 6681–6686.
13. Mattes, J., Yang, M., Mahalingam, S., et al. (2002) Intrinsic defect in T cell production of interleukin (IL)-13 in the absence of both IL-5 and eotaxin precludes the development of eosinophilia and airways hyperreactivity in experimental asthma. *J. Exp. Med.* **195,** 1433–1444.
14. Mould, A. W., Ramsay, A. J., Matthaei, K. I., Young, I. G., Rothenberg, M. E., and Foster, P. S. (1999) Role of IL-5, eotaxin, and T-lymphocytes in regulating eosinophil trafficking, degranulation, and airways hyperreactivity. *submitted.*
15. Mould, A. W., Ramsay, A. J., Matthaei, K. I., Young, I. G., Rothenberg, M. E., and Foster, P. S. (2000) The effect of IL-5 and eotaxin expression in the lung on eosinophil trafficking and degranulation and the induction of bronchial hyperreactivity. *J. Immunol.* **164,** 2142–2150.
16. Sanderson, C. J., Campbell, H. D., and Young, I. G. (1988) Molecular and cellular biology of eosinophil differentiation factor (interleukin-5) and its effects on human and mouse B cells. *Immunol. Rev.* **102,** 29–50.
17. Nishinakamura, R., Miyajima, A., Mee, P. J., Tybulewicz, V. L. J., and Murray, R. (1996) Hematopoiesis in mice lacking the entire granulocyte-macrophage colony-stimulating factor/interleukin-3/interleukin-5 functions. *Blood* **88,** 2458–2464.
18. Foster, P., Hogan, S., Ramsay, A., Matthaei, K., and Young, I. (1996) Interleukin-5 deficiency abolishes eosinophilia, airway hyperreactivity and lung damage in mouse asthma model. *J. Exp. Med.* **183,** 195–201.
19. Takamoto, M., Ovington, K. S., Behm, C. A., Sugane, K., Young, I. G., and Matthaei, K. I. (1997) Eosinophilia, parasite burden and lung damage in *Toxocara canis* infection in C57Bl/6 mice genetically deficient in IL-5. *Immunology* **90,** 511–517.
20. Robertson, S. A., Mau, V. J., Young, I. G., and Matthaei, K. I. (2000) Uterine eosinophils and reproductive performance in interleukin 5-deficient mice. *J. Reprod. Fertil.* **120,** 423–432.
21. Wang, J., Palmer, K., Lotvall, J., et al. (1998) Circulating, but not local lung, IL-5 is required for the development of antigen-induced airways eosinophilia. *J. Clin. Invest.* **102,** 1132–1141.
22. Coyle, A. J., Kohler, G., Tsuyuki, S., Brombacher, F., and Kopf, M. (1998) Eosinophils are not required to induce airway hyperresponsiveness after nematode infection. *Eur. J. Immunol.* **28,** 2640–2647.
23. Temelkovski, J., Hogan, S. P., Shepherd, D. P., Foster, P. S., and Kumar, R. K. (1998) An improved murine model of asthma: selective airway inflammation, epithelial lesions and increased methacholine responsiveness following chronic exposure to aerosolised allergen. *Thorax* **53,** 849–856.
24. Foster, P. S., Ming, Y., Matthei, K. I., Young, I. G., Temelkovski, J., and Kumar, R. K. (2000) Dissociation of inflammatory and epithelial responses in a murine model of chronic asthma. *Lab. Invest.* **80,** 655–662.
25. Saito, H., Matsumoto, K., Denburg, A. E., et al. (2002) Pathogenesis of murine experimental allergic rhinitis: a study of local and systemic consequences of IL-5 deficiency. *J. Immunol.* **168,** 3017–3023.
26. Spergel, J. M., Mizoguchi, E., Oettgen, H., Bhan, A. K., and Geha, R. S. (1999) Roles of TH1 and TH2 cytokines in a murine model of allergic dermatitis. *J. Clin. Invest.* **103,** 1103–1111.
27. Hogan, S. P., Mishra, A., Brandt, E. B., et al. (2001) A pathological role for eotaxin and eosinophils in eosinophilic gastrointestinal inflammation. *Nat. Immunol.* **2,** 353–360.
28. Hogan, S. P., Foster, P. S., and Rothenberg, M. E. (2002) Experimental analysis of eosinophil-associated gastrointestinal diseases. *Curr. Opin. Allergy Clin. Immunol.* **2,** 239–248.
29. Mishra, A., Hogan, S. P., Lee, J. J., Foster, P. S., and Rothenberg, M. E. (1999) Fundamental signals that regulate eosinophil homing to the gastrointestinal tract. *J. Clin. Invest.* **103,** 1719–1727.
30. Mishra, A., Hogan, S. P., Brandt, E. B., and Rothenberg, M. E. (2000) Peyer's patch eosinophils: identification, characterization, and regulation by mucosal allergen exposure, interleukin-5, and eotaxin. *Blood* **96.** 1538–1544.

31. Mishra, A., Hogan, S. P., Brandt, E. B., and Rothenberg, M. E. (2001) An etiological role for aeroallergens and eosinophils in experimental esophagitis. *J. Clin. Invest.* **107,** 83–90.
32. Mishra, A., Hogan, S. P., Brandt, E. B., et al. (2001) Enterocyte expression of the eotaxin and IL-5 transgenes induces compartmentalized dysregulation of eosinophil trafficking. *J. Biol. Chem.* **30,** 30.
33. Mishra, A., Hogan, S. P., and Rothenberg, M. E. (2002) Interleukin-5 promotes eosinophil trafficking to the esophagus. *J. Immunol.* **5,** 2464–2469.
34. Rothenberg, M. E., Mishra, A., Brandt, E. B., and Hogan, S. P. (2001) Gastrointestinal eosinophils. *Immunol. Rev.* **179,** 139–155.
35. Brunet, L. R., Sabin, E. A., Cheever, A. W., Kopf, M. A., and Pearce, E. J. (1999) Interleukin 5 (IL-5) is not required for expression of a Th2 response or host resistance mechanisms during murine *Schistosoma mansoni* but does play a role in development of IL-4-producing non-T, non-B cells. *Infect. Immun.* **67,** 3014–3018.
36. Sabin, E. A., Kopf, M. A., and Pearce, E. J. (1996) *Schistosoma mansoni* egg-induced early IL-4 production is dependent upon IL-5 and eosinophils. *J. Exp. Med.* **184,** 1871–1878.
37. Vallance, B. A., Blennerhassett, P. A., Deng, Y., Matthaei, K. I., Young, I. G., and Collins, S. M. (1999) IL-5 contributes to worm expulsion and muscle hypercontractility in a primary T. spiralis infection. *Am. J. Physiol.* **277,** G400–G408.
38. Vallance, B. A., Matthaei, K. I., Sanovic, S., Young, I. G., and Collins, S. M. (2000) Interleukin-5 deficient mice exhibit impaired host defence against challenge *Trichinella spiralis* infections. *Parasite Immunol.* **22,** 487–492.
39. Ovington, K. S., McKie, K., Matthaei, K. I., Young, I. G., and Behm, C. A. (1998) Regulation of primary *Strongyloides ratti* infections in mice: a role for interleukin-5. *Immunology* **95,** 488–493.
40. Nickdel, M. B., Roberts, F., Brombacher, F., Alexander, J., and Roberts, C. W. (2001) Counter-protective role for interleukin-5 during acute *Toxoplasma gondii* infection. *Infect. Immun.* **69,** 1044–1052.
41. Zhang, Y., and Denkers, E. Y. (1999) Protective role for interleukin-5 during chronic *Toxoplasma gondii* infection. *Infect. Immun.* **67,** 4383–4392.
42. Simeonovic, C. J., Townsend, M. J., Wilson, J. D., et al. (1997) Eosinophils are not required for the rejection of neovascularized fetal pig proislet xenografts in mice. *J. Immunol.* **158,** 2490–2499.
43. Surquin, M., Le Moine, A., Flamand, V., et al. (2002) Skin graft rejection elicited by beta 2-microglobulin as a minor transplantation antigen involves multiple effector pathways: role of Fas-Fas ligand interactions and Th2-dependent graft eosinophil infiltrates. *J. Immunol.* **169,** 500–506.
44. Stevceva, L., Pavli, P., Husband, A., Matthaei, K. I., Young, I. G., and Doe, W. F. (2000) Eosinophilia is attenuated in experimental colitis induced in IL-5 deficient mice. *Genes Immun.* **1,** 213–218.
45. Kinashi, T., Harada, N., Severinson, E., et al. (1986) Cloning of complementary DNA encoding T-cell replacing factor and identity with B-cell growth factor II. *Nature* **324,** 70–73.
46. Bao, S., Beagley, K. W., Murray, A. M., et al. (1998) Intestinal IgA plasma cells of the B1 lineage are IL-5 dependent. *Immunology* **94,** 181–188.
47. Takatsu, K., Kikuchi, Y., Takahashi, T., et al. (1987) Interleukin 5, a T-cell-derived B-cell differentiation factor also induces cytotoxic T lymphocytes. *Proc. Natl. Acad. Sci. USA* **84,** 4234–4238.
48. Apostolopoulos, V., McKenzie, I. F., Lees, C., Matthaei, K. I., and Young, I. G. (2000) A role for IL-5 in the induction of cytotoxic T lymphocytes in vivo. *Eur. J. Immunol.* **30,** 1733–1739.
49. MacKenzie, J. R., Mattes, J., Dent, L. A., and Foster, P. S. (2001) Eosinophils promote allergic disease of the lung by regulating CD4+ Th2 lymphocyte function. *J. Immunol.* **167,** 3146–3155.
50. Shi, H. Z., Humbles, A., Gerard, C., Jin, Z., and Weller, P. F. (2000) Lymph node trafficking and antigen presentation by endobronchial eosinophils. *J. Clin. Invest.* **105,** 945–953.

13

IL-6 Knockout Mice

Valeria Poli and Diego Maritano

Summary

Interleukin-6 (IL-6) is a pleiotropic cytokine thought to play important regulatory roles in immunity, hemopoiesis, and inflammation (reviewed in ref. *1*). The generation of IL-6-deficient mice by gene targeting has allowed direct testing of its role in a variety of physiological and pathological conditions. Thus, IL-6 has been shown to favour the resolution of infections and to promote optimal humoral responses to various antigens while at the same time being required for the development of immune-mediated diseases, such as CIA or EAE, as well as of diseases such as osteoporosis and plasmacytomas, caused by improper expansion of specific hematopietic compartments. In addition, IL-6-deficient mice display defective liver acute phase and regenerative responses, improper body weight regulation, impaired neuronal regeneration, and altered nociceptive responses, confirming the pleiotropic nature of this cytokine. This chapter attempts to review the ample literature in the field by trying to rationalize the main conclusions achieved and to highlight the open-ended problems.

Key words

IL-6, knockout mice, infections, arthritis, experimental autoimmune encephalomyelitis (EAE), plasmacytomas, osteoporosis, inflammation, acute phase response, liver regeneration, nociceptive responses, obesity

1. Introduction

Interleukin-6 (IL-6) was initially identified as a factor inducing the terminal maturation of B-lymphocytes into antibody-producing plasma cells. It has also been shown to trigger T-lymphocyte survival, to stimulate cytotoxic T-cell differentiation, to stimulate proliferation and/or differentiation of various hematopoietic stem cell lineages (reviewed in ref. *1*), and to mediate several host responses to acute inflammation, including the acute-phase reaction in the liver *(2)*. IL-6 can be produced by a variety of cells including T- and B-lymphocytes, phagocytic cells, fibroblasts, and endothelial cells. Its synthesis is normally tightly controlled and is rapidly increased in response to a wide range of stimuli such as bacterial or viral infection, inflammation, inflammatory cytokines, and different kinds of traumas. IL-6-disregulated production has been implicated in the pathogenesis of autoimmune disorders, plasma cell dyscrasias, and postmenopausal osteoporosis *(1)*.

IL-6 signaling occurs through the assembly of a receptor complex composed of two subunits, the ligand-binding IL-6 receptor α (IL-6Rα) and the signal-transducing gp130. gp130 also acts as a signaling subunit for a family of cytokines structurally related to IL-6: leukemia inhibitory factor (LIF), oncostatin M (OM), ciliary neurotrophic factor (CNTF), interleukin-11 (IL-11), and cardiotrophin-1 (recently reviewed in ref. *3*). In contrast to IL-6

From: *Contemporary Immunology: Cytokine Knockouts, 2nd Edition*
Edited by: Giamila Fantuzzi © Humana Press Inc., Totowa, NJ

and IL-11, which trigger gp130 homodimerization, LIF, OM, and CNTF assemble a heterodimeric complex between gp130 and a second signaling molecule, the LIFRβ or the OMRβ. The common sharing of gp130 and the differential involvement of the LIFRβ and OMRβ are likely explanations for the overlapping and diverging functions displayed by these cytokines. The IL-6Rα cytoplasmic domain is not required for signaling, and soluble IL-6Rα forms (sIL-6Rα) can act as agonists, conferring IL-6 responsiveness on cells that only harbor gp130 (recently reviewed in ref. *4*).

Circulating forms of IL-6Rα, generated by either alternative splicing or shedding from the cell surface, are naturally present in both humans and mice, and their production is highly regulated and specifically increased in a variety of pathologic conditions and during inflammation *(4)*. The interaction of IL-6 with its receptor complex triggers the activation of two different pathways *(5)*: the Ras-MAP kinase pathway, thought to culminate mainly in the activation of members of the C/EBP family of transcription factors, and the activation of Jak kinases and transcription factors belonging to the STAT family (signal transducers and activators of transcription). All members of the IL-6 cytokine family were shown to be able to activate STAT3 and to a lesser extent STAT1.

The complex functional interplay between different cytokines, which influence one another's synthesis and whose effects are unique or overlapping depending on the target tissue, has often made the unequivocal identification of the specific in vivo role of these molecules evasive. The development of mutant mice carrying null mutations in cytokine genes has recently provided the opportunity to characterize unambiguously the functions that are "unique" to certain cytokines, and those that are "redundant" and can be functionally complemented by other molecules.

With this goal in mind, we and other laboratories have generated IL-6-deficient ($IL\text{-}6^{-/-}$) mice by gene targeting *(6–8)*. Even though IL-6 is expressed during embryonic development, mice homozygous for the IL-6 mutation were born according to mendelian distribution and found to be perfectly viable and fertile, providing a valid model to study the pathophysiologic functions of this cytokine during adult life. During the 8 years since their first description, IL-6 null mice have been the object of hundreds of studies aimed at defining the role of this cytokine in regulating immune responses to soluble antigens or to infectious agents, the development of autoimmune disorders and of plasma cell dyscrasias, different aspects of inflammation including lymphocyte recruitment, activation of the hypothalamic-pituitary-adrenal (HPA) axis, fever and stimulation of acute-phase responses, liver and axonal regeneration, and body weight control. Although sometimes results have been impressively clear-cut and in substantial agreement, different studies have sometimes reached different conclusions. Here we would like to summarize this wealth of information by drawing the main firm conclusions possible and at the same time rationalizing the main discrepancies. Apologies to the many colleagues whose work it has not been possible to cite or describe in detail.

2. IL-6 and the Hematopoietic System

Despite the well-known in vivo capacity of IL-6 to stimulate stem cell proliferation and the formation of multilineage blast cell colonies, IL-6 knockout mice displayed normal steady-state hematologic parameters *(9)*. However, numbers of primitive clonal progenitors in the bone marrow and spleen were reduced and long-term repopulating functions compromised, suggesting that IL-6 promotes survival and self-renewal of hematopoietic stem cells and their early progenitors. In addition, the equilibrium between proliferation and final maturation of progenitor cells belonging to the myeloid and erythrocyte lineages was altered in the mutant mice.

3. T-Lymphocyte Functions

IL-6 is known to be able to mediate T-cell proliferation and survival and to induce the development of cytotoxic T-cells (CTLs) *(10–12)*. Indeed, the steady-state numbers of thymocytes and peripheral T-cells were found to be reduced by about 30% in the IL-$6^{-/-}$ mice *(6)*. However, T-cell subpopulations from the spleen, lymph nodes, and thymus showed a normal distribution and normal patterns of expression of the T-cell receptor chains and of CD4, CD8, CD44, and CD24 markers *(6,7,13)*. In addition, spleen or lymph node cells from naive mice displayed normal proliferative responses and IL-2 receptor expression, suggesting that IL-6 is not required for T-cell activation in vivo or in the presence of accessory cells *(6)*. In contrast, T-cell proliferative responses and cytokine production upon immunization with different antigens have been variably shown to be normal or defective depending on the route of immunization, the antigen, and the mouse strain (*see* Subheading 5), and production of T-cell-dependent antibodies was in several cases impaired in the IL-6 mutant mice *(6,14)*. Moreover, these mice have often shown skewed polarization of the T-helper response toward Th2 responses upon challenge with different infectious agents (*see* Subheading 5).

Also, the antiviral CTL responses do not require IL-6, as both CTL generation and their lytic activity were normal in the IL-$6^{-/-}$ mice infected with lymphocytic choriomeningitis virus (LCMV) or with an attenuated recombinant strain of vaccinia virus (VV) *(6)*. In contrast, CTL lytic activity was reduced upon infection with the strain Western Reserve of VV, with 10–1000-fold higher titers of virus recovered from ovaries and lungs. In the light of the normal CTL responses elicited by other viruses and dependent on viral strain and characteristics of the infection, this defect might in fact be secondary to the uncontrolled spread of the virus, in turn perhaps indirectly generated by impaired production or function of antiviral factors such as interferons *(15)*. In conclusion, the data reported so far do not support an essential role for IL-6 in determining the differentiation and function of T-lymphocytes, although specific T-cell responses may indeed be defective (*see* following sections).

4. B-Lymphocyte Development and Functions

IL-6 was originally identified as a potent growth factor for myeloma and plasmacytoma cells both in vitro and in vivo (reviewed in ref. *16*). It is a proliferation factor for early plasmablastic cells and also a potent inducer of the development of proliferating plasmablastic cells into mature high IgG-producing nondividing plasma cells *(17,18)*. Indeed, several pathologic conditions associated with disregulated IL-6 synthesis show IL-6-dependent overproduction of antibodies (reviewed in ref. *1*), and IL-6 transgenic mice develop splenomegaly and hypergammaglobulinemia *(19)*. Even so, not only did naive young IL-6 knockout mice display normal B-cell numbers and normal expression of markers like B220, IgM, IgD, and CD23, but also the numbers of plasma cells and the natural levels of circulating immunoglobulins were equivalent between mutant and wild-type littermates, suggesting that B-cell development and plasma cell differentiation are not impaired in the absence of IL-6 *(6)*. Further studies have confirmed that plasma cell maturation and antibody switching indeed occur normally in the IL-6 knockout mice. Interestingly, however, antibody titers in response to immunization with specific antigens were in many cases moderately to significantly decreased. In particular, T-cell-dependent IgG responses were decreased by 30% upon infection with vesicular stomatitis virus (VSV) *(6)*. Likewise, despite normal T-cell priming and cytokine production, immunization with the T-cell-dependent antigen DPN-ovalbumin (OVA) triggered normal IgM but reduced IgG1, IgG2a, and IgG2b levels. This correlated with arrested development of germinal centers, which were about five times smaller despite normal proliferation rates and no evident signs of apoptosis *(14)*.

This defect might be at least partially related to the totally impaired production of the complement protein C3 detected in the mutant mice. C3 is known to stimulate the humoral response and, similar to the IL-6$^{-/-}$ mice, C3-deficient mice show impaired germinal center formation and defective IgG2a and -2b responses *(14,20)*. Defective germinal center functions may at least partly explain the decreased antibody responses observed in the absence of IL-6. Impaired IgG antibody responses have also been reported upon challenge with a variety of other antigens or infectious agents, including *Schistosoma* eggs, collagen type II, methylated BSA (mBSA), the encephalitogenic peptide myelin oligodendrocyte glycoprotein (MOG), *Candida albicans*, and the pristane oil-induced anti-ds or ssDNA IgG *(21–31)*. Others have, however, reported either increased or normal IgG responses, as in the case of 129 IL-6 knockout mice immunized with OVA *(32)*, of repeated peroral immunization with OVA in the presence of cholera toxin *(33)*, or of infection with *Helicobacter felix* or with *Mycobacterium tuberculosis (33,34)*. In addition, Markine-Goryanoff and colleagues *(35)* have recently shown that, whereas polyclonal IgG2a responses to lactic dehydrogenase virus (LDV) or *Toxoplasma gondii* or even the T-cell-independent IgG3 response to lipopolysaccharide (LPS) were strongly reduced in the IL-6 knockout mice, antigen-specific antibody titers were normal. A possible explanation for this preferential defect in polyclonal cell expansion could be that the stimulation of preexisting, long-lived, already committed B-cells is IL-6-dependent *(35)*.

The heterogeneity of the results reported above might be partly owing to the capacity of particularly strong challenges to circumvent the loss of the IL-6-dependent pathway(s), consistent with the observation that antibody responses were less defective after secondary and tertiary immunization. In addition, it is likely that different antigen dosages, routes of administration, and adjuvants, together with differences in genetic background, may change the dependence on complement of the humoral response.

The development of mucosal immunity and IgA responses has been studied in detail in the IL-6$^{-/-}$ mice. Initial reports showed that the numbers of IgA+ plasma cells in mesenteric lymph nodes and in the gut of naive IL-6 knockout mice were decreased by 50% and that mucosal challenge with OVA generated very low levels of IgA-containing cells in the intestine *(36)*. Interestingly, two lineages of murine B-cells have been identified, distinguished by their tissue of origin, cell surface markers, antibody repertoire, and cytokine responsiveness. IgA+ B1-cells are selectively induced to secrete IgA by IL-5 and not by IL-6, whereas IgA+ B2-cells are mainly responsive to IL-6. Further work on the IL-6$^{-/-}$ mice has led to the observation that, although the overall numbers of B-cells in the gut were indeed reduced, the remaining population was enriched in IL-5-responsive B1-cells. Although natural IgA levels in the intestinal secretions were very low in the naive mutant mice, the anti-phosphorylcholine (PC) and anti-LPS antibody responses to a challenge with attenuated *Salmonella typhimurium* were increased *(37,38)*.

Taken together, these data suggest that the development of mucosal B2-cells is indeed impaired in the IL-$6^{-/-}$ mice but that intestinal B1-cells responding to microbial antigens develop normally and are fully functional. Other authors failed to detect any difference in the distribution of both B1- and B2-cells in the gut of naive mice *(33)* or in the naturally occurrying levels of IgA in fecal extracts, saliva, or serum *(39)*. The same authors showed normal IgA responses to oral or intranasal keyhole limpet hemocyanin (KLH) or OVA immunization (using cholera toxin as an adjuvant) or to infection with *H. felix* or rotavirus *(33,39)*. These discrepancies may partly reflect distinct processing steps triggered by the different antigens and suggest that mucosal immunity is not globally impaired in the absence of IL-6 but rather that specific responses to specific antigens require IL-6 for their optimal development.

5. Responses to Infectious Diseases

IL-6 is expressed early and abundantly during infections. However, because of its proinflammatory and pleiotropic effects, it has often not been clear whether its production is beneficial or detrimental for disease resolution.

Numerous studies have now demonstrated that in most cases IL-6 has a protective function during infections, although the exact mechanism(s) through which this protection is established are not perfectly understood and may vary depending on the infectious agent and the route of infection. Infection of IL-6 knockout mice with different agents leads in most cases to unbalanced T-helper responses, with increased production of Th2-type cytokines such as IL-10 and sometimes IL-4, and impaired production of Th1-type cytokines, particularly of interferon-γ (IFN-γ) (infection with *T. gondii, Chlamydia trachomatis, M. tuberculosis, Aspergillus fumigatus*, or *Candida albicans*) *(30,34,40–44)*. Infection with *Borrelia burgdoferi* represented an exception, correlating with decreased IL-4 and increased IFN-γ *(45)*. Sometimes, defective localized or blood neutrophilia were implied in the increased susceptibility (*Listeria monocytogenes, Escherichia coli,* and *Klebsiella pneumoniae*) *(8,46,47)*, in certain cases correlating and possibly explaining the unbalanced T-helper responses (*C. albicans* and *T. gondii*) *(30,40,41)*. Normal inflammatory cell recruitment but impaired phagocyte fungicidal function was instead demonstrated in response to *A. fumigatus* infection *(44)*. Increased microorganism burdens, consistent with defective clearance by inflammatory cells, have been shown in many cases *(8,30,34,40–46)*.

In contrast to the above studies, IL-6 did not play an important role in the responses to infection with *Leishmania major*, and IL-6 knockout mice on the C57Black6 background exhibited normal IFN-γ and low IL-4 levels *(48,49)*. Similar to *C. albicans* and *L. monocytogenes, L. major* represents a well-characterised example of T-cell-mediated control of an intracellular parasite. The different role of IL-6 in controlling these infections might be explained by a different requirement for efficient neutrophilia, which may be essential in candidiasis or listeriosis but inconsequential to the resolution of leishmaniasis, owing to the limited intramammalian habitat of the parasite. In addition, IL-$6^{-/-}$ mice could mount efficient responses to infection with *H. felix (33)*, rotavirus *(39)*, and scrapie *(50)*.

The different requirements for IL-6 in the responses to distinct infectious agents underline how this cytokine, rather than being required for specific fundamental functions of the immune cells, is important in the fine tuning of the delicate equilibrium among cellular, humoral, and inflammatory responses. The final outcome of infectious diseases in the IL-6 knockout mice is therefore likely to reflect the different strategies employed by the various microorganisms to affect this equilibrium.

6. IL-6 Knockout Mice Are Protected from the Development of Arthritides

Rheumatoid arthritis (RA) is a common human autoimmune disease characterized by chronic inflammation of the synovial joints and by subsequent progressive destruction of articular tissue; locally produced proinflammatory cytokines such as tumor necrosis factor-α (TNF-α) IL-1, and IL-6 are thought to play a central pathogenic role *(51)*. Serum and synovial fluids of RA and of juvenile rheumatoid arthritis patients display very high levels of IL-6 *(52,53)*, which are believed to be responsible for both local and systemic effects. In addition to stimulating B- and T-cell functions, in conjunction with sIL-6Rα, IL-6 can activate production of a subset of chemokines and adhesion molecules by endothelial cells *(54)* and induce synovial fibroblast proliferation *(55)* and osteoclast formation and activation *(56)*.

Several different models of arthritis have been established in the mouse. The one that perhaps resembles RA most closely is collagen-induced arthritis (CIA) because it elicits an autoimmune response against cartilage components *(57)*. CIA is triggered by immunization with type II collagen (CII) which is thought to break tolerance against murine collagen, thus initiating the disease, which resembles RA in a number of features including chronic inflammation of synovial tissue, pannus formation, cartilage destruction, and bone erosion. Antigen-induced arthritis (AIA) *(58)* is a monoarticular chronic form of immunologic arthritis triggered by intraarticular injection of mBSA in mice previously sensitized by immunisation with the same antigen. It also reproduces many of the characteristics of RA such as synovial lining hyperplasia, proliferation of sublining cells, infiltration of inflammatory cells, neovascularization, pannus formation, and articular cartilage destruction. Both CIA and AIA are considered T-cell-dependent arthritides. Zymosan-induced arthritis (ZIA) is, in contrast, a purely inflammatory model, triggered by direct injection of the inflammatory compund zymosan into the knee joint cavity *(59)*.

Mice carrying the IL-6 mutation on a DBA1/J or a C57Black6 background have been shown to be either totally or partially protected from the development of arthritic lesions in CIA *(22,24)* and AIA models, respectively *(23,25)*. Protection from the disease in CIA correlated with lower anti-CII IgG antibody levels *(22,24)*, with decreased proliferative responses of lymph node cells from immunized mice to both CII and concanavalin A (ConA) *(24)*, and with increased production of both IL-10 and IL-4 in response to ConA *(24)*. In AIA, the incidence of arthritis and arthritic score were strongly decreased in the mutant mice, with reduced cartilage destruction and no signs of osteaoclast activation *(23, 25)*. As in CIA, proliferation of lymph node cells and splenocytes in response to mBSA as well as anti-mBSA antibody titers in the serum were decreased. Subcutaneous injection of recombinant IL-6 reconstituted sensitivity to AIA, arguing for an important systemic role of the cytokine *(25)*. In addition, coadministration of IL-6 together with mBSA in the knee joint was also partially effective in conferring AIA sensitivity, suggesting that local production of IL-6 also plays a pathogenic role.

A recent report demonstrates that bone marrow transfer from a sensitized donor can also confer AIA to mice in which B- and T-cells have been depleted, arguing for the importance of bone marrow cells/stem cells in the pathogenesis of this disease *(60)*. Interestingly, bone marrow cells from a sensitized IL-6 knockout donor cannot confer AIA to a wild-type recipient, suggesting that IL-6 is important at levels other than the mere response to antigen. The role of IL-6 in ZIA is less defined: whereas the IL-6$^{-/-}$ mice present initially increased cartilage destruction, wild-type mice develop more severe joint inflammation and osteophyte formation during the chronic phase *(61,62)*.

In conclusion, there is general agreement that IL-6 plays a pathogenic role in all three models of arthritis examined, with particularly clear-cut results obtained in the two models of immunologic arthritides that resemble RA more closely. Although the exact mechanism through which IL-6 exerts its pathogenic role is still not completely elucidated, it is likely to occur at multiple levels including stimulation and amplification of the T-cell-dependent B-cell responses to arthritogenic antigens, promotion and maintenance of the chronic inflammatory response both systemically and locally, induction of osteoclastogenesis and osteoclasts activity, and possibly direct enhancement of the production of molecules contributing to tissue destruction such as prostaglandins and nitric oxide by monocytes and synovial fibroblasts. On the other hand, TNF-α and IL-1β are both amply recognized as important players in the pathogenesis of RA and of other forms of arthritis, and both are potent inducers of IL-6 synthesis. It is thus not surprising that IL-6 may mediate at least some of their arthritogenic effects. Interestingly, the inflammatory polyarthritis caused by expression of an abnormally stable form of human TNF-α in transgenic mice develops normally in IL-6$^{-/-}$ mice *(22)*, suggesting that IL-6 is not required for the establishment of an arthritic response when the inflammatory stimulus is without physiologic means of control.

7. IL-6 Knockout Mice are Protected from the Development of Autoimmune Encephalomyelitis

Autoimmune reactivity against minor components of myelin is thought to play an important role in the pathogenesis of multiple sclerosis (MS). In particular, MS patients exhibit a predominant T-cell response to MOG, which is rarely observed in the serum of healthy controls *(63)*. Synthetic MOG peptides (pMOG) are encephalitogenic in H-2^{b} strains of mice such as C57/Black6 and 129, in which they can induce experimental autoimmune encephalomyelitis (EAE) characterized by ascending paralysis associated with inflammatory cell infiltration foci in the brain and spinal cord and demyelinating lesions *(64)*. EAE can be adoptively transferred by pMOG-reactive T-cell lines, and anti-MOG antibodies show demyelinating activity. Cytokines, including IL-6, are key mediators in the pathogenesis of inflammatory lesions of the central nervous system and are likely to play a central pathogenic role in both MS and EAE.

IL-6 knockout mice have been the object of numerous studies aimed at determining the role of this cytokine in the pathogenesis of EAE; remarkably, all the studies have unanimously indicated complete protection from the disease in different genetic backgrounds, with complete absence of clinical symptoms and perivascular inflammatory infiltrate in brain and spinal cord *(26–29)*. Serum titers of anti-MOG antibodies were decreased, but this was not considered sufficient to warrant protection, as B-cell-deficient mice were shown to be able to develop the disease *(26)*. Moreover, injection of recombinant IL-6 could partially rescue disease development without increasing antibody production *(27)*. T-cell priming was normal in the (C57Black/6 × 129) F1 strain *(27)* but was impaired when the mutation was on the pure C57Black/6 background *(28,29)*, suggesting that mere low reactivity of T-cells could not be the basis of the protection. In addition, T-cell lines exhibiting high proliferative responses to MOG could equally well be derived from mutant and wild-type mice *(27)*. However, although the wild-type lines could successfully transfer EAE to a wild-type recipient mouse, they failed to do so in a knockout recipient, strongly implying that other mechanisms in addition to the impaired T-cell-mediated responses are involved in protection from the disease. On the other hand, knockout T-cell lines were unable to confer EAE to a wild-type recipient despite their strong reactivity against pMOG *(27)*.

The elucidation of the molecular bases for this difference will represent an important step forward in the understanding of the establishment of anti-myelin autoimmunity. Which other players are involved in addition to T-cells? IL-6 may be important to establish the local perivascular inflammatory process characteristic of the disease. First, wild-type T-cells elicit no signs of cell infiltrate in the brain or spinal cord when transferred into IL-6 knockout recipients *(27)*. Second, injection with IL-8, an important chemoattractant whose secretion by endothelial cells is induced by IL-6 in combination with its sIL-6R, causes 25% of the IL-6 knockout mice to develop EAE *(27)*. Third, both infiltration of leukocytes and endothelial expression of vascular cell adhesion molecule-1 (VCAM-1) and intercellular adhesion molecule-1 (ICAM-1) were dramatically reduced in the IL-6$^{-/-}$ mice *(26)*. Finally, injection of superantigen (staphylococcal enterotoxin B) partially reversed the resistance of IL-6$^{-/-}$ mice to MOG-induced EAE, correlating with increased VCAM-1 expression in brain endothelium *(65)*.

In conclusion, IL-6 plays a fundamental role in the pathogenesis of autoimmune encephalomyelitis, both by stimulating an encephalitogenic T-cell response and by establishing the local inflammatory response, probably through induction of chemokines and endothelium activation, and possibly by increasing the permeability of the blood-brain barrier *(66)*. Although these observations cannot be directly translated into equivalent human diseases, these findings make IL-6 and its pathway a target worth exploring for the cure of autoimmune and inflammatory disorders of the central nervous system such as multiple sclerosis and Alzheimer's disease.

8. IL-6 Participates in Bone Mass Regulation

Loss of estrogens or androgens is known to cause bone loss, often leading to debilitating osteoporosis (reviewed in ref. *67*). IL-6 levels increase under these conditions, and this cytokine was proposed to participate in the pathogenesis of osteoporosis via its ability to stimulate osteoclastogenesis (reviewed in ref. *68*). Indeed, IL-6$^{-/-}$ mice were shown to be protected from bone loss following estrogen or androgen depletion caused by ovariectomy or orchidectomy, respectively *(7,69)*. No changes in parameters of bone turnover were detected in the mutant mice following hormone depletion; remarkably, the numbers of granulocyte/macrophage colony-forming units (GM-CFUs; the osteoclast progenitors) and osteoclasts formed in bone marrow cultures from hormone-depleted mice failed to show the typical increase observed in wild-type mice. These results point toward a central role of IL-6 in mediating the effects of hormonal depletion on bone metabolism and suggest its participation in regulating bone homeostasis.

9. IL-6 Plays an Important Role in Plasma Cell Hyperplasia and the Establishment of B-Cell Lineage Neoplasms

IL-6 is known to be an important growth factor for a number of neoplastic cell types, in particular myeloma-plasmacytoma cells. Human patients with multiple myeloma have high circulating levels of this cytokine, and both primary myeloma explants and myeloma-derived cell lines are dependent on IL-6 for their growth (recently reviewed in ref. *70*). The high levels of IL-6 found in myeloma patients are also thought to play an important role in the development of the kidney and bone damage associated with the disease, and clinical studies have recently shown that treatment with IL-6-neutralizing monoclonal antibodies can improve several disease parameters in late-stage patients *(71)*.

In mouse, intraperitoneal injections with pristane oil cause the formation of granulomas and give rise to plasma cell hyperplasia in most strains of mice and in the BalbC strain to the development of plasmacytomas, a form of plasma cell tumor analogous to multiple myeloma (reviewed in ref. *72*). IL-6 is an essential factor for the in vitro and in vivo growth of primary plasmacytoma cells and plasmacytoma cell lines (*see* ref. *73* and references therein). Through studies on the IL-6$^{-/-}$ mice, IL-6 or the activation of its signaling pathway have been unequivocally demonstrated to be essential for plasma cell hyperplasias and/or plasmacytoma development *(74–78)*. Thus, the Castleman's-like disease developing in mice carrying a null mutation of the transcription factor C/EBPβ does not occur in the absence of IL-6 *(75)*, and IL-6$^{-/-}$ mice on the C57/Black6 × 129 background do not show any sign of plasma cell hyperplasia in the lymph nodes and spleen upon pristane oil injection *(74)*. IL-6$^{-/-}$ mice infected with a myc/raf-expressing retrovirus failed to develop B-cell lineage tumors, whereas myeloid tumors developed at normal frequencies *(77)*. Even in the more classical pristane oil model of plasmacytomagenesis that is thought to resemble the process of myeloma formation in humans more closely, IL-6$^{-/-}$ mice were found to be completely resistant to the development of plasmacytomas, although granuloma formation and B-cell activation in the lymph nodes was apparently unchanged *(76)*. Finally, plasmacytomas induced in the absence of IL-6 by an abl/myc-encoding retrovirus showed constitutive activation of STAT3, the main mediator of IL-6 functions, confirming the centrality of the IL-6-mediated pathway in B-cell tumoral growth *(78)*.

Taken together, all these findings unanimously indicate that IL-6, although not strictly required for the normal process of plasma cell maturation and antibody switching (*see* Subheading 4), is instead a crucial growth factor for triggering uncontrolled proliferation and expansion of plasmablastic cells.

10. IL-6 is an Important Stimulator of Hepatocyte Proliferation Following Injury

The liver has the unique property of regenerating its original mass after removal or destruction of part of the organ, owing to the capacity of differentiated, quiescent hepatocytes to reenter the cell cycle and undergo a controlled number of cell divisions (recently reviewed in ref. *79*). This ability is important in preserving organ functionality following different types of injury such as surgical removal of part of the tissue, liver transplantation, and chemical damage to the parenchyma. IL-6 is induced along with other proinflammatory cytokines and growth factors in response to these injuries. Indeed, whereas overexpression of IL-6 alone in transgenic mice has limited effects on hepatocyte proliferation and liver mass, coexpression of IL-6 with its soluble IL-6R leads to increased hepatocyte proliferation and the formation of nodular hyperplasia *(80)*. IL-6 knockout mice displayed impaired hepatocyte proliferation in distinct models of liver injury. Following partial hepatectomy (PH), DNA synthesis was decreased and delayed only in the parenchymal cells, although the liver returned eventually to its original mass *(81,82)*. Interestingly, proliferation of hepatocytes in response to mitogens was, in contrast, normal *(83)*, suggesting that IL-6 is not a universal requirement for adult liver cell proliferation. Liver damage was correspondently worstened in the mutant mice, which showed increased mortality, necrosis *(81)*, and steatosis *(82)*. These defects correlated with impaired expression of a number of immediate early genes normally induced by PH, including c-myc, c-fos, cyclin D1 and D2, Egr1, and IGFBP1 *(84)*.

Defective proliferation of hepatocytes also correlated with increased liver damage upon acute liver injury induced by the hepatotoxin CCl_4 *(85,86)*. Remarkably, chronic CCl_4-mediated injury triggered increased liver fibrosis and prolonged stellate cell activation in the knockout mice. Biliary fibrosis and mortality were also enhanced in the mutant mice upon bile duct ligation *(87)*, correlating with decreased proliferation of hepatocytes but increased proliferation of biliary epithelial cells, suggesting that IL-6 contributes to biliary tree integrity and maintenance of hepatocyte mass during chronic obstructive cholangiopathy. Liver damage was also worsened in the absence of IL-6 following warm ischemia/reperfusion *(88)*.

All together, these results indicate a fundamental role for IL-6 in maintaining liver homeostasis and functionality following different kinds of injuries and in limiting acute and chronic damage to the organ. Correct expression of IL-6 appears to be required to direct efficient healing processes and thus limit fibrosis, probably by maintaining the correct equilibrium between the different cell populations of the liver.

11. IL-6$^{-/-}$ Mice in Inflammatory Responses: Pro- or Antiinflammatory?

Acute inflammation triggered by different stimuli such as infection, endotoxemia, and sterile tissue damage elicits a number of systemic host responses including fever, anorexia, loss of body weight, hypoglycemia, and changes in the serum concentration of several plasma proteins produced by the hepatocytes, the so-called liver acute-phase response (reviewed in ref. *89*). Experimentally, intraperitoneal subministration of bacterial LPS is commonly used to mimic systemically induced inflammation, whereas subcutaneous injection of turpentine causes the formation of sterile abscesses and peripheral tissue damage *(90)*.

Circulating mediators such as proinflammatory cytokines (mainly IL-1β, TNF-α, and IL-6) and corticosteroid hormones (for review, *see* ref. *91*) play a fundamental role in regulating host responses to inflammation. Although production of IL-1 and IL-6 is rapidly induced by both LPS and turpentine, TNF-α is induced by LPS but not by turpentine, and it plays a major role in lethality following endotoxic shock *(92)*. Both compounds rapidly induce corticosterone (CS) production through the activation of the HPA axis and the release of adrenocorticotropic hormone (ACTH; reviewed in ref. *91*). Corticosteroid hormones synergize with inflammatory cytokines (IL-6, IL-1, and TNF-α) to induce most acute-phase proteins while at the same time suppressing cytokine production, hence playing an important role in the termination of the inflammatory responses *(91)*. The same proinflammatory cytokines have also been identified as main mediators of the fever response *(93)*, which is believed to be controlled by the preoptic area of the brain.

11.1 Systemic Responses to Localized Inflammation Require IL-6 Production

We and others have shown that IL-6 is an essential mediator of host responses to inflammation triggered by a localized insult such as turpentine or tissue infection with Gram-positive bacteria *(6,94)*. Induction of several acute-phase mRNAs was almost completely abolished in IL-6$^{-/-}$ mice either treated with turpentine or infected with *L. monocytogenes*. In addition, common clinical manifestations of acute inflammation such as anorexia, body weight loss, and hypoglycemia were extremely attenuated in the mutant mice in response to turpentine *(94)*, whereas the same responses were almost normal upon LPS treatment, suggesting functional complementation by other cytokines in response to LPS but not to turpentine oil *(94)*. In agreement with the knowledge that IL-6 can repress TNF-α production, LPS induced severalfold higher levels of TNF-α in the absence of IL-6 *(94,95)*. This upregulation may well contribute to the normal acute-phase response induction observed in the IL-6 knockout mice, possibly by inducing higher levels of other members of the gp130 family. Indeed, all gp130 family members have been shown to activate STAT3 and to be able to induce acute-phase response genes on hepatic cells *(96)*. Accordingly, normal or defective acute-phase response in the IL-6 knockout mice correlated with efficient or impaired activation of STAT3, respectively *(97)*, and a functional STAT3 gene was recently shown to be absolutely required for efficient acute-phase response genes induction *(98)*. Interestingly, whereas IL-6-deficient mice exhibited a partially impaired acute-phase response induction in response to recombinant TNF-α, they were neither more susceptible to nor protected from its lethal effects *(99)*, indicating that IL-6 is not involved in protection against TNF-induced shock.

11.2 Activation of the HPA Axis Is Not Strictly Dependent on IL-6

In contrast to the acute-phase responses discussed above, activation of the HPA axis was found to be independent of IL-6, as judged by normal CS production following restraint stress or treatment with LPS, turpentine oil, or IL-1β *(94,100–102)*. In contrast, CS production was found to be impaired upon injection with TNF-α *(99)* or, exclusively in female mice, upon LPS injection or restraint stress *(103)*. In addition, IL-6 was found to act in synergy with corticotropin-releasing hormone (CRH) to activate adrenal functions in response to immune stimuli *(47,103,104)*. These data suggest that during immune-mediated inflammatory responses, IL-6 may exert its role at least partly by contributing to establish optimal adrenal functions.

11.3 The Fever Response Requires IL-6 Production in the Central Nervous System

IL-6, IL-1β, and TNF-α are considered endogenous pyrogens as they can all elicit a fever response that is dependent on prostaglandin production *(105)*. Strikingly, fever responses to LPS, turpentine oil, IL-1β, or TNF-α all require the presence of IL-6 *(105–107)* and can be rescued in the IL-6$^{-/-}$ mice by intracerebroventricular (icv), but not intraperitoneal, injection of rIL-6 *(105,107)*. In addition, IL-6 is also required for development of fever in a sepsis model triggered by cecal ligation and puncture *(108)*. Thus, IL-6 is an essential mediator of fever in the central nervous system, where it acts downstream of other known endogenous pyrogens such as IL-1β and TNF-α, both strong inducers of IL-6 synthesis.

11.4 IL-6 Knockout Mice Show Both Defective and Augmented Inflammatory Responses as Measured by Cytokine Production and/or Infiltration of Inflammatory Cells

As detailed above, IL-6 production is always associated with inflammatory conditions and is strongly induced by recombinant IL-1β and TNF-α. IL-6 levels correlate with the degree of inflammation in several chronic inflammatory diseases, and the presence of an inflammatory reaction is often evaluated through measuring the levels of the major human acute-phase response C-reactive protein (CRP), whose synthesis is IL-6-dependent. However, the exact role of this cytokine during inflammation has been and still is an object of debate, as IL-6 has been reported to play both proinflammatory and antiinflammatory roles under different conditions. The studies on the IL-6 knockout mice have perpetuated this ambiguity, showing both augmented and decreased inflammatory reactions to a variety of stimuli in different models, as detailed in Table 1. The models have been divided into inflammatory responses to infectious agents, responses triggered by antigen immunization (immune-mediated), responses triggered by exposure to different inflammatory agents, and other models of inflammation. The data summarized in the table argue for a differential final role of IL-6 in regulating the balance between antiinflammatory and proinflammatory responses (with particular reference to the recruitment of inflammatory cells) depending on the inflammatory agent, the site, and the mechanism of the insult.

In general, IL-6 appears in most cases to be required for immune-mediated inflammation and for responses to inflammatory agents such as carrageenan and zymosan, whereas it can act as both a pro- and antiinflammatory agent in the responses to bacterial toxins. Recruitment of leukocytes to the site of inflammation is mainly directed by the production of specific chemokines and by the induction of adhesion molecules on the endothelium. Perhaps the apparently paradoxic results obtained with the IL-6 knockout mice can be explained by the observation that cells involved in regulating lymphocytic trafficking such as endothelial or mesothelial cells do not express the IL-6Rα and therefore cannot respond to IL-6. In the presence of soluble IL-6Rα, however, IL-6 can upregulate the expression of specific chemokine subsets and adhesion molecules such as VCAM-1 and ICAM-1 *(4,54)*. In turn, it has been shown that neutrophils can be stimulated to release high amounts of soluble receptor *(109)*. Therefore, the net effect of IL-6 on lymphocyte infiltration will vary according to the site of insult and the ancillary cell types involved, the availability of cells able to produce the sIL-6R, and the relative potency of the different stimuli to induce its release.

11.5 IL-6 Plays Essentially Proinflammatory Roles in the Central Nervous System

Proinflammatory cytokines are produced in the brain, where they are thought to play important roles in determining the activation of astrocytes and glial cells. One of the main antiinflammatory effects of IL-6 is thought to be its capacity to downregulate TNF-α production. Interestingly, this inhibitory role appears to be limited to the periphery, as IL-6$^{-/-}$ mice injected with LPS icv displayed TNF-α levels higher than the wild-type controls in the periphery but not in the central nervous system *(110)*. Indeed, constitutive expression of IL-6 in neurons led to increased rather than decreased brain expression of IL-6, IL-1β, and TNF-α upon icv injection of LPS, and IL-6 was able to downregulate LPS-induced TNF-α production in macrophages but not in microglial cells *(111)*. In agreement with these findings, IL-6 knockout mice have been consistently reported to mount reduced inflammatory responses generally associated with impaired repair processes in the brain after various insults. Thus, cryoinjury to the parietal cortex that disrupts the blood-brain barrier caused reduced recruitment of macrophages and decreased reactive astrocytosis, associated with heightened oxidative stress and neuronal apoptosis *(112,113)*. In agreement with this, IL-6 knockout mice exhibited slower tissue repair associated with reduced revascularization upon aseptic injury to the parietal cortex *(114)*, decreased neuroglial activation

Table 1
Analysis of Distinct Inflammatory Models Supports Both Pro- and Antiinflammatory Roles for Interleukin-6 (IL-6)[a]

A. Infectious agents

Agent	Route	Target tissue	Micro-organism burden	Recruitment of inflammatory cells	Blood neutrophilia	Cytokines/ chemokines, inflammatory mediators	Other	Ref.
T. gondii	ip	Brain	↑	↓	↓	↓ IFN-γ, ↓ IL-10		*40,41*
T. gondii	ip	Eye	↑	↑	n/r	↑ TNF-α		*122*
HSV	Intracorneal	Eye	↑	↓	n/r	↓ MIP-2, ↓ MIP-1α		*123*
C. albicans	ip/ig	Multiple	↑	↑ (inflammatory foci)	↓	↑ IL-10, TNF-α, IL-1 ↓ IFN-γ, IL-12	↑ Mortality ↑ Necrosis	*30,124*
L. monocytogenes	iv	Multiple	↑	↑ (inflammatory foci)	↓	⇔ IFN-γ	↑ Mortality ↑ Lesions	*8*
E. coli	ip	Multiple	↑	n/r	↓	n/d	↑ Mortality	*46*
K. pneumoniae	iv	Multiple	↑	↓	n/r	↑ TNF-α		*47*
A. fumigatus	Intranasal	Lung	↑	⇔ (PMN, MNC)	n/r	↑ IL-10, IL-4, IL-13 ↑ MCP-1, IL-17 ↓ IFN-γ, IL-12	↓ Phagocytic functions	*44*
S. pneumoniae	Intranasal	Lung	↑	n/r	n/r ↑ IL-10	↑ TNF-α, IL-1, IFN-γ	↑ Mortality	*125*
Pulpal pathogens	Intrapulpal	Dental pulpa	n/r	n/r	n/r	↑ IL-1 ↓ IL-10	↑ Bone resorp. ↑ Osteoclast no.	*126*

(continued)

Table 1 (Continued)

B. Immune-mediated

Antigen	Route	Target tissue	Recruitment of inflammatory cells	Cytokines/chemokines, inflammatory mediators	Other	Ref.
MOG peptide (EAE)	sc + CFA	Brain	↓	↑ Th2 (IL-4, IL-10) by LNC	Protection from EAE	*26–29*
Collagen type II (CIA)	id + CFA	Joints	↓	↑ Th2 (IL-4, IL-10) by LNC ⇔ Th1 (IFN-γ) by LNC	Protection from CIA	*22,24*
mBSA (AIA)	id (+ CFA) + intra-knee	Joints	↓	⇔ IL-1 and TNF-α in joints	Protection from AIA	*23, 25*
Ovalbumin	ip (+alum) + aerosol OVA	Lung	↑	↑ Th2 (IL-4, IL-5, IL-13) ↑ MCP-1, MIP-1α, MIP-2, ↑ TGF-β	↑ Eosinophils	*127*

C. Inflammatory agents

Agent	Route	Target tissue	Recruitment of inflammatory cells	Cytokines/chemokines, inflammatory mediators	Other	Ref.
LTA (100 mg)	Intranasal	Lung	⇔	↓ TNF-α, MCP-1, KC		*128*
LTA (10 mg)	Intranasal	Lung	↑	↑ TNF-α, MIP-1α, KC		*128*
PEPG	Intranasal	Lung	↓	n/r		*128*
PLY	Intranasal	Lung	↓	n/r		*129*
LPS	Aerosol	Lung	↑	↑ TNF-α, MIP-2		*95*
LPS	ip	Multiple	n/r	↑ TNF-α, MIP-2, GM-CSF, IFN-γ	↑ Mortality	*95*
LPS	ip	Multiple	n/r	n/r	⇔ Mortality	*46*
LPS	Corneal	Eye	n/r	n/r	⇔ Uveitis	*130*
SES	ip	Peritoneum	↑ PMN ↓ MNC	↑ KC, MIP-2 ↓ MCP-1		*131*
Carrageenan	Pleural	lung	↓	↓ COX-2, iNOS	↓ Injury ↓ Exudate	*134*
Carrageenan	Paw	Paw	↓	n/r	↓ Exudate	*119*
Carrageenan	Air pouch	Air pouch	↓ PMN ↓ MNC	↓ MCP-1	Rescued by IL-8	*54*
IL-1β	Air pouch	Air pouch	↓ PMN ↓ MNC	n/r		*54*
Zymosan	ip	Multiple	↓	↓ IL-1-β, TNF-α		*135*

Model	Target tissue	Recruitment of inflammatory cells	Cytokines/chemokines, inflammatory mediators	Other	Ref.
D. Other inflammatory models					
Splanchnic artery occlusion	Gut	↓	↓ ICAM, P-selectin	↓ Mortality	*132*
Hemorrhagic shock	Multiple	↓	n/r	↓ Liver necrosis	*133*

[a]The results obtained by challenging IL-6 knockout mice and their wild-type littermates with different inflammatory stimuli are reported (*see* Subheading 11.4. for a discussion). The inflammatory agent/model used, the route of administration, the eventual tissue targeted by the inflammatory response, and other relevant features (Other) are indicated. The inflammatory infiltrate, systemic blood neutrophilia, and production of cytokines, chemokines, and/or inflammatory mediators detected in the IL-6 knockout mice relative to the same parameters evaluated in the wild-type controls are indicated (↓, ↑, ⇔, decreased, increased, or unchanged with respect to the wild-type mice). n/r, not reported; ip, intraperitoneal; ig, intragastric; iv, intravenous; sc, subcutaneous; id, intradermic. **Infectious agents:** the features of the inflammatory response to infections are correlated with susceptibility as judged by microorganism burden and, when reported, mortality. **Immune-mediated:** inflammation triggered by immune responses to an antigen. Antigen and disease model are indicated. CFA, complete Freund's adjuvant. **Inflammatory agents:** inflammation triggered by exposure to various inflammatory agents (bacterial toxins, components of bacterial walls, polysaccharides, inactivated yeast cells). LTA, lipotheoic acid; PEPG, peptidoglycans; PLY, pneumolysin; LPS, lipopolysaccharide; SES, cell-free supernatant of *Staphylococcus epidermidis*. **Other inflammatory models:** the features of the inflammatory responses to splanchnic artery occlusion and to hemorrhagic shock are presented. AIA, adjuvant-induced arthritis; CIA, collagen-induced arthritis; COX-2, cyclooxygenase-2; EAE, experimental autoimmune encephalomyelitis; GM-CSF, granulocyte/macrophage colony-stimulating factor; HSV, herpes simplex virus; ICAM, intercellular adhesion molecule; IFN, interferon; iNOS, inducible nitric oxide synthase; KC, Kapffer cells; LNC, lymph node cells; MCP, macrophage chemottractant protein; MNC, mononuclear cells; MOG, myclin-oligodendrocyte protein; OVA, ovalbumin; PMN, polymorphonuclear leukocyte; TNF, tumor necrosis factor.

upon facial motor nucleus axotomy *(115)*, and increased neuronal death upon sciatic nerve axotomy *(116)*. Facial nerve axotomy led to recruitment of normal numbers of granulocytes and macrophages but reduced numbers of CD3+ T-cells, associated with impaired neuronal regeneration *(117)*. Finally, sciatic nerve crushing led to delayed recovery of the sensory branch but not of the motor branch, with no differences in macrophage recruitment *(118)*.

In addition to the already reported absence of inflammatory infiltrate in the brain of mice immunized with the MOG peptide in the EAE model (*see* Subheading 7), these results strongly indicate a central role for IL-6 in promoting inflammatory responses in the central nervous system, probably through the stimulation of proliferation and activity of astrocytes and microglial cells. Through these inflammatory responses, IL-6 appears to be involved in neuronal protection and tissue repair during acute nerve injury, probably by favoring the production of specific growth factors involved in promoting neuronal survival and regeneration by activated astrocytes and microglial cells. In contrast, these inflammatory responses contribute to tissue destruction once they become chronic, thus explaining the protection from EAE displayed by the IL-6$^{-/-}$ mice.

12. Other Central Nervous System Functions of IL-6

12.1 IL-6 Inactivation Affects Nociceptive Responses and Aggressive Behavior

Nociceptive responses, hyperalgesia, and analgesic effects of opioids are regulated by complex interactions among hormones, cytokines, and opioid peptides. IL-6 knockout mice have been reported to have decreased, normal, or increased thresholds to thermal and/or mechanical stimulation, perhaps owing to the different genetic backgrounds of the mice tested *(118–120)*. Interestingly, decreased inflammatory hyperalgesia and decreased hypersensitivity to heat and pressure upon constriction nerve injury have also been reported, consistent with reduced inflammatory reactions *(118,119)*. The IL-6 knockout mice also showed decreased analgesic responses to low doses of morphine and to restraint stress and more rapid development of tolerance to the analgesic effects of morphine, correlating with increased spleen and hypothalamic levels of β-endorphins and with decreased number of opioid receptors in the midbrain *(102,120)*. These findings suggest that lack of IL-6 induces an opioid tolerant-like status, possibly by affecting brain development. In line with this idea, IL-6$^{-/-}$ males also showed increased aggressive behavior correlating with decreased dopamine levels. Although not conclusive about the specific role played by IL-6 in the central nervous system development, these results suggest that loss of IL-6 causes profound alterations in several of its specific functions.

12.2 IL-6 Participates in Body Weight Control

Of particular relevance along this line is the observation that IL-6 knockout mice develop mature-onset obesity *(121)*, with a 20% increase in body weight and a 50–60% increase in the total weight of dissected fat pads at 9 mo of age. The obese mice displayed disturbed carbohydrate and lipid metabolism in conjunction with increased leptin levels and leptin resistance. Food intake was enhanced but proportional to body mass, and treatment with rIL-6 decreased body weight and leptin levels in the obese IL-6 knockout mice only. In addition, icv, but not ip, injection of low doses of rIL-6 in rats caused increased energy expenditure but not decreased food intake. All together, these observations suggest that IL-6 exerts a tonic central suppression of the fat mass most likely at the level of the hypothalamic nuclei that express IL-6 and its receptors and that are known to be involved in metabolism control. In contrast to ciliary neurophilic factor (CNTF), which has been shown to ameliorate obesity in mice and humans by suppressing food intake, IL-6 appears to act mainly via stimulating energy expenditure.

13. Concluding Remarks and Perspectives

The numerous studies performed so far on the IL-6 knockout mice have not only confirmed but even extended the pleiotropic functions of this cytokine. From these data we see that IL-6 plays subtle but important functions in regulating the balance among the cell types involved in naive and acquired immunity and that its synthesis, when following the appropriate pattern of induction, is beneficial in the resolution of infections and promotes an optimal humoral response to antigens. On the other hand, inappropriate or chronically induced IL-6 production participates in the pathogenesis of immune-mediated diseases such as CIA or EAE, as well as diseases caused by improper expansion of specific hematopietic compartments such as osteoclasts and their GM-CFU precursors (osteoporosis) and plasma cells (plasmacytosis). These experiments have indicated that IL-6 or its signaling pathway is a potentially useful therapeutic target, although inhibition of its activity should be considered immunosuppressive and consequently addressed with due care. It is worth noting that sometimes functional compensation by other cytokines belonging to the same or different families could have masked further IL-6 functions. In addition, the emerging central role of the sIL-6Rα in mediating IL-6 functions indicates how the functional cytokine is often the complex between IL-6 and sIL-6R. Future studies involving inducible or tissue-specific inactivation of either the IL-6 or the IL-6R gene may help to define better the precise role of this multifaceted cytokine.

References

1. Kishimoto, T. (1989) The biology of interleukin-6. *Blood* **74,** 1–10.
2. Gauldie, J., Richards, C., Harnish, D., Lansdorp, P., and Baumann, H. (1987) Interferon beta 2/B-cell stimulatory factor type 2 shares identity with monocyte-derived hepatocyte-stimulating factor and regulates the major acute phase protein response in liver cells. *Proc. Natl. Acad. Sci. USA* **84,** 7251–7255.
3. Behrmann, I., Hermanns, H. M., Haan, C., et al. (2000) Signalling of interleukin-6 type cytokines via gp130, leukemia inhibitory factor (LIF) receptor and oncostatin M receptor. *Eur. Cytokine Netw.* **11,** 491–492.
4. Jones, S. A., Horiuchi, S., Topley, N., Yamamoto, N., and Fuller, G. M. (2001) The soluble interleukin 6 receptor: mechanisms of production and implications in disease. *FASEB J.* **15,** 43–58.
5. Hirano, T., Nakajima, K., and Hibi, M. (1997) Signaling mechanisms through gp130: a model of the cytokine system. *Cytokine Growth Factor Rev.* **8,** 241–252.
6. Kopf, M., Baumann, H., Freer, G., et al. (1994) Impaired immune and acute-phase responses in interleukin-6-deficient mice. *Nature* **368,** 339–342.
7. Poli, V., Balena, R., Fattori, E., et al. (1994) Interleukin-6 deficient mice are protected from bone loss caused by estrogen depletion. *EMBO J.* **13,** 1189–1196.
8. Dalrymple, S. A., Lucian, L. A., Slattery, R., et al. (1995) Interleukin-6-deficient mice are highly susceptible to *Listeria monocytogenes* infection: correlation with inefficient neutrophilia. *Infect. Immun.* **63,** 2262–2268.
9. Bernad, A., Kopf, M., Kulbacki, R., Weich, N., Koehler, G., and Gutierrez-Ramos, J. C. (1994) Interleukin-6 is required in vivo for the regulation of stem cells and committed progenitors of the hematopoietic system. *Immunity* **1,** 725–731.

10. Houssiau, F. and Van Snick, J. (1992) IL6 and the T-cell response. *Res. Immunol.* **143,** 740–743.
11. Uyttenhove, C., Coulie, P. G., and Van Snick, J. (1988) T cell growth and differentiation induced by interleukin-HP1/IL-6, the murine hybridoma/plasmacytoma growth factor. *J. Exp. Med.* **167,** 1417–1427.
12. Lotz, M., Jirik, F., Kabouridis, P., et al. (1988) B cell stimulating factor 2/interleukin 6 is a costimulant for human thymocytes and T lymphocytes. *J. Exp. Med.* **167,** 1253–1258.
13. Ramsay, A. J. and Kopf, M. (1998) IL-6 knockout mice. In: Durum, S., Kopf, M., and Muegge, K., ed. *Cytokine Knockouts*. Humana, Totowa, NJ, pp. 227–236.
14. Kopf, M., Herren, S., Wiles, M. V., Pepys, M. B., and Kosco-Vilbois, M. H. (1998) Interleukin 6 influences germinal center development and antibody production via a contribution of C3 complement component. *J. Exp. Med.* **188,** 1895–1906.
15. Ramsay, A. J., Ruby, J., and Ramshaw, I. A. (1993) A case for cytokines as effector molecules in the resolution of virus infection. *Immunol. Today* **14,** 155–157.
16. Kishimoto, T. and Hirano, T. (1988) Molecular regulation of B lymphocyte response. *Annu. Rev. Immunol.* **6,** 485–512.
17. Jourdan, M., Bataille, R., Seguin, J., Zhang, X. G., Chaptal, P. A., and Klein, B. (1990) Constitutive production of interleukin-6 and immunologic features in cardiac myxomas. *Arthritis Rheum.* **33,** 398–402.
18. Suematsu, S., Matsusaka, T., Matsuda, T., et al. (1992) Generation of plasmacytomas with the chromosomal translocation t(12;15) in interleukin 6 transgenic mice. *Proc. Natl. Acad. Sci. USA* **89,** 232–235.
19. Fattori, E., Della Rocca, C., Costa, P., et al. (1994) Development of progressive kidney damage and myeloma kidney in interleukin-6 transgenic mice. *Blood* **83,** 2570–2579.
20. Fischer, M. B., Ma, M., Goerg, S., et al. (1996) Regulation of the B cell response to T-dependent antigens by classical pathway complement. *J. Immunol.* **157,** 549–556.
21. La Flamme, A. C. and Pearce, E. J. (1999) The absence of IL-6 does not affect Th2 cell development in vivo, but does lead to impaired proliferation, IL-2 receptor expression, and B cell responses. *J. Immunol.* **162,** 5829–5837.
22. Alonzi, T., Fattori, E., Lazzaro, D., et al. (1998) Interleukin 6 is required for the development of collagen-induced arthritis. *J. Exp. Med.* **187,** 461–468.
23. Ohshima, S., Saeki, Y., Mima, T., et al. (1998) Interleukin 6 plays a key role in the development of antigen-induced arthritis. *Proc. Natl. Acad. Sci. USA* **95,** 8222–8226.
24. Sasai, M., Saeki, Y., Ohshima, S., et al. (1999) Delayed onset and reduced severity of collagen-induced arthritis in interleukin-6-deficient mice. *Arthritis Rheum.* **42,** 1635–1643.
25. Boe, A., Baiocchi, M., Carbonatto, M., Papoian, R., and Serlupi-Crescenzi, O. (1999) Interleukin 6 knock-out mice are resistant to antigen-induced experimental arthritis. *Cytokine* **11,** 1057–1064.
26. Eugster, H. P., Frei, K., Kopf, M., Lassmann, H., and Fontana, A. (1998) IL-6-deficient mice resist myelin oligodendrocyte glycoprotein-induced autoimmune encephalomyelitis. *Eur. J. Immunol.* **28,** 2178–2187.
27. Mendel, I., Katz, A., Kozak, N., Ben-Nun, A., and Revel, M. (1998) Interleukin-6 functions in autoimmune encephalomyelitis: a study in gene-targeted mice. *Eur. J. Immunol.* **28,** 1727–1737.
28. Okuda, Y., Sakoda, S., Bernard, C. C., et al. (1998) IL-6-deficient mice are resistant to the induction of experimental autoimmune encephalomyelitis provoked by myelin oligodendrocyte glycoprotein. *Int. Immunol.* **10,** 703–708.
29. Samoilova, E. B., Horton, J. L., Hilliard, B., Liu, T. S., and Chen, Y. (1998) IL-6-deficient mice are resistant to experimental autoimmune encephalomyelitis: roles of IL-6 in the activation and differentiation of autoreactive T cells. *J. Immunol.* **161,** 6480–6486.
30. Romani, L., Mencacci, A., Cenci, E., et al. (1996) Impaired neutrophil response and CD4+ T helper cell 1 development in interleukin 6-deficient mice infected with *Candida albicans. J. Exp. Med.* **183,** 1345–1355.
31. Richards, H. B., Satoh, M., Shaw, M., Libert, C., Poli, V., and Reeves, W. H. (1998) Interleukin 6 dependence of anti-DNA antibody production: evidence for two pathways of autoantibody formation in pristane-induced lupus. *J. Exp. Med.* **188,** 985–990.

32. Brewer, J. M., Conacher, M., Gaffney, M., Douglas, M., Bluethmann, H., and Alexander, J. (1998) Neither interleukin-6 nor signalling via tumour necrosis factor receptor-1 contribute to the adjuvant activity of alum and Freund's adjuvant. *Immunology* **93,** 41–48.
33. Bromander, A. K., Ekman, L., Kopf, M., Nedrud, J. G., and Lycke, N. Y. (1996) IL-6-deficient mice exhibit normal mucosal IgA responses to local immunizations and *Helicobacter felis* infection. *J. Immunol.* **156,** 4290–4297.
34. Ladel, C. H., Blum, C., Dreher, A., Reifenberg, K., Kopf, M., and Kaufmann, S. H. (1997) Lethal tuberculosis in interleukin-6-deficient mutant mice. *Infect. Immun.* **65,** 4843–4849.
35. Markine-Goriaynoff, D., Nguyen, T. D., Bigaignon, G., Van Snick, J., and Coutelier, J. P. (2001) Distinct requirements for IL-6 in polyclonal and specific Ig production induced by microorganisms. *Int. Immunol.* **13,** 1185–1192.
36. Ramsay, A. J., Husband, A. J., Ramshaw, I. A., et al. (1994) The role of interleukin-6 in mucosal IgA antibody responses in vivo. *Science* **264,** 561–563.
37. Beagley, K. W., Bao, S., Ramsay, A. J., Eldridge, J. H., and Husband, A. J. (1995) IgA production by peritoneal cavity B cells is IL-6 independent: implications for intestinal IgA responses. *Eur. J. Immunol.* **25,** 2123–2126.
38. Bao, S., Husband, A. J., and Beagley, K. W. (1999) B1 B cell numbers and antibodies against phosphorylcholine and LPS are increased in IL-6 gene knockout mice. *Cell Immunol.* **198,** 139–142.
39. VanCott, J. L., Franco, M. A., Greenberg, H. B., et al. (2000) Protective immunity to rotavirus shedding in the absence of interleukin-6: Th1 cells and immunoglobulin A develop normally. *J. Virol.* **74,** 5250–5256.
40. Suzuki, Y., Rani, S., Liesenfeld, O., et al. (1997) Impaired resistance to the development of toxoplasmic encephalitis in interleukin-6-deficient mice. *Infect. Immun.* **65,** 2339–2345.
41. Jebbari, H., Roberts, C. W., Ferguson, D. J., Bluethmann, H., and Alexander, J. (1998) A protective role for IL-6 during early infection with *Toxoplasma gondii. Parasite Immunol.* **20,** 231–239.
42. Williams, D. M., Grubbs, B. G., Darville, T., Kelly, K., and Rank, R. G. (1998) A role for interleukin-6 in host defense against murine *Chlamydia trachomatis* infection. *Infect. Immun.* **66,** 4564–4567.
43. Saunders, B. M., Frank, A. A., Orme, I. M., and Cooper, A. M. (2000) Interleukin-6 induces early gamma interferon production in the infected lung but is not required for generation of specific immunity to *Mycobacterium tuberculosis* infection. *Infect. Immun.* **68,** 3322–3326.
44. Cenci, E., Mencacci, A., Casagrande, A., Mosci, P., Bistoni, F., and Romani, L. (2001) Impaired antifungal effector activity but not inflammatory cell recruitment in interleukin-6-deficient mice with invasive pulmonary aspergillosis. *J. Infect. Dis.* **184,** 610–617.
45. Anguita, J., Rincon, M., Samanta, S., Barthold, S. W., Flavell, R. A., and Fikrig, E. (1998) *Borrelia burgdorferi*-infected, interleukin-6-deficient mice have decreased Th2 responses and increased Lyme arthritis. *J. Infect. Dis.* **178,** 1512–1515.
46. Dalrymple, S. A., Slattery, R., Aud, D. M., Krishna, M., Lucian, L. A., and Murray, R. (1996) Interleukin-6 is required for a protective immune response to systemic *Escherichia coli* infection. *Infect. Immun.* **64,** 3231–3235.
47. van Enckevort, F. H., Sweep, C. G., Span, P. N., Netea, M. G., Hermus, A. R., and Kullberg, B. J. (2001) Reduced adrenal response and increased mortality after systemic *Klebsiella pneumoniae* infection in interleukin-6-deficient mice. *Eur. Cytokine Netw.* **12,** 581–586.
48. Moskowitz, N. H., Brown, D. R., and Reiner, S. L. (1997) Efficient immunity against *Leishmania major* in the absence of interleukin-6. *Infect. Immun.* **65,** 2448–2450.
49. Titus, R. G., DeKrey, G. K., Morris, R. V., and Soares, M. B. (2001) Interleukin-6 deficiency influences cytokine expression in susceptible BALB mice infected with *Leishmania major* but does not alter the outcome of disease. *Infect. Immun.* **69,** 5189–5192.
50. Mabbott, N. A., Williams, A., Farquhar, C. F., Pasparakis, M., Kollias, G., and Bruce, M. E. (2000) Tumor necrosis factor alpha-deficient, but not interleukin-6-deficient, mice resist peripheral infection with scrapie. *J. Virol.* **74,** 3338–3344.
51. Feldmann, M., Brennan, F. M., and Maini, R. N. (1996) Rheumatoid arthritis. *Cell* **85,** 307–310.

52. Houssiau, F. A., Devogelaer, J. P., Van Damme, J., de Deuxchaisnes, C. N., and Van Snick, J. (1988) Interleukin-6 in synovial fluid and serum of patients with rheumatoid arthritis and other inflammatory arthritides. *Arthritis Rheum.* **31,** 784–788.
53. De Benedetti, F., Massa, M., Robbioni, P., Ravelli, A., Burgio, G. R., and Martini, A. (1991) Correlation of serum interleukin-6 levels with joint involvement and thrombocytosis in systemic juvenile rheumatoid arthritis. *Arthritis Rheum.* **34,** 1158–1163.
54. Romano, M., Sironi, M., Toniatti, C., et al. (1997) Role of IL-6 and its soluble receptor in induction of chemokines and leukocyte recruitment. *Immunity* **6,** 315–325.
55. Mihara, M., Moriya, Y., Kishimoto, T., and Ohsugi, Y. (1995) Interleukin-6 (IL-6) induces the proliferation of synovial fibroblastic cells in the presence of soluble IL-6 receptor. *Br. J. Rheumatol.* **34,** 321–325.
56. Tamura, T., Udagawa, N., Takahashi, N., et al. (1993) Soluble interleukin-6 receptor triggers osteoclast formation by interleukin 6. *Proc. Natl. Acad. Sci. USA* **90,** 11924–11928.
57. Trentham, D. E., Townes, A. S., and Kang, A. H. (1977) Autoimmunity to type II collagen an experimental model of arthritis. *J. Exp. Med.* **146,** 857–868.
58. Brackertz, D., Mitchell, G. F., and Mackay, I. R. (1977) Antigen-induced arthritis in mice. I. Induction of arthritis in various strains of mice. *Arthritis Rheum.* **20,** 841–8450.
59. Keystone, E. C., Schorlemmer, H. U., Pope, C., and Allison, A. C. (1977) Zymosan-induced arthritis: a model of chronic proliferative arthritis following activation of the alternative pathway of complement. *Arthritis Rheum.* **20,** 1396–1401.
60. Kobayashi, H., Ohshima, S., Nishioka, K., et al. (2002) Antigen induced arthritis (AIA) can be transferred by bone marrow transplantation: evidence that interleukin 6 is essential for induction of AIA. *J. Rheumatol.* **29,** 1176–1182.
61. van de Loo, F. A., Arntz, O. J., and Van den Berg, W. B. (1997) Effect of interleukin 1 and leukaemia inhibitory factor on chondrocyte metabolism in articular cartilage from normal and interleukin-6-deficient mice: role of nitric oxide and IL-6 in the suppression of proteoglycan synthesis. *Cytokine* **9,** 453–462.
62. de Hooge, A. S., van De Loo, F. A., Arntz, O. J., and van Den Berg, W. B. (2000) Involvement of IL-6, apart from its role in immunity, in mediating a chronic response during experimental arthritis. *Am. J. Pathol.* **157,** 2081–2091.
63. Kerlero de Rosbo, N., Milo, R., Lees, M. B., Burger, D., Bernard, C. C., and Ben-Nun, A. (1993) Reactivity to myelin antigens in multiple sclerosis. Peripheral blood lymphocytes respond predominantly to myelin oligodendrocyte glycoprotein. *J. Clin. Invest.* **92,** 2602–2608.
64. Mendel, I., Kerlero de Rosbo, N., and Ben-Nun, A. (1995) A myelin oligodendrocyte glycoprotein peptide induces typical chronic experimental autoimmune encephalomyelitis in H-2b mice: fine specificity and T cell receptor V beta expression of encephalitogenic T cells. *Eur. J. Immunol.* **25,** 1951–1959.
65. Eugster, H. P., Frei, K., Winkler, F., et al. (2001) Superantigen overcomes resistance of IL-6-deficient mice towards MOG-induced EAE by a TNFR1 controlled pathway. *Eur. J. Immunol.* **31,** 2302–2312.
66. Campbell, I. L., Abraham, C. R., Masliah, E., et al. (1993) Neurologic disease induced in transgenic mice by cerebral overexpression of interleukin 6. *Proc. Natl. Acad. Sci. USA* **90,** 10061–10065.
67. Raisz, L. G. (1988) Local and systemic factors in the pathogenesis of osteoporosis. *N. Engl. J. Med.* **318,** 818–828.
68. Horowitz, M. C. (1993) Cytokines and estrogen in bone: anti-osteoporotic effects. *Science* **260,** 626–627.
69. Bellido, T., Jilka, R. L., Boyce, B. F., et al. (1995) Regulation of interleukin-6, osteoclastogenesis, and bone mass by androgens. The role of the androgen receptor. *J. Clin. Invest.* **95,** 2886–2895.
70. Klein, B., Zhang, X. G., Lu, Z. Y., and Bataille, R. (1995) Interleukin-6 in human multiple myeloma. *Blood* **85,** 863–872.
71. Klein, B., Wijdenes, J., Zhang, X. G., et al. (1991) Murine anti-interleukin-6 monoclonal antibody therapy for a patient with plasma cell leukemia. *Blood* **78,** 1198–1204.
72. Potter, M., and Wiener, F. (1992) Plasmacytomagenesis in mice: model of neoplastic development dependent upon chromosomal translocations. *Carcinogenesis* **13,** 1681–1697.

73. Degrassi, A., Hilbert, D. M., Rudikoff, S., Anderson, A. O., Potter, M., and Coon, H. G. (1993) In vitro culture of primary plasmacytomas requires stromal cell feeder layers. *Proc. Natl. Acad. Sci. USA* **90,** 2060–2064.
74. Dedera, D. A., Urashima, M., Chauhan, D., LeBrun, D. P., Bronson, R. T., and Anderson, K. C. (1996) Interleukin-6 is required for pristane-induced plasma cell hyperplasia in mice. *Br. J. Haematol.* **94,** 53–61.
75. Screpanti, I., Musiani, P., Bellavia, D., et al. (1996) Inactivation of the IL-6 gene prevents development of multicentric Castleman's disease in C/EBP beta-deficient mice. *J. Exp. Med.* **184,** 1561–1566.
76. Lattanzio, G., Libert, C., Aquilina, M., et al. (1997) Defective development of pristane-oil-induced plasmacytomas in interleukin-6-deficient BALB/c mice. *Am. J. Pathol.* **151,** 689–696.
77. Hilbert, D. M., Kopf, M., Mock, B. A., Kohler, G., and Rudikoff, S. (1995) Interleukin 6 is essential for in vivo development of B lineage neoplasms. *J. Exp. Med.* **182,** 243–248.
78. Hilbert, D. M., Migone, T. S., Kopf, M., Leonard, W. J., and Rudikoff, S. (1996) Distinct tumorigenic potential of abl and raf in B cell neoplasia: abl activates the IL-6 signaling pathway. *Immunity* **5,** 81–89.
79. Fausto, N. (2000) Liver regeneration. *J. Hepatol.* **32,** 19–31.
80. Maione, D., Di Carlo, E., Li, W., et al. (1998) Coexpression of IL-6 and soluble IL-6R causes nodular regenerative hyperplasia and adenomas of the liver. *EMBO J.* **17,** 5588–5597.
81. Cressman, D. E., Greenbaum, L. E., DeAngelis, R. A., et al. (1996) Liver failure and defective hepatocyte regeneration in interleukin-6-deficient mice. *Science* **274,** 1379–1383.
82. Sakamoto, T., Liu, Z., Murase, N., et al. (1999) Mitosis and apoptosis in the liver of interleukin-6-deficient mice after partial hepatectomy. *Hepatology* **29,** 403–411.
83. Ledda-Columbano, G. M., Curto, M., Piga, R., et al. (1998) In vivo hepatocyte proliferation is inducible through a TNF and IL-6-independent pathway. *Oncogene* **17,** 1039–1044.
84. Li, W., Liang, X., Leu, J. I., Kovalovich, K., Ciliberto, G., and Taub, R. (2001) Global changes in interleukin-6-dependent gene expression patterns in mouse livers after partial hepatectomy. *Hepatology* **33,** 1377–1386.
85. Kovalovich, K., DeAngelis, R. A., Li, W., Furth, E. E., Ciliberto, G., and Taub, R. (2000) Increased toxin-induced liver injury and fibrosis in interleukin-6-deficient mice. *Hepatology* **31,** 149–159.
86. Katz, A., Chebath, J., Friedman, J., and Revel, M. (1998) Increased sensitivity of IL-6-deficient mice to carbon tetrachloride hepatotoxicity and protection with an IL-6 receptor-IL-6 chimera. *Cytokines Cell. Mol. Ther.* **4,** 221–227.
87. Ezure, T., Sakamoto, T., Tsuji, H., et al. (2000) The development and compensation of biliary cirrhosis in interleukin-6-deficient mice. *Am. J. Pathol.* **156,** 1627–1639.
88. Camargo, C. A., Jr., Madden, J. F., Gao, W., Selvan, R. S., and Clavien, P. A. (1997) Interleukin-6 protects liver against warm ischemia/reperfusion injury and promotes hepatocyte proliferation in the rodent. *Hepatology* **26,** 1513–1520.
89. Kushner, I. (1982) The phenomenon of the acute phase response. *Ann. NY Acad. Sci.* **389,** 39–48.
90. Won, K., Campos, S.P., and Baumann, H. (1993) Experimental systems for studying hepatic acute phase response. In: Mackiewicz, A., Kushner, I., and Baumann, H., ed. *Acute Phase Protein.* CRC Press, Boca Raton FL, pp. 255-271.
91. Koj, A., Gauldie, J., and Baumann, H. (1993) Biological perspectives of cytokine and hormone networks. In: Mackiewicz, A., Kushner, I., and Baumann, H., ed. *Acute Phase Protein.* CRC Press, Boca Raton, FL, pp. 275–287.
92. Beutler, B., Milsark, I. W., and Cerami, A. C. (1985) Passive immunization against cachectin/tumor necrosis factor protects mice from lethal effect of endotoxin. *Science* **229,** 869–871.
93. Zetterstrom, M., Sundgren-Andersson, A. K., Ostlund, P., and Bartfai, T. (1998) Delineation of the proinflammatory cytokine cascade in fever induction. *Ann. NY Acad. Sci.* **856,** 48–52.
94. Fattori, E., Cappelletti, M., Costa, P., et al. (1994) Defective inflammatory response in interleukin 6-deficient mice. *J. Exp. Med.* **180,** 1243–1250.
95. Xing, Z., Gauldie, J., Cox, G., et al. (1998) IL-6 is an antiinflammatory cytokine required for controlling local or systemic acute inflammatory responses. *J. Clin. Invest.* **101,** 311–320.

96. Baumann, H., Ziegler, S. F., Mosley, B., Morella, K. K., Pajovic, S., and Gearing, D. P. (1993) Reconstitution of the response to leukemia inhibitory factor, oncostatin M, and ciliary neurotrophic factor in hepatoma cells. *J. Biol. Chem.* **268,** 8414–8417.
97. Alonzi, T., Fattori, E., Cappelletti, M., Ciliberto, G., and Poli, V. (1998) Impaired Stat3 activation following localized inflammatory stimulus in IL-6-deficient mice. *Cytokine* **10,** 13–18.
98. Alonzi, T., Maritano, D., Gorgoni, B., Rizzuto, G., Libert, C., and Poli, V. (2001) Essential role of STAT3 in the control of the acute-phase response as revealed by inducible gene inactivation [correction of activation] in the liver. *Mol. Cell Biol.* **21,** 1621–1632.
99. Libert, C., Takahashi, N., Cauwels, A., Brouckaert, P., Bluethmann, H., and Fiers, W. (1994) Response of interleukin-6-deficient mice to tumor necrosis factor-induced metabolic changes and lethality. *Eur. J. Immunol.* **24,** 2237–2242.
100. Benigni, F., Fantuzzi, G., Sacco, S., et al. (1996) Six different cytokines that share GP130 as a receptor subunit, induce serum amyloid A and potentiate the induction of interleukin-6 and the activation of the hypothalamus-pituitary-adrenal axis by interleukin-1. *Blood* **87,** 1851–1854.
101. Kozak, W., Kluger, M. J., Soszynski, D., et al. (1998) IL-6 and IL-1 beta in fever. Studies using cytokine-deficient (knockout) mice. *Ann. NY Acad. Sci.* **856,** 33–47.
102. Manfredi, B., Sacerdote, P., Gaspani, L., Poli, V., and Panerai, A. E. (1998) IL-6 knock-out mice show modified basal immune functions, but normal immune responses to stress. *Brain Behav. Immun.* **12,** 201–211.
103. Bethin, K. E., Vogt, S. K., and Muglia, L. J. (2000) Interleukin-6 is an essential, corticotropin-releasing hormone-independent stimulator of the adrenal axis during immune system activation. *Proc. Natl. Acad. Sci. USA* **97,** 9317–9322.
104. Venihaki, M., Dikkes, P., Carrigan, A., and Karalis, K. P. (2001) Corticotropin-releasing hormone regulates IL-6 expression during inflammation. *J. Clin. Invest.* **108,** 1159–1166.
105. Andersson, B., Jobin, M., and Olsson, K. (1966) Serotonin and temperature control. *Acta Physiol. Scand.* **67,** 50–56.
106. Kozak, W., Poli, V., Soszynski, D., Conn, C. A., Leon, L. R., and Kluger, M. J. (1997) Sickness behavior in mice deficient in interleukin-6 during turpentine abscess and influenza pneumonitis. *Am. J. Physiol.* **272,** R621–R630.
107. Chai, Z., Gatti, S., Toniatti, C., Poli, V., and Bartfai, T. (1996) Interleukin (IL)-6 gene expression in the central nervous system is necessary for fever response to lipopolysaccharide or IL-1 beta: a study on IL-6-deficient mice. *J. Exp. Med.* **183,** 311–316.
108. Leon, L. R., White, A. A., and Kluger, M. J. (1998) Role of IL-6 and TNF in thermoregulation and survival during sepsis in mice. *Am. J. Physiol.* **275,** R269–R277.
109. Jones, S. A., Novick, D., Horiuchi, S., Yamamoto, N., Szalai, A. J., and Fuller, G. M. (1999) C-reactive protein: a physiological activator of interleukin 6 receptor shedding. *J. Exp. Med.* **189,** 599–604.
110. Di Santo, E., Alonzi, T., Poli, V., et al. (1997) Differential effects of IL-6 on systemic and central production of TNF: a study with IL-6-deficient mice. *Cytokine* **9,** 300–306.
111. Di Santo, E., Alonzi, T., Fattori, E., et al. (1996) Overexpression of interleukin-6 in the central nervous system of transgenic mice increases central but not systemic proinflammatory cytokine production. *Brain Res.* **740,** 239–244.
112. Penkowa, M., Moos, T., Carrasco, J., et al. (1999) Strongly compromised inflammatory response to brain injury in interleukin-6-deficient mice. *Glia* **25,** 343–357.
113. Penkowa, M., Giralt, M., Carrasco, J., Hadberg, H., and Hidalgo, J. (2000) Impaired inflammatory response and increased oxidative stress and neurodegeneration after brain injury in interleukin-6-deficient mice. *Glia* **32,** 271–285.
114. Swartz, K. R., Liu, F., Sewell, D., et al. (2001) Interleukin-6 promotes post-traumatic healing in the central nervous system. *Brain Res.* **896,** 86–95.
115. Klein, M. A., Moller, J. C., Jones, L. L., Bluethmann, H., Kreutzberg, G. W., and Raivich, G. (1997) Impaired neuroglial activation in interleukin-6 deficient mice. *Glia* **19,** 227–233.
116. Murphy, P. G., Borthwick, L. S., Johnston, R. S., Kuchel, G., and Richardson, P. M. (1999) Nature of the retrograde signal from injured nerves that induces interleukin-6 mRNA in neurons. *J. Neurosci.* **19,** 3791–3800.

117. Galiano, M., Liu, Z. Q., Kalla, R., et al. (2001) Interleukin-6 (IL6) and cellular response to facial nerve injury: effects on lymphocyte recruitment, early microglial activation and axonal outgrowth in IL6-deficient mice. *Eur. J. Neurosci.* **14,** 327–341.
118. Zhong, J., Dietzel, I. D., Wahle, P., Kopf, M., and Heumann, R. (1999) Sensory impairments and delayed regeneration of sensory axons in interleukin-6-deficient mice. *J. Neurosci.* **19,** 4305–4313.
119. Xu, X. J., Hao, J. X., Andell-Jonsson, S., Poli, V., Bartfai, T., and Wiesenfeld-Hallin, Z. (1997) Nociceptive responses in interleukin-6-deficient mice to peripheral inflammation and peripheral nerve section. *Cytokine* **9,** 1028–1033.
120. Bianchi, M., Maggi, R., Pimpinelli, F., et al. (1999) Presence of a reduced opioid response in interleukin-6 knock out mice. *Eur. J. Neurosci.* **11,** 1501–1507.
121. Wallenius, V., Wallenius, K., Ahren, B., et al. (2002) Interleukin-6-deficient mice develop mature-onset obesity. *Nat. Med.* **8,** 75–79.
122. Lyons, R. E., Anthony, J. P., Ferguson, D. J., et al. (2001) Immunological studies of chronic ocular toxoplasmosis: up-regulation of major histocompatibility complex class I and transforming growth factor beta and a protective role for interleukin-6. *Infect. Immun.* **69,** 2589–2595.
123. Fenton, R. R., Molesworth-Kenyon, S., Oakes, J. E., and Lausch, R. N. (2002) Linkage of IL-6 with neutrophil chemoattractant expression in virus-induced ocular inflammation. *Invest. Ophthalmol. Vis. Sci.* **43,** 737–743.
124. van Enckevort, F. H., Netea, M. G., Hermus, A. R., et al. (1999) Increased susceptibility to systemic candidiasis in interleukin-6 deficient mice. *Med. Mycol.* **37,** 419–426.
125. van der Poll, T., Keogh, C. V., Guirao, X., Buurman, W. A., Kopf, M., and Lowry, S. F. (1997) Interleukin-6 gene-deficient mice show impaired defense against pneumococcal pneumonia. *J. Infect. Dis.* **176,** 439–444.
126. Balto, K., Sasaki, H., and Stashenko, P. (2001) Interleukin-6 deficiency increases inflammatory bone destruction. *Infect. Immun.* **69,** 744–750.
127. Wang, J., Homer, R. J., Chen, Q., and Elias, J. A. (2000) Endogenous and exogenous IL-6 inhibit aeroallergen-induced Th2 inflammation. *J. Immunol.* **165,** 4051–4061.
128. Leemans, J. C., Vervoordeldonk, M. J., Florquin, S., Van Kessel, K. P., and Van Der Poll, T. (2002) Differential role of interleukin-6 in lung inflammation induced by lipoteichoic acid and peptidoglycan from *Staphylococcus aureus*. *Am. J. Respir. Crit. Care Med.* **165,** 1445–1450.
129. Rijneveld, A. W., van den Dobbelsteen, G. P., Florquin, S., et al. (2002) Roles of interleukin-6 and macrophage inflammatory protein-2 in pneumolysin-induced lung inflammation in mice. *J. Infect. Dis.* **185,** 123–126.
130. Rosenbaum, J. T., Kievit, P., Han, Y. B., Park, J. M., and Planck, S. R. (1998) Interleukin-6 does not mediate endotoxin-induced uveitis in mice: studies in gene deletion animals. *Invest. Ophthalmol. Vis. Sci.* **39,** 64–69.
131. Hurst, S. M., Wilkinson, T. S., McLoughlin, R. M., et al. (2001) Il-6 and its soluble receptor orchestrate a temporal switch in the pattern of leukocyte recruitment seen during acute inflammation. *Immunity* **14,** 705–714.
132. Cuzzocrea, S., De Sarro, G., Costantino, G., et al. (1999) IL-6 knock-out mice exhibit resistance to splanchnic artery occlusion shock. *J. Leukoc. Biol.* **66,** 471–480.
133. Meng, Z. H., Dyer, K., Billiar, T. R., and Tweardy, D. J. (2001) Essential role for IL-6 in post-resuscitation inflammation in hemorrhagic shock. *Am. J. Physiol. Cell. Physiol.* **280,** C343–C351.
134. Cuzzocrea, S., Sautebin, L., De Sarro, G., et al. (1999) Role of IL-6 in the pleurisy and lung injury caused by carrageenan. *J. Immunol.* **163,** 5094–5104.
135. Cuzzocrea, S., de Sarro, G., Costantino, G., et al. (1999) Role of interleukin-6 in a non-septic shock model induced by zymosan. *Eur. Cytokine Netw.* **10,** 191–203.

14

IL-10 and IL-2 Knockout Mice

Effect on Intestinal Inflammation

Karen L. Madsen and Humberto Jijon

Summary

The colitis in IL-10 deficient mice is characterized by immune system dysregulation, in that regulatory T cells either fail to develop or are functionally impaired in the absence of IL-10. This leads to an IL-12 and IFN-γ directed excessive generation and activation of Th1 cells directed towards luminal bacterial antigens and resultant immunopathology resembling human Crohn's disease. Intestinal inflammation is dependent upon the presence of luminal microflora, and can be modulated through antibiotics, probiotics, and antibodies directed at proinflammatory cytokines. Disease is highly dependent upon genetic background. IL-2-deficient mice develop a progressive inflammatory bowel disease with similarities to human ulcerative colitis. IL-2-deficient mice initially have normal numbers of B and T lymphocytes; however, the lamina propria of inflamed colons in older mice contain elevated levels of CD4+ and CD8+ T cells, as well as B220+ B cells, suggesting that both T and B cells are spontaneously activated in the colonic immune response. As in the IL-10 deficient mouse, disease in the IL-2-deficient mouse is dependent upon the presence of luminal microflora and is modulated by the genetic background of the animal. Overall, findings in these two models of colitis suggest that genetically susceptible hosts can mount a pathogenic cellular immune response to specific nonpathogenic bacterial species as a consequence of defective immunologic tolerance.

Key words

microflora, colitis, Crohn's disease, cytokines, probiotics, antibiotics

1. Introduction

The advent of gene knockout and transgene technology has resulted in the discovery of various spontaneous models of chronic intestinal inflammation. In general, these models have involved either a dysregulation of the immune system or alterations in intestinal barrier function and require the presence of colonic microflora to develop disease. Two of the best characterized models of colitis are the interleukin-2 (IL-2) knockout *(1)* and the interleukin-10 knockout mouse *(2)*. However, although deletion of either of these cytokines renders mice susceptible to the development of intestinal inflammation, significant differences exist in disease phenotype between these two models. In the case of the IL-2-deficient mouse, the inflammation involves many features reminiscent of human ulcerative colitis, whereas in the IL-10-deficient mouse model, characteristics of the inflammatory disease more closely resemble Crohn's disease.

From: *Contemporary Immunology: Cytokine Knockouts, 2nd Edition*
Edited by: Giamila Fantuzzi © Humana Press Inc., Totowa, NJ

2. Interleukin-10

IL-10 is a potent antiinflammatory cytokine that inhibits gene expression and synthesis of T-cell and macrophage cytokines and suppresses the function of antigen-presenting cells *(3)*. IL-10 is produced as a monomer by T-cells, certain B-cells, macrophages, thymocytes, epithelial cells, and keratinocytes. IL-10 suppresses the production of IL-1α, IL-1β, tumor necrosis factor (TNF)-α, IL-6, IL-8, IL-12, IL-18, granulocyte-macrophage colony-stimulating factor, macrophage inflammatory protein-1α (MIP-1α), RANTES, leukemia-inhibiting factor, and IL-10 itself *(3)*. Importantly, IL-10 inhibits the production of IL-12 by macrophages and dendritic cells *(4)* and prevents dendritic cell maturation and antigen presentation; thus attenuating the development of interferon-γ (IFN-γ)-producing T-cells *(5,6)*. Evidence for a role for IL-10 in the upregulation of the chemokine receptor CCR7, which allows dendritic cells to move to the nearest lymphoid organ for antigen presentation, also exists *(7)*. In addition, in vitro studies have demonstrated that IL-10 is a strong stimulator of B-cell differentiation and immunoglobulin secretion *(3)*; thus IL-10 is implicated in the develoment of Th2-type immune responses. Following activation of the IL-10 receptor, intracellular signaling pathways involve the phosphorylation of JAK1, TYK2, and STAT3. There is some evidence to suggest that IL-10 can inhibit the translocation of nuclear factor-κB NF-κB), thus inhibiting the immediate-early proinflammatory response *(8)*.

2.1. The IL-10-Deficient Mouse

The original description of the IL-10-deficient mouse came from Kuhn et al. *(2)*, who initially made the observation that IL-10-deficient mice develop an enterocolitis similar to that seen in human Crohn's disease. The disease that develops appears largely to depend on an inappropriate immune response to intestinal bacterial antigens. The colitis in IL-10-deficient mice is characterized by immune system dysregulation, in that regulatory T-cells *(9)* either fail to develop or are functionally impaired in the absence of IL-10 *(10)*. This leads to an IL-12- and IFN-γ-directed excessive generation and activation of Th1 cells and resultant immunopathology. Although it is clear that T-cells are involved in the development of colitis and that colonic bacteria are important in this process, it is not known what specific bacteria antigens are involved.

2.2. Pathology and Histologic Abnormalities

Intestinal disease in the IL-10-deficient mouse is associated with weight loss, splenomegaly, high white blood cell counts, and anemia *(2)*. Under conventional conditions, some laboratories have described the development of an enterocolitis involving the duodenum, proximal jejunum, and proximal colon *(2)*. However, when animals are raised under specific pathogen-free conditions, the inflammation is generally limited to the terminal ileum, cecum, and colon, corresponding to those areas where microflora are found in highest concentrations. When mice are raised under sterile conditions, the animals remain disease-free *(11,12)*.

Histologic abnormalities in IL-10-deficient mice are limited to the intestinal tract and hematopoietic tissues *(2)*. In the intestine, inflammatory lesions begin as small multifocal infiltrates in the lamina propria. These changes progress, ultimately producing focal ulcerations and transmural lesions. IL-10-deficient mice also exhibit marked crypt hyperplasia, with only rare occurrences of granulomas, fibrosis, and lymphoid aggregates. The cellular infiltrate in these lesions comprises lymphocytes, plasma cells, macrophages, neutrophils, and the occasional multinucleated giant cell. Most of the plasma cells produce IgA. These histopathologic features of intestinal lesions, including the presence of discontinuous lesions affecting the mucosa and submucosa and occasionally extending into the serosa, most closely resemble lesions present in patients with Crohn's disease *(10)*. However, the marked crypt hyperplasia, the rare occurrence of granulomas and fibrosis, and the absence of fissures and fistulas are atypical of Crohn's disease; thus the IL-10-deficient mouse is not a perfect model for this disease.

2.3. Immunologic Abnormalities

IL-10-deficient mice exhibit abnormally high numbers of αβ T-cell receptor (αβTCR) +/CD4+ but not αβTCR+/CD8+ T-cells, resulting in a greater number of CD4+ compared with CD8+ cells. This is opposite to what is seen in wild-type mice *(10)*. In addition, in IL-10-deficient mice the CD4+ lamina propria lymphocytes are predominantly CD45RB^{low}, CD26L^{low}, and CD44^{high}, reflecting an activated or "memory" phenotype, whereas in wild-type mice both naive and activated phenotypes are found *(10)*. There are high numbers of F4/80+ macrophages and Ig+ B-cells in the lamina propria along with increased expression of MHC class II by epithelial cells *(10)*.

High levels of IL-1α, TNF-α, IL-6, IFN-γ, and nitric oxide are produced spontaneously in mucosae of IL-10-deficient mice *(10,12,13)*, whereas IL-4 is undetectable, suggesting that CD4+ T-cells in the colon of these mice have a polarized Th1 phenotype. Indeed, transfer of purified CD4+ Th1 cells from IL-10-deficient mice to immunodeficient RAG mice results in the development of chronic colitis *(13)*. The crucial role of T-cells, but not B-cells, in colitis pathogenesis in this model is evident from studies showing that IL-10-deficient mice bred to B-cell deficient mice, but not to T/B-cell-deficient mice still develop colitis *(13)*.

2.4. Species Variation and Time-Course of Colitis

The severity of disease in this model is highly dependent on the environment and genetic background. C57BL/6 mutants are relatively resistant to colitis, whereas BALB/c and 129 Sv/Ev strains develop a more severe colitis than do the original outbred strains (129/Ola × C57Bl/6) *(10)*. This would suggest the presence of an inheritable component in this model of colitis, and, indeed, work by Farmer et al. *(14)* has identified cytokine deficiency-induced colitis susceptibility modifiers in various strains of IL-10-deficient mice. This study has also revealed the extremely complex nature of the interactions among the various loci.

The age of onset and the progression of disease in the IL-10-deficient mouse model is also highly dependent on environment and strain. In 129 Sv/Ev mice, histologic abnormalities appear at 4–5 wk and progress in severity until 7–9 mo, at which time the mice die *(10,15)*. In other strains that demonstrate intermediate severity, disease appears between 7 and 9 wk. In IL-10-deficient mice bred on a C57BL/10 background, two distinct phases of colitis have been identified: an early phase that is distinguished by a progressive worsening of the histologic signs of inflammation and increases in mucosal IL-12 and IFN-γ production *(16)*. In the late phase of colitis in this strain, there is no further increase in severity of disease, but there is a dramatic drop in mucosal IL-12 and IFN-γ production, accompanied by an increase in IL-4 and IL-13 expression. As IL-10 has been shown to inhibit the production of both IL-4 and IL-13 in schistosome-infected mice *(17)*, it is plausible that the increase in production of these cytokines may be owing to the lack of IL-10.

These observations suggest that the molecular mechanisms that initiate inflammation may be distinct from those that drive chronic inflammation, a finding that may explain some of the variability of both animal and human responses to therapeutic modalities *(16)*. Interestingly, neither IL-1β nor TNF-α production was significantly different between pre-, early-, or late-stage disease in this mouse strain. In contrast, increased mucosal levels of both TNF-α and IFN-γ have been described to occur before the development of colitis in the 129 Sv/Ev strain *(15,18)*; thus it is not clear whether all strains exhibit similar differences between early and late disease.

In the 129 Sv/Ev IL-10-deficient mouse, a breakdown of intestinal barrier function precedes the development of inflammation by approximately 2–3 wk and is linked to increased colonic secretion of TNF-α and IFN-γ *(12)*. Enhanced colonic permeability is also present in IL-10-deficient C57/Black6 adult mice *(19)*. This breakdown in the intestinal barrier is associated with the presence of colonic microflora, as mice raised under sterile conditions do not demonstrate any alterations in barrier function or proinflammatory cytokine secretion *(12)*.

2.5. Colonic Microflora in the IL-10-Deficient Mouse

IL-10-deficient mice spontaneously develop colitis if raised in the presence of normal microflora but show no signs of disease under sterile conditions. Transfer of germ-free IL-10-deficient mice to conventional conditions results in the development of colitis within 1 wk of the mouse exposure to microbes *(11)*. IL-10-deficient mice have been shown to have significant alterations in the levels of bacteria adhering closely to the epithelium in the colon compared with control mice raised in the same environment *(15)*. Importantly, this altered bacterial colonization pattern is present within 24 h of birth, suggesting that the genetic background of the host can influence early bacterial colonization. Furthermore, as alterations in bacterial colonization precede the development of colitis, the idea that colitis is associated with an imbalance of colonic microflora is intriguing. Indeed, IL-10-deficient mice have reduced levels of probiotic bacteria (*Lactobacillus*) compared with controls, and furthermore, treating IL-10-deficient mice from birth with *Lactobacillus* actually prevents the development of colitis *(15)*. This would suggest that genetic factors may be critical in controlling which bacterial species are able to colonize the gastrointestinal tract.

2.6. Response to Therapeutics

Treatment of neonatal IL-10-deficient mice with a variety of therapies is effective in preventing the onset of disease; in contrast, once disease has become established, only a few therapeutic approaches have shown efficacy in attenuating disease. For disease prevention, injections of IL-10 are able to prevent the development of disease *(20)* (Table 1). However, the ability of IL-10 to prevent disease is dependent on continual administration; if treatment is stopped, intestinal inflammation immediately begins to develop, suggesting that the primary function of IL-10 is to suppress the activities of cells that produce cytokines involved in a Th1 response. Treatment of IL-10-deficient mice with anti-IL-12 or anti-IFN-γ are equally effective in preventing the onset of histologic inflammation (Table 1), clearly indicating a role for both cytokines in the initiation of disease. The finding that anti-IL-12 is able to prevent the development of disease completely suggests that antibodies to IL-12 may suppress the generation of pathogenic Th1 cells from a naive cell population. The efficacy of anti-IFN-γ in preventing disease, together with the known role of

Table 1
Prevention Therapies in IL-10-Deficient Mice

Treatment	Age at starting	Duration	Strain	Result	Reference
IL-10	21 d	8 wk	129 Sv/Ev	No colitis	*10,20*
Anti-IL-4	21 d	8 wk	129 Sv/Ev	No effect	*20*
Anti-IL-1	21 d	8 wk	129 Sv/Ev	No effect	*20*
Anti-IL-6	21 d	8 wk	129 Sv/Ev	No effect	*20*
Anti-IL-12	10 d	8 wk	129 Sv/Ev	No colitis	*13,20*
Anti-TNF-α	21 d	8 wk	129 Sv/Ev	No effect	*20*
Anti-IFN-γ	21 d	6 wk	129 Sv/Ev	Abolished MHC class II expression on epithelial cells Colitis in 30%	*10,20*
Lactobacillus sp.	7 d	4 wk	129 Sv/Ev	Attenuated colitis	*15*
	16 wk	16 wk	C57BL/6	Attenuated colitis and reduced colon cancer	*21*
	10–12 wk	4 wk	C57BL/6 × 129 Ola	Attenuated colitis	*22*
Lactulose	7 d	4 wk	129 Sv/Ev	Attenuated colitis	*15*
Metronidazole/ neomycin	7 d	4 wk	129 Sv/Ev	Attenuated colitis	*18*
Ciprofloxacin	7 d	4 wk	129 Sv/Ev	Attenuated colitis	*18*
Cross-fostering	24 h	3 wk	129 Sv/Ev	Attenuated colitis	*23*

IFN-γ, interferon-γ; IL, interleukin; TNF, tumor necrosis factor.

IFN-γ as a major Th1 differentiation factor, supports the concept that colitis in IL-10-deficient mice is driven by an unrestrained IL-12 driven expansion of certain subsets of Th1 cells. Neither anti-IL-1, anti-IL-6, or anti-TNF-α was effective in preventing disease in IL-10-deficient mice *(13)*.

Altering the microflora present during the neonatal period has also shown effectiveness in the prevention of disease. Treatment of mice with either neomycin/metronidazole or ciprofloxacin during the neonatal period resulted in a prevention of the development of colitis for up to 12 wk following removal of the antibiotics *(18)*. In a similar fashion, treating IL-10-deficient mice with *Lactobacillus sp.* from birth *(15,21,22)*, or feeding mice lactulose to stimulate the growth of *Lactobacillus* and *Bifidobacterium (15)* was also effective in preventing disease. Raising IL-10-deficient mice with a wild-type mother during the first 3 wk of life (cross-fostering) altered levels of adherent bacteria in the colon and prevented disease for up to 12 wk of age, suggesting a role for breast milk in controlling bacterial colonization *(23)*. Interestingly, the ability of breast milk from wild-type dams to prevent or protect from colitis was not dependent on IL-10 in the breast milk, as levels of IL-10 were undetectable in wild-type breast milk.

The chronic phase of colitis in IL-10-deficient mice appears to be perpetuated by different cytokines compared with the induction phase. Although both anti-IL12 and anti-IFN-γ are effective in preventing disease, only anti-IL-12 is able to reverse established colitis (Table 2). Interestingly, although antibodies against IL-12 were effective in ameliorating

Table 2
Treatment of Established Disease in IL-10-Deficient Mice

Treatment	Age at starting	Duration	Strain	Result	Reference
IL-10	12 wk	8 wk	129 Sv/Ev	No duodenitis Reduced incidence of colorectal carcinoma	*10*
Anti-IL-4	12 wk	8 wk	129 Sv/Ev	No effect	*20*
Anti-IL-1	12 wk	8 wk	129 Sv/Ev	No effect	*20*
Anti-IL-6	12 wk	8 wk	129 Sv/Ev	No effect	*20*
Anti-IL-12	12 wk	8 wk	129 Sv/Ev	Attenuated colitis	*12*
Anti-TNF-α	12 wk	8 wk	129 Sv/Ev	No effect	*20*
	24 wk	10 d		Attenuated colitis	*24*
Anti-IFN-γ	12 wk	6 wk	129 Sv/Ev	Abolished MHC class II expression on epithelial cells No effect on colitis	*10,13,20*
Nicotine	12 wk	2 wk	C57/BL10	Worse jejunal disease Attenuated colonic disease	*59*
3-Amino-benzamide	8 wk	4 wk	129 Sv/Ev	Attenuated disease	*25*
Lactobacillus sp.	8 wk	4 wk	129 Sv/Ev	Attenuated disease	*15*
	10–12 wk	16 wk	C57BL/6	Attenuated disease	*21*
	10–12 wk	4 wk	C57BL/6 × 129 Ola	Attenuated disease	*22*
VSL#3	8 wk	4 wk	129 Sv/Ev	Attenuated disease	*27*
Lactulose	8 wk	4 wk	129 Sv/Ev	Attenuated disease	*15*
Metronidazole/ neomycin	8 wk	4 wk	129 Sv/Ev	Attenuated disease	*18*
Ciprofloxacin	8 wk	4 wk	129 Sv/Ev	Attenuated disease	*18*

IFN-γ, interferon-γ; IL, interleukin; TNF, tumor necrosis factor.

established histologic disease, the improvement was independent of any effect of anti-IL-12 on IFN-γ production but did correlate with reduced CD4+ T-cell numbers in the colon *(20)*. Antibodies against IFN-γ are ineffective in the treatment of established disease *(20)*, supporting the idea that IFN-γ has a limited, if any, role in the perpetuation of colitis. In a similar fashion, IL-10 treatment is only mildly effective in treating established disease, and the combination of both IL-10 and anti-IL-12 is no more effective, suggesting that neither IL-10 or anti-IL12 are able to regulate the activity of pathogenic Th1 cells completely in IL-10-deficient mice *(20)*. Antibodies against TNF-α have been shown to either have no effect *(20)* or to have limited efficacy *(24)* in ameliorating colitis in IL-10-deficient mice. Inhibition of poly ADP-ribose polymerase (PARP) activity using 3-aminobenzamide *(25)* or antisense specific for PARP-2 *(26)* have shown efficacy in attenuating inflammation in adult IL-10-deficient mice. This beneficial effect of PARP inhibition may involve the normalization of epithelial permeability and a subsequent decrease in exposure of the mucosal immune system to bacterial antigens.

Likewise, altering the colonic microflora is effective in attenuating inflammation in IL-10-deficient mice, stressing the importance of the microflora in disease initiation and perpetuation in this model. Several studies using different species of lactobacilli to treat IL-10-deficient mice *(15,21,22)* were all equally efficacious in showing some attenuation of established disease. In contrast, a probiotic bacteria mixture (VSL#3) containing a combination of eight bacteria was much more effective in ameliorating colitis, restoring barrier function, and reducing proinflammatory cytokine secretion in adult 129 Sv/Ev IL-10-deficient mice with established disease *(27)*.

These studies provide a provocative message, in that the onset of inflammation in inflammatory bowel disorders may be associated with an imbalance in the intestinal microflora, with a relative predominance of "aggressive" bacteria and an insufficient concentration of "protective" species. Furthermore, reconditioning of the flora through either direct supplementation with protective bacteria or by indirect stimulation with dietary components may exert a protective role in inflammatory bowel disease.

3. Interleukin-2

IL-2 is a lymphokine originally described as a humoral factor required for the continual proliferation of activated T-cell clones. Originally discovered by Morgan et al. *(28)*, and cloned by Taniguchi et al. *(29)*, this T-cell-derived growth factor remains the focus of extensive research owing to the complexity underlying its mechanisms of action and its important role in T-cell homeostasis.

IL-2 exerts pleiotropic effects on T-cells, B-cells, and natural killer (NK) cells through its interaction with trimeric cell surface receptors composed of a high-affinity cytokine-binding IL-2-specific α-subunit (IL-2R α-chain, CD25), a β-subunit shared with the IL-15 receptor, and a common γ-chain (γc) that is shared with the IL-4, IL-7, IL-9, IL–15, and IL-21 receptors *(30)*. These receptors activate receptor-specific pathways including those transduced by the Janus kinases (JAKS) and signal transducers and activators of transcription (STATS) as well as general signaling pathways implicated in cell growth and differentiation *(31)*. IL-2 receptor activation has been shown to result in the activation of JAK1, JAK3, and STAT5, and to result in the recruitment of the adapter protein Shc, linking the IL-2 receptor to the Ras/MAP kinase and PI3K/AKT pathways *(32–34)*.

Although in vitro studies consistently point to a critical role for IL-2 in T-cell growth and survival *(35)*, in vivo studies have shown that T-cells can respond to antigen in the absence of this cytokine *(36)*. Thus, other growth factors must be able to support T-cell activation and expansion in vivo. Prime candidates for this function are cytokines that are related to IL-2 and also use the γc chain such as IL-4, IL-7, and IL-15. However, a function that is not shared by related cytokines is IL-2's role in the regulation of autoreactive T-cells *(1)*.

An important homeostatic mechanism for the maintenance of peripheral tolerance to self-antigens is apoptosis. One form of apoptosis is induced by repeated stimulation of lymphocytes and is called activation-induced cell death (AICD). IL-2 has been shown to promote T-cell survival through the activation of AKT and the induction of Bcl-2, through signals mediated via the β-subunit. Although other cytokines can induce T-cell proliferation and promote survival, IL-2 appears uniquely potent at sensitizing T-cells to AICD. A mechanistic basis for this observation is suggested by the demonstration that IL-2-mediated activation of STAT5 plays a role in potentiating AICD. STAT5 activation increases FasL expression following TCR crosslinking *(37)*. In addition, T-cell activation in the presence of IL-2 results in a reduction in the expression of the inhibitor of Fas-dependent apoptosis, FLIP *(38)*. In fact, IL-2 may be required for triggering this death pathway because T-cells from knockout mice lacking IL-2 *(39)* or the α-chain of the IL-2 receptor are resistant to AICD *(37)*. Thus, IL-2 may be involved in the maintenance of self-tolerance by promoting activated T-cells to undergo AICD *(37)*. Interestingly, Li et al. *(40)* have recently analyzed the relative roles of IL-15 and IL-2 in governing T-cell expansion in vivo. They provide evidence that IL-15 is a critical growth factor in initiating T-cell division in vivo, whereas IL-2 limits continued T-cell expansion via downregulation of the γc subunit. Decreased γc expression on cycling T-cells resulted in reduced levels of Bcl-2 expression and rendered T-cells more susceptible to apoptotic cell death *(40)*. Therefore, the paradoxic roles assigned to IL-2 in vitro may be better explained when one considers the partial overlap between IL-2 and IL-15 signaling and the differential expression of the cytokines both temporally and anatomically.

3.1. The IL-2-Deficient Mouse

Mice homozygous for the deletion of the IL-2 gene fail to produce IL-2 mRNA and completely lack IL-2 activity *(1,41)*. In 3–6-wk-old 129 Ola × C57BL/6 IL-2-deficient mice, immune responses are still relatively normal, and no intestinal or hepatic inflammation is evident *(36,41)*; however, between 4 and 9 wk after birth, about 50% of homozygous mutants on this genetic background die of a disease characterized by splenomegaly, lymphadenopathy, and severe anemia *(36)*. The remaining 50% develop a progressive inflammatory bowel disease with similarities to human ulcerative colitis that is first detectable between 6 and 15 wk of age if these animals are kept in a conventional environment *(1)*. IL-2-deficient mice initially have normal numbers of B- and T-lymphocytes; however, the lamina propria of inflamed colons in older mice contain elevated levels of CD4+ and CD8+ T-cells, as well as B220+ B-cells, suggesting that both T- and B-cells are spontaneously activated in the colonic immune response *(1,41)*.

3.2. Pathology and Histologic Abnormalities

Histologic features characteristic of this model include marked elongation of the crypts with epithelial cell proliferation, crypt branching, goblet cell depletion, occasional crypt abscesses, and the presence of inflammatory cells in the mucosa *(42)*. Signs of inflammatory bowel disease include diarrhea, intestinal bleeding, and frequent rectal prolapse. Microscopic examination of the spleen demonstrate increased amounts of red pulp, whereas the amount of white pulp is markedly decreased. The percentage of CD4+ T-cells is not changed relative to wild-type mice, but the percentage of CD8+ T-cells shows a significant decrease. Also, the number of CD11+ cells is elevated, suggesting an increased infiltration of macrophages *(42)*. Although virtually all organs examined have various degrees of mononuclear cell infiltrates, the digestive system (salivary glands, gastrointestinal tract, pancreas, and liver) is most severely affected *(1,36)*. Mononuclear inflammatory infiltrates are present in the lamina propria throughout the gastrointestinal tract with diffuse ulcerations in the colon. Livers have predominant periportal infiltrates.

The viability and disease development of IL-2-deficient mice is strongly dependent on the genetic background. Mutant mice crossed to a BALB/c background develop a generalized autoimmune disease and die within 5 wk of age *(43)*. Anemia and colitis are more delayed in C57BL/6 IL-2-deficient mice, compared with 129 Ola × C57BL/6 IL-2-deficient mice, occurring at 3 mo of age. However, although the time-course may differ, the pathology remains similar among the strains, namely, mononuclear cell infiltration, with the colon most severely affected.

Recently, animals deficient in both IL-2 and β_2-microglobulin were shown to develop colonic adenocarcinomas after 6–12 mo, analogous to humans with long- standing chronic colitis *(44)*. Thus, the IL-2-deficient mouse model more closely resembles human ulcerative colitis, as opposed to Crohn's disease.

3.3. Immunologic Abnormalities

Several studies have shown that the critical effector cells for the development of colitis in IL-2-deficient mice are the CD4+ T-cell subset. Mice with a double null mutation for IL-2 and B-cells (IL-2-deficient, JH-deficient) still develop colitis, demonstrating that neither B-cells nor autoantibodies are necessary for bowel inflammation in this model *(45)*. On the other hand, IL-2-deficient, JH-deficient mice experienced significantly reduced anemic symptoms, suggesting that B-cells are important for mediating the autoimmune hemolytic anemia in IL-2-deficient mice. The finding that IL-2-deficient, JH-deficient mice die at approximately the same age as IL-2-deficient, $JH^{+/-}$ mice despite retaining significantly higher hematocrits, indicates that bowel inflammation, as opposed to anemia, is likely to be the major cause of death in mice at this age. Interestingly, although elevations in serum immunoglobulins are observed early during the progression of disease in IL-2-deficient mice, there is a dramatic loss of B-cells and immunoglobulin secretion during progressive colitis, providing further evidence that B-cells are not involved in the pathogenesis of intestinal inflammation *(46)*.

On the other hand, the double deletion of both IL-2 and the recombinase activating gene-2 ($RAG\text{-}2^{-/-}$) results in a mouse with neither B- nor T-cells and subsequently no colitis *(45)*. Likewise, when IL-2-deficient animals were bred onto a nude mouse background, no colitis resulted *(47)*. However, when lymphocytes from conventional $IL\text{-}2^{-/-}$ mice were transferred into nude mice, disease was detected. Further evidence that CD4+ T-cells are the critical effectors include the finding that disease still develops in the double mutant model deficient in both IL-2 and β_2-microglobulin, in which mice lack both IL-2 and CD8+ cells *(48)*. Finally, Ehrhardt et al. *(49)* have shown that depletion of CD4+ cells (Th1 cells) abrogates gut inflammation in IL-2-deficient mice.

Several studies have analyzed the expression of cytokines and inflammatory mediators in IL-2-deficient mice. Autenrieth et al. *(50)* found detectable levels of IL-1α, IL-1β, IL-6, TNF-α, and IL-10 mRNAs as early as 10 d after birth in IL-2-deficient, but not wild-type control, mice. The levels of these mRNAs increased further at 13 and 23 wk post partum *(50)*. Notably, IL-4 was not expressed in the intestinal tissues of either IL-2-deficient or wild-type mice. These results suggest that bowel inflammation is both preceded and paralleled by an increase in mRNA expression of various cytokines in colonic tissue. This observation is consistent with the finding that treatment of IL-2-deficient mice with recombinant IL-2 prevents disorders of the immune system only when started during the first days of life *(50)*. Furthermore, 10-d-old, but not 6-d-old IL-2-deficient mice exhibit increased proliferation and polyclonal activation of lymphocytes, suggesting that IL-2 is required for the differentiation or maturation of regulatory cells *(50)*. Similar findings were reported by McDonald et al. *(51)*, who found elevated levels of TNF-α and IL-1β in IL-2-deficient mice over 35 d old compared with controls. In contrast, Garrelds et al. *(42)* found no difference in the levels of IL-6 or IL-10 between IL-2-deficient and wild-type mice, although they did observe elevated levels of IL-1β in the colons of IL-2-deficient mice *(42)*.

Finally, Meijssen et al. *(52)* analyzed expression of cytokines by colonic epithelial cells in IL-2-deficient mice before and after the onset of colitis. Interestingly, the levels of TGF-β, IL-15, and CD14 were found to be elevated in these cells prior to the onset of colitis, suggesting a possible role in the initiation of colitis in these mice. The expression of TNF-α, IL-6, KC (the mouse homolog of human GRO-α), and JE (the mouse homolog of human MCP-1) were only upregulated after the onset of colitis; thus, the expression of these cytokines was closely correlated with the histologic signs of inflammation. The finding that CD14 is upregulated prior to the onset of inflammation suggests a loss of tolerance to colonic bacteria in these mice, thus resulting in the activation of a proinflammatory cascade *(52)*. On the other hand, the elevated levels of IL-15 prior to, and during, inflammation in these mice suggest a compensatory mechanism by epithelial cells for the absence of IL-2. Together, these observations suggest that inflammation in IL-2-deficient mice is mediated by a Th1 response involving T-cells and macrophages *(50)*.

3.4. Role of Microflora in the IL-2-Deficient Mouse Model of Colitis

In the original description of colitis in IL-2-deficient mice, Sadlack et al. *(1)* demonstrated attenuated colitis in knockout mice raised in a specific pathogen-free environment and no clinical or histologic evidence of colitis in a limited number of germ-free (GF) IL-2-deficient mice. The absence of histologic evidence of colitis in young GF IL-2-deficient mice was confirmed by Contractor et al. *(53)*. However, anemia, generalized lymphoid hyperplasia, and hepatic inflammation in these mice was not dependent on bacterial colonization. These observations suggest that luminal microbial agents provide the persistent antigenic stimulus for the development of colitis. In contrast, Schultz et al. *(46)* report that older (up to 46 wk) IL-2-deficient mice housed under GF conditions developed a mild, focal, and nonlethal intestinal inflammation, whereas periportal hepatic inflammation was equal in the presence or absence of bacterial colonization. These authors suggest that exposure of GF IL-2-deficient mice to dead bacteria and bacterial constituents in autoclaved food and bedding may perhaps be enough to trigger a late inflammatory response. Finally, Autenrieth et al. *(50)* report that in preliminary experiments, colonization of IL-2-deficient mice with a single bacterial species is sufficient stimulus to induce colonic inflammation.

3.5. Loss of Tolerance in IL-2-Deficient Mice

Development of colitis in IL-2-deficient mice suggests that IL-2 plays a critical role in mucosal immunoregulatory pathways. These mice were originally believed to exhibit normal thymic development and thymocyte and peripheral T-cell subset composition, suggesting that other cytokines may compensate for the absence of IL-2. However, a later study found that IL-2-deficient mice have skewed single positive CD8+ thymocyte expression within the IL-2Rβ+ subset *(54)*. More recent data suggests that the immunopathology in IL-2-deficient mice depends on intrathymic T-cell differentiation and does not occur in the presence of thymus-derived IL-$2^{+/+}$ T-cells *(47)*. Finally, Ludviksson et al. *(55)* challenged IL-2-deficient mice with 2,4,6-trinitrophenol (TNP)-conjugated keyhole limpet hemocyanin (KLH) and showed that these mice exhibit a thymocyte maturation defect characterized by the presence of increased numbers of single positive CD4+ and CD8+

thymocytes. Concomitantly, they observed reduced thymocyte apoptosis in the thymus of these mice. These thymocytes had a cytokine profile skewed toward Th1 cell development and transferred disease to wild-type mice. Interestingly, disease in this model was ameliorated by the administration of anti-IL-12 antibodies, lending further support to the notion that colitis in this model is caused by a dysregulated Th1-like response *(55)*.

IL-2 was originally described as the major growth factor for T-cells, and, as a consequence, significant efforts have been made to understand the biochemical basis of this function. However, the more recent discovery of IL-15, which utilizes the IL-2 receptor β-chain and common γc subunits for signal transduction has led to a reevaluation of much of the original observations gathered using IL-2-deficient mice. In addition to IL-2-deficient mice, IL-2R$\alpha^{-/-}$ and more recently IL-2R$\beta^{-/-}$ mice have been shown also to develop colitis. The pathology observed in IL-2R$\alpha^{-/-}$ mice is easily reconciled, given the observed pathology in IL-2-deficient mice. On the other hand, colitis in IL-2R$\beta^{-/-}$ mice is not easily reconciled with the generally healthy, lymphopenic IL-15R$\alpha^{-/-}$ and IL-$15^{-/-}$ mice, which in addition lack NK cells, NK T-cells, and activated CD8+ cells. Poussier et al. *(56)* suggest that the development colitis in IL-2R$\beta^{-/-}$ mice is a result of the additional loss of CD8α+ regulatory cells, which suppress the activity of pathogenic T-cells. These investigators suggest that these cells are extrathymic in origin and require IL-2 signaling for their development *(56,57)*.

Naive T-cells express low levels of FasL and high levels of FLIP, which is strikingly similar to the situation in IL-2-deficient T-cells. This suggests that during T-cell activation, the critical factor that induces sensitivity to AICD is IL-2 itself. The finding is paradoxic considering that its first and most clearly established function is as a growth and survival factor. In any event, it is now clear that IL-2 is capable of inducing lymphocyte death as well as growth. It may be that the growth-promoting activity of this cytokine is dominant early during the immune response, and if T-cell stimulation is persistent or IL-2 concentrations increase above a threshold, the potentiation of AICD becomes dominant, leading to feedback regulation of the immune response *(40)*. The CD4+ T-cells that drive colitis in this model are believed to be thymus-derived, invading the colon and bone marrow to cause the observed colitis, anemia, and loss of B-cells. Although the extraintestinal manifestations appear to be independent of the microbial environment *(53)*, the early disturbances in cytokine secretion and lymphocyte function described above suggest a loss of tolerance to bacterial antigens in the colon. The fact that mice lacking IL-2 or a functional IL-2R accumulate activated T-cells and develop autoimmunity suggests that the dominant role of IL-2 in vivo is to terminate T-cell responses and maintain tolerance *(1,58)*. Thus, a possible mechanistic explanation for this function is provided by the observation that IL-2 renders activated T-cells susceptible to AICD, a pathway of cell death that serves to eliminate autoreactive T-cells *(30,35,38)*.

4. Conclusions

The mucosal immune system of the intestine achieves the remarkable task of maintaining tolerance in the face of an enormous bacterial load. It must, however, remain responsive to the threat of potential pathogens. Perhaps it is not surprising then that several alterations in the function of the mucosal immune system, such as those brought about by gene knockouts, result in the development of colitis. Contrary to previous thinking regarding the etiology of inflammatory bowel disease, these models suggest that no particular pathogen or antigenic stimulus is responsible for such development of inflammation, rather, the results in animal models of inflammatory bowel disease coupled with concurrent findings in patients with inflammatory bowel diseases suggest that genetically susceptible hosts can mount a pathogenic cellular immune response to specific nonpathogenic bacterial species as a consequence of defective immunologic tolerance and lack of appropriate mucosal defences.

The murine mucosal immune system has evolved in close association with its enteric flora. Likewise, the human enteric immune system has probably evolved unique mechanisms for dealing with intestinal pathogens and for the maintenance of tolerance to human commensal bacteria and dietary antigens. Thus it is important to keep in mind the many differences that no doubt exist between the murine models and humans. Nonetheless, these models have been critical in defining the role of bacteria in the development of colitis and have opened new avenues of inquiry regarding the ontogeny of the enteric immune system and the development of tolerance. When considering the "self versus non-self" education of the human immune system, it is becoming clear that these commensals may represent a unique "self" compartment. This compartment is acquired after birth and poses unique anatomic and temporal challenges to our immune system.

Questions that remain to be answered include investigations into how our genetic background influences the acquisition of enteric flora; how various components of our microflora alter the development of our immune system; and how we acquire tolerance toward our enteric flora. Collectively, knockout models of colitis including IL-2 and IL-10 gene-deficient mice have offered us insights into the possibility of altering our enteric flora in an attempt to restore immune tolerance to the bowel. It is likely that the elimination of some aggressive subsets of luminal bacteria, combined with a repopulation using beneficial probiotic bacteria, will lead to a selective blockade of proinflammatory cytokines and Th1 lymphocytes, while simultaneously enhancing antiinflammatory and protective immune responses. Thus, restoration of microbial balance may lead to a completely new avenue of therapy for inflammatory bowel diseases and complement therapies involving immunosuppression and immunomodulation.

References

1. Sadlack, B., Merz, H., Schorle, H., Schimpl, A., Feller, A. C., and Horak, I. (1993) Ulcerative colitis-like disease in mice with a disrupted interleukin-2 gene. *Cell* **75,** 253–261.
2. Kuhn, R., Lohler, J., Rennick, D., Rajewsky, K., and Muller, W. (1993) Interleukin-10-deficient mice develop chronic enterocolitis. *Cell* **75,** 263–274.
3. Moore, K. W., O'Garra, A., de Waal Malefyt, R., Vieira, P., and Mosmann, T. R. (1993) Interleukin-10. *Annu. Rev. Immunol.* **11,** 165–190.
4. D'Andrea, A., Aste-Amezaga, M., Valiante, N. M., Ma, X., Kubin, M., and Trinchieri, G. (1993) Interleukin 10 (IL-10) inhibits human lymphocyte interferon gamma production by suppressing natural killer cell stimulatory factor/IL-12 synthesis in accessory cells. *J. Exp. Med.* **178,** 1041–1048.
5. Faulkner, L., Buchan, G., and Baird, M. (2000) Interleukin-10 does not affect phagocytosis of particulate antigen by bone marrow-derived dendritic cells but does impair antigen presentation. *Immunology* **99,** 523–531.
6. De Smedt, T., Van Mechelen, M., De Becker, G., Urbain, J., Leo, O., and Moser, M. (1997) Effect of interleukin-10 on dendritic cell maturation and function. *Eur. J. Immunol.* **27,** 1229–1235.
7. Takayama, T., Morelli, A. E., Onai, N., et al. (2001) Mammalian and viral IL-10 enhance C-C chemokine receptor 5 but down-regulate C-C chemokine receptor 7 expression by myeloid dendritic cells: impact on chemotactic responses and in vivo homing ability. *J. Immunol.* **166,** 7136–7143.

8. Lentsch, A. B., Shanley, T. P., Sarma, V., and Ward, P. A. (1997) In vivo suppression of NF-kappa B and preservation of I kappa B alpha by interleukin-10 and interleukin-13. *J. Clin. Invest.* **100,** 2443–2448.
9. Groux, H., O'Garra, A., Bigler, M., et al. (1997) A CD4+ T-cell subset inhibits antigen-specific T-cell responses and prevents colitis. *Nature* **389,** 737–742.
10. Berg, D. J., Davidson, N., Kuhn, R., et al. (1996) Enterocolitis and colon cancer in interleukin-10-deficient mice are associated with aberrant cytokine production and CD4(+) TH1-like responses. *J. Clin. Invest.* **98,** 1010–1020.
11. Sellon, R. K., Tonkonogy, S., Schultz, M., et al. (1998) Resident enteric bacteria are necessary for development of spontaneous colitis and immune system activation in interleukin-10-deficient mice. *Infect. Immun.* **66,** 5224–5231.
12. Madsen, K. L., Malfair, D., Gray, D., Doyle, J. S., Jewell, L. D., and Fedorak, R. N. (1999) Interleukin-10 gene-deficient mice develop a primary intestinal permeability defect in response to enteric microflora. *Inflamm. Bowel Dis.* **5,** 262–270.
13. Davidson, N. J., Leach, M. W., Fort, M. M., et al. (1996) T helper cell 1-type CD4+ T cells, but not B cells, mediate colitis in interleukin 10-deficient mice. *J. Exp. Med.* **184,** 241–251.
14. Farmer, M. A., Sundberg, J. P., Bristol, I. J., et al. (2001) A major quantitative trait locus on chromosome 3 controls colitis severity in IL-10-deficient mice. *Proc. Natl. Acad. Sci. USA* **98,** 13820–13825.
15. Madsen, K. L., Doyle, J. S., Jewell, L. D., Tavernini, M. M., and Fedorak, R. N. (1999) *Lactobacillus* species prevents colitis in interleukin 10 gene-deficient mice. *Gastroenterology* **116,** 1107–1114.
16. Spencer, D. M., Veldman, G. M., Banerjee, S., Willis, J., and Levine, A. D. (2002) Distinct inflammatory mechanisms mediate early versus late colitis in mice. *Gastroenterology* **122,** 94–105.
17. Hoffmann, K. F., Cheever, A. W., and Wynn, T. A. (2000) IL-10 and the dangers of immune polarization: excessive type 1 and type 2 cytokine responses induce distinct forms of lethal immunopathology in murine schistosomiasis. *J. Immunol.* **164,** 6406–6416.
18. Madsen, K. L., Doyle, J. S., Tavernini, M. M., Jewell, L. D., Rennie, R. P., and Fedorak, R. N. (2000) Antibiotic therapy attenuates colitis in interleukin 10 gene-deficient mice. *Gastroenterology* **118,** 1094–1105.
19. Kennedy, R. J., Hoper, M., Deodhar, K., Erwin, P. J., Kirk, S. J., and Gardiner, K. R. (2000) Interleukin 10-deficient colitis: new similarities to human inflammatory bowel disease. *Br. J. Surg.* **87,** 1346–1351.
20. Rennick, D. M., Fort, M. M., and Davidson, N. J. (1997) Studies with IL-10–/– mice: an overview. *J. Leukoc. Biol.* **61,** 389–396.
21. O'Mahony, L., Feeney, M., O'Halloran, S., et al. (2001) Probiotic impact on microbial flora, inflammation and tumour development in IL-10 knockout mice. *Aliment Pharmacol. Ther.* **15,** 1219–1225.
22. Schultz, M., Veltkamp, C., Dieleman, L. A., et al. (2002) *Lactobacillus plantarum* 299V in the treatment and prevention of spontaneous colitis in interleukin-10-deficient mice. *Inflamm. Bowel Dis.* **8,** 71–80.
23. Madsen, K. L., Fedorak, R. N., Tavernini, M. M., and Doyle, J. S. (2002) Normal breast milk limits the development of colitis in IL-10 deficient mice. *Inflamm. Bowel Dis.* **6,** 390–398.
24. Gratz, R., Becker, S., Sokolowski, N., Schumann, M., Bass, D., Malnick, S. D. (2002) Murine monoclonal anti-tNF antibody administration has a beneficial effect on inflammatory bowel disease that develops in IL-10 knockout mice. *Dig. Dis. Sci.* **47,** 1723–1727.
25. Jijon, H. B., Churchill, T., Malfair, D., et al. (2000) Inhibition of poly(ADP-ribose) polymerase attenuates inflammation in a model of chronic colitis. *Am. J. Physiol. Gastrointest. Liver Physiol.* **279,** G641–G651.
26. Popoff, I., Jijon, H. B., Monia, B., et al. (2003) Antisense oligonucleotides to PARP-2 ameliorate colitis in IL-10 deficient mice. *J. Pharmacol. Exp. Ther.* **3,** 1145–1154.
27. Madsen, K., Cornish, A., Soper, P., et al. (2001) Probiotic bacteria enhance murine and human intestinal epithelial barrier function. *Gastroenterology* **121,** 580–591.
28. Morgan, D. A., Ruscetti, F. W., and Gallo, R. (1976) Selective in vitro growth of T lymphocytes from normal human bone marrows. *Science* **193,** 1007–1008.

29. Taniguchi, T., Matsui, H., Fujita, T., et al. (1983) Structure and expression of a cloned cDNA for human interleukin-2. *Nature* **302,** 305–310.
30. Leonard, W. J. (2001) Cytokines and immunodeficiency diseases. *Nat. Rev. Immunol.* **1,** 200–208.
31. Leonard, W. J. and O'Shea, J. J. (1998) Jaks and STATs: biological implications. *Annu. Rev. Immunol.* **16,** 293–322.
32. Johnston, J. A., Bacon, C. M., Finbloom, D. S., et al. (1995) Tyrosine phosphorylation and activation of STAT5, STAT3, and Janus kinases by interleukins 2 and 15. *Proc. Natl. Acad. Sci. USA* **92,** 8705–8709.
33. Friedmann, M. C., Migone, T. S., Russell, S. M., and Leonard, W. J. (1996) Different interleukin 2 receptor beta-chain tyrosines couple to at least two signalling pathways and synergistically mediate interleukin 2-induced proliferation. *Proc. Natl. Acad. Sci. USA* **93,** 2077–2082.
34. Lord, J. D., McIntosh, B. C., Greenberg, P. D., and Nelson, B. H. (1998) The IL-2 receptor promotes proliferation, bcl-2 and bcl-x induction, but not cell viability through the adapter molecule Shc. *J. Immunol.* **161,** 4627–4633.
35. Van Parijs, L., Biuckians, A., Ibragimov, A., Alt, F. W., Willerford, D. M., and Abbas, A. K. (1997) Functional responses and apoptosis of CD25 (IL-2R alpha)-deficient T cells expressing a transgenic antigen receptor. *J. Immunol.* **158,** 3738–3745.
36. Kundig, T. M., Schorle, H., Bachmann, M. F., Hengartner, H., Zinkernagel, R. M., and Horak, I. (1993) Immune responses in interleukin-2-deficient mice. *Science* **262,** 1059–1061.
37. Van Parijs, L., Refaeli, Y., Lord, J. D., Nelson, B. H., Abbas, A. K., and Baltimore, D. (1999) Uncoupling IL-2 signals that regulate T cell proliferation, survival, and Fas-mediated activation-induced cell death. *Immunity* **11,** 281–288.
38. Refaeli, Y., Van Parijs, L., London, C. A., Tschopp, J., and Abbas, A. K. (1998) Biochemical mechanisms of IL-2-regulated Fas-mediated T cell apoptosis. *Immunity* **8,** 615–623.
39. Kneitz, B., Herrmann, T., Yonehara, S., and Schimpl, A. (1995) Normal clonal expansion but impaired Fas-mediated cell death and anergy induction in interleukin-2-deficient mice. *Eur. J. Immunol.* **25,** 2572–2577.
40. Li, X. C., Demirci, G., Ferrari-Lacraz, S., et al. (2001) IL-15 and IL-2: a matter of life and death for T cells in vivo. *Nat. Med.* **7,** 114–118.
41. Schorle, H., Holtschke, T., Hunig, T., Schimpl, A., and Horak, I. (1991) Development and function of T cells in mice rendered interleukin-2 deficient by gene targeting. *Nature* **352,** 621–624.
42. Garrelds, I. M., van Meeteren, M. E., Meijssen, M. A., and Zijlstra, F. J. (2002) Interleukin-2-deficient mice: effect on cytokines and inflammatory cells in chronic colonic disease. *Dig. Dis. Sci.* **47,** 503–510.
43. Sadlack, B., Lohler, J., Schorle, H., et al. (1995) Generalized autoimmune disease in interleukin-2-deficient mice is triggered by an uncontrolled activation and proliferation of CD4+ T cells. *Eur. J. Immunol.* **25,** 3053–3059.
44. Shah, S. A., Simpson, S. J., Brown, L. F., et al. (1998) Development of colonic adenocarcinomas in a mouse model of ulcerative colitis. *Inflamm. Bowel Dis.* **4,** 196–202.
45. Ma, A., Datta, M., Margosian, E., Chen, J., and Horak, I. (1995) T cells, but not B cells, are required for bowel inflammation in interleukin 2-deficient mice. *J. Exp. Med.* **182,** 1567–1572.
46. Schultz, M., Tonkonogy, S. L., Sellon, R. K., et al. (1999) IL-2-deficient mice raised under germfree conditions develop delayed mild focal intestinal inflammation. *Am. J. Physiol.* **276,** G1461–G1472.
47. Kramer, S., Schimpl, A., and Hunig, T. (1995) Immunopathology of interleukin (IL) 2-deficient mice: thymus dependence and suppression by thymus-dependent cells with an intact IL-2 gene. *J. Exp. Med.* **182,** 1769–1776.
48. Simpson, S. J., Mizoguchi, E., Allen, D., Bhan, A. K., and Terhorst, C. (1995) Evidence that CD4+, but not CD8+ T cells are responsible for murine interleukin-2-deficient colitis. *Eur. J. Immunol.* **25,** 2618–2625.
49. Ehrhardt, R. O., Ludviksson, B. R., Gray, B., Neurath, M., and Strober, W. (1997) Induction and prevention of colonic inflammation in IL-2-deficient mice. *J. Immunol.* **158,** 566–573.
50. Autenrieth, I. B., Bucheler, N., Bohn, E., Heinze, G., and Horak, I. (1997) Cytokine mRNA expression in intestinal tissue of interleukin-2 deficient mice with bowel inflammation. *Gut* **41,** 793–800.

51. McDonald, S. A., Palmen, M. J., Van Rees, E. P., and MacDonald, T. T. (1997) Characterization of the mucosal cell-mediated immune response in IL-2 knockout mice before and after the onset of colitis. *Immunology* **91,** 73–80.
52. Meijssen, M. A., Brandwein, S. L., Reinecker, H. C., Bhan, A. K., and Podolsky, D. K. (1998) Alteration of gene expression by intestinal epithelial cells precedes colitis in interleukin-2-deficient mice. *Am. J. Physiol.* **274,** G472–G479.
53. Contractor, N. V., Bassiri, H., Reya, T., et al. (1998) Lymphoid hyperplasia, autoimmunity, and compromised intestinal intraepithelial lymphocyte development in colitis-free gnotobiotic IL-2-deficient mice. *J. Immunol.* **160,** 385–394.
54. Hanke, T., Mitnacht, R., Boyd, R., and Hunig, T. (1994) Induction of interleukin 2 receptor beta chain expression by self-recognition in the thymus. *J. Exp. Med.* **180,** 1629–1636.
55. Ludviksson, B. R., Gray, B., Strober, W., and Ehrhardt, R. O. (1997) Dysregulated intrathymic development in the IL-2-deficient mouse leads to colitis-inducing thymocytes. *J. Immunol.* **158,** 104–111.
56. Poussier, P., Ning, T., Chen, J., Banerjee, D., and Julius, M. (2000) Intestinal inflammation observed in IL-2R/IL-2 mutant mice is associated with impaired intestinal T lymphopoiesis. *Gastroenterology* **118,** 880–891.
57. Poussier, P., Ning, T., Banerjee, D., and Julius, M. (2000) A unique subset of self-specific intraintestinal T cells maintains gut integrity. *J. Exp. Med.* **195,** 1491–1497.
58. Willerford, D. M., Chen, J., Ferry, J. A., Davidson, L., Ma, A., and Alt, F. W. (1995) Interleukin-2 receptor alpha chain regulates the size and content of the peripheral lymphoid compartment. *Immunity* **3,** 521–530.
59. Eliakim, R., Fan, Q. X., and Babyatsky, M. W. (2002) Chronic nicotine administration differentially alters jejunal and colonic inflammation in interleukin-10 deficient mice. *Eur. J. Gastroenterol. Hepatol.* **14,** 607–614.

15

IL-12-Deficient Mice

Luciano Adorini

Summary

Interleukin 12 (IL-12) is a heterodimeric cytokine composed of two covalently linked chains, p35 and p40, produced primarily by antigen-presenting cells, which plays a key role in promoting type 1 T helper cell (Th1) responses. The powerful activity of IL-12 requires a tight control, which is exerted at different levels. The primary control is exerted on IL-12 production by antigen-presenting cells, a major factor driving the response toward the Th1 or Th2 phenotype. Another level of control regulates expression of the IL-12 receptor (R), which is composed of two subunits, β1 and β2. The IL-12Rβ2 subunit has signal-transducing capacity, and modulation of its expression is central to the control of IL-12 responsiveness. Endogenous IL-12 plays an important role in the host defence against infection by a variety of intracellular pathogens. Its Th1-promoting activity, however, also favors Th1-mediated immunopathology and, in particular, the induction of Th1-mediated autoimmune diseases. Both aspects of IL-12 activity have been extensively studied using IL-12-deficient mice, providing important information about the multifaceted role of this critical regulatory cytokine.

Key words

IL-12, Th1, Th2, autoimmune disease, infectious diseases, IL-12-deficient mice

1. Introduction

Interleukin-12 (IL-12) is a 75-kDa heterodimer composed of two covalently linked glycosylated chains, p35 and p40, encoded by distinct genes *(1,2)*. This cytokine, produced predominantly by activated monocytes and dendritic cells but also by other cell types such as neutrophils, enhances proliferation and cytolytic activity of natural killer (NK) and T-cells and stimulates their interferon-γ (IFN-γ) production *(3)*. Most importantly, IL-12 induces the development of type 1 T-helper (Th1) cells in vitro and is a potent cofactor stimulating growth, IFN-γ synthesis, and cell adhesion of already differentiated Th1 cells. Thus, IL-12 is a key cytokine in immunoregulation *(3)* and is intimately involved in the development of Th1-mediated autoimmune diseases *(4)*. This view is complicated by the fact that IL-12 is a member of a small family of dimeric cytokines that regulate IFN-γ production. Members of this family so far identified include, in addition to IL-12, IL-23 (composed of p40 and p19 subunits), IL-27 (composed of p28 and EBI3 subunits), and p35-EBI3, provisionally named after its subunits. To complicate matters further, the β1 receptor subunit is shared between IL-12 and IL-23. Because the characterization of the individual cytokines belonging to the IL-12 family is still in progress, some of the activities ascribed to IL-12 could actually be mediated by other family members *(4a)*.

From: Contemporary Immunology: Cytokine Knockouts, 2nd Edition
Edited by: Giamila Fantuzzi © *Humana Press Inc., Totowa, NJ*

Based on their pattern of cytokine production, CD4+ T-cells can be classed into three major subsets: Th1, Th2, and Th0 *(5,6)*. Th1 cells are characterized by secretion of IFN-γ, and they mainly promote cell-mediated immunity able to eliminate intracellular pathogens and the synthesis of complement-fixing antibody isotypes. Conversely, Th2 cells selectively produce IL-4 and are involved in the development of humoral immunity protecting against extracellular pathogens. Type 1 cytokines, associated primarily with Th1 responses, include, in addition to IFN-γ, IL-2, IL-15, and tumor necrosis factor-α (TNF-α). Type 2 cytokines, associated mainly with Th2 responses, include IL-5, IL-6, IL-10, and IL-13, in addition to IL-4. Th0 cells, which could represent either precursors of Th1/Th2 cells or a terminally differentiated subset, are not restricted in their lymphokine production.

Polarized Th1 and Th2 subsets can be generated from CD4+ populations in vitro *(7)*, can be recovered from primed animals *(8)*, and are found in patients suffering from autoimmune or allergic diseases *(9)*. However, polarized Th1 and Th2 cells represent extremes in a spectrum. Detection of intracytoplasmic cytokine production by polarized Th1 and Th2 cell populations analyzed at the single-cell level has confirmed the existence of defined Th1 and Th2 cells, selectively producing IFN-γ or IL-4, respectively, but has also revealed intermediate patterns *(10)*. Within this spectrum, discrete subsets of differentiated T-cells secreting a mixture of Th1 and Th2 cytokines, for example IFN-γ and IL-10, have been identified *(11)*.

Despite functional and phenotypic differences, both subsets of Th cells are derived from the same precursor Th (Thp) cell. The fate of differentiating Th cells is influenced by several factors, including cytokine milieu, type of antigen-presenting cell, type, amount and delivery route of antigens, and mode of costimulation *(12)*. The cytokine milieu is critical for both the initiation and the expansion of the Th1 and Th2 subsets. Mice lacking IFN-γ, IL-12 or their receptors, or the signal transducer and activator of infection (STAT) signaling molecule STAT4 downstream of the IL-12 receptor, fail to develop a robust Th1 compartment, whereas mice that lack IL-4, IL-4R, or STAT6 have severely compromised Th2 development *(13)*.

IFN-γ and IL-4 exert their effects through controlling the expression of subset-specific transcription factors in a bidirectional, positive feedback loop. For example, when a Thp cell is stimulated in the presence of IL-4 and antibodies against IL-12 or IFN-γ, the IL-4 signaling factor STAT6 is activated, translocates into the nucleus, and rapidly induces the expression of GATA-3, a Th2 cell-specific transcription factor that is a master regulator of the Th2 differentiation pathway *(14)*. The expression of GATA-3 is followed by the induction of the transcription factor c-Maf, also preferentially expressed in Th2 cells, which is a potent IL-4 gene-specific activator. In synergy with other transcription factors or coactivators, such as nuclear factor of activated T-cells (NFAT) and NIP45, c-Maf and GATA-3 control the expression of IL-4, further reinforcing the IL-4R/STAT6 signal *(13)*.

Conversely, if a Thp cell is stimulated in the presence of IL-12 and IFN-γ and antibody against IL-4, IL-12 binds to IL-12R and signals through STAT4, whereas IFN-γ signals through the IFN-γ receptor to activate STAT1, which leads to upregulated expression of the Th1 cell-specific transcription factor, T-bet *(15)*. T-bet is a potent transactivator of the IFN-γ gene and was recently demonstrated to be the master regulator of Th1 lineage commitment *(16)*. The expression of T-bet is followed by secretion of IFN-γ and upregulation of the IL-12Rβ2 chain, which further strengthens the IFN-γ and IL-12 signals.

The decision of naive CD4+ T-cells to develop into Th1 or Th2 effector cells is not simply related to whether the priming conditions include high levels of inflammatory cytokines such as IL-12. In the *Leishmania major* model, it has been suggested that the T-cell response that occurs in the absence of strong pathogen-driven signals may reflect a strain-specific intrinsic propensity to develop CD4+ cells along the Th1 or Th2 pathway *(17)*. Genetic differences have been demonstrated between T-cells of BALB/c versus B10.D2 mice in their Th phenotype acquisition under neutral condition in vitro, suggesting that the susceptibility of BALB/c mice to *L. major* infection may reside, at least in part, in their inability to sustain IL-12-dependent Th1 development rather than in the intrinsic capacity of BALB/c T-cells to differentiate toward the Th2 phenotype *(18)*. The difference in maintenance of IL-12 responsiveness between BALB/c and B10.D2 T-cells in vitro and the subsequent Th1/Th2 development is controlled by a single dominant genetic locus named T-cell phenotype modulator 1 (*Tmp-1*) Although the precise gene(s) involved has yet to be determined, this locus has been mapped to a region of chromosome 11 containing a cluster of genes important for T-cell differentiation, including IL-4, IL-5, IL-3, and other genes, such as interferon regulatory factor-1, that may influence Th1/Th2 development *(19)*. This region is syntenic with the homologous gene cluster in human chromosome 5 previously linked to several phenotypic markers of atopy.

Molecular mechanisms to explain the polarization of Th1 and Th2 subsets, based on the differential expression of the receptors for IFN-γ and IL-12, do exist. The ability of IFN-γ to inhibit the proliferation of Th2 but not of Th1 cells may be related to the lack of IFN-γRβ chain expression in Th1 cells *(20)*. However, IFN-γRβ chain loss also occurs in IFN-γ-treated Th2 cells and therefore does not appear to represent a Th1 cell-specific differentiation event *(21)*. Conversely, developmental commitment to the Th2 lineage results from rapid loss of IL-12 signaling in Th2 cells *(18)*. The inability of Th2 cells to respond to IL-12 appears to be owing to selective downregulation of IL-12Rβ2 subunit *(22–24)*. Inhibition of Th1 and induction of Th2 in vivo is also related to downregulation of the IL-12Rβ2 subunit expression *(25)*. These findings are therefore consistent with a general model in which selective modulation of IL-12 signaling plays an important role in the acquisition of polarized Th cell phenotypes.

The reciprocal regulation between Th cell subsets is another driving force polarizing CD4+ T-cells into differentiated Th1 or Th2 cells *(12)*. IL-12 promotes the development of Th1 cells and inhibits IL-4-induced IgE synthesis. IFN-γ amplifies the IL-12-dependent development of Th1 cells and inhibits Th2 cell proliferation. Conversely, IL-4 and IL-10 inhibit lymphokine production by Th1 clones. In addition, IL-10, IL-4, and IL-13 suppress the development of Th1 cells through downregulation of IL-12 production by monocytes. However, the reciprocal regulation of IL-12 and IL-4 is not only negative. For example, IL-12 administered to mice after the establishment of an *L. major*-specific Th2 response actually enhances rather than suppresses IL-4 production *(26,27)*.

2. The Role of IL-12 in Th1-Mediated Responses as Assessed by Analysis of IL-12-Deficient Mice

The important and related role of IL-12 cytokines in the induction of Th1 responses has been demonstrated in mice deficient for IL-12 *(28)*, IL-12Rβ1 *(29)*, IL-12Rβ2 *(30)*, or STAT4 *(31)*. The role of IL-12 is specifically defined by IL-12Rβ2-deficient mice, because

Table 1
Th1-Mediated Autoimmune Diseases in IL-12p40-Deficient Mice

Absent	
	Experimental allergic encephalomyelitis *(42,44a)*
	Experimental autoimmune uveoretinitis *(40)*
Reduced	
	Collagen-induced arthritis *(38)*
	Experimental autoimmune myasthenia gravis *(39)*
	Autoimmune thyroiditis *(41)*
Unmodified	
	Type 1 diabetes mellitus *(57)*
Enhanced	
	TNBS-induced colitis *(43)*

TNBS, 2,4,6-trinitrobenzene sulfonic acid.

the IL-12Rβ2 chain is expressed only by the IL-12R and it does not appear to be shared with receptors for other IL-12 family members. Mice that develop a Th1-type response to *L. major* are resistant to infection, but in the absence of IL-12 they mount a polarized Th2 cell response and succumb to infection *(32)*. IL-12-deficient mice also fail to control mycobacterial infections owing to a decreased ability to develop Th1-mediated protective immunity *(33)*. Similarly, humans with genetic deficiency of IL-12 or the IL-12 receptor demonstrate systemic dissemination of otherwise poorly pathogenic bacteria *(34–36)*. In contrast, IL-12 deficiency does not alter the control of viral infections, indicating that alternative pathways for the generation of type 1 responses may be induced *(37)*.

2.1. Autoimmune Diseases in IL-12p40-Deficient Mice

Several studies have addressed the role of IL-12 in autoimmune diseases by using IL-12-deficient mice. In general, induced autoimmune diseases are reduced or absent in IL-12p40-deficient mice, whereas type 1 diabetes mellitus, a spontaneous Th1-mediated autoimmune disease, does develop in IL-12p40-deficient mice.

IL-12p40 deficiency consistently leads to decreased autoantigen-specific Th1 responses in induced autoimmune diseases and prevents experimental allergic encephalomyelitis (EAE) *(42)* (Table 1). Strikingly, in 2,4,6-trinitrobenzene sulfonic acid (TNBS)-induced colitis, disruption of the IL-12p35 gene ameliorates disease, but inactivation of the IL-12p40 gene results in exacerbated disease *(43)*, probably because of the capacity of IL-12p40 monomer or dimer to inhibit binding competitively to the IL-12R of IL-12-like cytokines such as IL-23 *(44)*. IL-23 is composed of the p40 subunit of IL-12 linked to p19, and therefore IL-12p40-deficient mice lack both IL-12 and IL-23. As shown in the EAE model *(44a)*, IL-23 rather than IL-12 seems to be the critical cytokine for chronic inflammation of the brain. However, in all these models using IL-12p40-deficient mice, the concomitant induction of Th2-type responses or other immunoregulatory pathways is variable.

In collagen-induced arthritis (CIA), IL-12 deficiency is not associated with a significant modification of IL-5 levels, and IL-4 is still undetectable *(38)*. In experimental autoimmune myasthenia gravis (EAMG), autoantigen-specific cells from IL-12-deficient mice produce mainly IL-4 *(39)*. In experimental autoimmune uveoretinitis (EAU), antigen-specific T-cells from IL-12-deficient mice show increased production of IL-5 and IL-10 and no change in IL-4 levels *(40)*, whereas they fail to secrete IL-10 or IL-4 in the EAE model *(42)*. In the latter case, an immunoregulatory circuit involving IL-10 produced by antigen nonspecific CD4+ cells has been described. Interestingly, IL-12-deficient mice are only partially protected from CIA, experimental autoimmune thyroiditis, and EAMG, whereas they appear to be completely protected from EAE and EAU. Altogether, these results suggest that an impaired development of autoimmune Th1 cells may not be sufficient, and the induction of an immunoregulatory pathway could be necessary for complete inhibition of an autoimmune disease. This regulation could depend more on IL-10 than IL-4, as indicated by the observation that IL-4 transgenic mice do develop EAE but IL-10 transgenic mice are completely protected *(45)*, and by the capacity of IL-10-producing Tr1 cells to inhibit autoimmune colitis *(46)*.

Conversely, the nature of the autoantigen(s) and the chronicity of type 1 diabetes combined with a genetic deficiency in immunoregulation could lead, even in the absence of IL-12 and IL-23, to a diabetogenic Th1 development in the nonobese diabetic (NOD) mouse. IL-12p40-deficient NOD mice show a major reduction of purified protein derivative (PPD) or hen egg white lysozyme (HEL)-specific IFN-γ production but little enhancement of IL-4 and IL-10 secretion. Likewise, very few pancreas-infiltrating T-cells produce IL-4 or IL-10. A defective IL-4 production by NOD CD4+ cells has been implicated in type 1 diabetes development *(47)*, and it has been associated with an impairment of NK1.1 CD4+ cells, which could be involved in early IL-4 production *(48)*. It is possible that immunoregulatory pathways involving IL-10 are impaired in NOD mice as well. Consistent with this assumption, administration of a noncytolitic IL-10 fusion protein to NOD mice completely protects from type 1 diabetes *(49)*. The absence of IL-12 and IL-23, combined with a lack of immunoregulatory circuits, could still allow the development of autoimmune Th1 cells in a chronic progressive autoimmune disease under polygenic control, such as type 1 diabetes. Although IL-10 is clearly an immunosuppressive factor in the late phase of type 1 diabetes in NOD mice *(49,50)*, its presence before 2 wk of age in NOD mice favors the generation of effector CD8+ T-cells leading to pancreatitis and accelerated type 1 diabetes *(51)*.

Overall, these results point to the fact that multiple mediators and effector mechanisms contribute to autoimmune diseases and that disruption of genes encoding a single mediator may not necessarily affect the natural course of disease, as noted for EAE *(52)*. The observation that IL-12 and IFN-γ are dispensable for type 1 diabetes development is consistent with the notion that CD8+ T-cells, which are required for type 1 diabetes development in NOD mice, are unaffected in mice genetically deficient in IL-12 *(28)* or IFN-γ. In addition, it is likely that the genetic absence of IL-12 or IFN-γ allows the development of compensatory mechanisms not available in unmanipulated NOD mice, which do respond to treatment with cytokine antagonists. Conditional gene targeting, which offers the possibility of inactivating a gene at the desired time, should be able to clarify these issues.

2.1.1. Type 1 Diabetes Mellitus

Administration of IL-12 induces rapid onset of type 1 diabetes in 100% of NOD female mice, whereas only about 60–70% of control littermates eventually develop this disease *(53)*. This effect is not because of toxicity of IL-12 for pancreatic β-cells, as shown by the normal appearance of islet cells and by the absence of type 1 diabetes in BALB/c mice treated with IL-12. Acceleration of type 1 diabetes in genetically susceptible NOD mice is accompanied by increased Th1 cytokine production by islet-infiltrating CD4+ and CD8+ T-cells and by selective destruction of islet β-cells, suggesting a causal link among IL-12, Th1 cell induction, and development of type 1 diabetes *(54)*.

To study the role of Th1 and Th2 cells in type 1 diabetes, we first targeted endogenous IL-12 in NOD mice by administration of the IL-12 antagonist $(p40)_2$ *(55)*. Administration of $(p40)_2$ from 3 wk of age, before the onset of insulitis, results in the deviation of pancreas-infiltrating CD4+ but not CD8+ cells to the type 2 phenotype as well as in the reduction of spontaneous and cyclophosphamide-accelerated type 1 diabetes *(55)*. After treating NOD mice with $(p40)_2$ from 9 wk of age, when insulitis is well established, few Th2 and a reduced percentage of Th1 cells are found in the pancreas. This is associated with a slightly decreased incidence of spontaneous type 1 diabetes, but, at variance with another report *(56)*, no protection from cyclophosphamide-accelerated type 1 diabetes. IL-12$(p40)_2$ can inhibit in vitro the default Th1 development of naive T-cell receptor (TCR) transgenic CD4+ cells to the Th2 pathway but does not modify the cytokine profile of polarized Th1 cells, although it prevents further recruitment of CD4+ cells into the Th1 subset. Thus, when polarized Th1 cells infiltrate the pancreas, targeting endogenous IL-12 has a marginal effect on type 1 diabetes incidence *(55)*.

To evaluate the role of endogenous IL-12 and IL-23 in type 1 diabetes development, mice with targeted disruption of the gene encoding the p40 subunit *(28)* were backcrossed to the NOD background *(57)*. IL-12p40-deficient NOD mice show profoundly reduced antigen-specific Th1 responses in draining lymph nodes, and addition of IL-12 but not IL-18 restores Th1 development in vitro, demonstrating the nonredundant role of IL-12. Unexpectedly, IL-12p40-deficient NOD mice develop pancreas-infiltrating Th1 cells and autoimmune diabetes similar to controls *(57)*. T-cell recruitment in the pancreas seems to be favored in IL-12p40-deficient NOD mice, as revealed by increased P-selectin ligand expression on pancreas-infiltrating T-cells, and this can compensate for the defective Th1 cell pool recruitable from peripheral lymphoid organs. In addition, residual Th1 cells could accumulate in the pancreas of IL-12p40-deficient NOD mice because Th2 cells are not induced, in contrast to wild-type NOD mice treated with an IL-12 antagonist *(57)*. Therefore, targeting endogenous IL-12 does prevent type 1 diabetes *(55)*, but its genetic absence does not *(57)*. It is possible that in IL-12p40-deficient NOD mice other cytokines may compensate for the lack of IL-12 and IL-23.

A candidate potentially able to replace IL-12 and IL-23 could be the IFN-γ-inducing factor IL-18. A rise in both IL-18 and IL-12 p40 mRNA levels has been detected in the adherent cell population of cyclophosphamide-treated NOD mice *(58)*. IL-18 synergizes with IL-12 but is not able to restore the production of IFN-γ by HEL or PPD-specific T-cells from IL-12-deficient NOD mice *(57)*. Thus, IL-18 only acts on IL-12-primed Th1-developing cells, stimulating them to produce more IFN-γ, but in the absence of IL-12 it is inefficient in inducing the differentiation of Th1 cells. These data are consistent with results indicating that IL-12 is sufficient for normal Th1 development in the absence of IL-18 *(59)* and that IL-18 by itself does not induce Th1 cell development *(60,61)*. However, mice deficient in both IL-12 and IL-18 display a more profound impairment in the bacille Calmette-Guérin (BCG)-induced Th1 response compared with IL-12-deficient mice, suggesting that IL-12-independent Th1 development could be induced by the cooperative action of IL-18 and other, as yet unidentified, factor(s) *(59)*. This pathway could account for the residual Th1 development in IL-12-deficient NOD mice, but accumulation of diabetogenic Th1 cells in their pancreata is likely to depend on alternative mechanisms.

Several studies have implicated IFN-γ in type 1 diabetes development. Blockade of IFN-γ by specific antibodies *(62–64)* or by IFN-γ receptor-Ig fusion proteins *(64)* significantly reduces the incidence of diabetes. IFN-γ seems to play an important role in the homing of diabetogenic T-cells to the pancreas *(65)*, and IFN-γ in synergy with TNF-α can contribute to β-cell death. Surprisingly, diabetes develops in IFN-γ-deficient NOD mice, although with a slightly delayed onset *(66)*. Type 1 diabetes also develops in IFN-γ-receptor β-chain-deficient mice, as in control mice *(67)*. The absence of the IFN-γ receptor α *(68)*, in contrast to the IFN-γ receptor β-chain *(67)*, has been reported to lead to disease protection, probably because adjacent non-NOD genes were inherited during the backcrosses *(69)*. Thus, IFN-γ and the IFN-γR appear to be dispensable for type 1 diabetes development in the NOD mouse. IL-12-deficient NOD mice also develop type 1 diabetes with a similar incidence and time-course as in controls *(57)*. The genetic absence of IL-12 or IFN-γ may favor the early development of compensatory pathways, which are not induced in genetically unmanipulated NOD mice. Indeed, the NOD mouse, with at least 20 susceptibility loci contributing to diabetes *(70)*, presents multiple gene defects involved in the preferential development of Th1 cells that also affect regulatory mechanisms, which might overcome the absence of IFN-γ or IL-12 alone.

2.1.2. Experimental Allergic Encephalomyelitis

IL-12 administration significantly increases the severity of EAE *(71)*. Similarly, mice treated with IL-12 in vivo following the transfer of proteolipid protein (PLP)-stimulated lymph node cells (LNCs) develop a more severe and prolonged form of EAE, compared with vehicle-treated controls. Most importantly, administration of anti-IL-12 antibodies substantially reduces the incidence and severity of adoptively transferred EAE, suggesting that endogenous IL-12 plays a key role in its pathogenesis *(72)*. In addition, IL-12p40-deficient B6 mice are completely protected from myelin basic protein (MBP)-induced EAE *(42)*. However, this appears to be induced by a deficiency in IL-23 rather than IL-12, because $p19^{-/-}$ (lacking IL-23) and $p40^{-/-}$ (lacking both IL-12 and IL-23) fail to develop EAE induced by myelin oligodendrocyte glycoprotein (MOG) peptide 35-55, but $p35^{-/-}$ mice (lacking only IL-12) do develop EAE *(44a)*. Consistent with its role in promoting the activation and differentiation of pathogenic Th1 cells, IL-12 was detected in the brain of rats with EAE just before the development of clinical signs *(73)*. IL-12 can promote EAE via IFN-γ-dependent as well as independent pathways, as predicted by the separate but complementary roles of IL-12 and IFN-γ in the regulation of IL-12Rβ2 expression on antigen-specific CD4+ cells *(42)*. The important role of IL-12Rβ2 expression in the pathogenesis of EAE is also shown by the observation that B10.S mice fail to upregulate the IL-12Rβ2 subunit and are resistant to disease induction. Interestingly, the defective expression of the IL-12Rβ2 subunit is not secondary to the production of suppressive cytokines but reflects a failure of B10.S MBP-specific T-cells to upregulate CD40L expression and to induce IL-12 production *(74)*.

2.1.3. Collagen-Induced Arthritis

Treatment of DBA/1 mice with IL-12 enhances the autoimmune response to type II collagen, resulting in severe, destructive CIA. IFN-γ production by collagen-specific CD4+

T-cells as well as synthesis of complement-fixing antibodies of IgG2a and IgG2b isotypes is strongly upregulated, suggesting that IL-12-induced Th1 cells may have a crucial role in the pathogenesis of this form of arthritis *(75)*. This conversion by IL-12 of a weak autoimmunogenic stimulus into a strongly pathogenic one inducing severe arthritis is associated with a pronounced anti-type II collagen humoral immune response as well as a markedly enhanced type II collagen-specific IFN-γ production by CD4+ T-cells. This suggests that IL-12 unmasks latent autoimmunity by inducing pathogenic Th1 cells. This view is confirmed by the reduced incidence of CIA in IL-12-deficient DBA/1 mice, although a few mice developed severe disease in spite of a highly reduced Th1 response *(38)*. Surprisingly, injection of high doses of IL-12 into DBA/1 mice with established CIA profoundly ameliorates disease *(76)*. It is possible that owing to a supraoptimal induction of IFN-γ by high endogenous levels of IL-12, a gene activation program involving regulation of apoptosis could be initiated, leading to apoptotic deletion of autoaggressive T-cells. Suppressive effects of IL-12 treatment may also be mediated by a counterregulatory circuit driven by IL-10.

2.1.4. Experimental Colitis

A Th1-mediated experimental colitis can be induced by rectal administration of the haptenizing reagent TNBS *(77)*. This disease can be treated by administration of anti-IL-12 antibodies even late after onset, suggesting that endogenous IL-12 may be required not only for induction but also for progression of experimental colitis *(77)*. Surprisingly, IL-12p40-deficient mice develop patterns of TNBS-induced colitis characterized by distortion of crypts, loss of goblet cells, and mononuclear cell infiltration with fibrosis of the mucosal layer *(78)*. The role of IL-12 in the development of TNBS-induced colitis has been further dissected by studying mice deficient in IL-12p40, IL-12p35, or IL-12Rβ1 *(43)*. TNBS-treated IL-12Rβ1$^{-/-}$ and IL-12p35$^{-/-}$ mice develop only a mild disease associated with low-level IL-18 expression in IL-12p35$^{-/-}$ mice. In contrast, IL-12p40$^{-/-}$ mice lacking both IL-12 and IL-23, develop more severe colitis than wild-type mice associated with high-level colonic IL-18 expression. Administration of IL-12p40 neutralizing mononuclear antibody markedly increased pathology in IL-12p35$^{-/-}$ mice, similar to the disease seen in IL-12p40$^{-/-}$ mice. This indicates that IL-12p40, in contrast to IL-12p70, inhibits TNBS-induced colitis and IL-18 expression, probably by competitive binding to the IL-12R.

2.1.5. Experimental Autoimmune Myasthenia Gravis, an Antibody-Mediated Disease

IL-12 has been clearly shown to be involved in the pathogenesis of Th1-mediated autoimmune diseases, but its role in antibody-mediated autoimmune pathologies has not been extensively addressed. We have investigated the effects of exogenous and endogenous IL-12 in EAMG *(39)*, an animal model for MG, a T-cell-dependent, autoantibody-mediated disorder of neuromuscular transmission caused by antibodies to the muscle nicotinic acetylcholine receptor (AChR). Administration of IL-12 with *Torpedo* AChR (ToAChR) to C57BL/6 (B6) mice results in increased ToAChR-specific IFN-γ production and increased anti-ToAChR IgG2a serum antibodies compared with B6 mice primed with ToAChR alone *(39)*. These changes are associated with earlier and greater neurophysiologic evidence of EAMG in the IL-12 treated mice, as well as reduced numbers of AChRs. In contrast, when IL-12-deficient mice were immunized with ToAChR, ToAChR-specific Th1 cells and anti-ToAChR IgG2a serum antibodies were reduced compared with ToAChR-primed normal B6 mice, and the IL-12-deficient mice showed almost no neurophysiologic evidence of

EAMG and less reduction in AChR *(39)*. These results indicate an important role of IL-12 in the induction of an antibody-mediated autoimmune disease, suggest that Th1-dependent complement-fixing IgG2a anti-AChR antibodies are involved in the pathogenesis of EAMG, and help to account for the lack of correlation between anti-AChR levels and clinical disease seen in many earlier studies.

It is possible that Th1 cells can directly attack the neuromuscular junction in IL-12-treated mice. IFN-γ-deficient mice were resistant to EAMG, and this is associated with greatly reduced levels of both IgG1 and IgG2a antibodies specific for mouse AChR *(79)*. Conversely, transgenic expression of IFN-γ at the neuromuscular junction provokes an autoimmune humoral response resembling MG, characterized by infiltration of mononuclear cells and by autoantibody deposition at motor end plates, but these mice did not have detectable antibodies to mouse AChR *(80)*. In sera from our B6 mice injected with ToAChR and IL-12, however, there were raised levels of antibodies to ToAChR and to mouse AChR, and muscle AChRs had IgG bound to them consistent with a pathogenic role for antibodies. A possible explanation for the pathogenicity of IL-12-induced Th1 cells in EAMG, therefore, is that they induce increased production of complement-fixing anti-ToAChR IgG2a antibodies. In IL-12-deficient mice, the serum anti-ToAChR antibodies were predominantly of the IgG1 isotype; only IgG1 was found at the neuromuscular junctions, and AChRs were not so reduced. Thus, the deficit in neuromuscular transmission correlates with the Th1-dependent IgG2a anti-ToAChR antibodies rather than the Th2-dependent IgG1 antibodies *(39)*. These results are important because they may explain the lack of correlation between antibody levels and clinical severity that has been reported in many previous studies of EAMG *(81)*, which have not usually investigated IgG subclasses. In conclusion, EAMG involves, as determined using Il-12p40-deficient mice, an IL-12-dependent autoimmune response mediated by AChR-specific Th1 cells that promote the synthesis of pathogenic, complement-fixing, Th1-driven anti-AChR antibody isotypes.

2.2. Infectious Diseases in IL-12-Deficient Mice

The generation of Th1 responses and IFN-γ production has been shown to be important in promoting immunity to a number of infectious pathogens and to play a critical role in resistance to these pathogens *(82)*. Studies in IL-12-deficient mice have been particularly informative in this respect, documenting the role of IL-12 in the resistance to a variety of pathogens, mostly intracellular, including bacteria, fungi, and protozoa. The following section focuses primarily on the role of endogenous IL-12 in the response to infectious pathogens, using mice made deficient in IL-12 production by introduction of a mutation into the IL-12p40 *(83)* or IL-12p35 *(32)* subunit, or through the use of neutralizing monoclonal antibodies (MAbs).

2.2.1. Leishmania major

Infection of mice with *L. major* provides a valuable model for the study of Th1 responses in parasitic infection *(8)*. The genetic background of the mice dictates their ability to mount an effective immune response against the infection. C57BL/6 mice, as well as 129/SvEv and C3H mice, selectively initiate a Th1 response upon infection with *L. major* and are able to resolve the infection. In contrast, BALB/c mice respond to *L. major* infection by generation of a predominant Th2 response and subsequently succumb to the infection. IL-12 has been shown to be critical for the protective Th1 response since elimination of IL-12 in otherwise genetically resistant mice results in failure to generate a Th1 response and, consequently, in susceptibility to *L. major*. This was shown by the use of anti-IL-12 MAbs *(84,85)* and confirmed with IL-12-deficient mice *(32)*. Interestingly, deletion of either the p40 or the p35 subunit conferred susceptibility, suggesting a key role of IL-12 *(32)*. Indeed, both subunits of IL-12, p40 and p35, are required for continued resistance to *L. major*, but rather than modulating Th2 responses or optimizing IFN-γ production, the critical role for IL-12 in maintaining cell-mediated immunity may be to prevent the loss of Th1 cells during a challenge infection *(86)*. Experiments with IL-12-deficient mice have also shown that IL-12 is critical for the development of protective immunity to *Leishmania donovani*, although this cytokine is also responsible for inducing the significant immunopathology associated with visceral leishmaniasis *(87)*.

2.2.2. Toxoplasma gondii

Endogenous IL-12 is required for resistance to infection with *Toxoplasma gondii*, but this resistance is mediated by both IL-12-dependent and -independent events *(88)*. The IL-12-dependent events critical to resistance occur early during the infection, since administration of anti-IL-12 antibodies during the acute but not the chronic phase, results in death *(89)*. Impaired IFN-γ production and susceptibility to infection have been confirmed in parasite-infected IL-12p40$^{-/-}$ mice *(90)*. CD8+ T-cells isolated from IFN-γ-treated IL-12p40$^{-/-}$ mice exhibit an increase in both precursor cytotoxic T-lymphocyte (CTL) frequency and IFN-γ production and induce protective immunity against a lethal challenge when adoptively transferred into naive IL-12p40$^{-/-}$ and IFN-γ$^{-/-}$ mice, suggesting that IFN-γ can regulate the CD8+ T-cell response during *T. gondii* infection *(90)*.

2.2.3. Mycobacteria

IL-12 also appears to contribute to the ability to control infection by *Mycobacterium avium (91)* or by *Mycobacterium tuberculosis (92)*, since neutralization of IL-12 with MAbs suppressed resistance to infection with these pathogens. Data using IL-12-deficient mice further demonstrate the requirement for IL-12 in protective immunity to *M. avium (93)* or *M. tuberculosis (33)*. To compare the role of the IL-12p40 and p35 subunits, both IL-12p35 and p40 knockout mice were infected with *M. tuberculosis (94)*. Mice lacking the p40 subunit were highly susceptible to increased bacterial growth, exhibited reduced production of IFN-γ, and had increased mortality. In contrast, mice lacking the p35 subunit exhibited a moderate ability to control bacterial growth, were able to generate antigen-specific IFN-γ responses, and survived infection longer *(94)*. The superior antigen-specific responses of the p35 gene-disrupted, compared with the p40 gene-disrupted mice, suggest that the p40 subunit may act other than as a component of IL-12. A candidate molecule capable of driving the protective responses in the p35 gene-disrupted mice is the IL-23 *(44)*, a cytokine composed of the IL-12p40 and a p19 subunit that is induced in the lungs of mice infected with *M. tuberculosis (94)*.

2.2.4. Listeria

Resistance to a *Listeria monocytogenes* infection also involves both IL-12-mediated and IL-12-independent responses. Although neutralization of IL-12 during the primary response results in an increased susceptibility to *L. monocytogenes* infection, neutralization during the secondary response has significantly less effect *(95)*. Experiments using IL-12p40- or IL-12p35-deficient mice substantiate the requirement for IL-12 in resistance to *L. monocytogenes*, since IL-12 deficient mice die at normally sublethal doses of this pathogen *(96)*. Nevertheless, in contrast to the susceptibility of IL-12p40-deficient mice, IL-12p35-deficient mice can respond to intermediate doses of *L. monocytogenes* by sterile elimination of the bacteria despite the mouse's inability to produce biologically active IL-12. Interestingly, these IL-12p35-deficient mice produce normal levels of IL-12p40 dimer and monomer, suggesting that IL-12(p40)$_2$ or IL-12p40 monomer, alone or associated with a polypeptide distinct from IL-12p35, such as p19 in IL-23, can play a pivotal role in the elimination of *L. monocytogenes*. This is intriguing in light of the agonistic activity of IL-12(p40)$_2$ in a cardiac allograft model *(97)*. However, in contrast to the IFN-γ-inducing activity observed on CD8+ T-cells in the transplantation studies, no such effect on CD8+ T-cells was observed in these experiments *(96)*.

2.2.5. Cryptococcus neoformans

IL-12-deficient mice infected with *Cryptococcus neoformans* are also differentially susceptible to infection depending on which subunit of IL-12 was mutated, as shown by a chronic infection model in mice with targeted disruptions of the genes for the IL-12p35 and IL-12p40 subunits, as well as in mice with a targeted disruption of the IL-4 gene *(98)*. Long-term application of exogenous IL-12 could prevent death of infected wild-type mice for but did not resolve the infection. Infected IL-12p35$^{-/-}$ and IL-12p40$^{-/-}$ mice die significantly earlier than infected wild-type mice, whereas infection of IL-4-deficient mice leads to prolonged survival *(98)*. Interestingly, infected IL-12p40$^{-/-}$ mice die earlier and develop higher organ burdens than IL-12p35$^{-/-}$ mice, suggesting a protective role of the IL-12p40 subunit independent of the IL-12 heterodimer, possibly due to IL-23.

References

1. Wolf, S. F., Temple, P. A., Kobayashi, M., et al. (1991) Cloning of cDNA for natural killer stimulatory factor, a heterodimeric cytokine with multiple biological effects on T and natural killer cells. *J. Immunol.* **146,** 3074–3081.
2. Gubler, U., Chua, A. O., Schoenhaut, D. S., et al. (1991) Coexpression of two distinct genes is required to generate secreted, bioactive cytotoxic lymphocyte maturation factor. *Proc. Natl. Acad. Sci. USA* **88,** 4143–4147.
3. Gately, M. K., Renzetti, L. M., Magram, J., et al. (1998) The interleukin-12/interleukin-12-receptor system: role in normal and pathologic immune responses. *Annu. Rev. Immunol.* **16,** 495–512.
4. Trembleau, S., Germann, T., Gately, M. K., and Adorini, L. (1995) The role of IL-12 in the induction of organ-specific autoimmune diseases. *Immunol. Today* **16,** 383–386.

4a. Watford, W. T. and O'Shea, J. J. (2003) A case of mistaken identity. *Nature* **421,** 706–708.

5. Mosmann, T. R., Cherwinski, H., Bond, M. W., Giedlin, M. A., and Coffmann, R. L. (1986) Two types of murine helper T cell clone. I. Definition according to profile of lymphokine activities and secreted proteins. *J. Immunol.* **136,** 2348–2357.
6. Del Prete, G., De Carli, M., Mastromauro, C., et al. (1991) Purified protein derivative of *Mycobacterium tuberculosis* and escretory-secretory antigen(s) of *Toxocara canis* expand in vitro human T cells with stable and opposite (type 1 T helper or type 2 T helper) profile of cytokine production. *J. Clin. Invest.* **88,** 346–350.
7. Hsieh, C.-S., Macatonia, S. E., Tripp, C. S., Wolf, S. F., O'Garra, A., and Murphy, K. M. (1993) Development of Th1 CD4$^+$ T cells through IL-12 produced by *Listeria*-induced macrophages. *Science* **260,** 547–549.
8. Reiner, S. L. and Locksley, R. M. (1995) The regulation of immunity to *Leishmania major*. *Annu. Rev. Immunol.* **13,** 151–177.
9. Romagnani, S. (1994) Lymphokine production by human T cells in disease states. *Annu. Rev. Immunol.* **12,** 227–257.

10. Openshaw, P., Murphy, E. E., Hosken, N. A., et al. (1995) Heterogeneity of intracellular cytokine synthesis at the single-cell level in polarized T helper 1 and T helper 2 populations. *J. Exp. Med.* **182,** 1357–1367.
11. Mosmann, T. R. and Sad, S. (1996) The expanding universe of T-cell subsets: Th1, Th2 and more. *Immunol. Today* **17,** 138–146.
12. Farrar, J. D., Asnagli, H., and Murphy, K. M. (2002) T helper subset development: roles of instruction, selection, and transcription. *J. Clin. Invest.* **109,** 431–435.
13. Ho, I. C. and Glimcher, L. H. (2002) Transcription: tantalizing times for T cells. *Cell* **109(Suppl.),** S109–S120.
14. Ouyang, W., Ranganath, S., Weindel, K., et al. (1998) Inhibition of Th1 development by GATA-3 through an IL-4-independent mechanism. *Immunity* **9,** 745–755.
15. Lighvani, A. A., Frucht, D. M., Jankovic, D., et al. (2001) T-bet is rapidly induced by interferon-gamma in lymphoid and myeloid cells. *Proc. Natl. Acad. Sci. USA* **98,** 15137–15142.
16. Szabo, S. J., Sullivan, B. M., Stemmann, C., Satoskar, A. R., Sleckman, B. P., and Glimcher, L. H. (2002) Distinct effects of T-bet in TH1 lineage commitment and IFN-gamma production in CD4 and CD8 T cells. *Science* **295,** 338–342.
17. Hsieh, C., Macatonia, S. E., O'Garra, A., and Murphy, K. M. (1995) T cell genetic background determines default T helper phenotype development in vitro. *J. Exp. Med.* **181,** 713–731.
18. Szabo, S. J., Jacobson, A. G., Gubler, U., and Murphy, K. M. (1995) Developmental commitment to the Th2 lineage by extinction of IL-12 signaling. *Immunity* **2,** 665–675.
19. Gorham, J. D., Guler, M. L., Steen, R. G., et al. (1996) Genetic mapping of a murine locus controlling development of T helper 1/T helper 2 type responses. *Proc. Natl. Acad. Sci. USA* **93,** 12467–12471.
20. Pernis, A., Gupta, S., Gollob, K. J., et al. (1995) Lack of interferon γ receptor β chain and the prevention of interferon γ signaling in Th1 cells. *Science* **269,** 245–247.
21. Bach, E. A., Szabo, S., Dighe, A. S., et al. (1995) Ligand-induced autoregulation of IFN-γ receptor β chain expression in T helper cell subsets. *Science* **270,** 1215–1218.
22. Rogge, L., Barberis-Maino, L., Biffi, M., et al. (1997) Selective expression of an interleukin-12 receptor component by human T helper 1 cells. *J. Exp. Med.* **185,** 825–831.
23. Szabo, S. J., Dighe, A. S., Gubler, U., and Murphy, K. M. (1997) Regulation of the interleukin (IL)-12R β2 subunit expression in developing T helper 1 (Th1) and Th2 cells. *J. Exp. Med.* **185,** 817–824.
24. Rogge, L., D'Ambrosio, D., Biffi, M., et al. (1998) The role of STAT-4 in species-specific regulation of Th cell development by type I IFNs. *J. Immunol.* **161,** 6567–6574.
25. Galbiati, F., Rogge, L., Guéry, J.-C., Smiroldo, S., and Adorini, L. (1998) Regulation of the interleukin (IL)-12 receptor β2 subunit by soluble antigen and IL-12 in vivo. *Eur. J. Immunol.* **28,** 209–220.
26. Wang, Z. E., Zheng, S., Corry, D. B., et al. (1994) Interferon gamma-independent effects of interleukin-12 administered during acute or established infection due to *Leishmania major*. *Proc. Natl. Acad. Sci. USA* **91,** 12932–12936.
27. Schmitt, E., Hoehn, P., Germann, T., and Ruede, E. (1994) Differential effects of IL-12 on the development of naive mouse CD4+ T cells. *Eur. J. Immunol.* **24,** 343–347.
28. Magram, J., Connaughton, S., Warrier, R., et al. (1996) IL-12 deficient mice are defective in IFN-γ production and type 1 cytokine responses. *Immunity* **4,** 471–482.
29. Wu, C.-Y., Ferrante, J., Gately, M. K., and Magram, J. (1997) Characterization of IL-12 receptor β1 chain (IL-12Rβ1)-deficient mice: IL-12Rβ1 is an essential component of the functional mouse IL-12R. *J. Immunol.* **159,** 1658–1665.
30. Wu, C., Wang, X., Gadina, M., O'Shea, J. J., Presky, D. H., and Magram, J. (2000) IL-12 receptor beta 2 (IL-12R beta 2)-deficient mice are defective in IL-12-mediated signaling despite the presence of high affinity IL-12 binding sites. *J. Immunol.* **165,** 6221–6228.
31. Kaplan, M. H., Sun, Y.-L., Hoey, T., and Grusby, M. J. (1996) Impaired IL-12 responses and enhanced development of Th2 cells in Stat4-deficient mice. *Nature* **382,** 174–177.
32. Mattner, F., Magram, J., Ferrante, J., et al. (1996) Genetically resistant mice lacking interleukin-12 are susceptible to infection with *Leishmania major* and mount a polarized Th2 response. *Eur. J. Immunol.* **26,** 1553–1559.

33. Cooper, A. M., Magram, J., Ferrante, J., and Orme, I. M. (1997) Interleukin 12 (IL-12) is crucial to the development of protective immunity in mice intravenously infected with *Mycobacterium tuberculosis*. *J. Exp. Med.* **186,** 39–45.
34. Ottenhoff, T. H. M., Kumararatne, D., and Casanova, J.-L. (1998) Novel human immunodeficiencies reveal the essential role of type-1 cytokines in immunity to intracellular bacteria. *Immunol. Today* **19,** 491–494.
35. Schijns, V. E., Haagmans, B. L., Wierda, C. M., et al. (1998) Mice lacking IL-12 develop polarized Thl cells during viral infection. *J. Immunol.* **160,** 3958–3964.
36. de Jong, R., Altare, F., Haagen, I.-A., et al. (1998) Severe mycobacterial and *Salmonella* infections in interleukin-12 receptor-deficient patients. *Science* **280,** 1435–1438.
37. Adorini, L. (1999) Interleukin-12, a key cytokine in Thl-mediated autoimmune diseases. *Cell. Mol. Life Sci.* **55,** 1610–1625.
38. McIntyre, K. W., Shuster, D. J., Gillooly, K. M., et al. (1996) Reduced incidence and severity of collagen-induced arthritis in interleukin-12-deficient mice. *Eur. J. Immunol.* **26,** 2933–2938.
39. Moiola, L., Galbiati, F., Martino, G., et al. (1998) IL-12 is involved in the induction of experimental autoimmune myasthenia gravis, an antibody-mediated disease. *Eur. J. Immunol.* **28,** 2487–2497.
40. Tarrant, T. K., Silver, P. B., Chan, C.-C., Wiggert, B., and Caspi, R. R. (1998) Endogenous IL-12 is required for induction and expression of experimental autoimmune uveitis. *J. Immunol.* **161,** 122–127.
41. Zaccone, P., Hutchings, P., Nicoletti, F., Penna, G., Adorini, L., and Cooke, A. (1999) The involvement of IL-12 in experimentally induced autoimmune thyroid disease. *Eur. J. Immunol.* **29,** 1933–1942.
42. Segal, B. M., Dwyer, B. K., and Shevach, E. M. (1998) An interleukin (IL)-10/IL-12 immunoregulatory circuit controls susceptibility to autoimmune disease. *J. Exp. Med.* **187,** 537–546.
43. Camoglio, L., Juffermans, N. P., Peppelenbosch, M., et al. (2002) Contrasting roles of IL-12p40 and IL-12p35 in the development of hapten-induced colitis. *Eur. J. Immunol.* **32,** 261–269.
44. Oppmann, B., Lesley, R., Blom, B., et al. (2000) Novel p19 protein engages IL-12p40 to form a cytokine, IL-23, with biological activities similar as well as distinct from IL-12. *Immunity* **13,** 715–725.
44a. Cua, D. J., Sherlock, J., Chen, Y., et al. (2003) Interleukin-23, rather than interleukin-12, is the critical cytokine for autoimmune inflammation of the brain. *Nature* **421,** 744–748.
45. Bettelli, E., Prabhu Das, M., Howard, E. D., Weiner, H. L., Sobel, R. A., and Kuchroo, V. K. (1998) IL-10 is critical in the regulation of autoimmune encephalomyelitis as demonstrated by studies of IL-10- and IL-4-deficient and transgenic mice. *J. Immunol.* **161,** 3299–3306.
46. Groux, H., O'Garra, A., Bigler, M., et al. (1997) A $CD4^+$ T-cell subset inhibits antigen-specific T-cell responses and prevents colitis. *Nature* **389,** 737–742.
47. Rapoport, M. J., Jaramillo, A., Zipris, D., et al. (1993) Interleukin 4 reverses T cell proliferative unresponsiveness and prevents the onset of diabetes in nonobese diabetic mice. *J. Exp. Med.* **178,** 87–99.
48. Lehuen, A., Lantz, O., Beaudoin, L., et al. (1998) Overexpression of natural killer T cells protects $V\alpha14$-$J\alpha281$ transgenic nonobese diabetic mice against diabetes. *J. Exp. Med.* **188,** 1–9.
49. Zheng, X. X., Steele, A. W., Hancock, W. W., et al. (1997) A noncytolytic IL-10/Fc fusion protein prevents diabetes, blocks autoimmunity, and promotes suppressor phenomena in NOD mice. *J. Immunol.* **158,** 4507–4513.
50. Pennline, K. J., Roquegaffney, E., and Monahan, M. (1994) Recombinant human IL-10 prevents the onset of diabetes in the nonobese diabetic mouse. *Clin. Immunol. Immunopathol.* **71,** 169–175.
51. Balasa, B., Davies, J. D., Lee, J., Good, A., Yeung, B. T., and Sarvetnick, N. (1998) IL-10 impacts autoimmune diabetes via a $CD8^+$ T cell pathway circumventing the requirement for $CD4^+$ T and B lymphocytes. *J. Immunol.* **161,** 4420–4427.
52. Steinman, L. (1997) Some misconception about understanding autoimmunity through experiments with knockouts. *J. Exp. Med.* **185,** 2039–2041.
53. Trembleau, S., Penna, G., Bosi, E., Mortara, A., Gately, M. K., and Adorini, L. (1995) IL-12 administration induces Thl cells and accelerates autoimmune diabetes in NOD mice. *J. Exp. Med.* **181,** 817–821.

54. Adorini, L. (2001) Interleukin 12 and autoimmune diabetes. *Nat. Genet.* **27,** 131–132.
55. Trembleau, S., Penna, G., Gregori, S., Gately, M. K., and Adorini, L. (1997) Deviation of pancreas-infiltrating cells to Th2 by interleukin-12 antagonist administration inhibits autoimmune diabetes. *Eur. J. Immunol.* **27,** 2230–2239.
56. Rothe, H., O'Hara, R. M., Martin, S., and Kolb, H. (1997) Suppression of cyclophosphamide induced diabetes development and pancreatic Th1 reactivity in NOD mice treated with the interleukin (IL)-12 antagonist IL-12(p40)$_2$. *Diabetologia* **40,** 641–646.
57. Trembleau, S., Penna, G., Gregori, S., et al. (1999) Pancreas-infiltrating Th1 cells and diabetes develop in IL-12-deficient nonobese diabetic mice. *J. Immunol.* **163,** 2960–2968.
58. Rothe, H., Jenkins, N. A., Copeland, N. G., and Kolb, H. (1997) Active stage of autoimmune diabetes is associated with the expression of a novel cytokine, IGIF, which is located near Idd2. *J. Clin. Invest.* **99,** 469–474.
59. Takeda, K., Tsutsui, H., Yoshimoto, T., et al. (1998) Defective NK cell activity and Th1 response in IL-18-deficient mice. *Immunity* **8,** 383–390.
60. Matsui, K., Yoshimoto, T., Tsutsui, H., et al. (1997) *Propionibacterium acnes* treatment diminished CD4$^+$NK1.1$^+$T cells but induces type 1 T cells in the liver by induction of IL-12 and IL-18 production from Kupffer cells. *J. Immunol.* **159,** 97–106.
61. Robinson, D., Shibuya, K., Mui, A., et al. (1997) IGIF does not drive Th1 development but synergizes with IL-12 for interferon-γ production and activates IRAK and NFκB. *Immunity* **7,** 571–581.
62. Debray-Sachs, M., Carnaud, C., Boitard, C., et al. (1991) Prevention of diabetes in NOD mice treated with antibody to murine IFN-γ. *J. Autoimmun.* **4,** 237–248.
63. Campbell, I. L., Kay, T. W., Oxbrow, L., and Harrison, L. C. (1991) Essential role for interferon-gamma and interleukin-6 in autoimmune insulin-dependent diabetes in NOD/Wehi mice. *J. Clin. Invest.* **87,** 739–742.
64. Nicoletti, F., Zaccone, P., Di Marco, R., et al. (1996) The effects of a nonimmunogenic form of murine soluble interferon-γ receptor on the development of autoimmune diabetes in the NOD mouse. *Endocrinology* **137,** 5567–5575.
65. Savinov, A. Y., Wong, F. S., and Chervonsky, A. V. (2001) IFN-gamma affects homing of diabetogenic T cells. *J. Immunol.* **167,** 6637–6643.
66. Hultgren, B., Huang, X., Dybdal, N., and Stewart, T. A. (1996) Genetic absence of γ-interferon delays but does not prevent diabetes in NOD mice. *Diabetes* **45,** 812–817.
67. Serreze, D. V., Post, C. M., Chapman, H. D., Johnson, E. A., Lu, B., and Rothman, P. B. (2000) Interferon-gamma receptor signaling is dispensable in the development of autoimmune type 1 diabetes in NOD mice. *Diabetes* **49,** 2007–2011.
68. Wang, B., Andre, I., Gonzales, A., et al. (1997) Interferon-γ impacts at multiple points during the progression of autoimmune diabetes. *Proc. Natl. Acad. Sci. USA* **94,** 13844–13849.
69. Kanagawa, O., Xu, G., Tevaarwerk, A., and Vaupel, B. A. (2000) Protection of nonobese diabetic mice from diabetes by gene(s) closely linked to IFN-gamma receptor loci. *J. Immunol.* **164,** 3919–3923.
70. Wicker, L. S., Todd, J. A., and Peterson, L. B. (1995) Genetic control of autoimmune diabetes in the NOD mouse. *Annu. Rev. Immunol.* **13,** 179–200.
71. Santambrogio, L., Crisi, G. M., Leu, J., Hochwald, G. M., Ryan, T., and Thorbecke, G. J. (1995) Tolerogenic forms of auto-antigens and cytokines in the induction of resistance to experimental allergic encephalomyelitis. *J. Neuroimmunol.* **58,** 211–222.
72. Leonard, J. P., Waldburger, K. E., and Goldman, S. J. (1995) Prevention of experimental autoimmune encephalomyelitis by antibodies against interleukin-12. *J. Exp. Med.* **181,** 381–386.
73. Issazadeh, S., Ljungdahl, A., Hoejeberg, B., Mustafa, M., and Olsson, T. (1995) Cytokine production in the central nervous system of Lewis rats with experimental autoimmune encephalomyelitis: dynamics of mRNA expression for interleukin-10, interleukin-12, tumor necrosis factor α and tumor necrosis factor β. *J. Neuroimmunol.* **61,** 205–212.
74. Chang, J., Shevach, E., and Segal, B. (1999) Regulation of interleukin (IL)-12 receptor β2 subunit expression by endogenous IL-12: a critical step in the differentiation of pathogenic autoreactive T cells. *J. Exp. Med.* **189,** 969–978.

75. Germann, T., Szeliga, J., Hess, H., et al. (1995) Administration of IL-12 in combination with type II collagen induces severe arthritis in DBA/1 mice. *Proc. Natl. Acad. Sci. USA* **92,** 4823–4827.
76. Hess, H., Gately, M. K., Ruede, E., Schmitt, E., Szeliga, J., and Germann, T. (1996) High doses of interleukin-12 inhibit the development of joint disease in DBA/1 mice immunized with type II collagen in complete Freund's adjuvant. *Eur. J. Immunol.* **26,** 187–191.
77. Neurath, M. F., Fuss, I., Kelsall, B. L., Stueber, E., and Strober, W. (1995) Antibodies to interleukin 12 abrogate established experimental colitis in mice. *J. Exp. Med.* **182,** 1281–1290.
78. Dohi, T., Fujihashi, K., Kiyono, H., Elson, C. O., and McGhee, J. R. (2000) Mice deficient in Th1- and Th2-type cytokines develop distinct forms of hapten-induced colitis. *Gastroenterology* **119,** 724–733.
79. Balasa, B., Deng, C., Lee, J., et al. (1997) Interferon γ (IFN-γ) is necessary for the genesis of acetylcholine receptor-induced clinical experimental autoimmune myasthenia gravis in mice. *J. Exp. Med.* **186,** 385–391.
80. Gu, D., Wogesen, L., Calcutt, N. A., et al. (1995) Myasthenia gravis-like syndrome induced by expression of IFN-γ in the neuromuscular junction. *J. Exp. Med.* **181,** 547–557.
81. Vincent, A. (1994) Experimental autoimmune myasthenia gravis. In: Cohen, I., ed. *Autoimmune Disease Models: A Guidebook.* Academic Press, San Diego, pp. 83–106.
82. Trinchieri, G. (1995) Interleukin 12: a proinflammatory cytokine with immunoregulatory functions that bridge innate resistance and antigen-specific adaptive immunity. *Annu. Rev. Immunol.* **13,** 251–276.
83. Magram, J., Connaughton, S. E., Warrier, R. R., et al. (1996) IL-12 deficient mice are defective in IFN-γ production and type 1 cytokine responses. *Immunity* **4,** 471–481.
84. Scharton-Kersten, T., Afonso, L. C. C., Wysocka, M., Trinchieri, G., and Scott, P. (1995) IL-12 is required for natural killer cell activation and subsequent T helper 1 cell development in experimental leishmaniasis. *J. Immunol.* **154,** 5320–5330.
85. Heinzel, F. P., Rerko, R. M., Ahmed, F., and Pearlman, E. (1995) Endogenous IL-12 is required for control of Th2 cytokine responses capable of exacerbating leishmaniasis in normally resistant mice. *J. Immunol.* **155,** 730–739.
86. Park, A. Y., Hondowicz, B., Kopf, M., and Scott, P. (2002) The role of IL-12 in maintaining resistance to *Leishmania major*. *J. Immunol.* **168,** 5771–5777.
87. Satoskar, A. R., Rodig, S., Telford, S. R. 3rd, et al. (2000) IL-12 gene-deficient C57BL/6 mice are susceptible to *Leishmania donovani* but have diminished hepatic immunopathology. *Eur. J. Immunol.* **30,** 834–839.
88. Scharton-Kersten, T. M., Yap, G., Magram, J., and Sher, A. (1997) Inducible nitric oxide is essential for host control of persistent but not acute infection with the intracellular pathogen *Toxoplasma gondii*. *J. Exp. Med.* **185,** 1261–1273.
89. Gazzinelli, R. T., Wysocka, M., Hayasi, S., et al. (1994) Parasite-induced IL-12 stimulates early IFN-γ synthesis and resistance during acute infection with *Toxoplasma gondii*. *J. Immunol.* **153,** 2533–2543.
90. Ely, K. H., Kasper, L. H., and Khan, I. A. (1999) Augmentation of the CD8+ T cell response by IFN-gamma in IL-12-deficient mice during *Toxoplasma gondii* infection. *J. Immunol.* **162,** 5449–5454.
91. Castro, A. G., Silva, R. A., and Appelberg, R. (1995) Endogenously produced IL-12 is required for the induction of protective T cells during *Mycobacterium avium* infections in mice. *J. Immunol.* **155,** 2013–2019.
92. Cooper, A. M., Roberts, A. D., Rhoades, E. R., Callahan, J. E., Getzy, D. M., and Orme, I. M. (1995) The role of interleukin-12 in acquired immunity to *Mycobacterium tuberculosis* infection. *Immunology* **84,** 423–432.
93. Silva, R. A., Florido, M., and Appelberg, R. (2001) Interleukin-12 primes CD4+ T cells for interferon-gamma production and protective immunity during *Mycobacterium avium* infection. *Immunology* **103,** 368–374.
94. Cooper, A. M., Kipnis, A., Turner, J., Magram, J., Ferrante, J., and Orme, I. M. (2002) Mice lacking bioactive IL-12 can generate protective, antigen-specific cellular responses to mycobacterial infection only if the IL-12 p40 subunit is present. *J. Immunol.* **168,** 1322–1327.

95. Tripp, C. S., Kanagawa, O., and Unanue, E. R. (1995) Secondary response to *Listeria infection* requires IFN-gamma but is partially independent of IL-12. *J. Immunol.* **155,** 3427–3432.
96. Brombacher, F., Dorfmuller, A., Magram, J., et al. (1999) IL-12 is dispensable for innate and adaptive immunity against low doses of *Listeria monocytogenes. Int. Immunol.* **11,** 325–332.
97. Piccotti, J. R., Chan, S. Y., Li, K., Eichwald, E. J., and Bishop, D. K. (1997) Differential effects of IL-12 receptor blockade with IL-12 p40 homodimer on the induction of $CD4^+$ and $CD8^+$ IFN-gamma-producing cells. *J. Immunol.* **158,** 643–648.
98. Decken, K., Kohler, G., Palmer-Lehmann, K., et al. (1998) Interleukin-12 is essential for a protective Th1 response in mice infected with *Cryptococcus neoformans. Infect. Immun.* **66,** 4994–5000.

16

IL-13 and Double IL-4/IL-13 Knockout Mice

Duncan R. Hewett and Andrew N. J. McKenzie

Summary

Although early studies suggested that IL-4 and IL-13 would have redundant functions, it is becoming clear that even though their biologic activities may overlap, these cytokines perform more specific roles in vivo. It is apparent that in some circumstances IL-4 and IL-13 act in conjunction to ensure the rapid onset of a Th2-like response and that in their combined absence the vestiges of the Th2 response are abolished or significantly delayed. However, it is also evident that these cytokines can specifically modify individual immunologic functions depending on the nature of the antigenic challenge. For example, in the context of schistosome infection, IL-4 is beneficial, whereas IL-13 is detrimental, and IL-13 plays a more dominant role than IL-4 in the expulsion of certain worm infections. Furthermore, in asthma models, IL-13, rather than IL-4, has been shown to play a key role in the generation of AHR. The roles of IL-4 and IL-13 have obvious implications for the development of therapeutic strategies for cytokine/anti-cytokine modulation of immune reactions. The use of conventional transgenic mice and gene knockout mice has already provided important functional information regarding these molecules. The future development of conditional and cell-specific gene ablation models should further extend our understanding of this system.

Key words

interleukin-4, interleukin-13, cytokine, knockout, Th2, Helminth, Trichuris muris, Nippostrongylus brasiliensis, Schistosoma mansoni, Leishmania, asthma, airways hypereactivity (AHR), neonatal tolerance

1. Interleukin-13

In 1989 Brown et al. *(1)* reported several novel cDNA sequences induced upon activation of mouse lymphocytes in vitro. One of these sequences was termed P600, and it represents the first cloning of an interleukin-13 (IL-13) cDNA *(1)*. However, it was not until the human homolog was cloned and its activities on cells of the immune system identified that it was given the designation IL-13 *(2,3)*.

T-helper type 2 cell-driven responses, particularly IgE and eosinophilia, are instrumental in disease processes including allergies, asthma, and helminth infection *(4,5)*. Both IL-4 and IL-13 are produced primarily by Th2-like cells *(2,6)* and mast cells *(7)*, and in vitro assay systems have demonstrated that they share a number of biologic functions.

IL-13 shares approximately 30% homology with IL-4 and appears to have certain overlapping biologic activities *(8)*. Such convergence occurs at least partly because both of these cytokines utilize the IL-4 receptor α (IL-4Rα) chain as a component of their receptor

From: *Contemporary Immunology: Cytokine Knockouts, 2nd Edition*
Edited by: Giamila Fantuzzi © Humana Press Inc., Totowa, NJ

complexes *(9,10)* and signaling through a shared signal-transducer and activator of infection (STAT)6-dependent pathway *(11)*. Indeed, IL-4R$\alpha^{-/-}$ and STAT6$^{-/-}$ mice display phenotypes with a number of similarities to those observed in the IL-4$^{-/-}$/IL-13$^{-/-}$ mice *(12,13)*. Interestingly, the genes encoding IL-4 and IL-13 are closely linked on human chromosome 5 and the syntenic region of mouse chromosome 11 and map to a cytokine gene cluster that also includes IL-5, IL-3, and granulocyte/macrophage-colony-stimulating factor (GM-CSF) *(14,15)*.

To investigate the in vivo roles of IL-13, and IL-13 in combination with IL-4, gene deletion strategies have been employed to generate IL-13$^{-/-}$ and IL-4$^{-/-}$/IL-13$^{-/-}$ mice. These animals have proved extremely useful in examining the varied functions of these molecules in complex biologic responses such as those initiated during asthma and allergy and the immune response to helminth infection.

2. Transgenic Mouse Generation

2.1. IL-13$^{-/-}$ Mice

To generate IL-13$^{-/-}$ mice, exon 1 of the IL-13 gene was interrupted by the insertion of a cassette containing stop codons, a retroviral internal ribosome entry site (IRES) fused to a lacZ reporter gene, and a neomycin resistance gene flanked by loxP sites *(16,17)*. These were maintained on a 129Ola × C57BL/6 (F2) background but have since been backcrossed onto the BALB/c strain to facilitate studies into asthma-like phenotypes. These mice are the IL-13$^{-/-}$ mice distributed to the academic community by A. McKenzie and are the ones used in the studies described in this review. Subsequent investigators have backcrossed these mice on different strain backgrounds to suit their individual requirements. Two further lines of IL-13$^{-/-}$ mice have been generated by McKenzie et al. *(17)*, one of which is as outlined above, but with the neomycin cassette removed by cre-mediated recombination, and another in which a neomycin selection cassette was inserted into exon 3.

2.2. IL-4$^{-/-}$/IL-13$^{-/-}$ Mice

A single targeting strategy was used to disrupt both the IL-4 and IL-13 genes. The two genes are only some 11 kb apart on mouse chromosome 11. Homologous recombination of the targeting vector replaced the 15 kb between exon 3 of IL-13 and intron 3 of IL-4 with the neomycin selectable marker *(18)*. These animals were maintained on a 129Ola × C57BL/6 (F2) background, but have since been backcrossed on to the BALB/c strain to facilitate studies into asthma-like phenotypes. These mice are the ones disseminated to all the investigators whose work is referenced in this review. Neither IL-4 nor IL-13 transcripts could be detected in activated lymphocytes from IL-4$^{-/-}$/IL-13$^{-/-}$ mice by reverse transcriptase polymerase chain reaction (RT-PCR) and spleen-derived CD4+ T-cells cultured under Th2 cell differentiation conditions failed to produce IL-4 or IL-13 as detected using enzyme-linked immunosorbent assays (ELISA) *(18)*.

2.3. Overt Phenotypes

Homozygous IL-13$^{-/-}$ animals were healthy and displayed no obvious phenotypic abnormalities. Lymphoid organs had a normal appearance, and no differences were seen either in the numbers of lymphoid/myeloid cells or in the expression of a number of cell surface markers on these cells *(16)*. Similarly, the IL4$^{-/-}$/IL-13$^{-/-}$ mice were healthy and displayed no overt phenotypic abnormalities.

2.4. Impaired Development of Th2 Cells in IL-13-Deficient Mice

Initial characterization of the IL-$13^{-/-}$ mice verified that IL-13 production had been ablated *(17)*. No IL-13 mRNA or protein could be detected in concanavalin A (Con A)-stimulated cultured splenocytes derived from the IL-$13^{-/-}$ mice. However, these splenocytes also produced lower levels of IL-4 and IL-5 than wild-type controls, a pattern that was also observed in purified CD4+ T-cells. IL-4 and IL-5 are produced predominantly by Th2 cells, so the effect of IL-13 gene ablation on the development of Th2 cells was investigated further.

Purified CD4+ T-cell cultures from IL-$13^{-/-}$ and wild-type mice were stimulated to differentiate into either Th1 or Th2 cells. Th1 cells from wild-type mice had characteristic low levels of IL-4, IL-5, IL-10, and IL-13 expression, but high levels of interferon-γ (IFN-γ). Th2 cells generated from wild-type mice produced high levels of IL-4, IL-5, IL-10, and IL-13 and little IFN-γ. In contrast, Th2 cells cultured from the IL-$13^{-/-}$ mice produced significantly reduced levels of Th2 cytokines. The impaired in vitro development of Th2 cells was also seen when total splenocytes from IL-$13^{-/-}$ mice were cultured under Th2-promoting conditions, indicating that the presence of other cell types could not rescue this phenotype. Similarly, the addition of recombinant IL-13 to the Th2 cultures also failed to reverse this phenotype.

Intracellular cytokine staining indicated that populations of IL-4- and IL-5-producing cells were present in IL-$13^{-/-}$ mice but were much reduced in numbers compared with wild-type mice. The impairment in Th2 development was also seen upon challenge of the IL-$13^{-/-}$ mice with the complex schistosome egg antigen, an antigen known to induce a Th2-type immune response in wild-type mice. Mesenteric lymph node cells removed from IL-$13^{-/-}$ mice, previously vaccinated with schistosome eggs, were cultured in Th2 differentiation conditions and, as previously, reduced levels of IL-4 and IL-5 were produced compared with cells from wild-type mice.

Infection of IL-$13^{-/-}$ mice with the intestinal parasitic nematode *Nippostrongylus brasiliensis* had a profound effect on this impaired Th2 development phenotype. Mesenteric lymph node cells were removed at various time points post infection and cultured under Th2-promoting conditions, followed by analysis of cytokine production. Interestingly, by d 6 post infection, the Th2 cells from IL-$13^{-/-}$ mice generated amounts of IL-4, IL-5, and IL-10 comparable to those from wild-type mice and by d 10 post infection, the Th2 lines from the IL-$13^{-/-}$ mice produced significantly more IL-4 and IL-5 than wild-type Th2 lines. Sustained antigenic challenge was thus able to overcome the impairment of Th2 development.

The genes for IL-13, IL-4, and IL-5 are closely clustered on mouse chromosome 11, so it was possible that the presence of a strong promoter-driven neomycin resistance gene in the IL-$13^{-/-}$ mice might effect transcriptional control of the neighboring IL-4 and IL-5 genes. To eliminate this possibility, separate knockout mice were generated with an interruption of exon 1 of the IL-13 gene (*see* previous section). In these mice the neomycin resistance gene, used as the selection cassette for homologous recombination in embryonic stem cells, was removed by cre-mediated recombination prior to generation of the IL-$13^{-/-}$ mice *(17)*. The in vitro impairment of IL-4 and IL-5 production was still evident in Th2 cells established from these mice.

IL-13 is produced by cells other than T-cells, including mast cells. Interestingly, mast cells taken from the spleen and bone marrow of the IL-$13^{-/-}$ mice, stimulated and cultured in vitro, produce levels of IL-4 and IL-5 mRNA and protein equivalent to those cells taken from wild-type animals. These data indicated that the impaired production of IL-4 and IL-5 by Th2 cells from IL-$13^{-/-}$ mice is a T-cell-specific effect *(17)*.

A recent study has indicated that targeting of the IL-13 locus has disrupted the normal transcriptional control of the linked IL-4 gene *(19)*. This study involved the intercrossing of mice harboring a knockin green fluorescent protein gene in the IL-4 locus with the IL-$13^{-/-}$ mice. Comparison was then made of the levels of IL-4 expression and green fluorescent protein expression dependent on the presence or absence of the targeted IL-13 allele or the wild-type allele. Thus, in the in vitro cultures, the IL-$13^{-/-}$ cells produced reduced levels of IL-4 and failed to commit to the Th2 lineage. However, results from IL-$4R^{-/-}$ and IL-$4^{-/-}$/IL-$13^{-/-}$ mice suggest that IL-13 does play a role in driving the Th2 response in vivo *(12,18,20)* (*see* below).

2.5. Antigen-Specific Antibody Responses

Antibody responses in the IL-$13^{-/-}$ and IL-$4^{-/-}$/IL-$13^{-/-}$ animals have been investigated by assessment of the antigen-specific immunoglobulin isotype response generated against ovalbumin (OVA) in the presence of the Th2-inducing alum adjuvant *(17,18)*. Repeated intraperitoneal administration of OVA was followed by measurement of serum levels of Ig isotypes by ELISA. High IgG1 levels are characteristic of a Th2-biased response, whereas elevated IgG2a or IgG2b are characteristic of a Th1-biased response. $IL13^{-/-}$ animals developed a normal IgG1 response to antigen, whereas IL-$4^{-/-}$ or IL-$4^{-/-}$/IL-$13^{-/-}$ animals had impaired IgG1 induction. Similarly, IL-$13^{-/-}$ and wild-type animals produced little antigen-specific IgG2a or IgG2b, whereas IL-$4^{-/-}$ and IL-$4^{-/-}$/IL-$13^{-/-}$ animals had highly elevated levels of these Th1-response-associated isotypes. These results all suggest that IL-4 rather than IL-13 is important in the production of a Th2-characteristic antigen-specific IgG1 humoral response.

Analysis of IgE levels indicated that naive IL-$13^{-/-}$ mice produced levels of total serum IgE that were 5–20-fold lower than those seen in wild-type mice. Interestingly, reduced levels of CD23 (the low-affinity receptor for IgE) were also observed on IL-$13^{-/-}$-derived B220+ splenocytes compared with those from wild-type mice *(17)*. Although IL-13 has been demonstrated to induce human B-cells to switch to IgE production *(21)*, in vitro assays have failed to show a similar event in the mouse *(8)*. However, expression of IL-13 from a transgene in mice does preferentially induce IgE secretion, supporting a role for IL-13 in switching to IgE *(22)*.

3. Parasite Infection Responses

3.1. Helminth Infections

Protective immunity to helminth infections is associated with a strong Th2-type response *(4)*. Several helminth models have been studied using IL-$13^{-/-}$ mice and IL-$4^{-/-}$/IL-$13^{-/-}$ mice, and these have highlighted the importance of IL-13 in the immune response to worm infections. Significantly, these studies have also demonstrated that IL-4 and IL-13 are not completely redundant molecules and that both play important specific roles in worm expulsion.

3.2. Trichuris muris

The first IL-13 knockout studies that highlighted a role for IL-13 in immunity to helminth infection utilized the intestinal nematode *Trichuris muris (23)*. Wild-type mice normally expel *T. muris* from the intestine by d 35 post infection. In contrast, IL-13$^{-/-}$ mice retained significant numbers of *T. muris* parasites in their intestines 35 d after infection. Thus, removing IL-13 results in an inability to expel *T. muris* efficiently. Analysis of the cytokine profile produced by the IL-13$^{-/-}$ mice demonstrated that worms remained in the intestine despite the induction of other Th2 cytokines such as IL-4, IL-5, and IL-9 and the onset of several Th2 effector functions. Indeed, infected IL-13$^{-/-}$ mice developed elevated mast cell numbers in the cecum (measured at d 35 post infection) comparable to those seen in infected wild-type mice and very high levels of antigen-specific IgG1 and IgG2a. The infected IL-13$^{-/-}$ mice also displayed increased levels of total serum IgE (at d 35 post infection) compared with uninfected IL-13$^{-/-}$ mice, although both these levels were much lower than those detected in uninfected wild-type mice. Thus IL-13$^{-/-}$ mice are unable to expel *T. muris* worms despite the presence of many Th2 effectors. Interestingly, IL4$^{-/-}$ mice are also more susceptible to *T. muris*, which can be explained by their inability to make a sufficient Th2 response including IL-13 *(23,24)*.

3.3. Nippostrongylus brasiliensis

Further insight into the role of IL-13 in worm expulsion was obtained by infecting IL-4$^{-/-}$, IL-13$^{-/-}$, and IL-4$^{-/-}$/IL-13$^{-/-}$ mice with the parasitic gastrointestinal nematode *N. brasiliensis*. Wild-type and IL-4$^{-/-}$ mice normally mount an immune response that successfully clears *N. brasiliensis* from their intestines within 6–10 d of infection. In contrast, IL-13$^{-/-}$ mice demonstrated impaired expulsion of these parasites, with substantial numbers of worms still present at d 10 post infection *(16)*. This impairment of expulsion was partly reversed by administration of recombinant IL-13 at the time of infection.

Expulsion of *N. brasiliensis* worms was even further impaired in IL-4$^{-/-}$/IL-13$^{-/-}$ mice. These mice still harbored a substantial number of worms 14 d after parasite injection, whereas IL-13$^{-/-}$ mice had effectively cleared all parasites by this stage *(18)*. Thus, although the single knockout studies suggested that IL-13 is the primary cytokine regulating *N. brasiliensis* expulsion, IL-4 does play an additive role in his process.

Cytokine profiles from the infected IL-13$^{-/-}$ mice demonstrated that substantial levels of IL-4 and IL-5 were still produced at d 6 post infection, and eosinophilia and IgE expression were similar to infected wild-types. However, at d 6 post infection, IL-13$^{-/-}$ mice demonstrated none of the goblet cell hyperplasia or changes in goblet cell size and morphology that occurred in infected wild-type mice *(16)*. This represented the first report of a role for IL-13 in the regulation of goblet cell hyperplasia and proposed a mechanism by which helminth expulsion might be impaired through the absence of intestinal mucus.

Interestingly, even in the absence of IL-4 and IL-13, *N. brasiliensis* worms were still expelled from IL-4$^{-/-}$/IL-13$^{-/-}$ mice. Significantly, although these animals also failed to upregulate goblet cell production, elevated levels of IL-5 were detected, and these correlated with blood eosinophilia. Recent experiments undertaken in our laboratory using mice with a combined deficiency in IL-4, IL-5, and IL-13 have demonstrated that the additional absence of IL-5 results in a further delay in worm expulsion *(25)*.

3.4. Schistosoma mansoni

IL-13$^{-/-}$ and IL-4$^{-/-}$/IL13$^{-/-}$ mice have been used to investigate the roles of these cytokines in two separate models utilizing *Schistosoma mansoni* challenge. One model involves the infection of mice with live *S. mansoni* cercariae and the monitoring of infection within the mice and is used as a model of human disease. (Schistosomiasis is a major third-world disease.) A second model utilizes the Th2 antigenic properties of dead schistosome eggs to study pulmonary Th2 responses to eggs that become trapped in the lungs of mice following intravenous administration. This latter model induces many allergic-type responses, facilitating the study of this phenotype in a mouse lung model.

3.4.1. Schistosome Infection Model

Fallon et al. *(26)* dissected the roles of IL-13 and IL-4 in the mouse immune response to *S. mansoni* infection by acutely infecting IL-4$^{-/-}$, IL-13$^{-/-}$, and IL-4$^{-/-}$/IL-13$^{-/-}$ mice with *S. mansoni* cercariae *(26)*. The effects of cytokine gene ablation on mortality, liver inflammation and fibrosis, intestinal pathology, and T-cell cytokine profiles were examined.

IL-4 deficiency had a profound effect on long-term survival of infected mice, with 80% of IL-4$^{-/-}$ or IL-4$^{-/-}$/IL-13$^{-/-}$ mice dying by d 56 post infection. This contrasts sharply with wild-type mice: only 13% had died by this point. Interestingly, IL-13$^{-/-}$ mice displayed prolonged survival, with 100% of animals surviving to d 56. Repeat experiments using a lower infectious dose of *S. mansoni* cercariae gave similar results. Thus, removal of IL-13 from the immune response to *S. mansoni* infection was beneficial to host survival.

The liver is the major organ normally affected by schistosome infection, with trapped schistosome eggs invoking a granulomatous inflammation, usually characterized by numerous infiltrating eosinophils and the deposition of collagen with attendant fibrosis. Deficiency of either IL-4 or IL-13 had no effect on hepatic granuloma size or the percentage of eosinophils, whereas the livers from infected IL-4$^{-/-}$/IL-13$^{-/-}$ mice were notably different, displaying very small granulomas devoid of eosinophils *(26)*. Notably, IL-13$^{-/-}$ and IL-4$^{-/-}$/IL-13$^{-/-}$ mice showed very little collagen deposition and fibrosis in comparison with IL-4$^{-/-}$ mice or wild-type controls, indicating an important role for IL-13 in the control of fibrosis *(26)*. Studies using an IL-13-antagonist also support this role for IL-13 in fibrosis *(27)*. The impact of cytokine deficiency on liver damage was also analyzed by measuring plasma aspartate aminotransferase (AST) levels as an indicator of hepatocyte damage. IL-13$^{-/-}$ mice displayed low AST levels, as did wild-type mice. By contrast, IL-4$^{-/-}$ mice showed AST levels fivefold higher than wild-type, whereas IL-4$^{-/-}$/IL-13$^{-/-}$ mice had AST levels 10-fold higher than wild-type mice. Thus, in contrast to IL-13, IL-4 is protective of liver integrity during *S. mansoni* infection *(26)*.

During the natural course of *S. mansoni* infection, adult worms lay eggs in the mesenteric venules, which then translocate across the intestinal wall into the gut lumen. The process is associated with localized granulomatous inflammation, eosinophilia, and a Th2 response. Infected IL-4-deficient mice (both IL-4$^{-/-}$ and IL-4$^{-/-}$/IL-13$^{-/-}$) had distension and inflammation of the ileum correlating with impaired egg secretion into the gut lumen. Instead, the eggs accumulated in the gut wall, where small granulomas with limited eosinophilia were seen. These pathologies were slightly more severe in the IL-4$^{-/-}$/IL-13$^{-/-}$ mice. Wild-type mice showed marked intestinal eosinophilia, no inflammation of the ileum, and normal egg secretion into the gut lumen. The degree of damage that the IL-4-deficient mice suffer as a result of intestinal inflammation was measured by analysis of bacterial lipopolysaccharide (LPS) levels in the plasma. LPS levels were some 20-fold higher in IL-4$^{-/-}$ mice and IL-4$^{-/-}$/IL-13$^{-/-}$ mice compared with IL-13$^{-/-}$ or wild-type mice. Furthermore ileum-derived lamina propria T-cells from infected IL-4$^{-/-}$ and IL-4$^{-/-}$/IL-13$^{-/-}$ mice showed an absence of IL-5-staining cells but a large number of IFN-γ-staining cells, indicative of an inadequate Th2 response in the absence of IL-4. Similar skewing toward a Th1 phenotype was also detected in splenocytes from the IL-4$^{-/-}$ and IL-4$^{-/-}$/IL-13$^{-/-}$ mice, compared with the Th2 response of the IL-13$^{-/-}$ and wild-type mice *(26)*.

IL-4 therefore plays a much more protective role than IL-13 in the response to *S. mansoni* infection. The absence of IL-4 is associated with depressed Th2 responses, increased liver damage, failure to excrete eggs, extensive intestinal inflammation with systemic LPS leakage, and a substantial reduction in life expectancy. In the absence of IL-13 alone, mice retain a Th2 phenotype and excrete the eggs efficiently without the development of any intestinal inflammation. IL-4 thus seems to be the more dominant of the two cytokines, in terms of driving the Th2 response to *S. mansoni* infection. Having said this, some aspects of the intestinal pathology and cytokine profiling suggest that IL-13 plays an additive role in this process.

3.4.2. Pulmonary Granuloma Model Induced Using Schistosome Eggs

This protocol induces a cellular granulomatous response around parasite eggs that have become lodged in the lungs of treated mice. In wild-type mice this is normally a Th2 cytokine-mediated inflammatory response, with characteristic elevated serum IgE, eosinophil-dominated granulomas, mastocytosis, and goblet cell hyperplasia. In the primary granuloma model, a single intravenous administration of *S. mansoni* eggs is given, and lungs are analyzed after 2 wk for granuloma formation. In the secondary granuloma model, the mice are first sensitized by intraperitoneal injection with *S. mansoni* eggs, followed 2 wk later by intravenous challenge with eggs. After a further 2 wk, the lungs are analyzed for granuloma formation *(18)*.

Schistosome egg challenge of IL-4$^{-/-}$ and IL-13$^{-/-}$ mice demonstrated that the individual absence of either of these cytokines resulted in a reduction in granuloma volume relative to wild-type. This decrease in granuloma size correlated with a reduction in the number of eosinophils. In vitro cytokine analysis showed that the IL-4$^{-/-}$ and IL-13$^{-/-}$ mice were still capable of mounting a Th2-like response, and antigen-specific serum IgE and IgG1 were both elevated in the single-cytokine-deficient mice (although not to the degree seen in wild-type mice). Significantly, doubly deficient IL-4$^{-/-}$/IL-13$^{-/-}$ mice failed to develop eosinophil-rich pulmonary granulomas, and IgE and IgG1 were virtually undetectable *(18)*. Stimulated mediastinal lymph node cells taken from infected wild-type mice showed high levels of the Th2 cytokines IL-4, IL-13, IL-10, and IL-5 and low levels of IFN-γ, again, typical of an intact Th2 response. By contrast, lymph node cells from IL-4$^{-/-}$/IL-13$^{-/-}$ mice secreted a cytokine profile deficient in the Th2 cytokines IL-5 and IL-10, but dominated by elevated levels of the Th1 cytokine IFN-γ. Thus ablation of both IL-4 and IL-13 is capable of virtually abolishing Th2-like granuloma formation and associated eosinophilia and IgE/IgG1 production.

3.5. Leishmania

Leishmaniasis is a common human disease, with some 15 million people world-wide infected by the *Leishmania* protozoan flagellates. There are 22 different recognized infectious species of *Leishmania* that can cause symptoms, ranging from self-healing ulcers to systemic fatal infections *(28)*. Studies using IL13$^{-/-}$ and IL-4$^{-/-}$/IL-13$^{-/-}$ mice have started to elucidate the functions of these cytokines in the development of the different disease states observed in the animal models of disease.

3.5.1. Leishmania major

Inbred strains of mice differ in their susceptibility to chronic *L. major* infection. Resistant strains such as C57BL/6 develop an IL-12-dependent parasite-specific Th1 response, with rapid healing of infection. In contrast, susceptible strains such as BALB/c develop a parasite-specific Th2 response, characterized by enhanced expression of IL-4; cutaneous lesions develop unchecked, and the mice eventually die. To investigate the role of IL-13 in the immune response to *L. major*, Matthews et al. *(29)* backcrossed IL-4$^{-/-}$, IL-13$^{-/-}$, and IL-4$^{-/-}$/IL-13$^{-/-}$ mice onto a BALB/c (susceptible strain) background and then followed the course of infection by measuring footpad inflammation. Whereas the wild-type BALB/c mice succumbed to disease with the development of uncontrolled footpad swelling, the BALB/c IL-13$^{-/-}$ mice were able to control parasite infection, as were the IL-4$^{-/-}$ mice. IL-4$^{-/-}$/IL-13$^{-/-}$ double knockout mice resolved infections faster than either single IL-4$^{-/-}$, IL13$^{-/-}$, or wild-type C57BL/6 resistant strain *(29)*.

Cytokine profiling of popliteal lymph node cells from a panel of infected mice failed to provide any clear correlation of Th1 or Th2 cytokine levels with the degree of disease progression. For example, cells from IL-13$^{-/-}$ mice produced elevated levels of IL-4 compared with C57BL/6, but these two sets of mice were equally susceptible to chronic infection. Significantly, the normally resistant C57BL/6 mouse strain when harboring an IL-13 transgene overexpressing IL-13 became susceptible to *L. major* infection *(29)*. These data clearly demonstrate the role of IL-13 in regulating the Th2 immune response and highlight the utility of cytokine-deficient and cytokine-overexpressing mice in understanding disease progression.

4. Studies Using Experimental Allergic Asthma Models

Th2 immune responses are characteristic of asthma and allergy, and IL-13 maps to a genomic region associated with asthma *(5)*. Studies using IL-13 antagonists in mice have also linked IL-13 with asthma *(30,31)*. A number of mouse models of experimental allergic asthma exist; they rely on the generation of Th2 immune responses to antigens in the lung and the induction of airway hyperreactivity (AHR) *(32)*. Often these responses are dependent on the genetic background of specific mouse strains. For instance, models using OVA as the sensitizing antigen generally utilize BALB/c mice since this strain generates a strong Th2-like response. The IL-13$^{-/-}$ and IL-4$^{-/-}$/IL-13$^{-/-}$ mice have been backcrossed onto the BALB/c background to facilitate these studies. To date, conflicting results have been reported for the involvement of IL-13 in the generation of AHR in experimental allergic asthma models.

4.1. Persistence of AHR in the Absence of IL-13

Webb et al. *(33)* were first to test IL-13$^{-/-}$ mice in a model of AHR. The IL-13$^{-/-}$ mice were backcrossed onto the BALB/c strain for five generations and their AHR compared with similarly backcrossed control mice. Mice were initially sensitized by intraperitoneal injection with OVA, followed by repeated aero-challenge with the same nebulized antigen. Aerosol challenge with the bronchoconstrictor methacholine was used to induce AHR, and this was measured by the effects on the expiration parameter P_{enh} (enhanced pause).

Wild-type and IL13$^{-/-}$ mice both developed strong AHR compared with nonsensitized mice. The dependence of this AHR on IL-4 and IL-5 was determined using pretreatment with either anti-IL-4 or anti-IL-5 monoclonal antibodies (MAbs). Such treatment had little effect on the AHR in wild-type mice. In contrast, the AHR displayed by IL13$^{-/-}$ mice was dependent on IL-4 and IL-5. Cytokine production by peribronchial lymph node cells, simulated with OVA antigen, showed that AHR in wild-type and IL13$^{-/-}$ mice was associated with elevated IL-4 and IL-5. OVA-specific IgE levels were also similar in wild-type and IL13$^{-/-}$ sensitized and challenged mice.

Even though IL-13 does not appear to have a critical role in AHR, it demonstrated a clear involvement in airway eosinophilia. The numbers of eosinophils were determined in three compartments: the vasculature, the peribronchial/perivascular region, and the airway lumen. AHR in IL13$^{-/-}$ mice was associated with strong eosinophilia in all three of these compartments, paralleling the responses seen in wild-type mice. Interestingly, pretreatment with MAb to IL-4 neutralized the tissue eosinophilia in IL13$^{-/-}$ mice while having no effect in the wild-type, suggesting that IL-4 and IL-13 have redundant roles associated with the transendothelial migration of eosinophils. By contrast, IL-4 ablation greatly reduced the numbers of airway lumen eosinophils in both wild-type and IL13$^{-/-}$ mice, indicating that IL-4 provides a key signal for permeation of eosinophils into the airway lumen and that this signal cannot be compensated for by IL-13 in the absence of IL-4. The decrease in eosinophil infiltration correlated with a reduction in the levels of expression of the eosinophil chemokine eotaxin.

Hypersecretion of mucus is also seen in allergic asthma. The link between IL-13 and mucus secretion was investigated using histologic staining of lung sections from sensitized, challenged mice. Large numbers of mucin-secreting goblet cells cells were seen in wild-type mice even with anti-IL-4 MAb treatment. In contrast, extremely low numbers of goblet cells were seen in the lungs of IL13$^{-/-}$ mice.

4.2. A Critical Role for IL-13 in the Development of AHR

In contrast to the results detailed above, Walter et al. *(34)* have demonstrated that IL-13$^{-/-}$ mice do not develop AHR. The knockout mice used in this study were essentially the same as those used in the previous study, with the exception that the knockouts had been backcrossed onto BALB/c mice for seven generations, rather than five. The measurement of AHR utilized a method similar to that of Webb et al. It is not clear why the two groups should get such different results.

Walter et al. *(34)* used a comparative panel of three knockout mice. AHR was measured in single IL-13 and IL-4 knockouts, as well as the double IL-4/IL-13 knockout. Sensitized and challenged IL-13$^{-/-}$ mice showed no AHR, whereas wild-type mice showed profound AHR. IL-4$^{-/-}$ mice had significant AHR, but less than the wild-type controls. IL-4$^{-/-}$/IL-13$^{-/-}$ mice showed no AHR. Together these results indicated that IL-13, but not IL-4, was critical for the development of AHR.

One consistency between this study and the previous one was the failure of mucus production in the lungs of IL-13$^{-/-}$ mice. The failure of IL-13$^{-/-}$ mice to develop AHR was not owing to a lack of airway inflammation, since histology revealed a dense eosinophil- and lymphocyte-rich infiltrate in the peribronchial and perivascular tissue spaces.

In vitro analysis of cytokine production by bronchial lymph node cells gave results consistent with those of Webb et al. *(33)*. Cells from IL-13$^{-/-}$ mice sensitized and challenged with OVA showed high levels of the Th2 cytokines IL-4 and IL-5 and induction of OVA-specific IgE and IgG1. Thus, despite the generation of this polarized OVA-specific Th2 response, these mice develop no AHR. A further compelling observation for a critical role of IL-13 in AHR is the fact that addition of recombinant IL-13 to the IL-$13^{-/-}$ mice during the immunization protocol was capable of restoring strong AHR. Indeed, recombinant IL-13 administration was capable of inducing AHR in all mice tested (regardless of knockout status), even in naive mice. Interestingly, AHR in naive mice that received the recombinant cytokine was marked by the absence in the lungs of any cellular infiltration or mucus production.

The capacity of Th2 lines purified from the spleens of IL-$13^{-/-}$ mice to induce AHR upon transfer into SCID mice was also investigated. Such Th2 cells did not induce AHR, unlike Th2 cells from wild-type mice. The lack of AHR in IL-$13^{-/-}$ mice is therefore not owing to a failure of the Th2 responses to develop optimally.

Further studies will be required to understand the nature of the differences in the results obtained in the two AHR studies published to date. It is possible that the immunization strategies used by the two groups may fall on either side of a threshold in which more or less IL-4 may be produced in the lungs. It may be that in the study by Webb et al. more IL-4 is produced and that this is able to compensate for the loss of IL-13. Recent studies in our laboratory have highlighted the compensatory roles of IL-4 in Th2 responses and the differential importance of its production in response to different antigens and in different tissues *(25)*.

4.3. Role of IL-13 in Neonatal Tolerance

Neonatal exposure to foreign antigen often results in the development of immunologic tolerance to the antigen. Th2 immunity has been implicated in the development of neonatal immunity since neonatally tolerized mice exhibit a strong Th2, but weak Th1, response upon subsequent antigen exposure. The role of IL4 and Th2 immunity in the development of neonatal tolerance was investigated by testing whether tolerance to a minor histocompatibility antigen, the HY male antigen, can be induced in newborn mice that were IL-$4^{-/-}$ or IL-$4^{-/-}$/IL-$13^{-/-}$ *(35)*. Newborn female mice were injected with syngeneic male splenocytes, and 4 wk later skin grafts from syngeneic males were transplanted onto the mice. The acceptance or rejection of these grafts was used as a measure of tolerance. Both wild-type and IL-$4^{-/-}$ mice accepted the skin grafts readily. However, IL-$4^{-/-}$/IL-$13^{-/-}$ mice rejected the grafts. These results implicate IL-13 (possibly in combination with IL-4) as a major factor in determining neonatal tolerance. Further evidence for lack of tolerance in the double knockout mice was the capability of isolated splenocytes to mount a cytotoxic T-lymphocyte response against male target splenocytes. Such a response was not seen in the wild-type or IL-$4^{-/-}$ mice. A measure of the Th2 response was obtained from the cytokine production profiles of cultured, restimulated splenocytes taken from the mice. The most striking of these profiles was in the IL-$4^{-/-}$/IL-$13^{-/-}$ mice, in which even though large amounts of the Th2 cytokines IL-5 and IL-10 were produced, there was also a large increase in the concentration of IFN-γ. This profile suggests that the failure to induce neonatal tolerance in the doubly deficient mice is not owing to a failure to produce a Th2 response *per se*, but to the prevention of the suppression of the Th1 response.

References

1. Brown, K., Zurawski, S., Mosmann, T., and Zurawski, G. (1989) A family of small inducible proteins secreted by leukocytes are members of a new super-family that includes leukocyte and fibroblast-derived inflammatory agents, growth factors and indicators of various activation processes. *J. Immunol.* **142,** 679–687.

2. Mckenzie, A., Culpepper, J., de Waal Malefyt, R., et al. (1993) Interleukin-13, a T-cell-derived cytokine that regulates human monocyte and B-cell function. *Proc. Natl. Acad. Sci. USA* **90,** 3735–3739.
3. Minty, A., Chalon, P., Derocq, J.-M., et al. (1993) Interleukin-13 is a new human lymphokine regulating inflammatory and immune responses. *Nature* **362,** 248–250.
4. Finkelman, F., Shea-Donohue, T., Goldhill, J., et al. (1997) Cytokine regulation of host defence against parasitic gastrointestinal nematodes: lessons from studies with rodent models. *Annu. Rev. Immunol.* **15,** 505–533.
5. Marsh, D. G., Neely, J. D., Breazeale, D. R., et al. (1994) Linkage analysis of IL4 and other chromosome 5q31.1 markers and total serum immunoglobulin E concentrations. *Science* **264,** 1152–1156.
6. Mosmann, T. and Coffman, R. (1989) TH1 and TH2 cells: different patterns of lymphokine secretion lead to different functional properties. *Annu. Rev. Immunol.* **5,** 429–459.
7. Burd, P. R., Thompson, W. C., Max, E. E., and Mills, F. C. (1995) Activated mast cells produce interleukin 13. *J. Exp. Med.* **181,** 1373–1380.
8. Zurawski, G. and de Vries, J. (1994) Interleukin 13, an interleukin 4-like cytokine that acts on monocytes and B-cells but not on T-cells. *Immunol. Today* **15,** 19–26.
9. Zurawski, S., Vega, F., Huyghe, B., and Zurawski, G. (1993) Receptors for interleukin-13 and interleukin-4 are complex and share a novel component that functions in signal transduction. *EMBO J.* **12,** 3899–3905.
10. Zurawski, S., Chomarat, P., Djossou, O., et al. (1995) The primary binding subunit of the human interleukin-4 receptor is also a component of the interleukin-13 receptor. *J. Biol. Chem.* **270,** 13869–13878.
11. Lin, J.-X., Migone, T.-S., Tsang, M., et al. (1995) The role of shared recptor motifs and common Stat proteins in the generation of cytokine pleiotropy and redundancy by IL-2, IL-4, IL-7, IL-13, and IL-5. *Immunity* **2,** 331–339.
12. Barner, M., Mohrs, M., Brombacher, F., and Kopf, M. (1998) Differences between IL-4R alpha-deficient and IL-4-deficient mice reveal a role for IL-13 in the regulation of Th2 responses. *Curr. Biol.* **8,** 669–672.
13. Takeda, K., Tanaka, T., Shi, W., et al. (1996) Essential role of Stat6 in IL-4 signalling. *Nature* **380,** 627–630.
14. McKenzie, A. N., Li, X., Largaespada, D. A., et al. (1993) Structural comparison and chromosomal localization of the human and mouse IL-13 genes. *J. Immunol.* **150,** 5436–5444.
15. Frazer, K. A., Ueda, Y., Zhu, Y., et al. (1997) Computational and biological analysis of 680 kb of DNA sequence from the human 5q31 cytokine gene cluster region. *Genome Res.* **7,** 495–512.
16. McKenzie, G. J., Bancroft, A., Grencis, R. K., and McKenzie, A. N. (1998) A distinct role for interleukin-13 in Th2-cell-mediated immune responses. *Curr. Biol.* **8,** 339–342.
17. McKenzie, G. J., Emson, C. L., Bell, S. E., et al. (1998) Impaired development of Th2 cells in IL-13-deficient mice. *Immunity* **9,** 423–432.
18. McKenzie, G. J., Fallon, P. G., Emson, C. L., Grencis, R. K., and McKenzie, A. N. (1999) Simultaneous disruption of interleukin (IL)-4 and IL-13 defines individual roles in T helper cell type 2-mediated responses. *J. Exp. Med.* **189,** 1565–1572.
19. Guo, L., Hu-Li, J., Zhu, J., et al. (2001) Disrupting IL-13 impairs production of IL-4 specified by the linked allele. *Nat. Immunol.* **2,** 461–466.
20. Fallon, P. G., Emson, C. L., Smith, P., and McKenzie, A. N. (2001) IL-13 overexpression predisposes to anaphylaxis following antigen sensitization. *J. Immunol.* **166,** 2712–2716.
21. Punnonen, J., Aversa, G., Cocks, B., et al. (1993) Interleukin-13 induces interleukin-4-independent IgG4 and IgE synthesis and CD23 expression by human B-cells. *Proc. Natl. Acad. Sci. USA* **90,** 3730–3734.
22. Emson, C. L., Bell, S. E., Jones, A., Wisden, W., and McKenzie, A. N. (1998) Interleukin (IL)-4-independent induction of immunoglobulin (Ig)E, and perturbation of T cell development in transgenic mice expressing IL-13. *J. Exp. Med.* **188,** 399–404.
23. Bancroft, A. J., McKenzie, A. N., and Grencis, R. K. (1998) A critical role for IL-13 in resistance to intestinal nematode infection. *J. Immunol.* **160,** 3453–3461.
24. Bancroft, A. J., Artis, D., Donaldson, D. D., Sypek, J. P., and Grencis, R. K. (2000) Gastrointestinal nematode expulsion in IL-4 knockout mice is IL-13 dependent. *Eur. J. Immunol.* **30,** 2083–2091.

25. Fallon, P. G., Jolin, H. E., Smith, P., et al. (2002) IL-4 induces characteristic Th2 responses even in the absence of IL-5, IL-9 and IL-13. *Immunity* **17,** 7–17.
26. Fallon, P. G., Richardson, E. J., McKenzie, G. J., and McKenzie, A. N. (2000) Schistosome infection of transgenic mice defines distinct and contrasting pathogenic roles for IL-4 and IL-13: IL-13 is a profibrotic agent. *J. Immunol.* **164,** 2585–2591.
27. Chiaramonte, M. G., Donaldson, D. D., Cheever, A. W., and Wynn, T. A. (1999) An IL-13 inhibitor blocks the development of hepatic fibrosis during a T-helper type 2-dominated inflammatory response. *J. Clin. Invest.* **104,** 777–785.
28. Brombacher, F. (2000) The role of interleukin-13 in infectious diseases and allergy. *Bioessays* **22,** 646–656.
29. Matthews, D. J., Emson, C. L., McKenzie, G. J., Jolin, H. E., Blackwell, J. M., and McKenzie, A. N. (2000) IL-13 is a susceptibility factor for *Leishmania major* infection. *J. Immunol.* **164,** 1458–1462.
30. Grunig, G., Warnock, M., Wakil, A. E., et al. (1998) Requirement for IL-13 independently of IL-4 in experimental asthma. *Science* **282,** 2261–2263.
31. Wills-Karp, M., Luyimbazi, J., Xu, X., et al. (1998) Interleukin-13: central mediator of allergic asthma. *Science* **282,** 2258–2261.
32. Lloyd, C. M., Gonzalo, J. A., Coyle, A. J., and Gutierrez-Ramos, J. C. (2001) Mouse models of allergic airway disease. *Adv. Immunol.* **77,** 263–295.
33. Webb, D. C., McKenzie, A. N., Koskinen, A. M., Yang, M., Mattes, J., and Foster, P. S. (2000) Integrated signals between IL-13, IL-4, and IL-5 regulate airways hyperreactivity. *J. Immunol.* **165,** 108–113.
34. Walter, D. M., McIntire, J. J., Berry, G., et al. (2001) Critical role for IL-13 in the development of allergen-induced airway hyperreactivity. *J. Immunol.* **167,** 4668–4675.
35. Inoue, Y., Konieczny, B. T., Wagener, M. E., McKenzie, A. N., and Lakkis, F. G. (2001) Failure to induce neonatal tolerance in mice that lack both IL-4 and IL-13 but not in those that lack IL-4 alone. *J. Immunol.* **167,** 1125–1128.

17

IL-15

Insights from Characterizing IL-15-Deficient Mice

Pallavur V. Sivakumar, Sandra N. Brown, Ananda W. Goldrath, Anne Renee Van der Vuurst de Vries, Joanne L. Viney, and Mary K. Kennedy

Summary

Interleukin-15 (IL-15) is a 4-helix bundle cytokine with similar biologic properties as IL-2, consistent with their shared receptor subunits. Specificity for IL-15 and IL-2 is provided by unique private α-chain subunits. Studies to date examining the biology of IL-15 have identified several roles for this cytokine in both the differentiation as well as function of immune cells. IL-15 is important for NK cell, NK-T-cell, CD8 T-cell, and intestinal epithelial lymphocyte (IEL) growth and function. Recently, overexpression of IL-15 in diseased tissue has provided evidence for a potential role for IL-15 in inflammation. Mice that are genetically deficient in IL-15 or its unique receptor subunit IL-15Rα have recently been generated. These mice provide us with valuable tools to address the importance of IL-15 in immune responses. This chapter focuses on studies with the IL-15 deficient mice to address specific roles for IL-15 in the generation and function of immune cells. Wherever applicable, comparisons are provided to studies in IL-15Rα deficient mice.

Analysis of IL-15 and IL-15Rα deficient mice has shown that IL-15 is a crucial factor for the maturation, survival, and activation of NK cells. Furthermore, IL-15 is important for the survival of NK-T cells, differentiation, and activation of IEL and dendritic epidermal T-cells (DETC). Although the generation of primary and memory CD8 T-cell responses were not compromised significantly in IL-15 deficient mice, IL-15 plays an important role in maintaining memory CD8 T-cell, but not memory CD4 T-cell, homeostasis. IL-15 is crucial for the long-term survival of memory CD8 T-cells and for the bystander proliferation of naïve CD8 T-cells. Furthermore, APC from both IL-15 and IL-15Rα deficient mice are defective in both IFNγ and NO production, suggesting that IL-15 is important for both innate (APC, NK) as well as adaptive immunity (CD8 T-cells). Characterization of the IL-15 deficient mice has also provided another surprising function of IL-15 in the survival of kidney epithelial cells. The chapter also provides a summary of in vivo inflammation experiments performed in IL-15 deficient mice to identify a potential role for IL-15 in inflammatory disease. Although IL-15 deficient mice have normal DTH and contact hypersensitivity responses, they are increasingly susceptible to colitis suggesting that IL-15 may play an anti-inflammatory role in gut responses. Based on these studies, IL-15 or its unique IL-15Rα chain could serve as targets for therapy in human disease.

Key words

IL-15, knockout, memory T-cells, NK cells, inflammation

1. Introduction

Interleukin (IL)-15 is a proinflammatory cytokine and growth factor initially identified as a proliferative factor for the IL-2-dependent CTLL-2 T-cell line *(1,2)*. Cloning of the full-length cDNA for IL-15 showed that IL-15 belonged to the four-helix bundle cytokine family *(2)*, which includes human growth hormone, IL-2, IL-3, IL-6, IL-7, granulocyte

From: *Contemporary Immunology: Cytokine Knockouts, 2nd Edition*
Edited by: Giamila Fantuzzi © Humana Press Inc., Totowa, NJ

colony stimulating factor (G-CSF), and granulocyte/macrophage colony-stimulating factor (GM-CSF) *(3)*. Although it was identified as a stimulatory factor for T-cells mimicking IL-2, comparisons of primary protein and cDNA sequences of IL-15 revealed little primary homology to IL-2. However, functional studies using antibodies that blocked the various IL-2 receptor (R) subunits showed that IL-15 and IL-2 shared the use of common receptor signaling subunits. IL-15 and IL-2 both interact with receptor complexes that contain the common γ (γc) and IL-2Rβ chains *(2,4–6)*. It is therefore not surprising that IL-2 and IL-15 share some similar in vitro properties. Binding studies indicated that IL-15 bound to the γc and IL-2Rβ complex with low affinity, suggesting the existence of a unique receptor subunit for IL-15. The mouse and human IL-15Rα subunits were subsequently cloned, characterized, and shown to be highly homologous to their IL-2Rα counterparts *(7,8)*. These α-subunits do not appear to be involved in signaling but are required for high-affinity binding of these cytokines. The ability of a cell to respond to IL-2 or IL-15 can therefore also be controlled by the presence or absence of their unique α-subunits. In addition, IL-2 and IL-15 are produced by different cells and in different tissues, suggesting distinct roles for these cytokines in vivo (reviewed in refs. *9* and *10*).

Because IL-15 was identified initially as a "IL-2-like" cytokine, the biochemical and functional similarities and differences between these two cytokines have been studied extensively. Specifically, studies of mice carrying induced mutations in IL-2 or within the IL-2/15R system have provided definitive evidence that IL-2 and IL-15 have unique roles in vivo *(11–16)*. Mice lacking IL-2, IL-2Rα, or IL-2Rβ develop similar spontaneous autoimmune disorders. However, there are additional defects in the IL-2Rβ-deficient mice that are absent in the IL-2- and IL-2Rα-deficient mice. These additional defects, attributable to the lack of IL-15-mediated signaling, include the absence of functional natural killer (NK) cells and reduced numbers of NK T-cells and intestinal intraepithelial lymphocytes (IELs). These observations led to the belief that IL-2 was important for T-cell homeostasis whereas IL-15 was essential for development of NK cells, NK T-cells, and IELs (reviewed in ref. *17*). Numerous laboratories provided in vitro observations suggesting IL-15 as a growth/survival factor for NK cells *(18,19)*, NK T-cells *(15,20)*, and IELs *(21)*. Furthermore, IL-15 was shown to support the growth and proliferation of memory, but not naive, CD8 T-cells *(22)*. These results show that IL-15 is important for the development and survival of multiple hematopoietic lineages. Furthermore, other studies reported that IL-15 is an anabolic factor for muscle cells *(23)*, a differentiation factor for osteoclast progenitors *(24)*, a growth factor for mast cells and intestinal epithelial cells *(25,26)*, and a general inhibitor of apoptosis in T-cells, B-cells, and fibroblasts *(27)*.

Recently, C57BL/6 mice that are genetically deficient in either IL-15 (IL-15 knockout) *(28)*, or IL-15Rα chain (IL-15Rα knockout) *(29)* were generated and characterized. The IL-15 knockout and the IL-15Rα knockout mice provide us with valuable tools to address the importance of IL-15 in immune responses. This review focuses on data obtained using the IL-15 knockout mice to address specific roles for IL-15 in the generation and function of immune cells. Whenever applicable, comparisons are provided using data available from the IL-15Rα knockout mice.

2. Phenotypic Characterization of IL-15-Deficient Mice

The IL-15 gene spans 34 kb or more, mapping to mouse chromosome 8 and human chromosome 4q31 *(30,31)*. The genomic structure of mouse IL-15 contains seven coding exons.

The construct for the IL-15 knockout mice was engineered to represent a null mutation, as it deleted the initiation codon, the leader sequence, and the first 17 amino acids of the mature protein *(28)*. IL-15 knockout mice ($^{-/-}$) were generated from IL-15$^{+/-}$ intercrosses at the expected mendelian frequency and did not display any gross phenotypic anomalies. The mice also had a normal life span in specific pathogen-free conditions. Serologic and histologic characterization of IL-15 knockout mice showed no abnormality compared with wild-type controls (data not shown). These analyses included absolute and relative body and organ weights, tissue morphology, and immunophenotyping. There were no signs of autoimmune diseases or inflammatory bowel disease (IBD). Furthermore, basal levels of serum IgA, IgG, and IgM were within normal ranges compared with heterozygote (+/–) or wild-type (+/+) littermates.

Because IL-15 had been shown to have a stimulatory effect on T-cells and NK cells, weights and cellularity of lymphoid organs, namely, thymus, lymph nodes, spleen, and bone marrow were studied. There were no consistent or marked differences in the weights of the spleens, thymi, or the bone marrow between age- and sex-matched IL-15 knockout or control mice. However, the average absolute weight and organ to body weight ratio of the peripheral lymph nodes from IL-15 knockout mice were significantly lower than those of controls *(28)*. When cellularity was analyzed, pooled data from multiple experiments revealed that there was a significant decrease in the average cellularity of the peripheral lymph nodes, but not the spleen or thymi, between IL-15 knockout mice and the controls.

The relative proportions and absolute numbers of CD4 and CD8 double-positive and CD4 and CD8 single-positive thymocytes were similar in control and IL-15 knockout mice. In contrast, thymic NK T-cells were significantly reduced in IL-15 knockout mice compared with controls. Decreases in the relative proportions and absolute numbers of NK T-cells were also observed in the spleen and liver of IL-15 knockout mice. This reduction in NK T-cells mirrors that seen in IL-15Rα knockout mice as well as in IL-2/I5Rβ knockout mice *(15,29)*. IL-15 is therefore important for the survival of these NK T-cells and not for their development, as Vβ+ NK T-cells were present, albeit in smaller numbers in IL-15 knockout mice.

Analysis of IEL populations in IL-15 knockout mice also revealed a dramatic reduction in the numbers of T-cell receptor (TCR)αβ+/CD4-/CD8αα+ IELs. This population is thought to arise or mature independent of the thymus. This decrease was reflected by an increase in the proportions of TCRαβ+/CD4+/CD8- and TCRαβ+/CD4+/CD8+ IELs. Furthermore, the relative proportions TCRγδ+ IELs were also reduced three to fourfold in IL-15 knockout mice compared with controls *(28)*. The selective defect in these subpopulations of IELs suggests a role for IL-15 in the development or maintenance of IEL populations that mature extrathymically.

Analysis of splenic cell populations revealed that IL-15 knockout mice have a severe reduction in NK1.1+/CD3- (NK) cells. Administration of IL-15 to the IL-15 knockout mice restored NK cell numbers to levels comparable to those seen in wild-type mice, indicating that this defect was reversible. Furthermore, culture of splenic cells in IL-15 for 4–6 d resulted in the presence of an NK1.1+/CD3- population with cytolytic properties against NK-sensitive YAC-1 target cells (data not shown). These results suggest that an IL-15-responsive NK1.1- NK-precursor cell is present in the spleens of these mice and can mature to a functional NK cell upon stimulation with IL-15. Such an IL-15-responsive NK precursor has been defined in the bone marrow *(32,33)*. Furthermore, the ability of IL-15 to reverse the defect in NK cell number and function shows that bone marrow-derived IL-15 is an NK cell differentiation and maturation factor that is absolutely essential for the development of mature functional NK cells.

In an interesting development, Cooper et al. *(34)* demonstrated that IL-15 is also an NK cell survival factor and is absolutely necessary for the survival of mature NK cells. Adoptively transferred mature NK cells survive longer in wild-type mice compared with IL-15 knockout mice. Furthermore, SCID mice treated with a blocking antibody against the IL-2/15Rβ chain show a significant loss of NK cells. Finally, NK cells from Bcl-2 transgenic mice survive longer than wild-type NK cells after transfer into IL-15 knockout mice, suggesting that IL-15-dependent survival of mature NK cells is mediated via Bcl-2.

Our initial characterization of IL-15 knockout mice also revealed a reduction in the relative proportion of peripheral CD8 T-cells compared with controls *(28)*. The reduction was specific to the CD8+/CD44^{hi} memory phenotype T-cells. Administration of IL-15 restored CD8+/CD44^{hi} T-cells to numbers comparable to those found in control mice. B-cells, granulocytes, and CD4 T-cell numbers and proportions were similar between IL-15 knockout and control mice, suggesting that cellular defects in the spleen were mainly in the NK and CD8 memory populations. A summary of the phenotypic characterization is found in Table 1. Similar defects in NK T-cells, NK cells, memory CD8 T-cells, and IELs are also observed in the IL-15Rα knockout mice *(29)*. Surprisingly, IL-15Rα knockout mice show slightly more severe defects than IL-15 knockout mice. Younger IL-15Rα knockout mice exhibit an increased ratio of single-positive CD4+ to CD8+ thymocytes and a slight thymic hypocellularity. In addition, IL-15Rα knockout mice are markedly more lymphopenic relative to controls (30–80% decreased cellularity in IL15Rα knockout mice versus 15% decreased cellularity in IL-15 knockout mice compared with their respective controls). Further analysis of these mice housed under identical conditions is necessary to understand the nature of these phenotypic differences.

Dendritic epidermal T-cells (DETCs) are a unique subset of γ/δ T-cells that reside in the skin and play an important role in immune responses associated with the skin. DETCs respond to IL-15 in vitro *(35)* and are absent in IL-2Rβ knockout mice *(36)*, suggesting that their development is dependent on IL-2 and/or IL-15. A significant proportion of DETCs express a T-cell receptor comprised of a Vγ3/Vδ1 TCR. To study the role played by IL-2Rβ signaling in the development of DETC, Ye et al. *(37)* introduced a Vγ3/Vδ1 TCR transgene into IL-2Rβ knockout mice. To their surprise, introduction of this transgene did not rescue the DETC in the skin of IL-2Rβ knockout mice. These results suggest that signaling via IL-2Rβ is essential for the proliferation and survival of DETC in the fetal thymus and skin. De Creus et al. *(38)* studied DETC in IL-15 knockout mice and interferon regulatory factor-1 (IRF-1) knockout mice. Vγ3 DETCs were absent in IL-15 knockout mice, and adoptive transfer of wild-type fetal thymocytes into the IL-15 knockout mice did not result in development of Vγ3 DETCs, whereas normal DETC development could be seen when fetal thymocytes were transferred into control mice. These data show that IL-15 is essential for the development of DETCs in the skin.

3. Immune Responses in IL-15-Deficient Mice

3.1. IL-15 Knockout Mice Have a Reversible NK Cell Defect

As described above, IL-15 knockout mice have a severe reduction in the numbers of NK1.1+/CD3- cells in the spleen. To test whether IL-15 knockout mice lacked functional NK

Table 1
Summary of Phenotypic Differences in IL-15 Knockout Mice

	B-cells	CD4	CD8	NK1.1
Spleen				
Control	39.0 ± 2.4	19.8 ± 0.4	10.4 ± 0.5	2.4 ± 0.5
IL-15 knockout	43.2 ± 2.8	22.0 ± 0.6	**5.8 ± 0.2**	**0.5 ± 0.4**
Lymph nodes				
Control	24.4 ± 1.0	33.2 ± 0.7	26.5 ± 0.9	
IL-15 knockout	30.9 ± 0.8	40.4 ± 0.8	**14.4 ± 0.4**	
	$CD44^{hi}$ cells within CD8 gate		$CD44^{hi}$ cells within CD4 gate	
Spleen				
Control	19.7 ± 1.3		21.3 ± 0.3	
IL-15 knockout	**9.5 ± 0.5**		20.2 ± 1.1	
Lymph nodes				
Control	12.4 ± 0.4		11.5 ± 1.2	
IL-15 knockout	**3.4 ± 0.1**		9.3 ± 0.6	
	CD4/CD8	CD4	CD8	NK T-cells
Thymus				
Control	85.3 ± 6.7	7.6 ± 2.3	2.3 ± 1.0	5.1 ± 1.2
IL15 knockout	85.6 ± 5.8	8.5 ± 1.9	2.4 ± 0.7	**1.3 ± 0.7**
	TCRαβ+/CD8αα+		thy1-TCRγδ+	
IELs				
Control	50.9 ± 4.5		31.5 ± 3.6	
IL-15 knockout	**13.8 ± 2.3**		**2.7 ± 0.9**	

IL, interleukin; NK, natural killer; TCR, T-cell receptor. Bold type indicates significant differences between control and knockouts.

cells, splenocytes from wild-type and IL-15 knockout mice were tested for cytolytic activity against NK-sensitive YAC-1 targets. Splenocytes from phosphate-buffered saline (PBS) treated control mice exhibited low to weak NK activity whereas poly I:C-treated control mice exhibited strong NK activity *(28)*. In contrast, splenocytes from IL-15 knockout mice exhibited no demonstrable spontaneous or poly I:C inducible NK activity. Treatment of IL-15 knockout mice with IL-15 for seven days restored NK cell numbers as well as cytolytic activity against YAC-1 targets comparable to controls *(28)*. These results suggest that IL-15 serves as a maturation and activation factor for NK cells.

3.2. IL-15 Knockout Mice Have Enhanced Susceptibility to Vaccinia Virus Infection

Although IL-15 knockout mice remain healthy when maintained under specific pathogen-free conditions and have a normal life span, the defect in NK and CD8 T-cell numbers suggested that immune responses in these mice may be compromised. The response of IL-15 knockout mice to vaccinia virus was tested, as both NK and CD8 T-cells are thought to play an important role in immunity against this virus *(39–41)*. Wild-type and IL-15 knockout mice were infected with 10^6 pfu of a neurotropic wild-type WR strain of vaccinia virus and assessed daily for morbidity and mortality. Whereas wild-type mice showed minimal clinical symptoms and cleared the infection, IL-15 knockout mice showed severe symptoms, were unable to resolve the infection, and died by d 9 after infection *(28)*. Thus IL-15 is necessary for the host response against vaccinia virus. The susceptibility of IL-15 knockout mice to vaccinia virus could be owing to a defect in the NK or CD8 T-cells or both. However, based on the data given below, it is likely that NK cells, rather than CD8 T-cells, play a crucial role in the susceptibility of the IL-15 knockout mice to vaccinia virus.

3.3. IL-15 Knockout Mice Have a Reduced Primary Response to Vesicular Stomatitis Virus But a Normal Primary Response to Lymphocytic Choriomeningitis Virus

Two other groups have studied anti-viral CD8 T-cell responses in IL-15 knockout and IL15Rα knockout mice. Schluns et al. *(42)* studied the primary and memory CD8 T-cell responses to vesicular stomatitis virus (VSV; 10^6 pfu, Indiana strain) in wild-type, IL-15 knockout, and IL-15Rα knockout mice. At the peak of the response, 7 d after infection, the percentage of CD8 T-cells that were reactive to the immunodominant VSV-derived nucleoprotein peptide was decreased 40–50% in secondary lymphoid and tertiary tissues of IL-15 knockout mice compared with controls. The decrease in the same population of cells in IL-15Rα knockout mice was less dramatic (10–20%), suggesting that IL-15 may be able to deliver some signals using the low-affinity IL-2/15Rβ chain in the absence of the IL-15Rα chain. The decreased expansion of VSV-specific CD8 T-cells in the IL-15 knockout and the IL-15Rα knockout mice was not owing to a lower initial precursor frequency in these mice relative to controls. Thus the authors concluded that IL-15 was influencing the expansion of the antiviral CD8 T-cell population.

Becker and colleagues *(43)* characterized lymphocytic choriomeningitis virus (LCMV)-specific T-cell responses in wild-type, IL-15 knockout and IL-15Rα knockout mice. In contrast to the results obtained by Schluns and colleagues, they observed no differences in the primary CD8 T-cell responses to LCMV among wild-type, IL-15 knockout, and IL-15Rα knockout mice. This analysis included quantitation of virus-specific T-cells generated against four different viral epitopes. In addition, they showed that IL-15 knockout and IL-15Rα knockout mice were as efficient as wild-type mice in clearing the viral infection. The results of these two groups show that the requirement for IL-15 in primary antiviral CD8 T-cell responses may vary depending on the type of virus, their tropism, and the immune response generated against the virus.

3.4. Memory T-Cell Responses in IL-15 Knockout Mice

The generation and maintenance of memory T-cells in immune responses has been studied extensively over recent years. However, the requirements for the production and persistence of a functional memory T-cell pool are still unclear. Although there exists compelling evidence that survival of memory cells does not require TCR-MHC interactions *(44,45)*, recent evidence indicates that such interactions may be needed to maintain functional activity of these cells *(46,47)*. However, it is increasingly clear that cytokines play a major role in both production and maintenance of memory T-cells.

A specialized role for IL-15 in the regulation of T-cell memory was suggested by the ability of IL-15 to stimulate proliferation of memory CD8 T-cells but not memory CD4 T-cells or naive CD4 or CD8 T-cells in vivo *(22)*. In addition, phenotypic analysis of IL-15 knockout mice *(28)* and IL-15Rα knockout mice *(29)* revealed reduced numbers of CD8 T-cells in the periphery, specifically in the CD44^{hi} memory phenotype pool. Morover, IL-15 transgenic mice have increased numbers of *Listeria*-specific memory CD8 T-cells after *Listeria* infection *(48)* and develop a fatal leukemia involving expansion of NK cells and memory phenotype CD8 T-cells *(49)*. However, the precise role for IL-15 in generating or maintaining memory CD8 T-cell responses was not addressed in these studies. More recently, multiple laboratories, including our own, have addressed this issue using different antigen-specific systems.

Schluns et al. *(42)* analyzed the generation and presence of the virus-specific memory T-cell population in tissues of IL-15 and IL-15Rα knockout mice infected with VSV. Virus-specific memory CD8 T-cell numbers were decreased by 60–80% when analyzed 38 d after infection in both IL-15 and IL-15Rα knockout mice compared with controls. These results suggest that although IL-15 is required for optimal generation of memory CD8 T-cells, a subset of IL-15-independent CD8 memory T-cells exists in these mice. In the LCMV model described above, Becker and colleagues *(43)* demonstrated that although virus-specific memory T-cells were generated in substantial numbers in the IL-15 and the IL-15Rα knockout mice, a decline in memory T-cell numbers occurs over time in both groups of knockout mice compared with controls. These results suggest that IL-15 is important in the maintenance, but not the generation, of CD8 T-cell memory T-cells. Nevertheless, the overall findings indicate that CD8 memory T-cells are generated in both IL-15 and IL-15Rα knockout mice and these cells are capable of responding normally.

Using a slightly different approach, we analyzed the role for IL-15 and IL-7 in the turnover of ovalbumin (OVA)-specific or polyclonal memory CD8 T-cells *(50)* in a full compartment (basal homeostasis) or a lymphopenic compartment (acute homeostasis). For these studies, we used CD8 T-cells obtained from normal mice or OTI mice that express a transgenic TCR specific for a peptide of OVA *(51)*. Carboxyfluorescein diacetate succinimidyl ester (CFSE)-labeled polyclonal naive CD8 T-cells (CD8+/CD44^{lo}) or OVA-specific naive CD8 T-cells were transferred into irradiated (lymphopenic) wild-type or IL-15 knockout mice, which were treated with control protein or anti-IL-7Rα monoclonal antibody (MAb). Both polyclonal and transgenic naive CD8 T-cells proliferated equally well in both wild-type and IL-15 knockout mice, suggesting that IL-15 is not required for the proliferation of naïve CD8 T-cells. Treatment with IL-7Rα MAb blocked proliferation in both wild-type and IL-15 knockout mice, suggesting an important role for IL-7 in the in vivo proliferation of naive CD8 T-cells. When CFSE-labeled polyclonal memory CD8-T-cells (CD8+/CD44^{hi}) or OVA-specific memory CD8 T-cells (CD8+/Vα2+/CD44^{hi}) were transferred into lymphopenic wild-type or IL-15 knockout mice, proliferation was delayed in the IL-15 knockout mice relative to controls and was blocked completely in the IL-15 knockout mice treated with anti-IL-7Rα MAb (Fig. 1A). In contrast, anti-IL-7Rα MAb delayed proliferation of memory CD8 T-cells in wild-type mice. These results indicate that IL-7 compensates partially for the proliferative defect in CD8 T-cells in IL-15 knockout mice but that in the absence of both IL-7- and IL-15-mediated signals, proliferation is blocked completely.

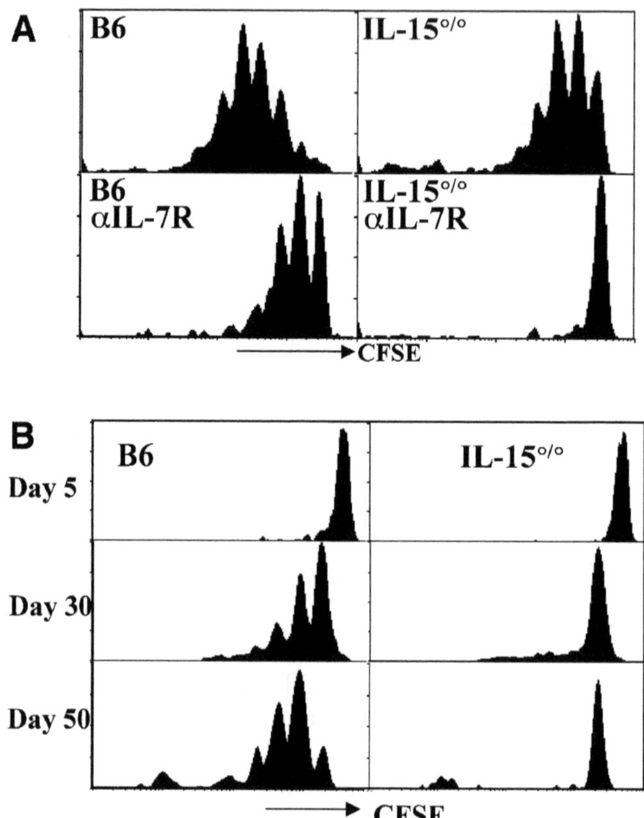

Fig. 1. (**A**) Both interleukin-7 receptor-α (IL-7Rα) and IL-15R-mediated signals contribute to acute homeostatic proliferation of CD8 memory T-cells in irradiated hosts. (**B**) Basal proliferation of memory CD8 T-cells requires IL-15. (**A**) OT-I memory CD8 T-cells were enriched, labeled with CFSE, and transferred intravenously into congenic irradiated (650 rads) C57BL/6 or IL-15 knockout hosts. Indicated recipients were given 1 mg anti-IL7Rα MAb intraperitoneally every other day beginning at the time of transfer. Histogram plots of CFSE intensity of memory OTI cells (Thy1.1+/CD8+/Vα2+) are shown 6 d after transfer. (**B**) OTI memory CD8 T-cells were enriched, labeled with CFSE, and transferred into unirradiated congenic C57BL/6 or IL-15 knockout hosts. Proliferation of transferred memory T-cells was monitored on d 5, 30, and 50 after transfer. CFSE, crystal field stabilization energy.

In contrast to these data, proliferation of OVA-specific memory CD8 T-cells was blocked completely after transfer into unirradiated (full compartment) IL-15 knockout mice compared with controls (Fig. 1B). Furthermore, the recovery of transferred memory CD8 T-cells from IL-15 knockout mice was always lower than from wild-type mice, suggesting that IL-15 is required for the proliferation of memory CD8 T-cells in a normal host. Thus IL-15-induced proliferation of CD8 T-cells may indirectly influence survival of memory CD8 T-cell population over time. Similar results have been reported recently by Tan et al. *(52)*.

The next set of experiments addressed maintenance of long-term CD8 T-cell memory in the IL-15 knockout mice. Transgenic OTI CD8 T-cells were transferred into wild-type or IL-15 knockout mice, and the mice were infected with a recombinant vaccinia virus expressing OVA. This recombinant vaccinia virus is less virulent than the strain used to

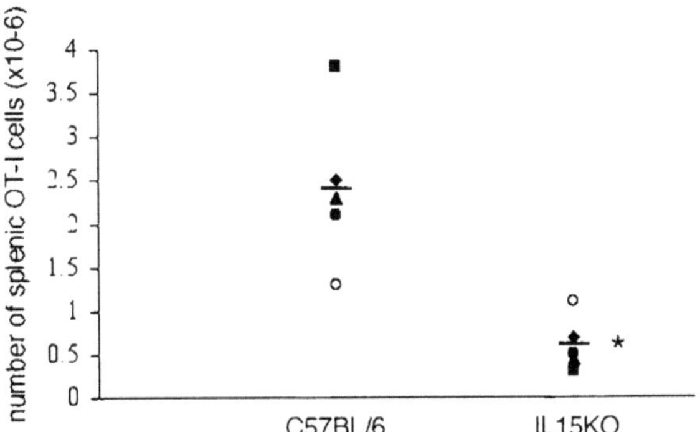

Fig. 2. IL-15 is necessary for the long-term survival of CD8 memory T-cells. Naive OTI CD8 T-cells (5×10^6) were transferred intravenously into congenic C57BL/6 or interleukin-15 (IL-15) knockout (KO) mice. Four hours after cell transfer, all mice were infected intravenously with 5×10^5 pfu recombinant vaccinia virus encoding ovalbumin. Spleen and lymph node cells were analyzed for the presence of OTI cells (Thy1.1+/CD8+/Vα2+) 18 mo after viral infection. Each symbol represents an individual mouse, and the mean for the group is depicted as a thick black line. $^*p < 0.0001$ compared with C57BL/6 mice.

infect the IL-15 knockout mice described above. OTI T-cells were monitored using flow cytometry. At the peak of the viral response (d 7), normal expansion of OTI T-cells was observed in wild-type and IL-15 knockout mice (P.V. Sivakumar and E. Butz, unpublished data). Mice were also characterized 4 and 18 mo after viral infection. No significant differences were found in the proportion of memory OTI T-cells at 4 mo after infection (data not shown). In contrast, IL-15 knockout mice had significantly lower numbers of memory OTI T-cells 18 mo after infection compared with controls (Fig. 2). This observation provides further evidence that IL-15 is required for the long-term survival of memory CD8 T-cells.

Interestingly, it has been reported recently that IL-15 is required for bystander proliferation of CD8 T-cells *(53)*. CD8 T-cells in IL-15Rα knockout mice fail to undergo poly I:C- or IL-15-driven bystander proliferation. Surprisingly, this defect in proliferation is owing to the absence of IL-15Rα on a radiosensitive, non-T-cell hematopoietic population. We made similar observations in the IL-15 knockout mice (P.V. Sivakumar, data not shown). These results indicate that IL-15 affects CD8 T-cell homeostasis via both direct and indirect mechanisms.

Summarizing all the data available, generation of primary and memory CD8 T-cell responses are largely independent of IL-15. However, in the absence of IL-15, there is a gradual decline in the numbers of memory CD8 T-cells. This decline can be attributed to the requirement for IL-15 for proliferation as well as survival of memory CD8 T-cells. It should be noted that there appears to be no defect in polyclonal or antigen-induced CD4 T-cell responses in IL-15 knockout mice *(52)* (P.V Sivakumar, unpublished data).

3.5. Antitumor Responses in IL-15 Knockout Mice

NK and CD8 T-cells play an important role in the generation of immune responses and clearance of tumors. Although the above experiments suggested that IL-15 knockout mice had normal primary CD8 T-cell responses to viral antigens, it was possible that CD8 T-cell responses to other type of immunogens may be affected in IL-15 knockout mice. Miller et

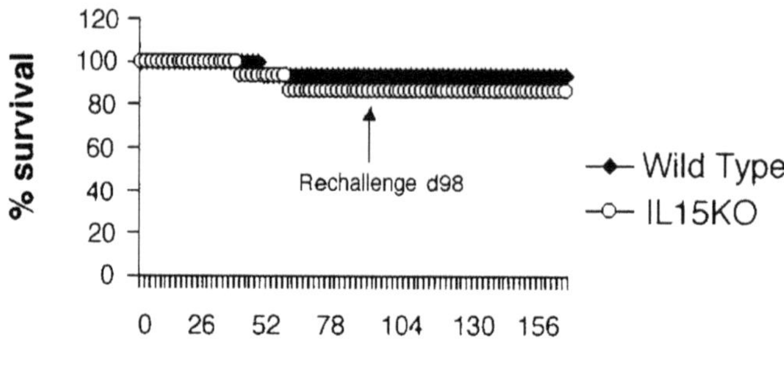

Fig. 3. Interleukin-15 knockout (IL-15 KO) mice mount an efficient memory response against syngeneic tumors. Wild-type (WT) BALB/c mice or IL-15 knockout mice (on the BALB/c background) were immunized with 8 × 10^6 irradiated syngeneic A20 tumor cells on d −14 and −7. Animals were challenged on d 0 with 1 × 10^5 live A20 cells. Surviving mice were rechallenged on d 98 with 1 × 10^5 live A20 cells. Survival of mice was monitored up to 5 mo. Unimmunized BALB/c or IL-15 knockout mice receiving A20 cells all died within 14 d (data not shown).

al. *(54)* demonstrated that C57BL/10 controls or IL-15 knockout mice were comparable in their ability to reject syngeneic B10.2 tumor cells, suggesting that IL-15 knockout mice were able to generate both primary and memory responses to the tumor. However, this study was complicated by the fact that all mice received antibodies against 41BB [a member of the tumor necrosis factor receptor (TNFR) superfamily], which activates CD8 T-cells. We therefore analyzed antitumor responses in wild-type BALB/c or IL-15 knockout (on the BALB/c background) against syngeneic A20 tumor cells. As shown in Fig. 3, A20-immunized wild-type and IL-15 knockout mice rejected the tumor challenge, whereas unimmunized mice were susceptible. Thus IL-15 knockout mice have a normal primary and memory response against tumor cells.

3.6. IL-15-Deficient Mice Have Normal Delayed-Type Hypersensitivity Responses

Delayed-type hypersensitivity (DTH) responses are characteristic of CD4 T-cell-initiated responses that require the trafficking of T-cells, neutrophils, and monocytes to the site of antigen challenge. To test whether IL-15 plays a role in DTH responses, Kim and colleagues *(55)* generated a receptor site-specific IL-15 antagonist by mutating glutamine residues within the C-terminus of IL-15 to aspartic acid and genetically linking this mutant to murine Fcγ2a. Treatment of immunized BALB/c mice with this antagonist inhibited a DTH response against methylated BSA. This inhibition was associated with a decreased infiltration of monocytes and CD4 T-cells to the site of antigen challenge. These results suggested that IL-15 was important for the inflammation associated with the DTH response.

To determine whether IL-15 knockout mice can develop a normal DTH response, we characterized their DTH response to OVA. The data in Fig. 4A show that the magnitude of the OVA-specific DTH response was similar in wild-type and IL-15 knockout mice. Our results indicate that IL-15 is not required for induction and elicitation of a DTH response or that IL-15 knockout mice have a compensatory mechanism to replace the need for IL-15 in this response.

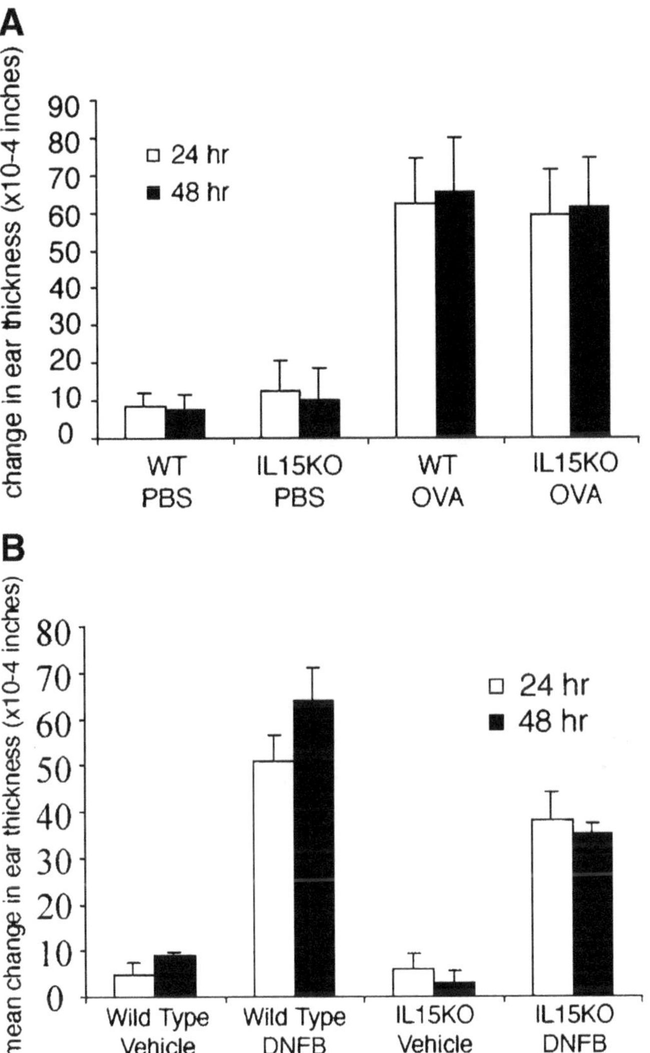

Fig. 4. Normal DTH and CH responses in interleukin-15 knockout (IL-15 KO) mice. (**A**) DTH responses: Groups of four C57BL/6 or IL-15 knockout mice were immunized subcutaneously in the base of the tail with 100 μg ovalbumin (OVA)/CFA. Six days later, groups of mice were challenged in the ear with phosphate-buffered saline (PBS; control) or 10 μg OVA in PBS. Ear thickness measurements were taken before and at 24 and 48 h after challenge. The results shown are representative of two experiments. (**B**) CH responses: Groups of four mice were painted on the back with olive oil/acetone (carrier alone) or 0.5% dinitrofluorobenzene (DNFB)/olive oil/acetone and challenged 5 d later by painting the ear with 0.25% DNFB. Data are shown from one of two experiments.

3.7. IL-15 Knockout Mice Have Normal Contact Hypersensitivity Responses

Contact hypersensitivity (CH) is a type IV hypersensitivity response and is thought to be different from classical DTH. In fact, there is evidence to indicate that cytolytic CD8+ T-cells are required for the expression of CH responses to dinitrofluorobenzene (DNFB) *(56)*. Furthermore, DETCs present in the skin also play a role in contact dermatitis *(57,58)*.

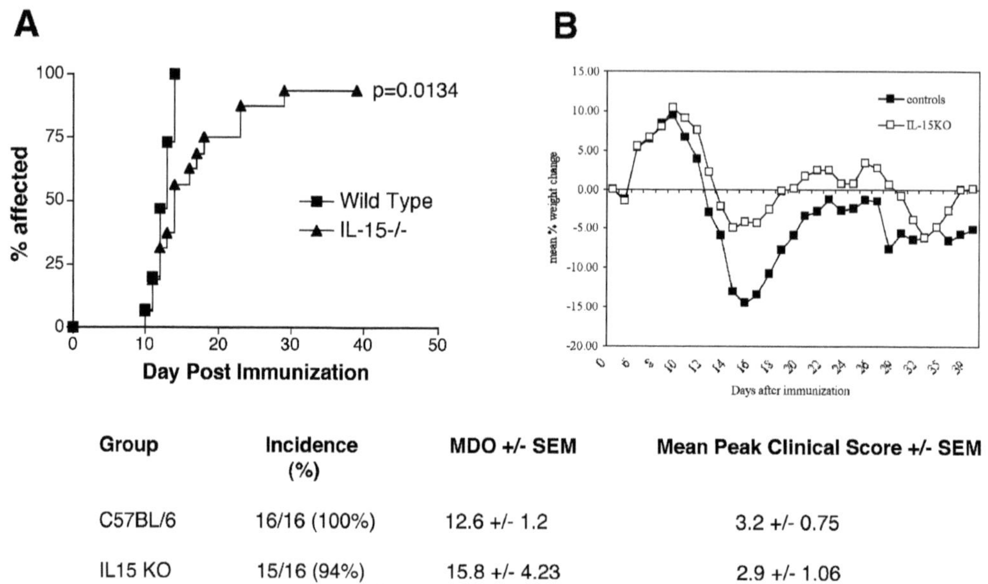

Group	Incidence (%)	MDO +/- SEM	Mean Peak Clinical Score +/- SEM
C57BL/6	16/16 (100%)	12.6 +/- 1.2	3.2 +/- 0.75
IL15 KO	15/16 (94%)	15.8 +/- 4.23	2.9 +/- 1.06

Fig. 5. Interleukin-15 knockout (IL-15 KO) mice have a slower rate of onset and reduced weight loss but a similar incidence of EAE compared with controls. Mice were immunized subcutaneously in the back on d 0 with 100 μg MOG_{35-55} in RIBI adjuvant. On d 2, all mice were injected intravenously with 200 ng pertussis toxin. Mice were weighed and graded per standard guidelines for the next 35–40 d. The data shown are pooled from two experiments. (**A**) Kaplan-Meier curves showing onset and incidence of EAE. The onset curves are significantly different ($p = 0.0134$). (**B**) Weight changes associated with EAE in C57BL/6 and IL-15 knockout mice (affected mice only). ($p = 0.0084$ on d 16, Student's t-test).

As described above, IL-15 knockout mice have a defect in development of DETCs. To study the functional consequence of the lack of DETC, we used the irritant DNFB to study CH responses in IL-15 knockout mice. Both IL-15 knockout and wild-type mice mounted specific responses to DNFB, which were of similar magnitude (Fig. 4B). These results indicate that IL-15 is not required for CH responses to DNFB. Furthermore, neither the defect in CD8 memory T-cells nor the absence of DETC in the skin of IL-15 knockout mice affects the ability of these mice to mount CH responses to DNFB.

3.8. Susceptibility of IL-15 Knockout Mice to EAE

Experimental autoimmune encephalomyelitis (EAE) is a T-cell-dependent inflammatory and demyelinating disease of the central nervous system (CNS) and is considered a model for multiple sclerosis (MS). In addition, it has been suggested that NK cells are important for the development of EAE, as depletion of NK cells caused a delay and reduced severity of EAE, induced by myelin oligodendrocyte glycoprotein (MOG) peptide (MOG_{35-55}) in C57BL/6 mice *(59,60)*. Furthermore, it has been shown by multiple groups that NK T-cell activation either potentiates or protects mice against MOG_{35-55}-induced EAE in C57BL/6 mice *(61–64)*.

Because IL-15 knockout mice have a functional defect in NK cells and also show decreased numbers of NK T-cells, we asked whether EAE induced by MOG_{35-55} would be altered in

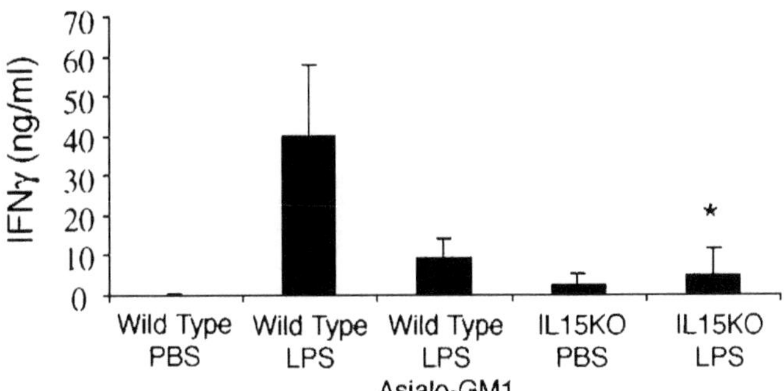

Fig. 6. Interleukin-15 knockout (IL-15 KO) mice are unable to make interferon-γ (IFN-γ) in response to acute lipopolysaccharide (LPS) challenge. C57BL/6 or IL-15 knockout mice were injected on d 0 with 200 μg LPS intraperitoneally. One group of C57BL/6 mice was injected with 200 μg asialo-GM1 intraperitoneally on d 1 and d 0 to deplete NK cells. Other mice received PBS injections. Serum from mice was isolated 7 h after LPS injection. The concentration of IFN-γ in serum of individual mice was analyzed using a standard ELISA protocol. $*p = 0.0406$ compared with C57BL/6, Student's *t*-test.

these mice. IL-15 knockout mice were susceptible to MOG_{35-55}-induced EAE and developed disease with a similar incidence and severity of clinical signs of paralysis compared with the controls (Fig. 5 and data not shown). However, the IL-15 knockout mice exhibited a slight delay in the onset of disease and lost less weight than the control mice. The observation that IL-15 knockout mice lost less weight despite having similar signs of paralysis compared with the control group suggests that weight loss is a more sensitive measure of disease activity and/or that weight loss and paralysis associated with EAE are regulated independently of one another *(65)*.

3.9. Defective IFN-γ Production in IL-15 Knockout Mice in Response to LPS

NK cells are important sources of interferon-γ (IFN-γ) during the initial stages of a bacterial infection *(66,67)*. It has also been suggested that NK cells are the main producers of IFN-γ in response to acute LPS challenge. Normal mice depleted of NK cells (using anti-asialoGM1 or anti-NK1.1) do not show an increase in IFN-γ in their serum in response to LPS injection *(68,69)*. We tested the IFN-γ response to LPS challenge in IL-15 knockout mice. As shown in Fig. 6, IFN-γ is increased in the serum of wild-type controls, but not IL-15 knockout mice, in response to challenge with LPS. These results are consistent with a requirement for NK cells in the innate immune response to bacterial antigens.

3.10. IL-15 Is Critical in Early Activation of APCs

Cytokines that are induced in response to infection may contribute to the initiation of immune responses through their ability to stimulate dendritic cells (DCs) and macrophages. Mattei et al. *(70)* reported that expression of both IL-15 and IL-15Rα chain are increased in splenic DCs from mice injected with dsRNA [poly(I:C)], LPS, or IFN-αβ and in purified mouse splenic DCs treated with IFN-αβ in vitro. Furthermore, IL-15 activates DCs in vitro and in vivo, as evidenced by an increase in their secretion of IFN-γ, upregulation of CD40, CD86, and MHC class II, and enhanced ability to stimulate Ag-specific proliferation of CD8

T-cells. Surprisingly, splenic DCs from IL-15-injected mice did not have an increased ability to stimulate Ag-specific proliferation of CD4 T-cells. The mechanism for the difference in the ability of IL-15-activated DCs to stimulate CD8 but not CD4 T-cells is unknown.

Ohteki et al. *(71)* analyzed DC number and function in IL-2-, IL-15-, IL-2Rβ-, and γc-deficient mice. Numbers of splenic CD8α+ and CD8α– DCs and macrophages are normal in IL-15-deficient mice. However, the production of IL-12p70 by splenic DCs and peritoneal macrophages is severely impaired in IL-15-, IL-2Rβ-, and γc-deficient, but not in IL-2-deficient mice. Exogenous IL-15 did not reverse the defect in IL-12p70 production by DCs from IL-15 knockout mice. In response to IL-12, IL-15 knockout DCs produced lower amounts of IFN-γ and nitric oxide (NO) compared with control or IL-2 knockout mice. However, the defect in IFN-γ and NO production by IL-15 knockout DC was restored by addition of IL-15. Furthermore, expression of IL-12Rβ RNA was significantly lower in DCs and peritoneal macrophages isolated from IL-15 knockout mice compared with controls, suggesting that the lower response to IL-12 by IL-15 knockout DCs may be owing in part to the lower expression of IL-12Rβ.

Based on these data, the authors propose that IL-15 plays a dual role in antigen-presenting cell (APC) maturation and function. The first role involves the exposure of DCs and macrophages to IL-15 during maturation. In normal mice, exposure of APCs to IL-15 during maturation leads to normal expression of IL-12Rβ. However, in IL-15 and IL-2Rβ knockout mice, APCs express lower levels of IL-12Rβ. Addition of IL-15 in vitro does not restore normal IL-12Rβ expression. A second role of IL-15 is in IL-12 production, which in turn controls IFN-γ and NO production by DCs and macrophages. The defect in IFN-γ and NO production by IL-15 knockout DCs is reversed by exogenous IL-15.

These data suggest that IL-15 is a crucial player in the innate immune response—it plays an important role in APC function and activation that leads to efficient adaptive immune responses, and it also plays an important role in NK cell maturation and function. It is possible that this defect in IL-15 knockout APCs is antigen- and immune response-dependent, as IL-15 knockout mice do show normal responses to some antigens, as specified above. However, it might account for the reduced primary antiviral response against VSV in the IL-15 knockout mice that has been demonstrated by Schluns et al. *(42)*. In preliminary experiments, we have been unable to show any differences in the ability of DCs isolated from IL-15 knockout mice to stimulate antigen-specific responses by CD4 and CD8 T-cells in vitro (data not shown).

3.11. Potential Protective Role for IL-15 in IBD

The pathology of IBD is dependent on multiple cell types, cytokines, and inflammatory mediators. It is hypothesized that the persistent inflammation and pathology observed in IBD may be a consequence of an increased or aberrant immune response to normal gut constituents or an overall dysregulation and imbalance of the immune system. Increased IL-15 mRNA has been reported in inflamed tissue from both Crohn's disease and ulcerative colitis patients *(72,73)*.

Both IL-15 and IL-15Rα knockout mice have reduced numbers of a specific CD8αα TCRαβ subset of IEL. Recent studies have shown that IL-15 is a growth factor for the CD8αα TCRαβ subset of IELs *(74)* and that this population of IELs is absent in IL-2Rβ knockout mice *(75)*. Furthermore subsets of IELs have been implicated in the maintenance of mucosal tolerance that is thought to be essential for preventing IBD *(76)*. Thus it is possible that

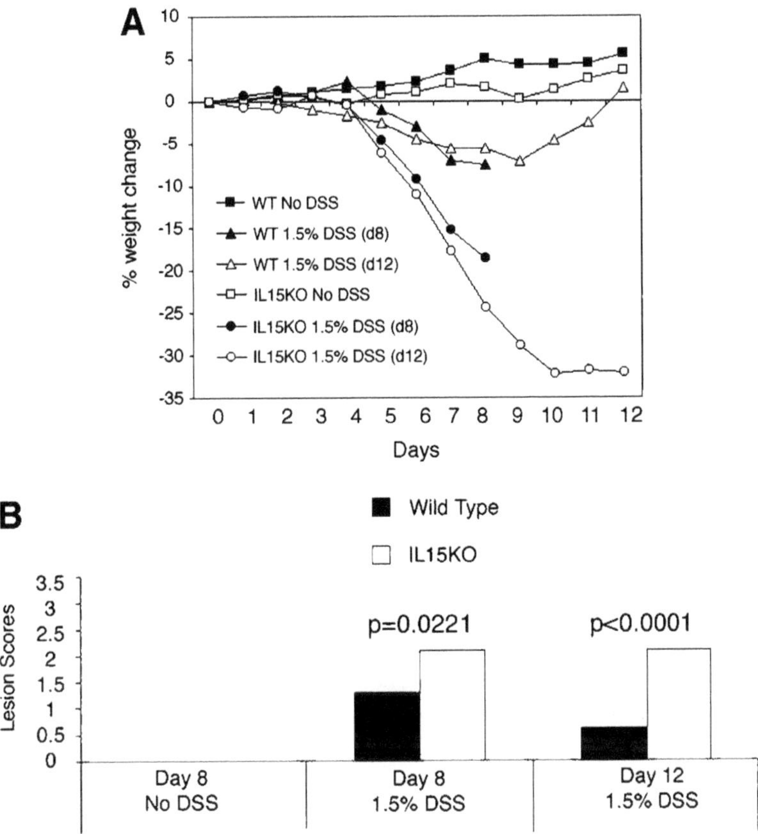

Fig. 7. Interleukin-15 knockout (IL-15 KO) mice show increased susceptibility to dextran sodium sulfate (DSS)-induced colitis. Wild-type C57BL/6 or IL-15 knockout mice were given water alone (squares) or 1.5% DSS in water (triangles and circles) from d 0 to 7. (**A**) Weights of individual mice were monitored on a daily basis. The data show the average percent weight change for each group ($n = 6$/group). The weight loss seen in the IL-15 knockout mice is statistically significant compared with control mice ($p < 0.01$ on d 8; $p < 0.0001$ on d 12). (**B**) Groups of six mice were sacrificed on d 8 and d 12. The ileum, cecum, and colon from individual mice were removed, fixed in formalin, paraffin-embedded, sectioned, and stained with hematoxylin and eosin. The histopathology was done in a blinded fashion using a standard scoring regimen. The total lesion scores shown are for the cecum and colon. No inflammation was seen in the ileum (data not shown).

IL-15 knockout and IL-15Rα knockout mice might have altered immune responses in the gut owing to the absence of specific IEL populations and/or to the absence of IL-15 during inflammatory responses within the gut.

To explore the role of IL-15 in a model of IBD, we used the dextran sodium sulfate (DSS)-induced model of colitis in wild-type and IL-15 knockout mice. As shown in Fig. 7A, control mice lose weight over the course of DSS administration (d 0–7) and regain weight after removal of DSS (d 8–12). In contrast, IL-15 knockout mice showed increased weight loss at the same DSS dose during the course of DSS administration and failed to regain weight after removal of DSS. This severity in weight loss is reflected in the histopathology scores of the colon and cecum. As shown in Fig. 7B, IL-15 knockout mice show increased lesion scores at both d 8 and d 12 of disease compared with controls. Wild-type mice given DSS had consistent mild to moderate changes in the distal colon and minimal to mild changes in the proximal colon and cecum on d 8. In contrast, IL-15 knockout mice developed moderate to severe lesions in the distal colon, often with severe necrosis and ulceration of the mucosa. By d 12, lesions in the wild-type mice were resolving, with evidence of regeneration of the crypt epithelium, reduced inflammation, and lack of ulceration. In contrast, lesions in IL-15 knockout mice remained moderate to severe, with a significant amount of ulceration and necrosis still present. Thus, IL-15 knockout mice are more susceptible to DSS-induced colitis and fail to recover after removal of DSS. This observation was independent of the strain of mice used, as IL-15 knockout mice on the BALB/c background also showed increased severity in colitis scores compared with their wild-type controls (data not shown).

It is possible that IL-15 acts directly on epithelial cells and induces regenerative factors for the epithelium during the recovery phase of colitis in this model. This theory is consistent with the recent observation by Shinozaki et al. described below. The protective effect of IL-15 on epithelial cells may also be responsible for the observation that IL-15 offers selective protection from irinotecan-induced intestinal toxicity in preclinical animal models *(77)*. Irinotecan (CPT-11) is a chemotherapeutic agent that is used in the treatment of a variety of solid tumor malignancies. Diarrhea represents the most common dose-limiting toxicity in these patients. In this model, IL-15 acts as an antiinflammatory agent, probably by acting directly on the epithelial cells.

3.12. IL-15 Knockout Mice Are More Susceptible to Nephrotoxic Serum Nephritis

Shinozaki and colleagues *(78)* induced nephrotoxic serum nephritis (NSN) in wild-type and IL-15 knockout mice and were surprised to find that IL-15 knockout mice had more damaging pathology and loss of renal function than wild-type controls. They showed that IL-2/IL-15R chains and IL-15 are expressed in tubular epithelial cells in wild-type mice and that IL-15 acts as an autocrine survival factor for these epithelial cells *(78)*. Furthermore, in vivo studies showed that IL-15 decreased induction of a nephritogenic chemokine, macrophage chemottractant protein-1 (MCP-1), in the kidney during NSN. IL-15 has also been shown to inhibit IL-1β-induced IL-8 and MCP-1 secretion in human colonic epithelial cells *(79)*.

4. Conclusions

The role of IL-15 in immune responses can be broadly classified into four major categories

- NK cell, IEL, DETC differentiation, survival, and activation
- Memory CD8 T-cell proliferation and survival
- Role in APC function
- Role in epithelial cell survival during inflammation

Characterization of both IL15 and IL-15Rα knockout mice revealed that IL-15 is a crucial factor in NK cell maturation and survival. The demonstration that APCs from IL-15 knockout mice are defective in IFN-γ and NO production compared with controls provides additional evidence that IL-15 is important for innate immunity.

Although the generation of primary and memory CD8 T-cell responses appears to be largely independent of IL-15, it is clear that IL-15 plays an important role in maintaining homeostasis of CD8, but not CD4, T-cells. IL-15 is crucial for the long-term survival of memory CD8 T-cells and for the bystander proliferation of naive CD8 T-cells. The differential effect of IL-15 on CD8 versus CD4 T-cells can be explained in part by the increased expression of IL-15Rα on CD8 compared with CD4 T-cells. However, the observation that IL-15-stimulated DCs have an enhanced ability to activate CD8, but not CD4, T-cells in vitro suggests that IL-15-induced effects on APC function in vivo may also contribute to the differential role of IL-15 with regard to CD8 versus CD4 T-cell responses.

More recent analyses of IL-15 knockout mice have changed our view of IL-15 as a proinflammatory cytokine that activates NK and CD8 T-cells to one that can also be characterized as antiinflammatory based on its protective effect on epithelial cells. IL-15 is a survival factor for kidney epithelial cells and inhibits IL-1β-induced chemokine production by intestinal epithelial cells. These observations suggest that during inflammation involving epithelial cells, IL-15 can inhibit inflammation by enhancing epithelial cell survival and by inhibiting the ability of epithelial cells to attract inflammatory cells.

IL-15 has emerged as a crucial cytokine affecting both innate and adaptive immune responses. Use of the IL-15 and IL-15Rα knockout mice has enabled us to understand the role for these molecules in immune responses and multiple disease models. Based on our current understanding, IL-15 and IL-15Rα could serve as targets for therapy in some human diseases. Blocking IL-15 functions may be beneficial in some models, whereas use of the cytokine itself as a therapeutic either as an antiinflammatory (IBD, kidney disease) or as an immune activator (vaccines, tumor therapy) may also prove to be beneficial. In conclusion, we suggest that targeting IL-15 or its receptor as a therapeutic should be strongly considered.

Acknowledgments

The authors would like to acknowledge the members of the Pathology Department at Amgen, specifically Suzanne Kanaly for histology analysis. We appreciate the helpful discussions provided by Eric Butz and Jacques Peschon on the characterization of these knockout mice. The authors thank Moira Glacuum for maintaining this line at Amgen. The IL-15 knockout mice are available commercially through the Taconic Emerging Models Program (http://www.taconic.com/emerging/004200.htm).

References

1. Burton, J. D., Bamford, R. N., Peters, C., et al. (1994) A lymphokine, provisionally designated interleukin T and produced by a human adult T-cell leukemia line, stimulates T-cell proliferation and the induction of lymphokine-activated killer cells. *Proc. Natl. Acad. Sci. USA* **91,** 4935–4939.
2. Grabstein, K. H., Eisenman, J., Shanebeck, K., et al. (1994) Cloning of a T cell growth factor that interacts with the β chain of the interleukin-2 receptor. *Science* **264,** 965–968.
3. Bazan, J. F. (1990) Haemopoietic receptors and helical cytokines. *Immunol. Today* **11,** 350–354.
4. Bamford, R. N., Grant, A. J., Burton, J. D., et al. (1994) The interleukin (IL) 2 receptor beta chain is shared by IL-2 and a cytokine, provisionally designated IL-T, that stimulates T-cell proliferation and the induction of lymphokine-activated killer cells. *Proc. Natl. Acad. Sci. USA* **91,** 4940–4944.
5. Carson, W. E., Giri, J. G., Lindemann, M. J., et al. (1994) Interleukin (IL) 15 is a novel cytokine that activates human natural killer cells via components of the IL-2 receptor. *J. Exp. Med.* **180,** 1395–1403.

6. Giri, J. G., Ahdieh, M., Eisenman, J., et al. (1994) Utilization of the β and γ chains of the IL-2 receptor by the novel cytokine IL-15. *EMBO J.* **13,** 2822–2830.
7. Giri, J. G., Kumaki, S., Ahdieh, M., et al. (1995) Identification and cloning of a novel IL-15 binding protein that is structurally related to the α chain of the IL-2 receptor. *EMBO J.* **14,** 3654–3663.
8. Anderson, D. M., Kumaki, S., Ahdieh, M., et al. (1995) Functional characterization of the human interleukin-15 receptor alpha chain and close linkage of IL15RA and IL2RA genes. *J. Biol. Chem.* **270,** 29862–29869.
9. Fehniger, T. A. and Caligiuri, M. A. (2001) Interleukin 15: biology and relevance to human disease. *Blood* **97,** 14–32.
10. Waldmann, T. A., Dubois, S., and Tagaya, Y. (2001) Contrasting roles of IL-2 and IL-15 in the life and death of lymphocytes: implications for immunotherapy. *Immunity* **14,** 105–110.
11. Kundig, T. M., Schorle, H., Bachmann, M. F., Hengartner, H., Zinkernagel, R. M., and Horak, I. (1993) Immune responses in interleukin-2-deficient mice. *Science* **262,** 1059–1061.
12. Suzuki, H., Kundig, T. M., Furlonger, C., et al. (1995) Deregulated T cell activation and autoimmunity in mice lacking interleukin-2 receptor beta. *Science* **268,** 1472–1476.
13. Willerford, D. M., Chen, J., Ferry, J. A., Davidson, L., Ma, A., and Alt, F. W. (1995) Interleukin-2 receptor α chain regulates the size and content of the peripheral lymphoid compartment. *Immunity* **3,** 521–530.
14. Suzuki, H., Duncan, G. S., Takimoto, H., and Mak, T. W. (1997) Abnormal development of intestinal intraepithelial lymphocytes and peripheral natural killer cells in mice lacking the IL-2 receptor β chain. *J. Exp. Med.* **185,** 499–505.
15. Ohteki, T., Ho, S., Suzuki, H., Mak, T. W., and Ohashi, P. S. (1997) Role for IL-15/IL-15 receptor beta-chain in natural killer 1.1+ T cell receptor-alpha beta+ cell development. *J. Immunol.* **159,** 5931–5935.
16. Boesteanu, A., De Silva, A. D., Nakajima, H., Leonard, W. J., Peschon, J. J., and Joyce, S. (1997) Distinct roles for signals relayed through the common cytokine receptor γ chain and interleukin 7 receptor α chain in natural T cell development. *J. Exp. Med.* **186,** 331–336.
17. Di Santo, J. P., Colucci, F., and Guy-Grand, D. (1998) Natural killer and T cells of innate and adaptive immunity: lymphoid compartments with different requirements for common gamma chain-dependent cytokines. *Immunol. Rev.* **165,** 29–38.
18. Mrozek, E., Anderson, P., and Caligiuri, M. A. (1996) Role of interleukin-15 in the development of human CD56+ natural killer cells from CD34+ hematopoietic progenitor cells. *Blood* **87,** 2632–2640.
19. Puzanov, I. J., Bennett, M., and Kumar, V. (1996) IL-15 can substitute for the marrow microenvironment in the differentiation of natural killer cells. *J. Immunol.* **157,** 4282–4285.
20. Ohteki, T., Yoshida, H., Matsuyama, T., Duncan, G. S., Mak, T. W., and Ohashi, P. S. (1998) The transcription factor interferon regulatory factor 1 (IRF-1) is important during the maturation of natural killer 1.1+ T cell receptor-alpha/beta+ (NK1+ T) cells, natural killer cells, and intestinal intraepithelial T cells. *J. Exp. Med.* **187,** 967–972.
21. Inagaki-Ohara, K., Nishimura, H., Mitani, A., and Yoshikai, Y. (1997) Interleukin-15 preferentially promotes the growth of intestinal intraepithelial lymphocytes bearing gamma delta T cell receptor in mice. *Eur. J. Immunol.* **27,** 2885–2891.
22. Zhang, X., Sun, S., Hwang, I., Tough, D. F., and Sprent, J. (1998) Potent and selective stimulation of memory-phenotype CD8+ T cells in vivo by IL-15. *Immunity* **8,** 591–599.
23. Quinn, L. S., Haugk, K. L., and Grabstein, K. H. (1995) Interleukin-15: a novel anabolic cytokine for skeletal muscle. *Endocrinology* **136,** 3669–3672.
24. Ogata, Y., Kukita, A., Kukita, T., et al. (1999) A novel role of IL-15 in the development of osteoclasts: inability to replace its activity with IL-2. *J. Immunol.* **162,** 2754–2760.
25. Tagaya, Y., Burton, J. D., Miyamoto, Y., and Waldmann, T. A. (1996) Identification of a novel receptor/signal transduction pathway for IL-15/T in mast cells. *EMBO J.* **15,** 4928–4939.
26. Reinecker, H. C., MacDermott, R. P., Mirau, S., Dignass, A., and Podolsky, D. K. (1996) Intestinal epithelial cells both express and respond to interleukin 15. *Gastroenterology* **111,** 1706–1713.
27. Bulfone-Pau, S. S., Bulanova, E., Pohl, T., et al. (1999) Death deflected: IL-15 inhibits TNF-alpha-mediated apoptosis in fibroblasts by TRAF2 recruitment to the IL-15Ralpha chain. *FASEB J.* **13,** 1575–1585.

28. Kennedy, M. K., Glaccum, M., Brown, S. N., et al. (2000) Reversible defects in natural killer and memory CD8 T cell lineages in interleukin 15-deficient mice [see comments]. *J. Exp. Med.* **191,** 771–780.
29. Lodolce, J. P., Boone, D. L., Chai, S., et al. (1998) IL-15 receptor maintains lymphoid homeostasis by supporting lymphocyte homing and proliferation. *Immunity* **9,** 669–676.
30. Anderson, D. M., Johnson, L., Glaccum, M. B., et al. (1995) Chromosomal assignment and genomic structure of Il15. *Genomics* **25,** 701–706.
31. Krause, H., Jandrig, B., Wernicke, C., Bulfone-Paus, S., Pohl, T., and Diamantstein, T. (1996) Genomic structure and chromosomal localization of the human interleukin 15 gene (IL-15). *Cytokine* **8,** 667–674.
32. Williams, N. S., Moore, T. A., Schatzle, J. D., et al. (1997) Generation of lytic natural killer 1.1$^+$, Ly-49$^-$ cells from multipotential murine bone marrow progenitors in a stroma-free culture: definition of cytokine requirements and developmental intermediates. *J. Exp. Med.* **186,** 1609–1614.
33. Williams, N. S., Klem, J., Puzanov, I. J., Sivakumar, P. V., Bennett, M., and Kumar, V. (1999) Differentiation of NK1.1+, Ly49+ NK cells from flt3+ multipotent marrow progenitor cells. *J. Immunol.* **163,** 2648–2656.
34. Cooper, M. A., Bush, J. E., Fehniger, T. A., et al. (2002) In vivo evidence for a dependence on interleukin-15 for natural killer cell survival. *Blood* **10,** 3633–3638.
35. Edelbaum, D., Mohamadzadeh, M., Bergstresser, P. R., Sugamura, K., and Takashima, A. (1995) Interleukin (IL)-15 promotes the growth of murine epidermal gamma delta T cells by a mechanism involving the beta- and gamma c-chains of the IL- 2 receptor. *J. Invest. Dermatol.* **105,** 837–843.
36. Kawai, K., Suzuki, H., Tomiyama, K., Minagawa, M., Mak, T. W., and Ohashi, P. S. (1998) Requirement of the IL-2 receptor beta chain for the development of Vgamma3 dendritic epidermal T cells. *J. Invest. Dermatol.* **110,** 961–965.
37. Ye, S. K., Maki, K., Lee, H. C., et al. (2001) Differential roles of cytokine receptors in the development of epidermal gamma delta T cells. *J. Immunol.* **167,** 1929–1934.
38. De Creus, A., Van Beneden, K., Stevenaert, F., Debacker, V., Plum, J., and Leclercq, G. (2002) Developmental and functional defects of thymic and epidermal V gamma 3 cells in IL-15-deficient and IFN regulatory factor-1-deficient mice. *J. Immunol.* **168,** 6486–6493.
39. Karupiah, G., Woodhams, C. E., Blanden, R. V., and Ramshaw, I. A. (1991) Immunobiology of infection with recombinant vaccinia virus encoding murine IL-2. Mechanisms of rapid viral clearance in immunocompetent mice. *J. Immunol.* **147,** 4327–4332.
40. Buller, R. M. and Palumbo, G. J. (1991) Poxvirus pathogenesis. *Microbiol. Rev.* **55,** 80–122.
41. Ruby, J. and Ramshaw, I. (1991) The antiviral activity of immune CD8+ T cells is dependent on interferon-gamma. *Lymphokine Cytokine Res.* **10,** 353–358.
42. Schluns, K. S., Williams, K., Ma, A., Zheng, X. X., and Lefrancois, L. (2002) Cutting edge: requirement for IL-15 in the generation of primary and memory antigen-specific CD8 T cells. *J. Immunol.* **168,** 4827–4831.
43. Becker, T. C., Wherry, E. J., Boone, D., et al. (2002) Interleukin 15 is required for proliferative renewal of virus-specific memory CD8 T cells. *J. Exp. Med.* **195,** 1541–1548.
44. Murali-Krishna, K., Lau, L. L., Sambhara, S., Lemonnier, F., Altman, J., and Ahmed, R. (1999) Persistence of memory CD8 T cells in MHC class I-deficient mice. *Science* **286,** 1377–1381.
45. Swain, S. L., Hu, H., and Huston, G. (1999) Class II-independent generation of CD4 memory T cells from effectors. *Science* **286,** 1381–1383.
46. Kassiotis, G., Garcia, S., Simpson, E., and Stockinger, B. (2002) Impairment of immunological memory in the absence of MHC despite survival of memory T cells. *Nat. Immunol.* **3,** 244–250.
47. Rocha, B. (2002) Requirements for memory maintenance. *Nat. Immunol.* **3,** 209–210.
48. Yajima, T., Nishimura, H., Ishimitsu, R., et al. (2002) Overexpression of IL-15 in vivo increases antigen-driven memory CD8+ T cells following a microbe exposure. *J. Immunol.* **168,** 1198–1203.
49. Fehniger, T. A., Suzuki, K., Ponnappan, A., et al. (2001) Fatal leukemia in interleukin 15 transgenic mice follows early expansions in natural killer and memory phenotype CD8+ T cells. *J. Exp. Med.* **193,** 219–231.
50. Goldrath, A. W., Sivakumar, P. V., Glaccum, M., et al. (2002) Cytokine requirements for acute and basal homeostatic proliferation of naive and memory CD8+ T cells. *J. Exp. Med.* **195,** 1515–1522.

51. Hogquist, K. A., Jameson, S. C., Heath, W. R., Howard, J. L., Bevan, M. J., and Carbone, F. R. (1994) T cell receptor antagonist peptides induce positive selection. *Cell* **76,** 17–27.
52. Tan, J. T., Ernst, B., Kieper, W. C., LeRoy, E., Sprent, J., and Surh, C. D. (2002) Interleukin (IL)-15 and IL-7 jointly regulate homeostatic proliferation of memory phenotype CD8+ cells but are not required for memory phenotype CD4+ cells. *J. Exp. Med.* **195,** 1523–1532.
53. Lodolce, J. P., Burkett, P. R., Boone, D. L., Chien, M., and Ma, A. (2001) T cell-independent interleukin 15Ralpha signals are required for bystander proliferation. *J. Exp. Med.* **194,** 1187–1194.
54. Miller, R. E., Jones, J., Le, T., et al. (2002) 4-1BB-specific monoclonal antibody promotes the generation of tumor-specific immune responses by direct activation of CD8 T cells in a CD40-dependent manner. *J. Immunol.* **169,** 1792–1800.
55. Kim, Y. S., Maslinski, W., Zheng, X. X., et al. (1998) Targeting the IL-15 receptor with an antagonist IL-15 mutant/Fc gamma2a protein blocks delayed-type hypersensitivity. *J. Immunol.* **160,** 5742–5748.
56. Kehren, J., Desvignes, C., Krasteva, M., et al. (1999) Cytotoxicity is mandatory for CD8(+) T cell-mediated contact hypersensitivity. *J. Exp. Med.* **189,** 779–786.
57. Kaminski, M. J., Bergstresser, P. R., and Takashima, A. (1993) In vivo activation of mouse dendritic epidermal T cells in sites of contact dermatitis. *Eur. J. Immunol.* **23,** 1715–1718.
58. Shiohara, T. and Moriya, N. (1997) Epidermal T cells: their functional role and disease relevance for dermatologists. *J. Invest. Dermatol.* **109,** 271–275.
59. Zhang, B., Yamamura, T., Kondo, T., Fujiwara, M., and Tabira, T. (1997) Regulation of experimental autoimmune encephalomyelitis by natural killer (NK) cells. *J. Exp. Med.* **186,** 1677–1687.
60. Shi, F. D., Takeda, K., Akira, S., Sarvetnick, N., and Ljunggren, H. G. (2000) IL-18 directs autoreactive T cells and promotes autodestruction in the central nervous system via induction of IFN-gamma by NK cells. *J. Immunol.* **165,** 3099–3104.
61. Singh, A. K., Wilson, M. T., Hong, S., et al. (2001) Natural killer T cell activation protects mice against experimental autoimmune encephalomyelitis. *J. Exp. Med.* **194,** 1801–1811.
62. Jahng, A. W., Maricic, I., Pedersen, B., et al. (2001) Activation of natural killer T cells potentiates or prevents experimental autoimmune encephalomyelitis. *J. Exp. Med.* **194,** 1789–1799.
63. Fritz, R. B. and Zhao, M. L. (2001) Regulation of experimental autoimmune encephalomyelitis in the C57BL/6J mouse by NK1.1+, DX5+, alpha beta+ T cells. *J. Immunol.* **166,** 4209–4215.
64. Pal, E., Tabira, T., Kawano, T., Taniguchi, M., Miyake, S., and Yamamura, T. (2001) Costimulation-dependent modulation of experimental autoimmune encephalomyelitis by ligand stimulation of V alpha 14 NK T cells. *J. Immunol.* **166,** 662–668.
65. Encinas, J. A., Lees, M. B., Sobel, R. A., et al. (2001) Identification of genetic loci associated with paralysis, inflammation and weight loss in mouse experimental autoimmune encephalomyelitis. *Int. Immunol.* **13,** 257–264.
66. Fehniger, T. A., Yu, H., Cooper, M. A., Suzuki, K., Shah, M. H., and Caligiuri, M. A. (2000) Cutting edge: IL-15 costimulates the generalized Shwartzman reaction and innate immune IFN-gamma production in vivo. *J. Immunol.* **164,** 1643–1647.
67. Seki, S., Habu, Y., Kawamura, T., et al. (2000) The liver as a crucial organ in the first line of host defense: the roles of Kupffer cells, natural killer (NK) cells and NK1.1 Ag+ T cells in T helper 1 immune responses. *Immunol. Rev.* **174,** 35–46.
68. Kim, S., Iizuka, K., Aguila, H. L., Weissman, I. L., and Yokoyama, W. M. (2000) In vivo natural killer cell activities revealed by natural killer cell-deficient mice. *Proc. Natl. Acad. Sci. USA* **97,** 2731–2736.
69. Lindemann, R. A. (1991) The regulatory effects of monocytes on human natural killer cells activated by lipopolysaccharides. *J. Periodontal Res.* **26,** 486–490.
70. Mattei, F., Schiavoni, G., Belardelli, F., and Tough, D. F. (2001) IL-15 is expressed by dendritic cells in response to type I IFN, double-stranded RNA, or lipopolysaccharide and promotes dendritic cell activation. *J. Immunol.* **167,** 1179–1187.
71. Ohteki, T., Suzue, K., Maki, C., Ota, T., and Koyasu, S. (2001) Critical role of IL-15-IL-15R for antigen-presenting cell functions in the innate immune response. *Nat. Immunol.* **2,** 1138–1143.
72. Kirman, I. and Nielsen, O. H. (1996) Increased numbers of interleukin-15-expressing cells in active ulcerative colitis. *Am. J. Gastroenterol.* **91,** 1789–1794.

73. Liu, Z., Geboes, K., Colpaert, S., D'Haens, G. R., Rutgeerts, P., and Ceuppens, J. L. (2000) IL-15 is highly expressed in inflammatory bowel disease and regulates local T cell-dependent cytokine production. *J. Immunol.* **164,** 3608–3615.
74. Lai, Y. G., Gelfanov, V., Gelfanova, V., et al. (1999) IL-15 promotes survival but not effector function differentiation of CD8+ TCRalphabeta+ intestinal intraepithelial lymphocytes. *J. Immunol.* **163,** 5843–5850.
75. Porter, B. O. and Malek, T. R. (1999) IL-2Rbeta/IL-7Ralpha doubly deficient mice recapitulate the thymic and intraepithelial lymphocyte (IEL) developmental defects of gammac-/- mice: roles for both IL-2 and IL-15 in CD8alphaalpha IEL development. *J. Immunol.* **163,** 5906–5912.
76. Nielsen, O. H., Vainer, B., Bregenholt, S., Claesson, M. H., Bishop, P. D., and Kirman, I. (1997) Inflammatory bowel disease: potential therapeutic strategies. *Cytokines Cell. Mol. Ther.* **3,** 267–281.
77. Cao, S., Black, J. D., Troutt, A. B., and Rustum, Y. M. (1998) Interleukin 15 offers selective protection from irinotecan-induced intestinal toxicity in a preclinical animal model. *Cancer Res.* **58,** 3270–3274.
78. Shinozaki, M., Hirahashi, J., Lebedeva, T., et al. (2002) IL-15, a survival factor for kidney epithelial cells, counteracts apoptosis and inflammation during nephritis. *J. Clin. Invest.* **109,** 951–960.
79. Lugering, N., Kucharzik, T., Maaser, C., Kraft, M., and Domschke, W. (1999) Interleukin-15 strongly inhibits interleukin-8 and monocyte chemoattractant protein-1 production in human colonic epithelial cells. *Immunology* **98,** 504–509.

18

IL-18 and IL-18 Receptor Knockout Mice

Hiroko Tsutsui, Tomohiro Yoshimoto,
Haruki Okamura, Shizuo Akira, and Kenji Nakanishi

1. Introduction

Interferon-γ (IFN-γ), a primary cytokine for the development of inflammatory responses, plays an essential role in host defense but has the potential to induce pathologic changes. Initially, IFN-γ was believed to be produced by limited sets of cells, such as T-cells and natural killer (NK) cells. T-cells need to develop into T-helper type 1 (Th1) cells to gain the capacity to produce IFN-γ in response to antigen (Ag) *(1)*. In contrast, NK cells can produce IFN-γ in response to IL-12 without such differentiation *(2)*. Discovery of IL-18 significantly changed this scenario for explaining IFN-γ production *(3–10)*. First, upon stimulation with IL-18 and IL-12 without T-cell receptor (TCR) engagement, freshly isolated Th cells and Th1 cells can produce higher levels of IFN-γ than Ag-stimulated Th1 cells. IL-18 only moderately upregulates IFN-γ production by Th1 cells stimulated with TCR engagement. Moreover, IL-18, unlike IL-12, has no activity to induce Th1 cell development in naive Th cells *per se (11)*. These findings suggest a minor role for IL-18 in adaptive immunity, but the importance of IL-18 in innate immunity. Second, IL-18 synergizes with IL-12 for IFN-γ production by a wide range of cell types, including NK cells, and B-cells, macrophages, dendritic cells, and smooth muscle cells *(9,12–15)*. This TCR engagement-independent IFN-γ induction is a unique property of IL-18/IL-12 biology (Fig. 1).

Recently, IL-23p19 was cloned as an IL-12p35 homolog *(16)*. IL-23 is composed of IL-12p40 and IL-23p19, the receptor of which is comprised of IL-12 receptor β1 (Rβ1) and a novel protein, IL-23R *(17)* (Fig. 1). IL-23 has the ability to induce clonal expansion and IFN-γ production by memory Th1 cells, but not naive Th cells, with simultaneous stimulation with TCR engagement (Fig. 1). In contrast to IL-23, IL-27, a recently identified ligand for an orphan receptor whose structure resembles that of IL-6R/IL-12R, together with the stimulation through TCR, can induce rapid clonal expansion and IFN-γ production in naive Th cells, but not in memory Th1 cells *(18–20)* (Fig. 1). Thus, IFN-γ production is guaranteed by the redundant function of these IL-12-related molecules and IL-18. Further study will definitely increase our understanding of their roles in host defense. In this chapter, we describe the biologic roles of endogenous IL-18 in immunity and diseases, with a particular focus on recent articles and experimental findings using IL-18- and/or IL-18R-deficient mice. Detailed information about IL-18 and its receptor is provided by recently published review articles by us and others *(3–10,21,22)*.

From: *Contemporary Immunology: Cytokine Knockouts, 2nd Edition*
Edited by: Giamila Fantuzzi © Humana Press Inc., Totowa, NJ

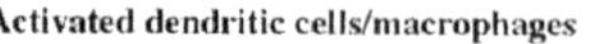

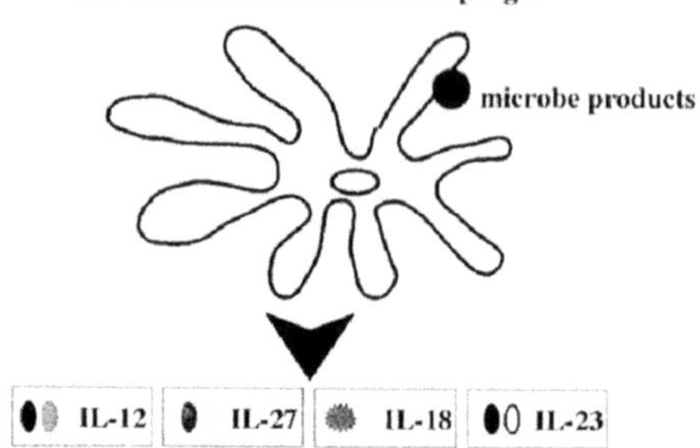

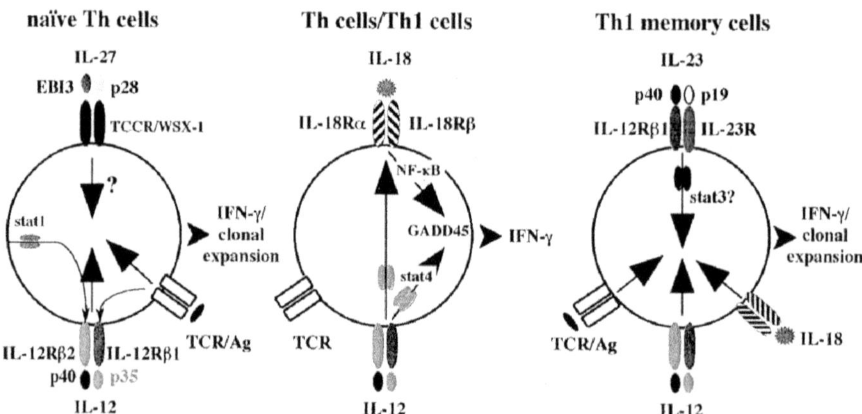

Fig. 1. Clonal expansion and acquirement of interferon-γ (IFN-γ)-producing activity of Th cells. Microbial products stimulate antigen-presenting cells such as dendritic cells to secrete interleukin-12 (IL-12) composed of IL-12p35 and IL-12p40 *(162)*, IL-18 *(163)*, IL-23 composed of p19 and IL-12p40 *(16)*, and IL-27 composed of p28 and Epstein-Barr virus-induced gene 3 (EBI3) *(18)* via the corresponding Toll-like receptor (TLR). IL-27 together with IL-12 stimulates naive Th cells, but not memory Th cells, to expand clonally and produce IFN-γ upon T-cell receptor (TCR) engagement *(18)*. During this activation process, Th cells express IL-12Rβ1 via TCR-mediated activation signals *(2,152)* and IL-12 Rβ2 via IFN-γ-induced stat1 activation *(164)*. IL-12 can induce Th1 cell development in naive Th cells upon TCR engagement even without signaling through IL-27R *(1,19)*, whereas IL-18 does not induce Th1 cell development *(11)*. IL-18 together with IL-12 activates Th and Th1 cells to produce a large amount of IFN-γ without TCR engagement *(44)*, which depends on nuclear factor-κB (NF-κB)/stat4 activation *(59)* and also partly on GADD45-mediated p38 activation *(67,68)*. Stimulation with IL-23 together with TCR engagement selectively activates Th1 memory cells to proliferate and produce IFN-γ via activation of stat3 rather than stat4 *(16)*. IL-12R consists of IL-12Rβ1 and IL-12 Rβ2 *(152)*. IL-18R consists of IL-18Rα and IL-18Rβ *(9)*. IL-27R consists of WSX-1/TCCR *(19,20)*. IL-23R consists of IL-12 Rβ1 and IL-23R *(17)*.

2. Overview of IL-18 and Its Signaling

2.1. Regulation of IL-18 Release

IL-18 has structural homology with IL-1β. Both IL-18 and IL-1β are produced as biologically inactive precursors and become active after cleavage by caspase-1 (originally termed IL-1β-converting enzyme) and other caspase members *(23–27)*. A wide range of cell types, including macrophages, dendritic cells, and keratinocytes, can produce IL-18 as well as IL-1β *(9,10,28)*. Unlike the secretory cytokines, IL-18 is stored intracellularly in these cells, presumably suggesting rapid secretion of biologic active IL-18 in response to stimuli, such as microbe products *(29,30)*. Therefore, the notion that IL-18 secretion is primarily regulated at the levels of its processing, whether by caspase-1 or other caspases, is convincing.

Upon stimulation with lipopolysaccharide (LPS), primary cultured Kupffer cells secrete IL-18 as well as IL-12 depending on Toll-like receptor-4 (TLR4), a signaling receptor for LPS *(29)*. In sharp contrast to IL-12, IL-18 secretion from LPS-stimulated Kupffer cells depends on caspase-1 and requires no *de novo* protein synthesis. Indeed, Kupffer cells constitutively express both proIL-18 and pro-caspase-1 and can secrete a substantial amount of IL-18 in response to LPS even in the presence of transcriptional or translational inhibitors *(29)*. Moreover, myeloid differentiation factor 88 (MyD88), an intracellular adaptor molecule required for signaling through TLRs *(31)*, IL-1R, and IL-18R *(32)* (described below; Fig. 2), is dispensable for LPS-induced IL-18 secretion, because MyD88-deficient Kupffer cells secrete IL-18 but not IL-12 in response to LPS *(29)*. These different pathways for secretion between IL-12 and IL-18 may provide a clue to the possible biologic outcomes caused by IL-18 without IL-12, such as IL-18-mediated Th2 cell responses (described below; Fig. 3).

We and others have demonstrated that stimulation with Fas ligand induces IL-18 and IL-1β release from macrophages and neutrophils, respectively, depending on caspases other than caspase-1 *(26,33)*. Since a broadly acting caspase inhibitor reduces the secretion of these cytokines from caspase-1-deficient cells, we assume that this secretion is also under the control of a caspase. The mechanism underlying IL-1β/IL-18 release via activation of Fas is still to be elucidated.

2.2. IL-18 Signaling

Like IL-1R, IL-18R is composed of a ligand-binding component, IL-18Rα, and a signaling component, IL-18Rβ (Figs. 1 and 2). Both of the components belong to the TLR/IL-1R family *(22)*. In particular, cytoplasmic domains of individual TLR/IL-1R family members, including IL-18Rα and IL-18Rβ, exhibit high homology with each other. Freshly isolated T-cells show binding to IL-18 but with low affinity *(34)*. However, IL-12-stimulated T-cells and Th1 cells express both components of IL-18R and bind to IL-18 with high affinity *(34)*, indicating that both IL-18R components are required for high-affinity binding to IL-18. Like signaling through various TLRs and IL-1R *(31,35)*, upon activation with IL-18, the cytoplasmic domains of both IL-18Rα and IL-18Rβ associate with MyD88, to activate IL-1R-associated kinase (IRAK) and/or perhaps IRAK4 *(36a,36b)* to relay a signal, leading to the activation of nuclear factor κB (NF-κB) and activation protein-1 (AP-1) (Fig. 2). Indeed, MyD88-deficient cells, IRAK-deficient cells, or IRAK-4-deficient cells do not respond to IL-18 as well as IL-1 *(32,36b,37)*. Lymphocytes constitutively express IL-18Rβ *(38)*, whereas IL-18Rα expression is strictly regulated by various stimuli. NK cells constitutively express IL-18Rα, whereas freshly isolated Th cells moderately express it *(34,39)*. Their IL-18Rα expression is upregulated by IL-12 or type 1 IFN in a signal transducer and activator of transcription 4 (STAT4)-dependent manner *(40–42)* and is down-regulated by IL-4 *(43,44)*. Expression is restored by IFN-γ *(45)*. Indeed, Th1 cells express high levels of IL-18Rα, whereas Th2 cells do not express IL-18Rα *(11,34,46,47)*.

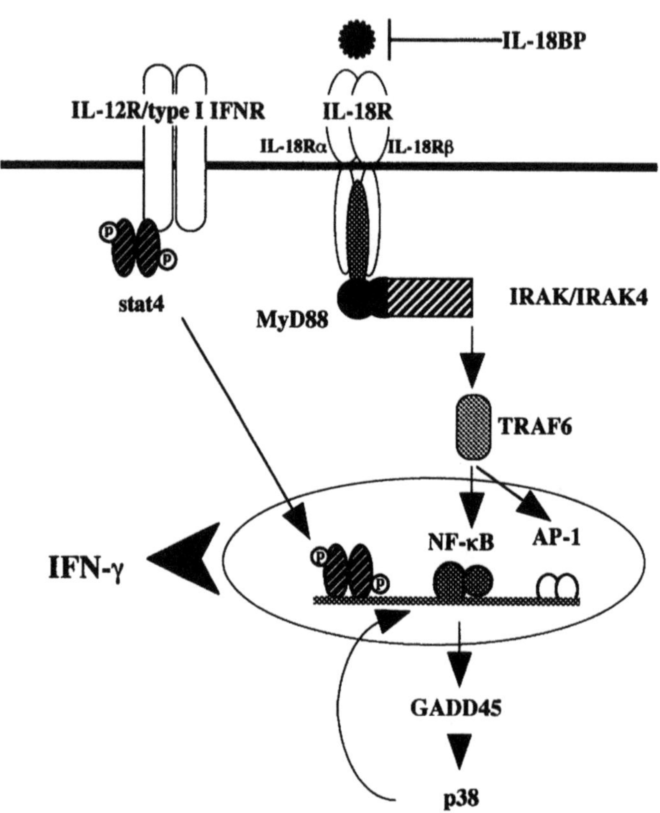

Fig. 2. Synergistic action of interleukin-12 (IL-12) and IL-18 signalings for interferon-γ (IFN-γ). After stimulation with IL-18, nuclear factor-κB (NF-κB) and activation protein-1 (AP-1) are activated depending on the recruitment and activation of the IL-18 signaling molecules, myeloid differentiation factor 88 (MyD88; *42*), IL-1R-associated kinase (IRAK; *37*), and TNF receptor-associated factor 6 (TRAF6; *165*). As with IL-1 signaling, IRAK4 seems to be essentially involved in the IL-18 signaling pathway *(36a,36b)*. Upon stimulation with IL-12 or type 1 interferon (IFN), stat4 is activated *(51,50)*. Phosphorylated stat4 enhances the binding capacity of AP-1 to the AP-1 binding site of the IFN-γ promoter region *(41)*. Simultaneously, GADD45β/γ-mediated p38 activation occurs after activation of both stat4 and NF-κB *(57,58)*. Collectively, a large amount of IFN-γ is produced. IL-18BP inhibits IL-18 binding to IL-18R. IL-18BP, IL-18 binding protein; stat4, signal transducer and activator of transcription 4.

IL-18 and IL-12 synergistically induce IFN-γ production by various types of cells including freshly isolated Th cells and NK cells, whereas stimulation with the single cytokines does not induce large amounts of IFN-γ. This synergy is explained by the upregulation of their receptor expression. IL-12 upregulates IL-18Rα expression *(34,43,48)*. Therefore, the synergistic IFN-γ production occurs on the basis of the upregulated responsiveness to IL-18 during Th cell culture with IL-12. Furthermore, the synergy also comes from the interaction of IL-18 and IL-12 signaling for IFN-γ production *(49)*. IL-12 and IL-18 have distinct signaling pathways. IL-12 signaling uses the STAT4 activation pathway *(50)*, whereas IL-18 activates NF-κB *(32)* and AP-1 *(41)*. Interestingly, the mouse IFN-γ promoter region has an AP-1-binding site but no obvious binding site for STAT4, whereas human AP-1 and STAT4 interact with the human IFN-γ promoter at distinct sites *(51)*. Thus, in mice, IL-12-activated STAT4 enhances the binding activity of AP-1 on its IFN-γ promoter instead of direct binding to the IFN-γ promoter *(49)*.

Recently, Tyk2, a member of the Janus kinase (JAK) family, has been demonstrated to be involved in the synergistic action of IL-12 and IL-18 for IFN-γ production and also in the upregulation of NK activity by IL-12 or IL-18 *(52)*. Tyk2-deficient NK cells produce much less IFN-γ or show less increase in cytotoxic activity in response to IL-18 and/or IL-12 than wild-type cells. As Tyk2 is required for IL-12-induced STAT4 activation *(53)*, the idea is convincing that Tyk2-deficient cells show poor response to IL-12 for IFN-γ production, elevation of NK activity, or increase in IL-18R expression. This may well explain the failure of Tyk2-deficient NK cells in synergistic IFN-γ production by IL-12 and IL-18. Interestingly, Tyk2-deficient NK cells cannot produce IFN-γ in response to IL-18, although they express substantial amounts of IL-18R on their surface. These observations strongly suggest that the IL-18 signal might be transduced via a Tyk2-dependent JAK/STAT pathway besides the MyD88/IRAK/IRAK4 pathway *(54,55)*.

Synergy of IL-12 and IL-18 for IFN-γ production is also explained by the GADD45 family protein-mediated p38 activation *(56–58)* (Figs. 1 and 2). The GADD45 family, composed of three members, GADD45α, GADD45β, and GADD45γ, was originally proposed to be involved in the maintenance of genome stability *(59)*. Indeed, a recent study of GADD45α-deficient mice revealed that GADD45α was a genome stabilizer *(60)*. Unlike GADD45α, however, GADD45β and GADD45γ have been implicated as regulators of cell cycle progression and differentiation, presumably in part via activation of both the p38 and JNK pathways *(61–63)*. In fact, both GADD45β and GADD45γ, but not GADD45α, are induced in Th1 cells after stimulation with TCR engagement or stimulation combined with IL-12 and IL-18 *(57,58)*. IL-12/IL-18-induced GADD45β, but not GADD45γ, then activates Th1 cells to produce IFN-γ through p38 activation *(57)* (Fig. 2). Interestingly, data from GADD45γ-deficient mice demonstrate that GADD45γ is important for both p38 activation and IFN-γ production by Th1 cells in response to TCR engagement *(58)*. Furthermore, GADD45γ-deficient Th1 cells also have partial impairment of IFN-γ production in response to IL-12 and IL-18 *(58)*. These findings suggest that both proteins are involved in IFN-γ production by IL-12/IL-18-stimulated Th1 cells. Data from GADD45β-deficient mice will elucidate the individual roles of GADD45β and/or GADD45γ in IL-12/IL-18-induced IFN-γ production pathways (Fig. 2).

IL-18R is a Th1 cell marker *(11,47)*, whereas T1/ST2, an orphan receptor of the IL-1R family, is a Th2 cell marker in mouse *(64)*. This is also the case for human Th cells *(65)*. In humans, IL-18Rα is selectively expressed on Th1 and Tc1 cells, whereas T1/ST2, but not IL-18Rα, is expressed on Th2 cells and Tc2 cells. However, we do not know whether IL-18R is stably expressed on Th1 cells or is expressed only transiently on freshly developed Th1 cells.

IL-18 binding protein (IL-18BP) is a natural IL-18 inhibitor present in serum and urine. IL-18BP is not a member of the TLR/IL-1R family but has homology with poxvirus products *(66–68)*. IL-18BP is constitutively produced and is upregulated by IFN-γ *(69)*. As IL-18BP has a high-affinity binding capacity to IL-18, IL-18BP might become a rational target for therapeutic regimens against various inflammatory diseases in which IL-18 is profoundly involved (see below; Fig. 2).

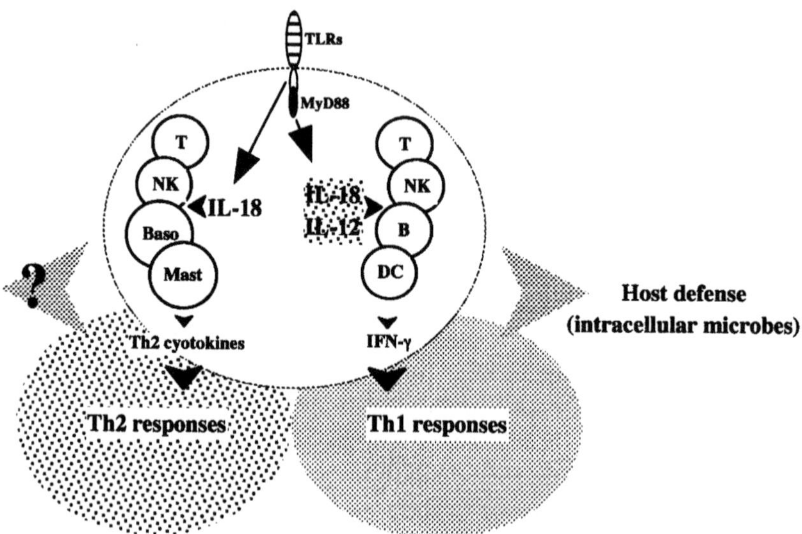

Fig. 3. Roles for interleukin-18 (IL-18) in immune responses *(9,10)*. After being stimulated with microbe products, macrophages and dendritic cells secrete IL-18 as well as IL-12. IL-18, in the presence of IL-12, stimulates T-cells (T), natural killer (NK) cells, B-cells (B), dendritic cells (DC), and other types of cells to produce large amounts of interferon-γ (IFN-γ), which triggers inflammatory and Th1 immune responses. This process is useful for host defense. When the cells secrete IL-18 without IL-12 production, T-cells, NK cells, basophils, and mast cells secrete Th2 cytokines such as IL-13 and IL-4, eventually leading to atopic inflammatory and Th2 immune responses. MyD88, myeloid differentiation factor 88; TLRs, Toll-like receptors.

2.3. Dual Immunologic Actions of IL-18

A prominent feature of IL-18 is its pleiotropy. As recent review articles describe the biologic functions of IL-18 in detail *(4,5,7–10,21)*, we will briefly review the dual actions of IL-18 on Th1/Th2 cell development. Th1 and Th2 immune responses are two faces of adaptive immunity *(70)*. Th1 cells and Th2 cells have distinct immunologic functions, to promote inflammatory responses and atopic inflammatory responses, respectively, based on their different cytokine profiles. Upon TCR engagement, Th cells develop into Th1 cells upon the action of T-bet, which is a Th1-specific transcription factor targeting chromatin remodeling to individual IFN-γ alleles and also inducing IL-12Rβ2 expression *(71,72)*, accelerated by IL-12 stimulation and/or IL-4 depletion. In contrast, upon TCR engagement Th cells can develop into Th2 cells in the presence of IL-4, in which STAT6 and GATA3 seem to be essential transcription factors for chromatin remodeling of the IL-4 locus *(73–77)*.

In general, cytokines responsible for Th1 or Th2 cell development have a cross-inhibitory action for the corresponding Th cell polarization. For example, IL-4 initiates Th2 cell development of naive Th cells and simultaneously inhibits their development into Th1 cells. Unexpectedly, IL-18 has the ability both to accelerate Th1 cell development and inversely to induce Th2 cell development depending on its cytokine microenvironment (Fig. 3). Indeed, IL-18 participates in acceleration of in vivo Th1 cell development after treatment with heat-killed *Propionibacterium acnes* and other Th1-promoting microbes *(78,79)* (described below). In contrast, daily administration of IL-18 induces increase in serum levels of IgE via elevation of expression of CD40 ligand and production of IL-4 by Th cells, which are essential for isotype-switching to IgE in B-cells *(80–82)*. This is also the case for various mutant mice that overrelease biologically active IL-18 *(81,83,84)*. As will be described below, IL-18- or IL-18R-deficient mice demonstrate important roles of endogenous IL-18 in Th1 cell development or Th1 responses. However, we have not yet had conclusive evidence that proves a contribution of endogenous IL-18 to Th2 responses in these mutant mice.

2.4. IL-18 in Host Defense

As expected from its immunologic roles as a potent IFN-γ-inducing factor, IL-18 is important for host defense against some types of pathogens *(85)*. Intracellular microbes cannot be eradicated by humoral immune responses, because of their infectious localization within the target cells, which antibodies cannot reach. The host developed cellular immunity against these microbes, in an innate and/or adaptive fashion. After viral infection, host cells recognize viral products via TLRs or other receptors to produce various proinflammatory cytokines, such as type 1 IFN, IL-12, tumor necrosis factor-α (TNF-α), IL-1, and IL-18, which in turn stimulate NK cells to produce IFN-γ *(86)*. IFN-γ together with TNF-α contributes to reduce, and possibly abolish, viral replication *(87,88)*. NK cells also participate in host defense against viruses. NK cells kill microbe-infected cells depending on their unusual expression of MHC class I, resulting in a supply of soluble viral antigens that evoke virus-specific Th responses. Cytotoxic T-lymphocytes (CTLs) are professional effector cells that contribute to the killing of virus-infected cells in an MHC class 1-restricted manner, although their cytotoxicity has not been widely accepted as the main action against viruses, rather, CTL-derived proinflammatory cytokines mostly contribute to virus eradication by abolishing viral replication *(87,88)*.

Intracellular bacteria, fungi, and protozoa are also mainly eradicated by the activation of the host cellular immunity, in which IFN-γ plays a central role as a potent macrophage-activating and inflammation-inducing element (Fig. 3). For example, *Listeria monocytogenes*, a Gram-positive, intracellular facultative bacterium, is expelled by the activation of innate immunity in the early infectious phase and later by anti-*L. monocytogenes* CTLs *(89)*. Upon *L. monocytogenes* infection, macrophages produce proinflammatory cytokines including TNF-α, IL-12, and IL-18 through TLRs, including TLR2 *(90–93)*. These proinflammatory cytokines seem to concentrate their potentials on IFN-γ induction *(89)*. A similar scenario is constructed against intracellular fungi such as *Cryptococcus neoformans (94,95)* and protozoa such as *Leishmania major (79,96–98)*, *Plasmodium yoelii (99)*, and *Toxoplasma gondii (100)*. Thus, IL-18 might play distinct roles in host defense depending on the species of the microbes and their virulence, and also on the genetic background of the host.

2.5. Antimetastatic Effect of IL-18

IL-18 can upregulate cytotoxic activity of both NK cells and CTLs *(3,4,6–10,21)*. Moreover, IL-18 is capable of inhibiting angiogenesis, which is required for tumor growth *(101)*. Therefore, it is plausible that IL-18 is an efficient antimetastatic factor. Indeed, many investigators have shown a suppressive effect of IL-18 on metastasis of various types of tumors in vivo via upregulation of perforin/granzyme- and/or Fas ligand-mediated killing actions of CTLs and/or NK cells *(4,9)*.

2.6. Pathologic Roles of IL-18

Based on its powerful biologic functions, IL-18 is involved in various pathologic disorders *(8,9)* including various inflammatory tissue diseases such as inflammatory bowel diseases *(102–105)*, acute graft-versus-host disease *(106–108)*, as well as inflammatory dermatitis *(84,109,110)* and autoimmune diseases such as rheumatoid arthritis *(111–115)*. Recent clinical data show a causative role of IL-18-induced IFN-γ in atherosclerotic lesions and in the development of lethal angina *(116–119)*. IL-18 is highly expressed in human atherosclerotic plaques of clinical specimens. In the plaque, macrophages are a major cell source of IL-18, and vascular endothelial cells express IL-18R. Moreover, serum levels of IL-18 parallel mortality by cardiovascular death in patients with angina independently of clinical manifestations *(120)*. Serum levels of IL-18 are thus a potent prognostic indicator for the lethal outcome of patients with coronary artery diseases. Furthermore, resent studies revealed that a diminished-function mutation in TLR4 is associated with a decreased risk of atherosclerosis *(121)*, suggesting the involvement of TLR-mediated innate immune responses in the development of atherosclerosis. IL-18 produced in the plaque together with IL-12, which might be induced after activation of TLRs, induce IFN-γ production by vascular smooth muscle cells *(15,122)*, subsequently leading to lethal angina, if produced in the coronary artery. These observations will provide a novel therapeutic regimen against atherosclerosis targeting IL-18 and IL-18R.

A second observation is the spontaneous development of atopic dermatitis in mutant mice that overexpress biologically active IL-18 in a keratinocyte-specific manner *(84,109)*. It has been a central dogma since the discovery of IgE that mast cells and basophils are activated to induce atopic manifestations upon crosslinkage of their surface FcεRI with allergen-specific IgE binding to multivalent allergens *(123,124)*. In fact, NC/Nga mice, which show intact skin under specific pathogen-free conditions, develop inflammatory skin lesions like atopic dermatitis with elevation of IgE when kept under conventional conditions, in which they have an opportunity to be exposed to mite antigens, a potent allergen *(125)*. However, recent studies have revealed that STAT6-deficient NC/Nga mice manifest skin lesions without an increase in serum IgE levels under conventional conditions *(126)*, strongly indicating a dispensable role of IgE in development of atopic dermatitis.

Furthermore, our recent studies revealed that IL-18 has the ability to induce directly the spontaneous development of pruritic cutaneous lesions like human atopic dermatitis as well as elevation of serum levels of IgE. In fact, caspase-1-transgenic mice that overexpress caspase-1 specifically in their keratinocytes, which constitutively express precursor IL-18, spontaneously suffer from chronic dermatitis with apparent itching *(84,109)*. Deletion of *il-18* but not *il*-1 protects them from skin alterations, indicating that overrelease of IL-18 in the skin is responsible for these cutaneous alterations. In addition, these mice manifest skin alterations without IgE induction, indicating that IgE is not essential for development of skin lesions *(84)*. In human cases, there is evidence for a substantial proportion of patients with atopic dermatitis without obvious elevation of allergen-specific IgE. These findings tell us that some types of atopic diseases might occur owing to exposure to high levels of IL-18 without triggering allergen-specific immune responses.

3. IL-18 and IL-18R Knockout Mice

IL-18-deficient mice and IL-18Rα-deficient mice were generated on a mixture of C57BL/6 and 129 backgrounds according to the technique of homologous recombination *(78,97,127,*

128). IL-18-deficient mice do not express or secrete IL-18 upon appropriate stimulation *(78,97,128)*. As expected from the requirement of IL-18Rα for IL-18 signaling (described above), IL-18Rα-deficient cells cannot bind to IL-18 or respond to IL-18 *(127)*. Both types of mutant mice were backcrossed with C57BL/6 mice, and F8 to F10 mice were used as IL-18-deficient and IL-18Rα-deficient mice with a C57BL/6 background, respectively. Both types of mutant mice are born healthy and grow normally. IL-18-deficient mice do not secrete IL-18 after LPS treatment *(78)*. There are no obvious differences in lymphocyte phenotypes, proliferative responses of T-cells and B-cells, or immunoglobulin isotype switching between wild-type mice and IL-18- or IL-18Rα-deficient mice. However, NK cells from both types of mutant mice equally show partial impairment in spontaneous NK killing activity, although they display normal responses to IL-12 and IL-2 by increase in their cytotoxicity *(78,127)*. Moreover, Th cells from both types of mutant mice have a partial impairment in Th1 cell development in vivo upon treatment with Th1-inducing substances, such as heat-killed *P. acnes* or Bacille Calmette-Guérin (BCG) *(78,127)*. Accumulated lines of evidence using these mutant mice have revealed important roles for endogenous IL-18 in host defense and various diseases.

3.1. Roles of Endogenous IL-18 in Inflammatory Diseases

IL-18-deficient mice are resistant to endotoxin (LPS)-induced liver injury. Mice are resistant to LPS compared with humans. However, treatment with heat-killed *P. acnes* renders mice highly susceptible to LPS-induced liver injury as well as lethal shock *(8,129)*. *P. acnes* treatment of mice reduces the median lethal dosey (LD_{50}) of LPS by a thousandth. LPS-induced proinflammatory cytokines are essential for this liver injury. *P. acnes*-elicited Kupffer cells, tissue macrophages in the liver, secrete hepatocytotoxic TNF-α- and IFN-γ-inducing cytokines, IL-12 and IL-18, in response to LPS in vitro, and *P. acnes*-elicited hepatic lymphocytes produce large amounts of IFN-γ in response to IL-12 and IL-18 and express Fas ligand in response to IL-18 but not IL-12. Administration of anti-IFN-γ inhibits induction of TNF-α expression but not Fas ligand in the liver of *P. acnes*-primed mice after LPS administration, whereas anti-IL-18 prevents induction of IFN-γ, TNF-α, and Fas ligand in the liver, indicating that LPS-triggered IL-18 induces all these hepatocytotoxic factors, leading to liver injury. Thus, IL-18-deficient mice evade liver injury induced by the sequential administration of *P. acnes* and LPS *(130)*. Interestingly, IL-18-deficient mice are resistant to this liver injury but highly susceptible to *P. acnes*/LPS shock, suggesting that distinct mechanisms underlie these two LPS pathologies.

In contrast to *P. acnes*/LPS shock, IL-18-deficient mice are moderately resistant to treatment with high-dose LPS plus D-galactosamine, a model of TNF-α-dependent lethal shock *(128)*. The LD_{50} of LPS for wild-type mice is 600 μg, whereas that for IL-18-deficient mice is 900 μg. Serum levels of IFN-γ are much lower in the mutant mice compared with wild-type mice after LPS challenge. However, IL-18-deficient mice are comparably sensitive to *Staphylococcus aureus* enterotoxin B (SEB), a superantigen selectively and directly activating a limited T-cell repertoire, with comparable increase in serum levels of IFN-γ as in wild-type mice *(128)*. Furthermore, treatment with IL-12 and IL-18 induces severe colitis in mice in an IFN-γ-dependent manner *(102)*. Thus, IL-18 seems to be dispensable for T-cell-dependent lethal shock.

IL-18-deficient mice are resistant to intestinal inflammatory disease induced by 2,4,6-trinitrobenzene sulfoinic acid (TNBS), a mouse model of Crohn's disease *(131)*. TNBS-treated wild-type mice show weight loss and severe inflammatory colitis with dense infiltration with macrophages, possible IL-18-releasing cells. In contrast, IL-18-deficient mice are relatively resistant to TNBS-induced colitis, indicating an essential role of IL-18 in this model of colitis. Indeed, selective in vivo depletion of macrophages protects mice from TNBS-induced colitis with reduced IL-18 expression, indicating the importance of macrophage-derived IL-18. Thus, IL-18 plays a causative role in some types of inflammatory bowel diseases.

IL-18 is also involved in ischemic tissue injuries *(132,133)*. Hypoxic ischemia induces brain injury in mice, in which IL-18 and caspase-1 are selectively expressed by microglia and macrophages, whereas IL-18R is expressed on neurons of the cerebral cortex and thalamus. IL-18-deficient mice show a reduced neuropathology score compared with wild-type mice, indicating a critical role for IL-18 in ischemia-induced brain injury *(132,133)*.

3.2. Pathologic Roles of IL-18 in Autoimmune Diseases

Tissue-specific autoimmune diseases such as rheumatoid arthritis and multiple sclerosis are believed to be associated with autoreactive Th1 cells, which are collagen- and myelin sheath-derived molecule-specific Th1 cell responses, respectively *(10,134)*. Patients with these autoimmune diseases frequently exhibit elevation of serum levels of IL-18 *(135–138)*. Type II collagen-induced arthritis is a mouse model of rheumatoid arthritis. Eighty percent of wild-type mice developed arthritis a month after treatment with collagen, whereas less than 40% of IL-18-deficient mice suffered from arthritis, with lower levels of proinflammatory cytokines in their serum and impaired histologic changes in their joints, indicating the importance of IL-18 in collagen-induced arthritis in mice *(139)*.

Experimental autoimmune encephalomyelitis (EAE) is an animal model of multiple sclerosis. Administration of various kinds of myelin sheath-derived substances, such as myelin basic protein and myelin-oligodendrocyte glycoprotein (MOG) in adjuvant can induce multiple sclerosis-like lesions in the central nervous system of wild-type C57BL/6 mice. However, IL-18-deficient mice with a C57BL/6 background are resistant to EAE and do not develop encephalitogenic Th1 cells, although they show similar proliferative response to MOG as in wild-type mice, indicating the importance of IL-18 in development of MOG-specific encephalitogenic Th1 cells *(140)*.

Experimental autoimmune uveitis (EAU) is a photoreceptor-associated antigen-specific Th1 cell-mediated eye disease that resembles human noninfective uveitis. Although EAU is associated with autoantigen-specific Th1 cell development, IL-18-deficient mice with a susceptible background, like wild-type littermates, are sensitive to this autoimmune disease, indicating a minor role of IL-18 in EAU *(141)*.

3.3. Role of Endogenous IL-18 in Host Defense

As expected from the accumulated lines of evidence demonstrating the importance of IL-18-mediated IFN-γ in host defense, IL-18-deficient mice are, in general, susceptible to various pathologic microbes.

3.3.1. Viral Infection

Upon infection of mice with cytomegalovirus, both liver and spleen are targeted, and IFN-γ plays a crucial role in the early phase clearance of cytomegalovirus *(2,142)*. Both IL-18-deficient mice and IL-12p35-deficient mice failed to increase IFN-γ in the circulation. However, IL-18-deficient mice are resistant to this infection, with comparable elevation of IFN-γ in the liver as in wild-type mice, whereas IL-12p35-deficient mice are susceptible, with impairment of IFN-γ induction in their liver *(143)*. Therefore, IL-18-dependent IFN-γ production in the liver plays an essential protective role in cytomegalovirus infection in mice.

Herpes simplex virus type 2 (HSV2) is a genital organ-tropic virus. IFN-γ also plays a critical role in its clearance *(144)*. IL-18-deficient mice are comparably susceptible to HSV2 as IFN-γ-deficient mice when infected with a sublethal titer of the virus, indicating the importance of endogenous IL-18 against HSV2 *(145)*. Interestingly, IL-18-deficient mice, unlike IFN-γ-deficient mice, successfully develop adaptive immunity against HSV2, indicating a minor role of IL-18 in memory T-cell development against HSV2.

IL-18 is also important for eradication of neurovirulent influenza A virus. Upon infection with this strain, IL-18-expressing microglia accumulate in the central nervous system, followed by the elevation of IFN-γ-expressing neurons. IL-18-deficient mice show impairment in eradication of neurovirulent influenza A virus compared with wild-type mice *(146)*. Moreover, exogenous IFN-γ improves the viral clearance in IL-18-deficient mice. Therefore, IL-18 is essential in the activation of microglia to expel neurovirulent influenza A virus through induction of IFN-γ.

3.3.2. Bacterial Infection

L. monocytogenes, an intracellular bacterium, preferentially invades and replicates in liver parenchymal and Kupffer cells in the host's liver. Early-phase clearance of *L. monocytogenes* is dependent on levels of IFN-γ and TNF-α produced by host innate immune cells such as NK cells, macrophages, and dendritic cells *(89,147)*. The role of endogenous proinflammatory cytokines is dependent on the mouse strain *(90,101)*. IL-18 is more important for listerial clearance in BALB/c susceptible mice *(90)*. However, in C57BL/6 resistant mice, IL-18 plays a substantial role in early-phase clearance of *L. monocytogenes,* but is not as important as IL-12, because IL-12p40-deficient mice have a larger bacterial burden in their liver than IL-18-deficient mice. The mutant mice lacking both IL-12 and IL-18 are more susceptible than IL-12-deficient mice but are more resistant than IFN-γ-deficient mice, indicating that some other IFN-γ-inducing factor might be involved in this clearance *(92)*. As IL-18 activates CTLs, a key effector in late-phase clearance, IL-18 is essential for listerial eradication in both the early and late infectious phases *(90)*.

Mycobacterium tuberculosis is also an intracellular facultative bacterium. IL-18 is important for eradication of *M. tuberculosis (148,149)*. Upon *M. tuberculosis* infection of mice, a similar hierarchy of proinflammatory cytokines for its eradication as in the early listerial clearance in resistant mice *(92)* is reported *(149)*. Analyses of bacterial numbers in the lung of infected mice post infection revealed that endogenous IL-12 plays a more important role in eradication of *M. tuberculosis* than IL-18. Interestingly, spleen cells from infected IL-18-deficient mice showed impaired IFN-γ production upon in vitro antigen stimulation compared with infected wild-type mice, whereas those from infected IL-12-deficient mice do not produce IFN-γ. These results indicate that IL-18 plays a role in eradication of *M. tuberculosis* by acceleration of bacterial antigen-specific Th1 cell development and that IL-12, in contrast, is essential to develop bacterial antigen-specific Th1 cells and to eradicate *M. tuberculosis.*

IL-18 is also critical for early eradication of some types of extracellular bacteria. Upon nasal infection with *Streptococcus pneumoniae*, the most common causative microbe of community-acquired pneumonia, IL-18-deficient mice exhibit more bacterial burden in their lung than wild-type mice. IL-12-deficient mice are more sensitive to this bacterium than wild-type mice but more resistant than IL-18-deficient mice *(150)*. Therefore, IL-18 plays an important role in the early antibacterial host response during pneumococcal pneumonia.

3.3.3. Fungal Infection

Cryptococcus neoformans, a widely spread fungal pathogen, causes severe central nervous system infection in immunocompromised hosts. Cellular immunity mediated by Th1 cells and by IFN-γ-dependent nitric oxide production plays an essential role for host defense against this fungus *(151)*. Upon intratracheal infection with *C. neoformans*, IL-18-deficient mice show impaired clearance in the lung compared with wild-type mice, but more successful clearance when compared with IL-12-deficient mice *(95)*. Interestingly, IL-12 and IL-18 double knockout mice have significantly higher and comparable titers of *C. neoformans* in their lung compared with IL-12-deficient mice and IFN-γ-deficient mice, respectively. IL-12-deficient mice lack the development of fungus-specific Th1 response, which is not improved by exogenous IL-18, indicating that IL-12 but not IL-18 is essential for Th1 cell development against this fungus *(95)*.

3.3.4. Protozoan Infection

IL-18 as well as IL-12 is important for anti-protozoa host response during some types of intracellular protozoa infection. Murine leishmaniasis is the prototype of Th1 and Th2 cell responses in vivo *(152)*. Most mouse strains spontaneously eradicate *Leishmania major* via induction of anti-leishmanial Th1 cell responses, whereas some mouse strains are susceptible owing to development of Th2 responses against *L. major*. IL-18-deficient mice with a resistant background show partial impairment in *L. major* clearance, with higher levels of leishmanial burden in the cutaneous lesion compared with wild-type littermates after initial infection *(79,97,98)*. Expectedly, although showing impairment in leishmanial eradication, IL-18-deficient mice develop normal Th1 cell response against *L. major*. Importantly, IL-18-deficient mice develop poor memory immunity against *L. major*. In fact, upon reinfection, IL-18-deficient mice have a comparable clinical course as in the initial infection *(79)*. Therefore, IL-18 seems to be essential for the clonal expansion and clonal maintenance of *L. major*-specific Th1 cells.

IL-18 is also important for host defense against attenuated strains of *Plasmodium*. *Plasmodium* has a complicated life cycle in the mosquito as the terminal host and in mice or humans as the intermediate host. In mice or humans, *Plasmodium* promptly invades and proliferates in the liver parenchymal cells. In this liver stage, the host shows few pathologic manifestations. After maturation and proliferation, the protozoa start to parasitize host erythrocytes, during which time the host shows various pathologic changes depending on the strain of the protozoa. *P. yoelii* is a causative protozoan of nonlethal mouse malaria. Upon inoculation with *P. yoelii*-parasitized erythrocytes, IL-18-deficient mice exhibit higher levels of parasitemia compared with wild-type mice, indicating the importance of IL-18 for eradication of *P. yoelii (99)*. In contrast, IL-18-deficient mice are comparably susceptible to *P. berghei*, a lethal mouse malaria strain, as wild-type mice *(153)*.

3.3.5. Helminth Infection

Gastrointestinal helminths are generally eradicated by activation of host Th2 responses *(154–156)*. Although IL-18 has the ability to induce Th2 cell development in naive Th cells in vitro *(81)*, IL-18-deficient mice comparably shift to the polarization into Th2 cells after infection with *Nippostrongylus braziliensis*, a gut-parasitizing nematode, compared with wild-type mice *(78)*. Moreover, endogenous IL-18 promotes the development of chronic infection with *Trichuris muris,* a gastrointestinal nematode via reduction of production of IL-13 that is essential for its eradication *(157)*. IL-18-deficient mice, like IL-12-deficient mice, more efficiently eradicate *T. muris* compared with wild-type mice with elevation of serum levels of IL-13. This is also the case for expulsion of *Trichinella spiralis*, a parasitic nematode *(158)*. Therefore, to date, IL-18 apparently seems to be a negative regulator for nematode eradication. Nevertheless, it is still important to keep in mind that IL-18 also stimulates Th2 responses in the absence of IL-12 *(9)*. We cannot exclude the possibility that IL-18 may contribute to eradication of helminths in some circumstances. We need further study to describe the precise role of IL-18 in helminth infection.

4. Conclusions

Based on its unique properties, IL-18 plays various biologic and pathologic roles in immune responses and various diseases, as described above. However, we do not yet fully understand the mechanism of activation of IL-18. Recent findings strongly suggest that macrophages secrete IL-18 depending on caspase-1 activation upon stimulation with microbial products such as LPS. However, similar to IL-1β release, various kinds of stimuli other than microbial products may induce IL-18 release. Indeed, proteinase 3, a potent protease stored in the granules within neutrophils *(159,160)*, induces IL-18 release from IFN-γ/LPS-primed human epithelial cells *(161)*, although the molecular mechanism of proteinase 3-triggered IL-18 secretion is unclear. Moreover, various types of cells, such as intestinal epithelial cells, keratinocytes, and chondrocytes constitutively express IL-18 and have the potential to release biologically active IL-18 *(9)*. IL-18 released from these cells might potently contribute to unknown pathophysiologic events.

Analysis of exogenous IL-18 revealed that IL-18 has the ability to induce Th2 cell responses. However, to date we do not know of situations in which endogenous IL-18 contributes to establishment of Th2 cell responses or polyclonal IgE induction. Does natural infection induce Th2 cell responses depending on endogenous IL-18? This is a second issue to be elucidated definitely.

References

1. Murphy, K. M., Ouyang, W., Farrar, D. J., et al. (2000) Signaling and transcription in T helper development. *Annu. Rev. Immunol.* **18,** 451–494.
2. Trinchieri, G. (1995) Interleukin-12: a proinflammatory cytokine with immunoregulatory functions that bridge innate resistance and antigen-specific and adaptive immunity. *Annu. Rev. Immunol.* **13,** 251–276.
3. Okamura, H., Tsutsui, H., Komatsu, T., et al. (1995) Cloning of a new cytokine that induces IFN-γ production by T cells. *Nature* **378,** 88–91.
4. Okamura, H., Tsutsui, H., Kashiwamura, S., Yoshimoto, T., and Nakanishi, K. (1998) Interleukin-18: a novel cytokine that augments both innate and acquired immunity. *Adv. Immunol.* **70,** 281–312.
5. Okamura, H., Kashiwamura, S., Tsutsui, H., Yoshimoto, T., and Nakanishi, K. (1998) Regulation of interferon-γ production by IL-12 and IL-18. *Curr. Opin. Immunol.* **10,** 259–264.
6. Fantuzzi, G. and Dinarello, C. A. (1999) Interleukin-18 and interleukin-1β: two cytokine substrates for ICE (caspase-1). *J. Clin. Immunol.* **19,** 1–11.
7. Dinarello, C. A. (2000) Interleukin-18, a proinflammatory cytokine. *Eur. Cytokine Netw.* **11,** 483–486.
8. Tsutsui, H., Matsui, K., Okamura, H., and Nakanishi, K. (2000) Pathophysiological roles of interleukin-18 for inflammatory liver diseases. *Immunol. Rev.* **174,** 192–209.

9. Nakanishi, K., Yoshimoto, T., Tsutsui, H., and Okamura, H. (2001) Interleukin-18 regulates both Th1 and Th2 responses. *Annu. Rev. Immunol.* **19,** 423–474.
10. Nakanishi, K., Yoshimoto, T., Tsutsui, H., and Okamura, H. (2001) Interleukin-18 is a unique cytokine that stimulates both Th1 and Th2 responses depending on its cytokine milieu. *Cytokine Growth Factor Rev.* **12,** 53–72.
11. Robinson, D., Shibuya, K., Mui, A., et al. (1997) IGIF does not drive Th1 development but synergizes with IL-12 for interferon-gamma production and activates IRAK and NF-κB. *Immunity* **7,** 571–581.
12. Yoshimoto, T., Okamura, H., Tagawa, Y., Iwakura, Y., and Nakanishi, K. (1997) Interleukin 18 together with interleukin 12 inhibits IgE production by induction of interferon-γ production from activated B cells. *Proc. Natl. Acad. Sci. USA* **94,** 3948–3953.
13. Munder, M., Mallo, M., Eichmann, K., and Modolell, M. (1998) Murine macrophages secrete interferon γ upon combined stimulation with interleukin (IL)-12 and IL-18: a novel pathway of autocrine macrophage activation. *J. Exp. Med.* **187,** 2103–2108.
14. Fukao, T., Matsuda, S., and Koyasu, S. (2000) Synergistic effects of IL-4 and IL-18 on IL-12-dependent IFN-γ production by dendritic cells. *J. Immunol.* **164,** 64–71.
15. Gerdes, N., Sukhova, G. K., Libby, P., Reynolds, R. S., Young, J. L., and Schönbeck, U. (2002) Expression of interleukin (IL)-18 and functional IL-18 receptor on human vascular endothelial cells, smooth muscle cells, and macrophages: implications for atherogenesis. *J. Exp. Med.* **195,** 245–257.
16. Oppmann, B., Lesley, R., Blom, B., et al. (2000) Novel p19 protein engages IL-12p40 to form a cytokine, IL-23, with biological activities similar as well as distinct from IL-12. *Immunity* **13,** 715–725.
17. Parham, C., Chirica, M., Timans, J., et al. (2002) A receptor for the heterodimeric cytokine IL-23 is composed of IL-12Rβ1 and a novel cytokine receptor subunit, IL-23R. *J. Immunol.* **168,** 5699–5708.
18. Pflanz, S., Timans, J. C., Cheung, J., et al. (2002) IL-27, a heterodimeric cytokine composed of EBI3 and p28 protein, induces proliferation of naive $CD4^+$ T cells. *Immunity* **16,** 779–790.
19. Yoshida, H., Hamano, S., Senaldi, G., et al. (2001) WSX-1 is required for the initiation of Th1 responses and resistance to *L. major* infection. *Immunity* **15,** 569–578.
20. Chen, Q., Ghilardi, N., Wang, H., et al. (2000) Development of Th1-type immune responses requires the type 1 cytokine receptor TCCR. *Nature* **07,** 916–920.
21. Dinarello, C. A. (1999) Interleukin-18. *Methods* **19,** 123–132.
22. Sims, J. E. (2002) IL-1 and IL-18 receptors, and their extended family. *Curr. Opin. Immunol.* **14,** 117–122.
23. Bazan, J. F., Timans, J. C., and Kastelein, R. A. (1996) A newly defined interleukin-1? *Nature* **379,** 591.
24. Gu, Y., Kuida, K., Tsutsui, H., et al. (1997) Activation of interferon-γ inducing factor mediated by interleukin-1β converting enzyme. *Science* **275,** 206–209.
25. Ghayur, T., Banerjee, S., Hugunin, M., et al. (1997) Caspase-1 processes IFN-γ-inducing factor and regulates LPS-induced IFN-γ production. *Nature* **386,** 619–623.
26. Tsutsui, H., Kayagaki, N., Kuida, K., et al. (1999) Caspase-1-independent, Fas/Fas ligand-mediated IL-18 secretion from macrophages causes acute liver injury in mice. *Immunity* **11,** 359–367.
27. Debets, R., Timans, J. C., Homey, B., et al. (2001) Two novel IL-1 family members, IL-1δ and IL-1ε, function as an antagonist and agonist of NF-κB activation through the orphan IL-1 receptor-related protein 2. *J. Immunol.* **167,** 1440–1446.
28. Stoll, S., Muller, G., Kurimoto, M., et al. (1997) Production of IL-18 (IFN-γ-inducing factor) messenger RNA and functional protein by murine keratinocytes. *J. Immunol.* **159,** 298–302.
29. Seki, E., Tsutsui, H., Nakano, H., et al. (2001) LPS-induced IL-18 secretion from murine Kupffer cells independently of MyD88 that is critically involved in induction of production of IL-12 and IL-1β. *J. Immunol.* **166,** 2651–2657.
30. Morelli, A. E., Zahorchak, A. F., Larregina, A. T., Colvin, B. L., Logar, A. J., and Takayama, T. (2001) Cytokine production by mouse myeloid dendritic cells in relation to differentiation and terminal maturation induced by lipopolysaccharide or CD40 ligation. *Blood* **98,** 1512–1523.
31. Akira, S., Takeda, K., and Kaisho, T. (2001) Toll-like receptors: critical proteins linking innate and acquired immunity. *Nat. Immunol.* **2,** 675–680.

32. Adachi, O., Kawai, T., Takeda, K., et al. (1998) Targeted disruption of the MyD88 gene results in loss of IL-1- and IL- 18-mediated function. *Immunity* **9,** 143–150.
33. Miwa, K., Asano, M., Horai, R., Iwakura, Y., Nagata, S., and Suda, T. (1998) Caspase-1-independent IL-1β release and inflammation induced by the apoptosis inducer Fas ligand. *Nat. Med.* **4,** 1287–1292.
34. Yoshimoto, T., Takeda, K., Tanaka, T., et al. (1998) IL-12 up-regulates IL-18 receptor expression on T cells, Th1 cells, and B cells: synergism with IL-18 for IFN-γ production. *J. Immunol.* **161,** 3400–3407.
35. O'Neill, L. A. and Dinarello, C. A. (2000) The IL-1 receptor/toll-like receptor superfamily: critical receptors for inflammation and host defense. *Immunol. Today* **21,** 206–209.
36a. Suzuki, N., Suzuki, S., Duncan, G. S., et al. (2002) Severe impairment of interleukin-1 and Toll-like receptor signaling in mice lacking IRAK-4. *Nature* **416,** 750–754.
36b. Suzuki, N., Chen, N.-J., Miller, D. G., et al. (2003) IRAK-4 is essential for interleukin-18-mediated natural killer and T helper cell type 1 response. *J. Immunol.* (in press).
37. Kanakaraj, P., Ngo, K., Wu, Y., et al. (1999) Defective interleukin (IL)-18-mediated natural killer and T helper cell type 1 responses in IL-1 receptor-associated kinase (IRAK)-deficient mice. *J. Exp. Med.* **189,** 1129–1138.
38. Born, T. L., Thomassen, E., Bird, T. A., and Sims, J. E. (1998) Cloning of a novel receptor subunit, AcPL, required for interleukin-18 signaling. *J. Biol. Chem.* **273,** 29445–29450.
39. Hyodo, Y., Matsui, K., Hayashi, N., et al. (1999) IL-18 up-regulates perforin-mediated NK activity without increasing perforin messenger RNA expression by binding to constitutively expressed IL-18 receptor. *J. Immunol.* **162,** 1662–1668.
40. Nakahira, M., Tomura, M., Iwasaki, M., et al. (2001) An absolute requirement for STAT4 and a role for IFN-γ as an amplifying factor in IL-12 induction for the functional IL-18 receptor complex. *J. Immunol.* **167,** 1306–1312.
41. Freudenberg, M. A., Merlin, T., Kalis, C., Chvatchko, Y., Stübig, H., and Galanos, C. (2002) A murine, IL-12-independent pathway of IFN-γ induction by gram-negative bacteria based on STAT4 activation by type 1 IFN and IL-18 signaling. *J. Immunol.* **169,** 1665–1668.
42. Matikainen, S., Paananen, A., Miettinen, M., et al. (2001) IFN-α and IL-18 synergistically enhance IFN-γ production in human NK cells: differential regulation of Stat4 activation and IFN-γ gene expression by IFN-α and IL-12. *Eur. J. Immunol.* **31,** 2236–2245.
43. Tominaga, K., Yoshimoto, T., Torigoe, K., et al. (2000) IL-12 synergizes with IL-18 or IL-1β for IFN-γ production from human T cells. *Int. Immunol.* **12,** 151–160.
44. Smeltz, R. B., Chen, J., Gu-Li, J., and Shevach, E. M. (2001) Regulation of interleukin (IL)-18 receptor α chain expression on $CD4^+$ T cells during T helper (Th) 1/Th2 differentiation: critical downregulatory role of IL-4. *J. Exp. Med.* **194,** 143–153.
45. Smeltz, R. B., Chen, J., Ehrhardt, R., and Shevach, E. M. (2002) Role of IFN-γ in Th1 differentiation: IFN-γ regulates IL-18Rα expression by preventing the negative effects of IL-4 and by inducing/maintaining IL-12 receptor β2 expression. *J. Immunol.* **168,** 6165–6172.
46. Kohno, K., Kataoka, J., Ohtsuki, T., et al. (1997) IFN-γ-inducing factor (IGIF) is a costimulatory factor on the activation of Th1 but not Th2 cells and exerts its effect independently of IL-12. *J. Immunol.* **158,** 1541–1550.
47. Xu, D., Chan, W. L., Leung, B. P., et al. (1998) Selective expression and functions of interleukin 18 receptor on T helper (Th) type 1 but not Th2 cells. *J. Exp. Med.* **188,** 1485–1492.
48. Ahn, H. J., Maruo, S., Tomura, M., et al. (1997) A mechanism underlying synergy between IL-12 and IFN-γ-inducing factor in enhanced production of IFN-γ. *J. Immunol.* **159,** 2125–2131.
49. Nakahira, M., Ahn, H.-J., Park, W.-R., et al. (2002) Synergy of IL-12 and IL-18 for IFN-γ gene expression: IL-12-induced STAT4 contributes to IFN-γ promoter activation by up-regulating the binding activity of IL-18-induced activator protein 1. *J. Immunol.* **168,** 1146–1153.
50. Kaplan, M. H., Sun, Y. L., Hoey, T., and Grusby, M. J. (1996) Impaired IL-12 responses and enhanced development of Th2 cells in Stat4-deficient mice. *Nature* **382,** 174–177.
51. Barbulescu, K., Becker, C., Schlaak, J. F., Schmitt, E., Meyer zum Büschenfelde, K., and Neurath, M. F. (1998) IL-12 and IL-18 differentially regulate the transcriptional activity of the human IFN-γ promoter in primary CD4+ T lymphocytes. *J. Immunol.* **160,** 3642–3647.

52. Shimoda, K., Tsutsui, H., Aoki, K., et al. (2002) Partial impairment of interleukin-12 (IL-12) and IL-18 signaling in Tyk2-deficient mice. *Blood* **99,** 2094–2099.
53. Shimoda, K., Kato, K., Aoki, K., et al. (2000) Tyk2 plays a restricted role in IFN-α signaling, although it is required for IL-12-mediated T cell function. *Immunity* **13,** 561–571.
54. Kalina, U., Kauschat, D., Koyama, N., et al. (2000) IL-18 activates STAT3 in the natural killer cell line 92, augments cytotoxic activity, and mediates IFN-γ production by the stress kinase p38 and by the extracellular regulated kinases $p44^{erk-1}$ and $p42^{erk-21}$. *J. Immunol.* **165,** 1307–1313.
55. Morel, J. C., Park, C. C., Zhu, K., Kumar, P., Roth, J. H., and Koch, A. E. (2002) Signal transduction pathways involved in rheumatoid arthritis synovial fibroblast IL-18-induced vascular cell adhesion molecule-1 expression. *J. Biol. Chem.* **277,** 34679–34691.
56. Nakanishi, K. (2001) Innate and acquired activation pathways in T cells. *Nat. Immunol.* **2,** 140–142.
57. Yang, J., Zhu, H., Murphy, T. L., Ouyang, W., and Murphy, K. M. (2001) IL-18-stimulated GADD45β required in cytokine-induced, but not TCR-induced, IFN-γ production. *Nat. Immunol.* **2,** 157–164.
58. Lu, B., Yu, H., Chow, C., et al. (2001) GADD45γ mediates the activation of the p38 and JNK MAP kinase pathways and cytokine production in effector Th1 cells. *Immunity* **14,** 583–590.
59. Fornace, A. J. Jr., Jackman, J., Hollander, M. C., Hoffman-Liebermann, B., and Liebermann, D. A. (1992) Genotoxic-stress-response genes and growth-arrest genes. *gadd, MyD,* and other genes induced by treatments eliciting growth arrest. *Ann. NY Acad. Sci.* **663,** 139–153.
60. Hollander, M. C., Sheikh, M. S., Bulavin, D. V., et al. (1999) Genomic instability in Gadd45α-deficient mice. *Nat. Genet.* **23,** 176–184.
61. Abdollahi, A., Lord, K. A., Hoffman-Liebermann, B., and Liebermann, D. A. (1991) Sequence and expression of a cDNA encoding MyD118: a novel myeloid differentiation primary response gene induced by multiple cytokines. *Oncogene* **6,** 165–167.
62. Beadling, C., Johnson, K. W., and Smith, K. A. (1993) Isolation of interleukin 2-induced immediate-early genes. *Proc. Natl. Acad. Sci. USA* **90,** 2719–2723.
63. Takekawa, M. and Saito, H. (1998) A family of stress-inducible GADD45-like proteins mediate activation of the stress-responsive MTK1/MEKK4/MAPKKK. *Cell* **95,** 521–530.
64. Hoshino, K., Kashiwamura, S., Kuribayashi, K., et al. (1999) The absence of interleukin 1 receptor-related T1/ST2 does not affect T helper cell type 2 development and its effector function. *J. Exp. Med.* **190,** 1541–1547.
65. Chan, W. L., Pejnovic, N., Lee, C. A., and Al-Ali, N. A. (2001) Human IL-18 receptor and ST2L are stable and selective markers for the respective type 1 and type 2 circulating lymphocytes. *J. Immunol.* **167,** 1238–1244.
66. Novick, D., Kim, S. H., Fantuzzi, G., Reznikov, L. L., Dinarello, C. A., and Rubinstein, M. (1999) Interleukin-18 binding protein: a novel modulator of the Th1 cytokine response. *Immunity* **10,** 127–136.
67. Kim, S.-H., Eisenstein, M., Reznikov, L., et al. (2000) Structural requirements of six naturally occurring isoforms of the IL-18 binding protein to inhibit IL-18. *Proc. Natl. Acad. Sci. USA* **97,** 1190–1195.
68. Xiang, Y. and Moss, B. (2001) Correspondence of the functional epitopes of poxvirus and human interleukin-18-binding protein, *J. Virol.* **75,** 9947–9954.
69. Paulukat, J., Bosmann, M., Nold, M., et al. (2001) Expression and release of IL-18 binding protein in response to IFN-γ. *J. Immunol.* **167,** 7038–7043.
70. Mosmann, T. R. and Coffman, R. L. (1989) TH1 and TH2 cells: different patterns of lymphokine secretion lead to different functional properties. *Annu. Rev. Immunol.* **7,** 145–173.
71. Szabo, S. J., Kim, S. T., Costa, G. L., Zhang, X., Fathman, C. G., and Glimcher, L. H. (2000) A novel transcription factor, T-bet, directs Th1 lineage commitment. *Cell* **100,** 655–669.
72. Mullen, A. C., High, F. A., Hutchins, A. S., et al. (2001) Role of T-bet in commitment of Th1 cells before IL-12-dependent selection. *Science* **298,** 1907–1910.
73. Zheng, W.-P. and Flavell, R. A. (1997) The transcription factor GATA-3 is necessary and sufficient for Th2 cytokine gene expression in $CD4^+$ T cells. *Cell* **89,** 587–596.
74. Ouyang, W., Ranganath, S. H., Weindel, K., et al. (1998) Inhibition of Th1 developmental mediated by GATA-3 through an IL-4 independent mechanism. *Immunity* **9,** 745–755.
75. Ferber, I. A., Lee, H. J., Zonin, F., et al. (1999) GATA-3 significantly downregulates IFN-γ production from developing Th1 cells in addition to inducing IL-4 and IL-5 levels. *Clin. Immunol.* **91,** 134–144.

76. Zhang, D.-H., Yang, L., Cohn, L., et al. (1999) Inhibition of allergic inflammation in a murine model of asthma by expression of a dominant-negative mutant of GATA-3 *Immunity* **11,** 473–482.
77. Agarwal, S. and Rao, A. (1998) Modulation of chromatin structure regulates cytokine gene expression during T cell differentiation. *Immunity* **9,** 765–775.
78. Takeda, K., Tsutsui, H., Yoshimoto, T., et al. (1998) Defective NK cell activity and Th1 response in IL-18-deficient mice. *Immunity* **8,** 383–390.
79. Ohkusu, K., Yoshimoto, T., Takeda, K., et al. (2000) Potentiality of interleukin-18 as a useful reagent for treatment and prevention of *Leishmania major* infection. *Infect. Immun.* **68,** 2449–2456.
80. Hoshino, T., Yagita, H., Ortldo, R. H., and Young, H. A. (2000) In vivo administration of IL-18 can induce IgE production through Th2 cytokine induction and up-regulation of CD40 ligand (CD154) expression on $CD4^+$ T cells. *Eur. J. Immunol.* **30,** 1998–2006.
81. Yoshimoto, T., Mizutani, H., Tsutsui, H., et al. (2000) IL-18 induction of IgE: dependence on CD4+ T cells, IL-4 and STAT6. *Nat. Immunol.* **1,** 132–137.
82. Xu, D., Trajkovic, V., Hunter, D., et al. (2000) IL-18 induces the differentiation of Th1 or Th2 cells depending upon cytokine milieu and genetic background. *Eur. J. Immunol.* **30,** 3147–3156.
83. Hoshino, T., Kawase, Y., Okamoto, M., et al. (2001) IL-18-transgenic mice: in vivo evidence of a broad role for IL-18 in modulating immune function. *J. Immunol.* **166,** 7014–7018.
84. Konishi, H., Tsutsui, H., Murakami, T., et al. (2002) IL-18 contributes to the spontaneous development of atopic dermatitis-like inflammatory skin lesion independently of IgE/stat6 under specific pathogen-free conditions. *Proc. Natl. Acad. Sci. USA* **99,** 11340–11345.
85. Nakanishi, K., Yoshimoto, T., Kashiwamura, S.-I., Tsutsui, H., and Okamura, H. (2000) Interleukin-18. In: Holland, S. M., ed. *Cytokine Therapeutic in Infectious Diseases.* Lippincott Williams & Wilkins, Philadelphia, pp. 119–144.
86. Sareneva, T., Julkunen, I., and Matikainen, S. (2000) IFN-α and IL-12 induce IL-18 receptor gene expression in human NK and T cells. *J. Immunol.* **165,** 1933–1938.
87. Guidotti, L. G., Rochford, R., Chung, J., Shapiro, M., Purcell, R., and Chisari, F. V. (1999) Viral clearance without destruction of infected cells during acute HBV infection. *Science* **284,** 825–829.
88. Guidotti, L. G. and Chisari, F. V. (2001) Noncytolytic control of viral infections by the innate and adaptive immune response. *Annu. Rev. Immunol.* **19,** 65–91.
89. Unanue, E. R. (1997) Studies in listeriosis show the strong symbiosis between the innate cellular system and the T-cell response. *Immunol. Rev.* **158,** 11–25.
90. Neighbors, M., Xu, X., Barrat, F., et al. (2001) A critical role for interleukin 18 in primary and memory effector responses to *Listeria monocytogenes* that extends beyond its effects on interferon γ production. *J. Exp. Med.* **194,** 343–354.
91. Edelson, B. T. and Unanue, E. R. (2002) MyD88-dependent but Toll-like receptor 2-independent innate immunity to *Listeria*: no role for either in macrophage listericidal activity. *J. Immunol.* **169,** 3869–3875.
92. Seki, E., Tsutsui, H., Tuji, N. M., et al. (2002) Critical roles of myeloid differentiation factor 88-dependent proinflammatory cytokine release in early phase clearance of *Listeria monocytogenes* in mice. *J. Immunol.* **169,** 3863–3868.
93. Swain, S. L. (2001) Interleukin 18: tipping the balance towards a T helper cell 1 response. *J. Exp. Med.* **194,** F11–F14.
94. Kawakami, K., Qureshi, M. H., Zhang, T., Okamura, H., Kurimoto, M., and Saito, A. (1997) IL-18 protects mice against pulmonary and disseminated infection with *Cryptococcus neoformans* by inducing IFN-γ production. *J. Immunol.* **159,** 5528–5534.
95. Kawakami, K., Koguchi, Y., Qureshi, M. H., et al. (2000) IL-18 contributes to host resistance against infection with *Cryptococcus neoformans* in mice with defective IL-12 synthesis through induction of IFN-γ production by NK cells. *J. Immunol.* **165,** 941–947.
96. Mattner, F., Magram, J., Ferrante, J., et al. (1996) Genetically resistant mice lacking interleukin-12 are susceptible to infection with *Leishmania major* and mount a polarized Th2 cell response. *Eur. J. Immunol.* **26,** 1553–1559.
97. Wei, X. Q., Leung, B. P., Niedbala, W., et al. (1999) Altered immune responses and susceptibility to *Leishmania major* and *Staphylococcus aureus* infection in IL-18-deficient mice. *J. Immunol.* **163,** 2821–2828.

98. Monteforte, G. M., Takeda, K., Rodriguez-Sosa, M., Akira, S., David, J. R., and Satoskar, A. R. (2000) Genetically resistant mice lacking IL-18 gene develop Th1 response and control cutaneous *Leishmania major* infection. *J. Immunol.* **164,** 5890–5893.
99. Singh, R. P., Kashiwamura, S., Rao, P., Okamura, H., Mukherjee, A., and Chauhan, V. S. (2002) The role of IL-18 in blood-stage immunity against murine malaria *Plasmodium yoelii 265* and *Plasmodium berghei ANKA*. *J. Immunol.* **168,** 4674–4681.
100. Yap, G. S., Ortmann, R., Sheavach, E., and Sher, A. (2001) A heritable defect in IL-12 signaling in B10.Q/J mice. II. Effect on acute resistance to *Toxoplasma gondii* and rescue by IL-18 treatment. *J. Immunol.* **166,** 5720–5725.
101. Coughlin, C. M., Salhany, K. E., Wysocka, M., et al. (1998) Interleukin-12 and interleukin-18 synergistically induce murine tumor regression which involves inhibition of angiogenesis. *J. Clin. Invest.* **101,** 1441–1452.
102. Chikano, S., Sawada, K., Shimoyama, T., et al. (2000) IL-18 and IL-12 induce intestinal inflammation and fatty liver in mice in an IFN-γ-dependent manner. *Gut* **47,** 779–786.
103. Siegmund, B., Lehr, H.-A., Fantuzzi, G., and Dinarello, C. A. (2001) IL-1β-converting enzyme (caspase-1) in intestinal inflammation. *Proc. Natl. Acad. Sci. USA* **96,** 13249–13254.
104. Wirtz, S., Becker, C., Blumberg, R., Galle, P. R., and Neurath, M. F. (2002) Treatment of T cell-dependent experimental colitis in SCID mice by local administration of an adenovirus expressing IL-18 antisense mRNA. *J. Immunol.* **168,** 411–420.
105. Sivakumar, P. V., Westich, G. M., Kanaly, S., et al. (2002) Interleukin 18 is a primary mediator of the inflammation associated with dextran sulfate sodium induced colitis: blocking interleukin 18 attenuates intestinal damage. *Gut* **50,** 812–820.
106. Fujimori, Y., Takatsuka, H., Takemoto, Y., et al. (2000) Elevated interleukin (IL)-18 levels during acute graft-versus-host disease after allogeneic bone marrow transplantation. *Br. J. Haematol.* **109,** 652–657.
107. Itoi, H., Fujimori, Y., Tsutsui, H., et al. (2001) Fas ligand-induced caspase-1-dependent accumulation of interleukin (IL)-18 in mice with acute graft-versus-host disease. *Blood* **98,** 235–237.
108. Reddy, P., Teshima, T., Kukuruga, M., et al. (2001) Interleukin-18 regulates acute graft-versus-host disease by enhancing Fas-mediated donor T cell apoptosis. *J. Exp. Med.* **194,** 1433–1440.
109. Yamanaka, K., Tanaka, M., Tsutsui, H., et al. (2000) Skin-specific caspase-1 transgenic mice show cutaneous apoptosis and pre-endotoxin shock condition with a high serum level of IL-18. *J. Immunol.* **165,** 997–1003.
110. Wang, B., Feliciani, C., Howell, B. G., et al. (2002) Contribution of Langerhans cell-derived IL-18 to contact hypersensitivity. *J. Immunol.* **168,** 3303–3308.
111. McInnes, I. B., Gracie, J. A., and Liew, F. Y. (2001) Interleukin-18: a novel cytokine in inflammatory rheumatic disease. *Arthritis Rheum.* **44,** 1481–1483.
112. Alaaeddine, N., Olee, T., Hashimoto, S., Creighton-Achermann, L., and Lotz, M. (2001) Production of the chemokine RANTES by articular chondrocytes and role in cartilage degradation. *Arthritis Rheum.* **44,** 1633–1643.
113. Morel, J. C., Park, C. C., Woods, J. M., and Koch, A. E. (2001) A novel role for interleukin-18 in adhesion molecule induction through NFκB and phosphatidylinositol (PI) 3-kinase-dependent signal transduction pathways. *J. Biol. Chem.* **276,** 37069–37075.
114. Plater-Zyberk, C., Joosten, L. A., Helsen, M. M., et al. (2001) Therapeutic effect of neutralizing endogenous IL-18 activity in the collagen-induced model of arthritis. *J. Clin. Invest.* **108,** 1825–1832.
115. Park, C. C., Morel, J. C., Amin, A. M., Connors, M. A., Harlow, L. A., and Koch, A. E. (2001) Evidence of IL-18 as a novel angiogenic mediator. *J. Immunol.* **167,** 1644–1653.
116. Mallat, Z., Corbaz, A., Scoazec, A., et al. (2001) Expression of interleukin-18 in human atherosclerotic plaque and relation to plaque instability. *Circulation* **104,** 1598–1603.
117. Libby, P., Ridker, P. M., and Maseri, A. (2002) Inflammation and atherosclerosis. *Circulation* **105,** 1135–1143.
118. Whitman, S. C., Ravisankar, P., and Daugherty, A. (2002) Interleukin-18 enhances atherosclerosis in apolipoprotein $E^{-/-}$ mice through release of interferon-γ. *Circ. Res.* **90,** e34–e38.
119. Kosco-Vilbois, M. H. (2002) IL-18-a destabilizer of atherosclerotic disease. *Trends Immunol.* **23,** 123.

120. Blackenberg, S., Tiret, L., Bickel, C., et al. (2002) Interlelukin-18 is a strong predictor of cardiovascular death in stable and unstable angina. *Circulation* **106,** 24–30.
121. Kiechl, S., Lorenz, E., Reindl, M., et al. (2002) Toll-like receptor 4 polymorphisms and atherosclerosis. *N. Engl. J. Med.* **347,** 185–192.
122. Young, J. L., Sukhova, G. K., Foster, D., Kisiel, W., Libby, P., and Schonbeck, U. (2000) The serpin proteinase inhibitor 9 is an endogenous inhibitor of interleukin-1β-converting enzyme (caspase-1) activity in human vascular smooth muscle cells. *J. Exp. Med.* **191,** 1535–1544.
123. Plaut, M., Pierce, J. H., Watson, C. J., Hanley-Hyde, J., Nordan, R. P., and Paul, W. E. (1989) Mast cell lines produce lymphocytes in response to cross-linkage of Fcε RI or to calcium ionophores. *Nature* **339,** 64–67.
124. Paul, W. E., Seder, R. A., and Plaut, M. (1993) Lymphokine and cytokine production by $Fc\varepsilon RI^+$ cells. *Adv. Immunol.* **53,** 1–29.
125. Matsuda, H., Watanabe, N., Geba, G. P., et al. (1996) Development of atopic dermatitis-like skin lesion with IgE hyperproduction in NC/Nga mice. *Int. Immunol.* **9,** 461–466.
126. Yagi, R., Nagai, H., Iigo, Y., Akimoto, T., Arai, T., and Kubo, M. (2002) Development of atopic dermatitis-like skin lesions in STAT6-deficient NC/Nga mice. *J. Immunol.* **168,** 2020–2027.
127. Hoshino, K., Tsutsui, H., Kawai, T., et al. (1999) Generation of IL-18 receptor-deficient mice: evidence for IL-1 receptor-related protein as an essential IL-18 binding receptor. *J. Immunol.* **162,** 5041–5044.
128. Hochholzer, P., Lipford, G. B., Wagner, H., Pfeffer, K., and Heeg, K. (2000) Role of interlukin-18 (IL-18) during lethal shock: decreased lipopolysaccharide sensitivity by normal superantigen reaction in IL-18-deficient mice. *Infect. Immun.* **68,** 3502–3508.
129. Tsutsui, H., Matsui, K., Kawada, N., et al. (1997) IL-18 accounts for both TNF-α- and Fas ligand-mediated hepatotoxic pathways in endotoxin-induced liver injury in mice. *J. Immunol.* **159,** 3961–3967.
130. Sakao, Y., Takeda, K., Tsutsui, H., et al. (1999) IL-18-deficient mice are resistant to endotoxin-induced liver injury but highly susceptible to endotoxin shock. *Int. Immunol.* **11,** 471–480.
131. Kanai, T., Watanabe, M., Oakazawa, A., et al. (2001) Macrophage-derived IL-18-mediated intestinal inflammation in the murine model of Crohn's disease. *Gastrotenterology* **121,** 875–888.
132. Melnikov, V. Y., Ecder, T., Fantuzzi, G., et al. (2001) Impaired IL-18 processing protects caspase-1-deficient mice from ischemic acute renal failure. *J. Clin. Invest.* **107,** 1145–1152.
133. Hedtjarn, M., Leverin, A. L., Eriksson, K., Blomgren, K., Mallard, C., and Hagberg, H. (2002) Interelukin-18 involvement in hypoxic-ischemic brain injury. *J. Neurosci.* **22,** 5910–5919.
134. Taneja, V. and David, C. S. (1999) HLA class II transgenic mice as models of human diseases. *Immunol. Rev.* **169,** 67-79.
135. Gracie, J. A., Forsey, R. J., Chan, W. L., et al. (1999) A proinflammatory role for IL-18 in rheumatoid arthritis. *J. Clin. Invest.* **104,** 1393–1401.
136. Dayer, J. M. (1999) Interleukin-18, rheumatoid arthritis, and tissue destruction. *J. Clin. Invest.* **104,** 1337–1339.
137. Wong, C. K., Li, E. K., Ho, C., and Lam, C. W. (2000) Elevation of plasma interleukin-18 concentration is correlated with disease activity in systemic lupus erythematosus. *Rheumatology* **39,** 1078–1081.
138. Nicoletti, F., Di Marco, R., Mangano, K., et al. (2000) Increased serum levels of interleukin-18 in patients with multiple sclerosis. *Neurology* **24,** 342–344.
139. Wei, X., Leung, B. P., Arthur, H. M., McInnes, I. B., and Liew, F. Y. (2001) Reduced incidence and severity of collagen-induced arthritis in mice lacking IL-18. *J. Immunol.* **166,** 517–521.
140. Shi, F.-D., Takeda, K., Akira, S., Sarvetnick, N., and Ljunggren, H.-G. (2000) IL-18 directs autoreactive T cells and promotes autodestruction in the central nervous system via induction of IFN-γ by NK cells. *J. Immunol.* **165,** 3099–3104.
141. Jiang, H.-R., Wei, Z., Niedbala, W., Lumsden, L., Liew, F. Y., and Forrester, J. V. (2001) IL-18 not required for IRBP peptide-induced EAU: studies in gene-deficient mice. *Invest. Ophthalmol. Vis. Sci.* **42,** 177–182.
142. Trinchieri, G. (1989) Biology of natural killer cells. *Adv. Immunol.* **47,** 187–376.
143. Pien, G. C., Satoskar, A. R., Takeda, K., Akira, S., and Biron, C. A. (2000) Selective IL-18 requirements for induction of compartmental IFN-γ responses during viral infection. *J. Immunol.* **165,** 4787–4791.

144. Parr, M. B. and Parr, E. L. (1999) The role of gamma interferon in immune resistance to vaginal infection by herpes simplex virus type 2 in mice. *Virology* **258,** 282–294.
145. Harandi, A. M., Svennerholm, B., Holmgren, J., and Eriksson, K. (2001) Interleukin-12 (IL-12) and IL-18 are important in innate defense against genital herpes simplex virus type 2 infection in mice but are not required for the development of acquired gamma interferon-mediated protective immunity. *J. Virology* **75,** 6705–6709.
146. Mori, I., Hossain, J., Takeda, K., et al. (2001) Impaired microglial activation in the brain of IL-18-gene-disrupted mice after neurovirulent influenza A virus infection. *Virology* **287,** 163–170.
147. Ohteki, T., Fukao, T., Suzue, K., et al. (1999) Interleukin 12-dependent interferon gamma production by CD8α^+ lymphoid dendritic cells. *J. Exp. Med.* **189,** 1981–1986.
148. Sugawara, I., Yamada, H., Kaneko, H., Mizuno, S., Takeda, K., and Akira, S. (1999) Role of interleukin-18 (IL-18) in mycobacterial infection in IL-18-gene-disrupted mice. *Infect. Immun.* **67,** 2585–2589.
149. Kinjo, Y., Kawakami, K., Uezu, K., et al. (2002) Contribution of IL-18 to Th1 response and host defense against infection by *Mycobacterium tuberculosis*: a comparative study with IL-12p40. *J. Immunol.* **169,** 323–329.
150. Lauw, F. N., Branger, J., Florquin, S., et al. (2002) IL-18 improves the early antimicrobial host response to pneumococcal pneumonia. *J. Immunol.* **168,** 372–378.
151. Lim, T. S. and Murphy, J. W. (1980) Transfer of immunity to criptococcosis by T-enriched splenic lymphocytes from *Cryptococcus neoformans*-sensitized mice. *Infect. Immun.* **30,** 5–15.
152. Afonso, L. C., Scharton, T. M., Vieira, L. Q., Wysocka, M., Trinchieri, G., and Scott, P. (1994) The adjuvant effect of interleukin-12 in a vaccine against *Leishmania major*. *Science* **263,** 235–237.
153. Adachi, K., Tsutsui, H., Kashiwamura, S., et al. (2001) *Plasmodium berghei* infection in mice induces liver injury by an IL-12- and Toll-like receptor/myeloid differentiation factor 88-dependent mechanism. *J. Immunol.* **167,** 5928–5934.
154. Finkelman, F. D., Pearce, E. J., Urban, J. F. J., and Sher, A. (1991) Regulation and biological function of helminth-induced cytokine responses. *Immunol. Today* **12,** A62–A66.
155. Urban, J. F. Jr., Madden, K. B., Svetíc, A., et al. (1992) The importance of Th2 cytokines in protective immunity to nematodes. *Immunol. Rev.* **127,** 205–220.
156. Locksley, R. M. (1994) Th2 cells: help for helminth. *J. Exp. Med.* **179,** 1405–1407.
157. Helmby, H., Takeda, K., Akira, S., and Grencis, R. K. (2001) Interleukin (IL)-18 promotes the development of chronic gastrointestinal helminth infection by downregulating IL-13. *J. Exp. Med.* **194,** 355–364.
158. Helmby, H. and Grencis, R. K. (2002) IL-18 regulates intestinal mastocytosis and Th2 cytokine production independently of IFN-γ during *Trichinella spiralis* infection. *J. Immunol.* **169,** 2553–2560.
159. Csernok, E., Lüdemann, J., Gross, W. L., and Bainton, D. F. (1990) Ultrastructural localization of proteinase 3, the target antigen of anti-cytoplasmic antibodies circulating in Wegener's granulomatosis. *Am. J. Pathol.* **137,** 1113–1120.
160. Dolman, K. M., van de Wiel, B. A., Kam, C.-M., et al. (1992) Determination of proteinase 3-α_1-antitrypsin complexes in inflammatory fluids. *FEBS Lett.* **2,** 117–121.
161. Sugawara, S., Uehara, A., Nochi, T., et al. (2001) Neutrophil proteinase 3-mediated induction of bioactive IL-18 secretion by human oral epithelial cells. *J. Immunol.* **167,** 6568–6575.
162. de Saint-Vis, B., Fugier, V. I., Massacrier, C., et al. (1998) The cytokine profile expressed by human dendritic cells is dependent on cell subtype and mode of activation. *J. Immunol.* **160,** 1666–1676.
163. Stoll, S., Jonuleit, H., Schmitt, E., et al. (1998) Production of functional IL-18 by different subtypes of murine and human dendritic cells (DC): DC-derived IL-18 enhances IL-12-dependent Th1 development. *Eur. J. Immunol.* **28,** 3231–3239.
164. Afkarian, M., Sedy, J. R., Yang, J., et al. (2002) T-bet is a stat1-induced regulator for IL-12R expression in naive CD4$^+$ T cells. *Nat. Immunol.* **3,** 549–557.
165. Kojima, H., Takeuchi, M., Ohta, T., et al. (1998) Interleukin-18 activates the IRAK-TRAF6 pathway in mouse EL-4 cells. *Biochem. Biophys. Res. Commun.* **244,** 183–186.

19

Mice Knockouts for Chemokines and Chemokine Receptors

Jane M. Schuh, Steven L. Kunkel, and Cory M. Hogaboam

Summary

Chemokines are small, mainly soluble cytokines that are chemotactic for leukocytes. In inflammation, they are integral to the activation of both immune and resident cells in addition to their function in leukocyte recruitment. The chemokine network is ostensibly both redundant and promiscuous, which would imply superfluous activities. However, gene-targeted chemokine and chemokine receptor mutants have revealed that chemokine regulation is incredibly intricate, incorporating temporal, spatial, and pathogen-specific expression. Studying the actions and interactions of chemokines in vivo has been invaluable in elucidating the contribution that these mediators impart on the immune response.

Key words

chemokine, knockout, inflammation, leukocytes, cytokine

1. Introduction

Cellular trafficking and interaction are essential aspects of a directed immune response. To provide host defense, intricate cellular complexes must be coordinated to counter invasion by pathogenic organisms. The orchestration of leukocyte movement is accomplished through chemoattractant cytokines, or chemokines, signaling through seven-membered transmembrane G-protein-coupled receptors. Chemokines are a group of small (7–16 kDa), mainly soluble, bioactive cytokines that are expressed by a number of immune and non-immune cells. They are the principal movers of leukocytes into sites of pathogenic challenge or injury. The role of chemokines is not limited to recruitment: they may also orchestrate the immune response by activation, degranulation, or differentiation of participating cells. Unfortunately, an overly aggressive chemokine response frequently perpetrates tissue injury, contributing to the pathogenesis of the primary disease. Indeed, elevated chemokine levels have been noted in a number of infectious, allergic, and autoimmune diseases, making these molecules and the receptors that bind them attractive targets for potential therapeutic intervention.

Chemokines contain conserved cysteine residues that form disulfide bonds essential to the quaternary protein structure. The number and spacing of the first two cysteines is used to characterize chemokine subfamilies (C, CC, CXC, CX_3C). For example, if the first two

From: *Contemporary Immunology: Cytokine Knockouts, 2nd Edition*
Edited by: Giamila Fantuzzi © Humana Press Inc., Totowa, NJ

cysteines are adjacent, they are classified in the CC family (also referred to as the β-subclass). The CXC family (α) has a single amino acid between the initial two cysteines. Within the CXC subfamily, the chemokines can be further divided into two groups, those having the defining three amino acid ELR (glutamic acid-leucine-arginine) sequence motif immediately preceding the first conserved cysteine and those that lack this domain. Two recently discovered chemokines, lymphotactin and fractalkine, represent the first members of the C and CX_3C subfamilies, respectively.

Initially, chemokines acquired names based on their function. This practice was confusing since many of these molecules have multiple functions. Recently, the nomeclature has been standardized for clarity (reviewed in ref. *1*). Many of the ELR-containing CXC chemokines are chemotactic for neutrophils, whereas non-ELR CXC chemokines recruit lymphocytes. In contrast, the CC chemokines are chemotactic for monocytes, T- and B-lymphocytes, dendritic cells, natural killer cells, eosinophils, and basophils, but rarely neutrophils. The unique C chemokine lymphotactin is chemotactic for lymphocytes. Fractalkine (CX_3C), whose chemokine domain is tethered on a mucin-like stalk, has been found to trigger the adhesion of T-cells and monocytes *(2,3)*. The activities of many of the more recently discovered chemokines are just being elucidated.

The chemokine receptors are similarly grouped according to the ligands that they bind. There are 10 known CC receptors and 6 CXC receptors. Based on in vitro binding assays, a single chemokine is often capable of binding multiple chemokine receptors, and one receptor may have more than one chemokine ligand. Knockout mice have been instrumental in showing that, although binding may be possible between multiple chemokines and multiple receptors, the spatial and temporal expressions of these molecules are probably responsible for one dominant chemokine:receptor binding pair in most situations. Chemokines with similar actions that are genetically clustered appear to be more promiscuous in their binding characteristics, which accounts for the putative redundancy in the system. Chemokines with isolated genes tend to exhibit affinity to only one receptor. Indeed, the trend in recently described chemokines seems to be that of one chemokine, one receptor (for example, CX3CR1:CX3CL1, XCR1:XCL1).

Knockout mice have increased our knowledge of the role that chemokines play in clinically relevant disease models. To generate the knockout genotype, the gene of interest is isolated from a murine HM-1 embryonic stem (ES) cell library by plaque hybridization using the target cDNA as a probe. The resulting genomic DNA is inserted into a construction vector where the coding sequence of the gene is replaced with an unrelated gene sequence. After a selection process, positive plasmid DNA is used to tranfsect an HM-1 ES cell line *(4)*. ES cell clones are then used to produce chimeric mice by blastocyst injection according to established procedures *(5)*. Most of our information on the biology of chemokines is based on knockout mice. However, it is important to note that genetic and phenotypic differences do exist between both human and murine chemokines as well as among mouse strains. For example, mice do not have an IL-8 homolog, one of the most important human CXC neutrophil chemoattractants. Therefore, neutrophil research requires careful interpretation of the performance of functional homologs and the realization that the experimental conditions do not ideally reflect the human disease. Another instance involves one of the primary asthma models used today, the ovalbumin (OVA) model. C57Bl/6 mice are resistant to the OVA-induced asthma phenotype *(6,7)*. Since many of the null mice are raised on a C57Bl/6 background, the appropriate use of this model in knockout systems is limited. Phenotypic differences are evident in the comparison of F2 (second filial generation) versus congenic mice. This controversy will, no doubt, raise discrepancies in the resulting literature. Still, knockout mice have been an invaluable tool for establishing a basic understanding of the roles that chemokines and their receptors play in diseases. In addition to knockout mice, transgenic mice have been used to elucidate the effect that overexpression of chemokines has on a model system. Use of chemokine and chemokine receptor knockout mice will continue to guide research in the appropriate applications to exploit these promising therapeutic targets.

2. Chemokine Knockout Mice

2.1. MIP-1α

Macrophage inflammatory protein-1α (MIP-1α/CCL3) is a CC chemokine that has proinflammatory and stem cell inhibitory properties. It is produced by a number of cells including lymphocytes, fibroblasts, epithelial cells, and both resident and recruited monocytes and macrophages *(8–12)*. MIP-1α is chemotactic for both monocytes and neutrophils in mice *(13,14)* but mainly directs monocytic cells in humans *(15)*, making it an important participant in the innate immune response. It is a ligand for CCR1 and CCR5. MIP-1α knockout mice have no overt anomalies in either peripheral or bone marrow cells, indicating that MIP-1α is not necessary for normal hematopoiesis *(16)*.

The initial characterization of the MIP-1α knockout mouse showed the importance of this chemokine in the mediation of virus-induced disease via the efferent, or cell recruitment stage. Reduced monocyte recruitment following viral infection significantly decreases the inflammatory pathology seen in coxsackievirus-induced myocarditis, influenza virus-induced pneumonitis, and paramyxovirus-induced pulmonary inflammation *(17,18)*. Along with decreased inflammation, a delay in viral clearance and /or an increase in viral burden were noted.

MIP-1α is also a critical factor in the afferent arm of the immune response. It is required for clearance of the Gram-negative bacterium *Klebsiella pneumoniae*; the alveolar macrophages from mice deficient in MIP-1α have significantly impaired phagocytic abilities *(19)*. MIP-1α prevents the switch to a Th2 response, which is not protective in a *Crytococcus neoformans* fungal infection *(20,21)*.

2.2. MCP-1

Monocyte chemotactic protein-1 (MCP-1/CCL2), also known as JE in the murine system, is expressed in most inflammatory conditions. Its expression correlates with monocyte infiltration into sites of inflammation. Lack of MCP-1 abrogates this recruitment. The chemokine binds exclusively to CCR2, which is found on monocytes, basophils, natural killer (NK) cells, and activated T-cells *(22)*. Disruption of the MCP-1 gene results in the inability to mount a strong Th2-type cytokine response *(23)*.

As an important innate immune chemokine, MCP-1 production has important implications in many diseases whose immunopathology can be attributed to recruitment of inflammatory monocytes to the site of injury. Atherosclerosis is such a disease. Peripheral blood monocytes are the precursors of lipid-bearing foam cells that are recruited to the walls of blood vessels, forming atherosclerotic lesions *(24)*. Disruption of the MCP-1 gene reduces susceptibility to atherosclerosis in transgenic mice that overexpress apolipoprotein B *(25)*, as well as those that were deficient in low-density lipoprotein receptor *(26)*. Ostensibly, this is owing to reduced recruitment of macrophages to the atherosclerotic lesions.

Chemokine induction, including MCP-1, has been implicated in the pathogenesis of brain injury following stroke. In an experimental model of stroke, MCP-1 deficiency was protective in both early and late events following focal ischemia. MCP-$1^{-/-}$ mice experienced significantly reduced infarction size at 24 h, reduced astrocyte hypertrophy at 2 wk, and reduced phagocytic macrophage accumulation at 2 wk after middle cerebral artery occlusion (experimental stroke). Although the late time point protection can be attributed to the reduction in macrophage recruitment, the acute protection seen in the knockout mice cannot. Interestingly, MCP-$1^{-/-}$ mice produced significantly less interleukin-1β (IL-1β) in the affected tissue, which may be tissue-protective *(27)*.

2.3. Eotaxin-1

Eosinophilia in the peripheral blood and tissues is a clinical feature of parasitic infection as well as several atopic disorders including allergy, asthma, and eczema; thus eusinophils are major players in a Th-2-type immune response *(28)*. Eotaxin-1 (CCL11) is a CC chemokine that binds CCR3 and selectively recruits eosinophils. Eotaxin has been implicated in asthma, as its expression is increased in the bronchoalveolar lavage fluid of asthmatics *(29)*, and both epithelial cells and plasma cells express eotaxin in chronic asthmatics *(30)*. Eotaxin is the main chemoattractant and a potent activator of eosinophils. It is capable of inducing both superoxide generation and degranulation *(31)*. IL-5 works synergistically with the chemokine to ensure the growth and survival of these cells. The only nonhematopoietic organs with constitutive eosinophil occupation are the thymus and the gastrointestinal tract. Eosinophils are conspicuously absent in these organs in eotaxin-deficient mice *(32,33)*. However, allergen-induced eosinophilia is only partially ablated in the lungs of the knockouts *(34,35)*, and airway hyperreactivity develops normally in eotaxin-deficient mice. In the *Aspergillus* asthma model, eotaxin$^{-/-}$ mice treated intratracheally with soluble antigen exhibited attenuated acute responses. Interestingly, knockout mice that were treated with live fungal spores intratracheally experienced no attenuation of disease *(36)*. Taken together, these studies suggest redundant pathways to recruit eosinophils and call into question the role that eosinophils play in airway hyperresponsiveness *(37)*.

2.4. Fractalkine

Fractalkine (CX_3CL1) is an unusual chemokine, as it is found in either a membrane-bound or a soluble form. It may be tethered to the membrane by a mucin-like stalk or cleaved, which results in a soluble mediator. Both forms are functional. It is the lone member of the CX_3C chemokine family. Fractalkine is found mainly on activated endothelial cells and is induced by proinflammatory signals including lipopolysaccharide, IL-1, tumor necrosis factor (TNF), interferon-γ (IFN-γ), and CD40 ligand *(38)*. Fractalkine's receptor CX_3CR1 is expressed on NK cells, Th-1-polarized cells, monocytes, dendritic cells, and murine neutrophils *(3,39,40)*. The Th2-type cytokines IL-4 and IL-13 dramatically reduce the induction of fractalkine by the synergistic action of TNF and IFN-γ, indicating that fractaline may help direct the polarization of a Th1-type response *(38)*. The fact that fractalkine is expressed on endothelial cells during a number of inflammatory vascular injury disease states has positioned it as a therapeutic target for allograft rejection, glomerulonephritis, and rheumatoid arthritis *(39,41,42)*.

Fractalkine is abundantly and constitutively expressed on the neurons of the brain. Its receptor is expressed constitutively on microglia, the resident macrophages of the brain *(43)*. Crosstalk between these two cell types acts as a survival factor for microglia cells. Indeed, treatment of these cells with fractalkine ensures survival by upregulating antiapoptotic factors and blocking Fas-mediated cell death *(43–45)*. Surprisingly, mice with disrupted fractalkine genes develop normally, with no neural defect. Unchallenged fractalkine knockout mice differ from their wild-type counterparts only in that they have a significant decrease in the F4/80-expressing monocyte population *(46)*. Even more surprising is that in several models of inflammation—delayed-type hypersensitivity, peritonitis, and enterocolitis—leukocytes traffic normally with no perceptible dysfunction *(46)*.

Fractalkine has a role in acetaminophen-induced liver injury. Initially, a liver enzyme typically used to assess damage (aspartate aminotransferase) is equivalent in knockout mice, wild-type mice, and transgenic mice that overproduce fractalkine. However, after acetaminophen challenge, necrosis and oxidative injury are considerably greater in the transgenic mice and to a lesser extent in the wild-type mice, whereas the fractalkine knockouts are largely protected. The mechanism of protection is the reduction of leukocytes, most notably neutrophils, trafficking into the liver *(47)*.

2.5. SDF-1 and CXCR4

Chemokines are not a new invention of the immune system. *Drosophila* has a chemokine receptor homologous to CXCR4, the receptor for stromal cell-derived factor-1 (SDF-1/CXCL12). This chemokine/receptor pair fulfills regulatory functions outside the immune response. In fact, disrupting the gene for either SDF-1 or CXCR4 results in an embryonic lethal condition. Mice deficient in either molecule have dramatic defects in brain and heart development, intestinal vascular organization, and B-cell hematopoiesis *(48,49)*. In instances when knockout mice are not viable, specific neutralizing antibodies or small-molecule antagonists may help define the roles for these important molecules in the mature system. CXCR4 is a coreceptor for T-cell-tropic HIV-1. In addition, it is highly expressed in a number of cancers, making its regulation a highly attractive target for clinicians.

2.6. Lungkine

Lungkine (CXCL15) is highly and selectively expressed on murine lung epithelial cells, which secrete it into the airway spaces to recruit neutrophils. It is upregulated in response to intratracheal inoculation with various fungal, parasitic, and bacterial components *(50)*. Mice deficient in this chemokine have a defective pulmonary host response *(51)*. When infected with *K. pneumoniae*, the knockout mice are more susceptible to infection, with an increase in bacterial burden and subsequent mortality *(51)*. Interestingly, although neutrophils seem to track normally to the parenchyma of the lung, they fail to reach the airspace *(51)*.

3. Chemokine Receptor Knockout Mice

3.1. CCR1

CCR1 is constitutively expressed on neutrophils, monocytes, lymphocytes, and eosinophils *(52–56)*. It binds MIP-1α, MIP-1γ, MIP-3, MIP-5, regulated on activation, noronal T-cell expressed and secreted (RANTES), MCP-3, and C10 in vitro, but MIP-1α is the major ligand in vivo. In the *Aspergillus* fungal allergy model, a Th2-mediated disease, the airway remodeling that is associated with chronic disease progression is absent in CCR1$^{-/-}$ mice owing to a skewing toward a Th1 response *(57)*. This Th1 skewing also has deleterious effects in nephritis: an enhanced Th1 response in the knockouts exacerbates glomerular injury. CCR1 is induced in both the early, neutrophil-dependent phase of nephritis and in later phases when mononuclear cell infiltration is the dominant characteristic *(58)*. The specificity of the chemokine system is hallmarked by the fact that whereas CCR1 binds both RANTES and MIP-1α, only MIP-1α is able to induce cell migration and at the same time change the effector phase of the disease *(58)*. In CCR1$^{-/-}$ mice, MIP-1α fails to recruit neutrophils to the peripheral blood in vivo. When injected intravenously with *Aspergillus fumigatus*, a fungus controlled mainly by neutrophils, the CCR1$^{-/-}$ mice rapidly proceed toward death *(59)*. These findings clearly show that CCR1's roles are not redundant and that this receptor impacts on the immune response not only through cell recruitment but also via modulation of predominant cytokine profiles.

CCR1 is important for viral clearance. Knockout mice have fewer neutrophils recruited into sites of inflammation and a greater viral load when infected with paramyxovirus *(18)*. Models of Th1-mediated pulmonary granuloma induced by purified protein derivative of *Mycobacterium bovis* have revealed that NK cell recruitment into the lesions of CCR1$^{-/-}$ mice is reduced by 60%, whereas the lesion size remains unchanged between knockout and wild-type mice *(60)*.

Heterotropic cardiac transplants across MHC class I and class II barriers survive, on average, twice as long in CCR1$^{-/-}$ mice as they do in wild-type mice *(61)*. When the knockout mice are treated with subtherapeutic dosages of cyclosporin A, the grafts survive permanently *(61)*. Two other conditions of long-term graft survival are also improved in CCR1$^{-/-}$ mice. Graft arteriosclerosis and chronic rejection are completely eliminated in the knockouts *(61)*.

3.2. CCR2

CCR2 is expressed on monocytes, dendritic cells, basophils, activated T-cells, NK cells, and B-lymphocytes *(22,62)*. CCR2 is the major receptor for MCP-1 and as such has been implicated in a number of inflammatory diseases. It also binds the other homologs of MCP (MCP-2 through MCP-5) *(22,63–66)*.

Consistent with its role in recruiting innate immune cells, CCR2-deficient mice have difficulty mounting a protective response to bacterial or fungal infection. CCR2$^{-/-}$ mice experience increased susceptibility to *Listeria monocytogenes (67)*, *Leishmania major (68)*, *C. neoformans (69)*, and *A. fumigatus (70)*. In leishmaniasis, reduced macrophage recruitment is accompanied by decreased Th2-inducing dendritic cells in the spleen and increased B-cell proliferation, probably causing a shift in the immune response to a nonprotective Th2-type *(68)*. It is interesting that this chemokine deficiency is so critical to macrophage recruitment in these infections. Macrophage and monocyte recruitment can be successfully accomplished via MIP-1α signaling through either CCR1 or CCR5, as well as other chemokine interactions. This fact suggests that the redundancy seen in the chemokine network may not be applicable in many in vivo situations and that the interactions between ligand and receptor are quite probably exquisitely regulated temporally, spatially, and through affinity and avidity of binding.

The asthma models of both OVA and *Aspergillus* show the importance of CCR2 in response to an allergen. Many of the major characteristics of asthma are exacerbated in the CCR2$^{-/-}$ mouse. Airway hyperresponsiveness in reaction to a spasmogen, eosinophilia in the bronchioaolveolar lavage fluid, peribronchial inflammation, immunoglobulin isotype switching, and Th2-type cytokine production are all significantly increased in these allergy models *(70,71)*. In this instance, an overly aggressive Th2 response is detrimental to the host.

In a Th1-mediated granulomatous reaction induced by purified protein derivative of *M. bovis*, CCR2$^{-/-}$ mice exhibit a defect in delayed-type hypersensitivity as well as a reduction in the ability to produce Th1-type cytokines. The CCR2 knockout mouse produces reduced amounts of IFN-γ *(72)*. The reduction in IFN-γ seems to be a trafficking defect. Macrophages, acting as antigen-presenting cells, do not migrate to the draining lymph nodes in CCR2$^{-/-}$ mice. As a result, the antigen-specific, IFN-γ-producing cells in the lymph node are reduced by as much as 70% *(73)*. This clearly demonstrates the important role of CCR2 in linking the innate and acquired immune response. In a Th2-mediated granulomatous reaction induced by *Schistosoma mansoni* eggs, CCR2$^{-/-}$ mice had only transient early monocyte recruitment impairment, which was abrogated by the fourth day, emphasizing the effect of CCR2 on Th1 responses, but not necessarily Th2 responses *(74)*. It is interesting to note that the chemokine knockout (MCP-1) and the receptor knockout (CCR2) mice have very different phenotypes. MCP-1$^{-/-}$ mice exhibit a Th2 defect, and the CCR2$^{-/-}$ knockouts have a Th1 defect.

CCR2-deficient mice crossed with mice deficient in the lipid clearance receptor, apolipoprotein E (ApoE), have reduced severity of atherosclerosis *(75,76)*. Macrophages are considered the major inflammatory cell in atherosclerosis, driving the subsequent progression of the developing plaque through intercellular mediators. ApoE-deficient mice are spontaneously hypercholesterolemic and develop atherosclerotic lesions similar to those seen in humans *(76)*. When backcrossed with CCR2$^{-/-}$ mice, the resulting mouse experiences a threefold reduction in mean aortic lesion size. Serum lipid levels and circulating monocyte numbers remain unchanged compared with controls, but noticeably fewer macrophages accumulate in the lesions, dramatically highlighting the importance of this receptor in atherosclerosis *(75)*.

CCR2$^{-/-}$ mice are almost completely resistant to myelin-oligodendrocyte glycoprotein-induced experimental autoimmune encephalomyelitis (EAE), a model of human multiple sclerosis *(77,78)*. After induction of EAE in CCR2$^{-/-}$ mice, there was a reduction in inflammatory mononuclear cell infiltrates in the central nervous system (CNS), and levels of the chemokines RANTES, MCP-1, IFN-inducible protein-10 (IP-10). There was a significant decrease in expression of the chemokine receptors CCR1, CCR2, and CCR5 *(78)*.

CCR2 is an important receptor in the context of liver injury owing to drug toxicity. MCP-1, CCR2's predominant ligand, is elevated after acetaminophen toxicity. This appears to be a host-protective mechanism, as CCR2$^{-/-}$ mice treated with acetaminophen have dramatically increased liver damage compared with CCR2$^{+/+}$ mice *(47)*. CCR2:MCP-1's role in liver injury appears to be owing to an alleviation of oxidative injury, not directly on cell recruitment *(47)*, which again highlights the multiple functions of chemokines in the immune response.

In other models in which macrophage infiltration has been associated with immunopathology (glomerulonephritis, EAE, and peripheral nervous system injury), the absence of CCR2 imparted protection from disease *(78–80)*. Taken as a whole, this research clearly indicates a critical role for CCR2 in macrophage recruitment in both health and disease, which makes this receptor a highly attractive target for potential therapeutic applications, but one that will need to be approached cautiously.

3.3 CCR3

The CCR3 receptor is expressed on eosinophils, mast cells, Th2-polarized cells, basophils, and neural tissue epithelia *(81)*. Eotaxin is the major ligand of CCR3, but the receptor also binds RANTES, MCP-2, MCP-3, and MCP-4.

Many individuals with atopic dermatitis develop asthma or allergies later in life. This suggests a link between allergic conditions in the skin and lung. CCR3's expression on eosinophils and mast cells make it a likely player in this interaction. Knockout mice sensitized with OVA in a model of atopic dermatitis have no eosinophil recruitment to the skin and little to the parenchyma of the lung *(81)*. Airway hyperresponsiveness does not develop as a result of the OVA sensitization *(81)*. However, CCR3 does not seem to have a major effect on mast cell recruitment to the skin or on the other Th2-dependent mechanisms in this model: mast cell numbers, IL-4 levels, and OVA-specific IgE were all equivalent to controls *(81)*. In a separate study, CCR3 was found to be important in basal eosinophil trafficking to the gut, but only induced eosinophilia in the gut after antigen challenge *(82)*. The majority of the eosinophils in the CCR3$^{-/-}$ mice never made it to the airway but were arrested in the subepithelial space *(82)*, suggesting a multistep process for eosinophil recruitment to the lung. Interestingly, increased number of mast cells were observed in the trachea of the sensitized CCR3$^{-/-}$ mice, but the implications of this fact for allergic inflammation remain unclear *(82)*.

3.4. CCR4

CCR4 is the receptor for thymus and activation-regulated chemokine (TARC/CCL17) *(83)* and macrophage-derived chemokine (MDC/CCL22) *(84)*. It is expressed in the thymus and spleen as well as on peripheral T-lymphocytes, macrophages, basophils, platelets, and monocytes *(85)*. CCR4$^{-/-}$ mice develop normally, and under unchallenged conditions are phenotypically similar to their wild-type littermates *(86)*.

During the characterization of the CCR4$^{-/-}$ mouse, it was discovered that when the mice are challenged with lipopolysaccharide, they exhibit significantly decreased mortality *(86)*. Initially, this was the only phenotypic difference noted between CCR4$^{-/-}$ and CCR4$^{+/+}$ mice, which was surprising considering that Th2-polarized cells express high levels of CCR4 *(87)*. Even so, sensitized CCR4$^{-/-}$ mice exhibit an asthmatic phenotype similar to that of CCR4$^{+/+}$ mice when challenged with a short course of OVA *(86)*. However, when sensitized CCR4$^{-/-}$ mice are challenged with fungal spores, their phenotype is markedly different from that of wild-type mice *(86a)*. After live spore challenge with *A. fumigatus*, CCR4$^{-/-}$ mice have increased neutrophil and macrophage influx into the lungs. This inflammation is accompanied by increased activation of these cells, resulting in the rapid clearance of the spores from the lungs. Cytokine production—both Th2-type and Th1-type—is up at d 3 along with airway hyperresponsiveness to a nonspecific spasmogen (methacholine), but these parameters are reduced to below wild-type levels from d 7 onward. Finally, the chronic aspects of asthma, represented by peribronchial fibrosis and goblet cell hyperplasia in this model, are comparable to those of controls *(86a)*. The differences observed between the two models of asthma (OVA and *Aspergillus*) are presumably owing to the chronicity of the models (5 versus 30 d). From these studies, CCR4 appears to be a link between the innate and acquired immune responses. When CCR4 is absent, the innate immune response is engaged but cannot proceed to an acquired response.

3.5. CCR5

CCR5 is a chemokine receptor that is expressed on monocytes, dendritic cells, activated T-lymphocytes, and NK cells *(88)*. Its ligands are MIP-1α (CCL3), MIP-1β (CCL4), and RANTES (CCL5), all of which are involved in the generation of a Th1-type immune responses *(88,89)*. CCR5 is a coreceptor for macrophage-tropic HIV-1 *(90)*. A natural mutation in the *ccr5* gene (CCR5Δ32) imparts resistance to HIV-1. Only a very few cases of HIV-1 infection have been documented in CCR5Δ32 homozygous individuals *(91)*. Heterozygosity is believed to prolong the time to seroconversion in HIV-1-infected persons *(92)*. Because CCR5 and its ligands, especially RANTES, have been implicated in other diseases, the CCR5Δ32 population has been examined to determine whether the mutation imparts resistance to asthma and allergy. Initially, studies examining adolescents carrying the CCR5Δ32 mutation revealed a reduced risk of asthma *(93)*. However, genetic linkage studies failed to substantiate this finding in adults *(94)*. It is possible that the protection seen in youth is eliminated as other pathways assume mediation of the allergic response.

In the *A. fumigatus* fungal asthma model, CCR5$^{-/-}$ mice show transient disease at the d-12 time point (after live spore challenge). However, at time points both before and after d 12, airway hyperresponsiveness, peribronchial inflammation, goblet cell hyperplasia, and fibrosis are significantly reduced in the knockouts. This short-lived manifestation of disease correlates with a peak in one of CCR5's major ligands, RANTES *(95)*. The research suggests that CCR5 is important in the immune response to fungus and further that RANTES is working through an alternate receptor to induce disease at d 12 but that this phenomenon is temporary. This model clearly demonstrates the dynamic nature of the chemokine system.

The CCR5 receptor is vital in mediating the immune response to a wide range of infectious agents. CCR5$^{-/-}$ mice have difficulty clearing *L. monocytogenes (96)*. When faced with a *C. neoformans* infection, CCR5$^{-/-}$ mice experience significant mortality. More than 90% of the wild-type mice challenged with *Cryptococcus* survived to 12 wk, but fewer than 25% of the knockouts were alive at the same time point *(97)*. Similarly, CCR5$^{-/-}$ mice are significantly more susceptible to a *Toxoplasma gondii* protozoan parasite infection than their wild-type counterparts *(98)*.

Expression of the CCR5 ligands MIP-1α and RANTES is amplified in inflammatory bowel disease *(99)*. Murine colitis models and human Crohn's disease are mediated through a predominant Th1-type response *(100,101)*. Since all the CCR5 ligands are thought to be involved to some extent in the generation of Th1 immunity, this chemokine:chemokine receptor interaction has been examined for possible therapeutic relevance. Indeed, in a colitis model induced by dextran sodium sulfate, the migration of macrophages into the lamina propria of the colon is not reduced in CCR5$^{-/-}$ mice. The CCR5$^{-/-}$ mice are also largely protected from the mucosal ulcerations and adhesions typical of this model *(102)*. However, the knockout mice do exhibit a decided switch from the immunopathologic Th1 response, highlighted by increased IFN-γ, to a host-protective Th2 response, which includes increased expression of IL-4, IL-5, and IL-10 *(102)*. This occurrence is mitigated by an increase in NK 1.1+ and CD4+ lymphocytes *(102)*.

3.6. CCR6

CCR6 is expressed on immature dendritic cells (DCs), B-lymphocytes, and memory T-cells *(103)*. Its ligand, MIP-3α (CCL20), is expressed constitutively in the spleen as well as follicle-associated epithelial cells in the mucosa, particularly in the subepithelial dome of murine Peyer's patches *(104,105)*. CCR6's role in positioning and recruiting cells for the initiation of memory responses and its role in promoting T-cell-dependent mucosal inflammation makes the CCR6 knockout particularly important for studying cutaneous and intestinal mucosal lymphocyte trafficking.

CCR6 and its ligand MIP-3α participate in the mucosal immune response in the lung. In the cockroach antigen model of allergic pulmonary inflammation, CCR6$^{-/-}$ mice exhibit reduced airway hyperresponsiveness when challenged with a spasmogen, less peribronchial eosinophilia, and decreased production of both IgE and IL-5 compared with their wild-type counterparts *(106)*.

CCR6 is a mucosa-specific regulator of humoral immunity and lymphocyte homeostasis in the small intestine. It is required for positioning of DCs in the Peyer's patches *(107)*. CCR6-deficient mice have underdeveloped Peyer's patches that lack DCs in the subepithelium *(108)*. The intestinal mucosa of these mice exhibit persistent, severe inflammation in a model of cutaneous hypersensitivity, but when challenged with allogenic spleen cells in a model of delayed-type hypersensitivity, CCR6$^{-/-}$ mice experienced no inflammatory response *(108)*. When challenged with rotavirus, an enteropathgen, or antigens given via an oral route, CCR6$^{-/-}$ mice have a diminished humoral response, although the systemic response to either oral or subcutaneous antigen is normal *(107)*. Although it has been shown that CCR6 is fully functional on quiescent T-lymphocytes, cellular activation is required before MIP-3α responsiveness can be detected in B lymphocytes *(62)*.

Although MIP-3α is not produced constitutively in the skin, its expression is significantly augmented in atopic dermatitis both in the skin lesions and in the plasma of atopic individuals *(104)*. The epidermal keratinocytes produce the chemokine when induced by proinflammatory cytokines such as IL-1α and TNF-α. Immature DCs and memory T-cells that express CCR6 are then recruited into the inflamed tissue. The CCR6 knockout mouse promises to be an interesting target to investigate further cutaneous inflammation in atopic individuals.

3.7. CCR7

CCR7 is expressed on B- and T-lymphocytes and on mature, activated DCs *(109–111)*. Its ligands are MIP-3β and secondary lymphoid tissue chemokine (SLC/CCL21). CCR7 directs immune function by instituting the microenvironments of the secondary lymphoid organs. Skin DCs from CCR7$^{-/-}$ mice fail to migrate to the draining lymph nodes after activation. Thus, T-lymphocyte priming is severely stunted in these mice *(112,113)*. In addition, humoral immune responses are altered in CCR7$^{-/-}$ mice. There is an inappropriate activation of B-lymphocytes, with subsequent elevations in IgG1, IgG2a, and IgE *(112)*. Interestingly, a significant delay in the onset of IgG isotype switching after immunization with a T-cell-dependent antigen is also noted *(112)*.

3.8. CCR8

CCR8 is preferentially expressed on Th2 lymphocytes *(114)*. Its ligand is the T-cell activation-specific gene 3 (TCA-3/CCL1), in the murine system, and I-309 in humans, which is the homolog of TCA-3 *(114)*. CCR8 knockout mice exhibit an atypical Th2 response. Production of Th2-type cytokines is significantly reduced in $CCR8^{-/-}$ mice in several models of Th2-associated disease (*S. mansoni* egg antigen-induced granuloma and ovalbumin- and cockroach antigen-induced pulmonary inflammation), but a Th1-driven model (*M. bovis* purified protein derivative-induced granuloma) was not affected *(115)*. CCR8 is not required for the normal development of Th2 cells, so the reduction in Th2-type cytokine production seems to be mediated solely by cell recruitment. Eosinophil migration into sites of lung inflammation is significantly impaired in $CCR8^{-/-}$ mice compared with their wild-type counterparts *(115)*. As eosinophils clearly do not migrate in response to TCA-3, the reason for this is unclear, but it may be related to inefficient eosinophil release into the circulating system or a defective maturation process in these mice *(115)*.

3.9. CCR9

CCR9 is selectively expressed on thymocytes and small intestine *(116)* and is maintained on mature on CD8+ T-lymphocytes *(117)*. Its only ligand is thymus-expressed chemokine (TECK/CCL25) *(118)*, which is expressed by most thymic epithelial cortical cells, thymic DCs, and the epithelial lining of the intestine *(119)*. As its expression pattern would suggest, CCR9:TECK has a role in intrathymic T-cell maturation. However, this function is not required for normal T-cell development, as $CCR9^{-/-}$ mice lag by only 1 d in the production of CD4+/CD8+ double-positive cells in the thymus *(119)*. CCR9 is lost on CD4+ cells before their exit from the thymus. In addition, CCR9 may have an additional role in the extravasation of T-lymphocytes into areas of inflammation in the gut *(119)*.

3.10. CCX CKR

A putative chemokine receptor, CCX CKR, was investigated for binding to known chemokines. Its characterization revealed that Epstein-Barr virus-induced molecule 1 ligand chemokine (ELC/CCL19), SLC/CCL21, and TECK bind with high affinity, but no signaling was evident in any of the three interactions *(120)*. All these ligands had previously been assigned to bind only one receptor—CCR7, CCR7, and CCR9, respectively. The molecule was designated CCR10 by Gosling et al. *(120)* and alternatively CCR11 by Schweickart et al. *(121)*. In accordance with the International Union of Pharmacology Committee on Receptor Nomenclature and Drug Classification, the CCR designation has been removed from this receptor, since binding of the receptor causes no in vivo signaling *(122)*. Returning to the original designation, CCX CKR is expressed on DCs, T-lymphocytes, spleen, lymph node, and several nonhematopoietic organs *(120)*. Intuitively, a receptor that binds chemokines with high affinity yet causes no migration or activation in the cell would be considered a decoy receptor. It is conceivable that this receptor is used as a sink to eliminate extra soluble chemokines in the vicinity and is yet another mechanism for orchestrating a finely tuned immune response.

The absence of this receptor has dramatic effects in vivo. In the *A. fumigatus* model of fungal asthma, these knockout mice have significantly elevated airway hyperresponsiveness 14 d after challenge with live spores and remain hyperresponsive 30 d after the challenge compared with wild-type mice (Fig. 1). Dramatic eosinophilia is noted in the knockout mice at d 14 (Fig. 2A) but is resolved to normal limits by the d-30 time point (Fig. 2B). At d 30, the Th2 cytokine IL-4 level is twice that of control mice (Fig. 3), and collagen, a measure of airway remodeling, is significantly increased in the knockout mice (Fig. 4).

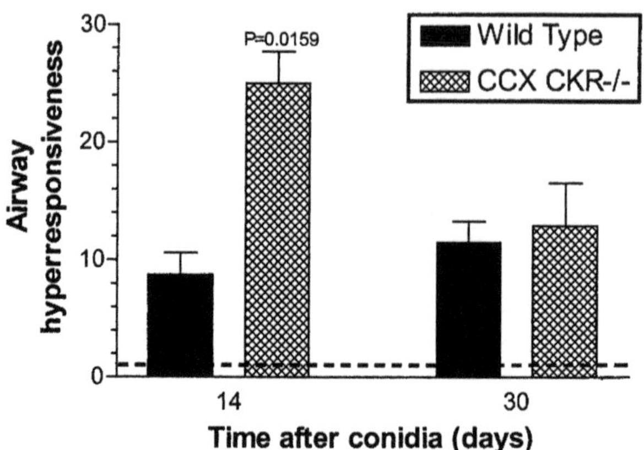

Fig. 1. Airway hyperresponsiveness in *Aspergillus fumigatus*-sensitized wild-type and CCX CKR knockout mice at d 14 and 30 after an intrapulmonary challenge with live *A. fumigatus* conidia. Peak increases in airway resistance or hyperresponsiveness (units = cm H_2O/mL/s) were determined at each time point after the intravenous injection of methacholine. Values are expressed as mean ± SE; n = 4–7/group/time point.

3.11. Duffy Antigen/Receptor for Chemokines (DARC)

DARC is a second receptor that binds chemokines yet fails to induce signaling events. DARC is found primarily on erythrocytes, so it is not surprising that it does not induce intracellular signaling. Thus, it does not warrant a chemokine receptor designation in the new nomenclature. However, these regulatory receptors do deserve examination since their function may be one of critical importance in ensuring a precise response to the eliciting stimulus. DARC was first noted as a receptor for *Plasmodium vivax* but was soon recognized as an erythrocyte chemokine receptor that can bind multiple chemokines. The receptor is also expressed on a subset of endothelial cells *(123)*. DARC$^{-/-}$ mice have no overt developmental abnormalities, although they do present an exaggerated inflammatory response to lipopolysaccharide *(124)*. These knockouts lose all chemokine binding capability on their erythrocytes, demonstrating that DARC is the only erythrocyte chemokine receptor *(124)*.

3.12. CXCR2

CXCR2 is expressed on neutrophils *(125,126)*, mast cells *(127)*, IL-5-treated eosinophils *(128)*, monocytes *(129)*, astrocytes *(130)* keratinocytes *(131)*, and epithelial cells *(131,132)*. It is important in neutrophil migration, innate immune responses, acute inflammation, and angiogenesis. Lipopolysaccharide-induced CXC chemokine (LIX/CXCL5), MIP-2 (CXCL2), and KC (CXCL1) bind CXCR2. Mice do not have an IL-8 homolog, but CXCR2 binds the ligands that act as the functional homolog of this important proinflammatory chemokine in humans. CXCR2 ligands have been associated with neovascularization in the context of a number of disease conditions including cancerous tumor growth *(133–135)*, psoriasis *(136)*, idiopathic pulmonary fibrosis *(137)*, and wound healing *(131)*. In addition, CXCR2 promotes asthma and is necessary for its maintenance *(138)*. CXCR2 mice appear outwardly healthy even though they present with a hematopoietic defect. CXCR2$^{-/-}$ mice

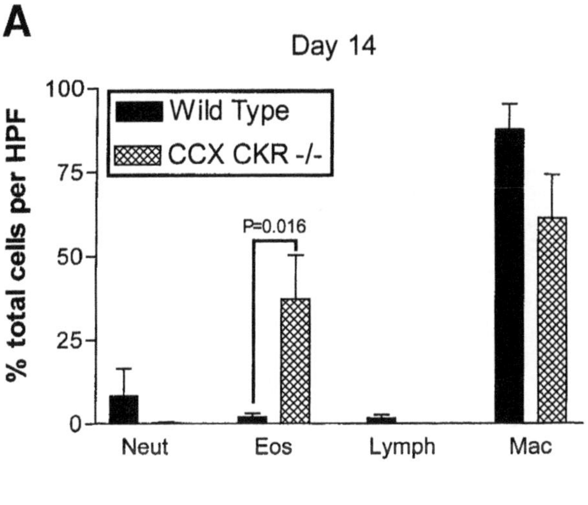

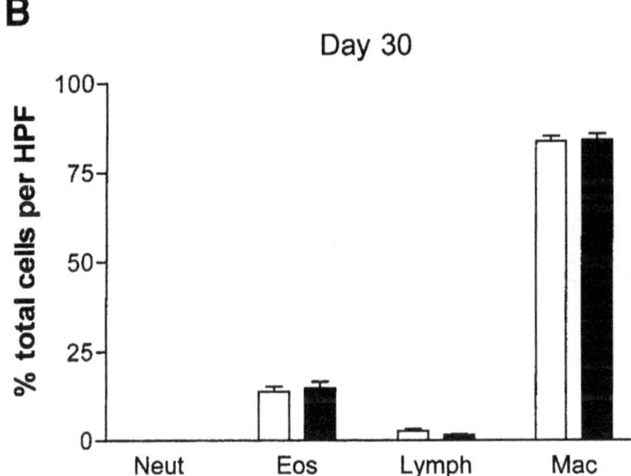

Fig. 2. Leukocyte counts in bronchoalveolar lavage (BAL) fluid from *Aspergillus fumigatus*-sensitized wild-type and CCX CKR knockout mice at d 14 (**A**) and 30 (**B**) after a live *A. fumigatus* conidia challenge. BAL cells were dispersed onto microscope slides by using a cytospin, and eosinophils, neutrophils, T-lymphocytes, and macrophages were stained differentially with Wright-Giesma stain. A minimum of 10–20 high-powered fields (hpf) was examined in each cytosine. Values are expressed as percent of total cells per high powered field (hpf) ± SE.

exhibit both lymphadenopathy, owing to an increased B-cell population, and splenomegaly, owing to an increase of both immature and mature neutrophils *(139)*.

In response to pathogenic challenge with *T. gondii*, impaired neutrophil recruitment causes increased susceptibility in the CXCR2$^{-/-}$ mice compared with the wild-type mice *(140)*. In this model, it is believed that the mast cell is the major chemokine source used to engage neutrophils *(140)*. When treated with lipopolysaccharide via an intraperitoneal or intratracheal route, there is a significant reduction in neutrophil recruitment in the knockout mice. Surprisingly, there is no reduction in neutrophil recruitment when CXCR2$^{-/-}$ mice are infected intraperitoneally with *Mycobacterium avium (141)*. In the *Aspergillus* allergy

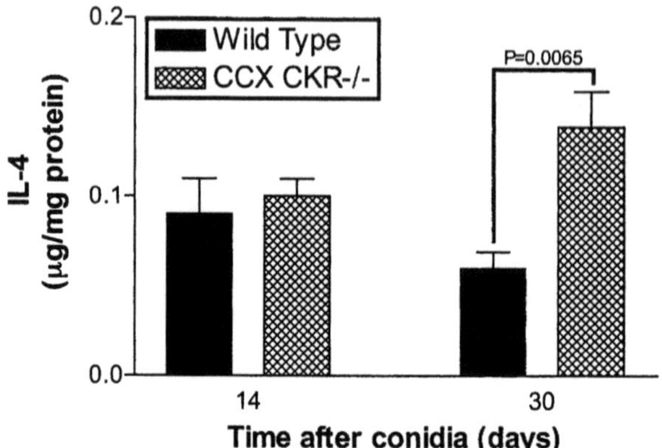

Fig. 3. Interleukin-4 (IL-4) levels in whole lung homogenates from *Aspergillus fumigatus*-sensitized wild-type and CCX CKR knockout mice at d 14 and 30 after a live *A. fumigatus* conidia challenge. Cytokine levels were measured by using a specific ELISA following standard protocols. Values are expressed as mean ± SE; *n* = 4–7 mice/group/time point.

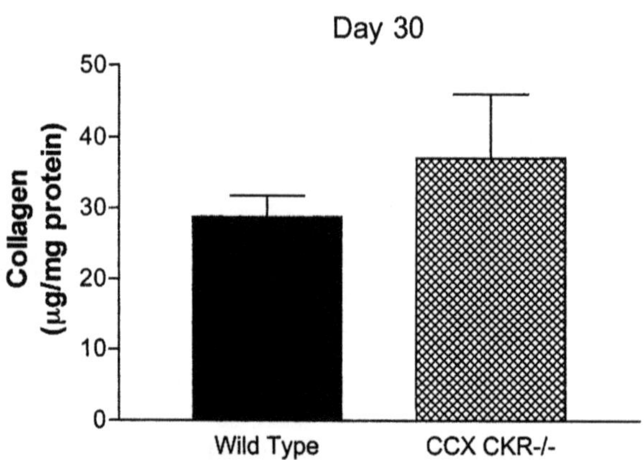

Fig. 4. Total collagen levels in whole lung homogenates from *Aspergillus fumigatus*-sensitized wild-type and CCX CKR knockout mice at d 30 after a live *A. fumigatus* conidia challenge. Total collagen levels were measured with the Sircol Collagen Assay (Biocolor Ltd., Belfast, Ireland) per the manufacturer's protocol. Values are expressed as mean ± SE; *n* = 4–7/group/time point.

model, neutrophil recruitment into the lungs is not only undiminished in the CXCR2$^{-/-}$ mice, the phenomenon is dependent on the presence of monokine induced by IFN-γ (MIG/CXCL9) and interferon-inducible protein-10 (IP-10/CXCL10) *(138)*. These chemokines bind to CXCR3, which has not been detected on neutrophils. Clearly, there are many intricacies in the chemokine network that have not been elucidated.

CXCR2 has been detected in the atherosclerotic lesions of humans. CXCR2$^{-/-}$ mice backcrossed with low-density lipoprotein (LDL) receptor-deficient mice show significantly fewer macrophages in their resulting atherosclerotic lesions *(142)*. Furthermore, the CXCR2 ligand KC was noted in all the experimental aortic atherosclerotic lesions, suggesting that this chemokine:receptor pair functions to mediate pathologic recruitment of macrophages in this disease *(142)*.

CXCR2 and its ligand growth-regulated protein (GRO-α/CXCL) are expressed during wound healing and have been found to be important to the necessary construction of new blood vessels and epithelium *(131)*. Both neutrophil and monocyte recruitment are altered in CXCR2$^{-/-}$ mice in the wound-healing model *(131)*. Interestingly, keratinocytes from CXCR2$^{-/-}$ mice display a significant delay in wound closure parameters when they are examined in vitro *(131)*. In addition, the use of the CXCR2 knockout mouse has allowed the identification of this molecule as the endothelial cell receptor responsible for neutrophil recruitment in chemokine-induced angiogenesis *(132)*.

3.13. CXCR3

CXCR3 is expressed on activated Th1 lymphocytes, eosinophils, and murine microglial cells. The receptor binds IP-10, MIG, and interferon-inducible T-cell α chemoattractant (I-TAC/CXCL11). CXCR3 has an emerging role in Th1-mediated inflammation, T-cell migration, and the adaptive immune response. Unlike some of the other chemokine receptor pairs, CXCR3 and its ligands do not seem to have a role in homeostatic lymphocyte movement, rather, they are expressed predominantly in inflammatory conditions in a number of diseases.

Acute human cardiac allografts express high levels of all three CXCR3 ligands. As a result, CXCR3 was examined for possible therapeutic intervention. CXCR3$^{-/-}$ mice show profound resistance to rejection of cardiac allografts. Additionally, knockout mice that were treatment with a short, subtherapeutic course of cyclosporin A maintained their grafts permanently *(143)*.

Recent research focusing on CXCR3's role in brain microglial cells has challenged some commonly held beliefs about chemokine binding. It has been established that a single chemokine may have multiple receptors and that a single receptor frequently binds multiple chemokines. However, SLC/CCL21, a CC chemokine, binds and triggers chemotaxis through the CXC receptor CXCR3 *(144)*. Isolated microglial cells from CCR7$^{-/-}$ mice, SLC's normal receptor, respond normally to the chemokine whereas CXCR3 deficiency results in defective microglial cell signaling. This is the first reported instance of a CXC receptor binding a CC ligand and may be limited to the murine system. Further research will be needed before this result can be extrapolated to the human system, but it does exemplify the dynamic nature of the chemokine network.

3.14. CXCR5

The CXCR5 receptor is found on B-lymphocytes and is thought to be essential for the positioning of B-cells in the DC network in the follicles of the spleen. As such, it is critical for proper lymphoid development. CXCR5's only known ligand is B-lymphocyte chemoattractant (BLC/CXCL13). Mice lacking CXCR5 lack inguinal lymph nodes and normal Peyer's patches *(145)*. Although mice deficient in CXCR5 have severely impaired organization of the primary follicles of the spleen, they are still able to construct a microenvironment that allows affinity maturation to proceed *(146)*.

3.15. CX$_3$CR1

CX$_3$CR1 is the sole member of the CX$_3$CR subfamily. It binds fractalkine and is important in T-cell and NK cell movement and adhesion. Furthermore, it fulfills roles in both the innate and acquired immune response, including Th1-type inflammation. CX$_3$CR1$^{-/-}$ mice develop normally in a pathogen-free environment.

In an antibody-induced glomerulonephritis model, the knockout mice closely resemble their wild-type littermates *(147)*. Similarly, a model of multiple sclerosis (EAE induced with myelin-oligodendrocyte glycoprotein) showed comparable levels of disease in the $CX_3CR1^{-/-}$ and $CX_3CR1^{+/+}$ mice *(147)*. This lack of a neural phenotype is surprising, given that fractalkine is known as a neurotactin in the mouse and is believed to be important in regulating microglia *(45)*. However, when a subtherapeutic dose of cyclosporin A was used to treat the mice after heterotopic cardiac transplant, the $CX3CR1^{-/-}$ mice showed a marked reduction in graft rejection *(147)*.

4. Conclusions

Genetically engineered knockout animals are incredibly valuable in the study of a myriad of diseases from the central nervous system to the gut, and this technology continues to evolve. It is becoming evident that the chemokine network that was once thought to be exceedingly redundant is, in fact, rarely so. Furthermore, it is becoming clear that the expression of these molecules is both temporally and spatially regulated. We look forward to the time when traditional knockout mice will give way to a new generation of animals in which genes are not deleted but turned off at the whim of the investigator. This will allow time- and tissue-dependent expression of chemokines and receptors to be examined in detail. At the present, we have only begun to investigate the relative role of single chemokines and single receptors. In the future, we will move toward targeting groups of receptors and/or ligands to manipulate immune responses. Finally, in a relatively new field such as chemokine biology, there is always the possibility of new chemokines on the horizon, which will undoubtedly give rise to more questions and more knockout mice to help answer these questions.

References

1. Zlotnik, A. and Yoshie, O. (2000) Chemokines: a new classification system and their role in immunity. *Immunity* **12,** 121–127.
2. Bazan, J. F., Bacon, K. B., Hardiman, G., et al. (1997) A new class of membrane-bound chemokine with a CX3C motif. *Nature* **385,** 640–644.
3. Pan, Y., Lloyd, C., Zhou, H., et al. (1997) Neurotactin, a membrane-anchored chemokine upregulated in brain inflammation. *Nature* **387,** 611–617.
4. Thomas, K. R. and Capecchi, M. R. (1987) Site-directed mutagenesis by gene targeting in mouse embryo-derived stem cells. *Cell* **51,** 503–512.
5. McMahon, A. P. and Bradley, A. (1990) The Wnt-1 (int-1) proto-oncogene is required for development of a large region of the mouse brain. *Cell* **62,** 1073–1085.
6. Corry, D. B., Rishi, K., Kanellis, J., et al. (2002) Decreased allergic lung inflammatory cell egression and increased susceptibility to asphyxiation in MMP2-deficiency. *Nat. Immunol.* **3,** 347–353.
7. Corry, D. B., Folkesson, H. G., Warnock, M. L., et al. (1996) Interleukin 4, but not interleukin 5 or eosinophils, is required in a murine model of acute airway hyperreactivity. *J. Exp. Med.* **183,** 109–117.
8. Broxmeyer, H. E., Sherry, B., Cooper, S., et al. (1993) Comparative analysis of the human macrophage inflammatory protein family of cytokines (chemokines) on proliferation of human myeloid progenitor cells. Interacting effects involving suppression, synergistic suppression, and blocking of suppression. *J. Immunol.* **150,** 3448–3458.
9. Broxmeyer, H. E., Sherry, B., Lu, L., et al. (1989) Myelopoietic enhancing effects of murine macrophage inflammatory proteins 1 and 2 on colony formation in vitro by murine and human bone marrow granulocyte/macrophage progenitor cells. *J. Exp. Med.* **170,** 1583–1594.

10. Cipriani, B., Borsellino, G., Poccia, F., et al. (2000) Activation of C-C beta-chemokines in human peripheral blood gammadelta T cells by isopentenyl pyrophosphate and regulation by cytokines. *Blood* **95,** 39–47.
11. Danforth, J. M., Strieter, R. M., Kunkel, S. L., Arenberg, D. A., VanOtteren, G. M., and Standiford, T. J. (1995) Macrophage inflammatory protein-1 alpha expression in vivo and in vitro: the role of lipoteichoic acid. *Clin. Immunol. Immunopathol.* **74,** 77–83.
12. Graham, G. J., Wright, E. G., Hewick, R., et al. (1990) Identification and characterization of an inhibitor of haemopoietic stem cell proliferation. *Nature* **344,** 442–444.
13. Sherry, B., Tekamp-Olson, P., Gallegos, C., et al. (1988) Resolution of the two components of macrophage inflammatory protein 1, and cloning and characterization of one of those components, macrophage inflammatory protein 1 beta. *J. Exp. Med.* **168,** 2251–2259.
14. Davatelis, G., Tekamp-Olson, P., Wolpe, S. D., et al. (1988) Cloning and characterization of a cDNA for murine macrophage inflammatory protein (MIP), a novel monokine with inflammatory and chemokinetic properties. *J. Exp. Med.* **167,** 1939–1944.
15. Didier, P. J., Paradis, T. J., and Gladue, R. P. (1999) The CC chemokine MIP-1alpha induces a selective monocyte infiltration following intradermal injection into nonhuman primates. *Inflammation* **23,** 75–86.
16. Cook, D. N. (1996) The role of MIP-1 alpha in inflammation and hematopoiesis. *J. Leukoc. Biol.* **59,** 61–66.
17. Cook, D. N., Beck, M. A., Coffman, T. M., et al. (1995) Requirement of MIP-1 alpha for an inflammatory response to viral infection. *Science* **269,** 1583–1585.
18. Domachowske, J. B., Bonville, C. A., Gao, J. L., Murphy, P. M., Easton, A. J., and Rosenberg, H. F. (2000) The chemokine macrophage-inflammatory protein-1 alpha and its receptor CCR1 control pulmonary inflammation and antiviral host defense in paramyxovirus infection. *J. Immunol.* **165,** 2677–2682.
19. Lindell, D. M., Standiford, T. J., Mancuso, P., Leshen, Z. J., and Huffnagle, G. B. (2001) Macrophage inflammatory protein 1alpha/CCL3 is required for clearance of an acute *Klebsiella pneumoniae* pulmonary infection. *Infect. Immun.* **69,** 6364–6369.
20. Olszewski, M. A., Huffnagle, G. B., Traynor, T. R., McDonald, R. A., Cook, D. N., and Toews, G. B. (2001) Regulatory effects of macrophage inflammatory protein 1alpha/CCL3 on the development of immunity to *Cryptococcus neoformans* depend on expression of early inflammatory cytokines. *Infect. Immun.* **69,** 6256–6263.
21. Olszewski, M. A., Huffnagle, G. B., McDonald, R. A., et al. (2000) The role of macrophage inflammatory protein-1 α/CCL3 in regulation of T cell-mediated immunity to *Cryptococcus neoformans* infection. *J. Immunol.* **165,** 6429–6436.
22. Franci, C., Wong, L. M., Van Damme, J., Proost, P., and Charo, I. F. (1995) Monocyte chemoattractant protein-3, but not monocyte chemoattractant protein-2, is a functional ligand of the human monocyte chemoattractant protein-1 receptor. *J. Immunol.* **154,** 6511–6517.
23. Gu, L., Tseng, S., Horner, R. M., Tam, C., Loda, M., and Rollins, B. J. (2000) Control of Th2 polarization by the chemokine monocyte chemoattractant protein-1. *Nature* **23,** 407–411.
24. Peters, W. and Charo, I. F. (2001) Involvement of chemokine receptor 2 and its ligand, monocyte chemoattractant protein-1, in the development of atherosclerosis: lessons from knockout mice. *Curr. Opin. Lipidol.* **12,** 175–180.
25. Gosling, J., Slaymaker, S., Gu, L., et al. (1999) MCP-1 deficiency reduces susceptibility to atherosclerosis in mice that overexpress human apolipoprotein B. *J. Clin. Invest.* **103,** 773–778.
26. Gu, L., Okada, Y., Clinton, S. K., et al. (1998) Absence of monocyte chemoattractant protein-1 reduces atherosclerosis in low density lipoprotein receptor-deficient mice. *Mol. Cell.* **2,** 275–281.
27. Hughes, P. M., Allegrini, P. R., Rudin, M., Perry, V. H., Mir, A. K., and Wiessner, C. (2002) Monocyte chemoattractant protein-1 deficiency is protective in a murine stroke model. *J. Cereb. Blood Flow Metab.* **22,** 308–317.
28. Rothenberg, M. E. (1999) Eotaxin. An essential mediator of eosinophil trafficking into mucosal tissues. *Am. J. Respir. Cell Mol. Biol.* **21,** 291–295.
29. Lamkhioued, B., Renzi, P. M., Abi-Younes, S., et al. (1997) Increased expression of eotaxin in bronchoalveolar lavage and airways of asthmatics contributes to the chemotaxis of eosinophils to the site of inflammation. *J. Immunol.* **159,** 4593–4601.

30. Kumar, R. K., Thomas, P. S., Seetoo, D. Q., et al. (2002) Eotaxin expression by epithelial cells and plasma cells in chronic asthma. *Lab. Invest.* **82,** 495–504.
31. Uguccioni, M., Mackay, C. R., Ochensberger, B., et al. (1997) High expression of the chemokine receptor CCR3 in human blood basophils. Role in activation by eotaxin, MCP-4, and other chemokines. *J. Clin. Invest.* **100,** 1137–1143.
32. Matthews, A. N., Friend, D. S., Zimmermann, N., et al. (1998) Eotaxin is required for the baseline level of tissue eosinophils. *Proc. Natl. Acad. Sci. USA* **95,** 6273–6278.
33. Mishra, A., Hogan, S. P., Lee, J. J., Foster, P. S., and Rothenberg, M. E. (1999) Fundamental signals that regulate eosinophil homing to the gastrointestinal tract. *J. Clin. Invest.* **103,** 1719–1727.
34. Rothenberg, M. E., MacLean, J. A., Pearlman, E., Luster, A. D., and Leder, P. (1997) Targeted disruption of the chemokine eotaxin partially reduces antigen-induced tissue eosinophilia. *J. Exp. Med.* **185,** 785–790.
35. Yang, Y., Loy, J., Ryseck, R. P., Carrasco, D., and Bravo, R. (1998) Antigen-induced eosinophilic lung inflammation develops in mice deficient in chemokine eotaxin. *Blood* **92,** 3912–3923.
36. Schuh, J. M., Blease, K., Kunkel, S. L., and Hogaboam, C. M. (2002) Eotaxin/CCL11 is involved in acute, but not chronic, allergic airway responses to *Aspergillus fumigatus. Am. J. Physiol. Lung Cell. Mol. Physiol.* **283,** L198–L204.
37. Tomkinson, A., Duez, C., Cieslewicz, G., and Gelfand, E. W. (2001) Eotaxin-1-deficient mice develop airway eosinophilia and airway hyperresponsiveness. *Int. Arch. Allergy Immunol.* **126,** 119–125.
38. Fraticelli, P., Sironi, M., Bianchi, G., et al. (2001) Fractalkine (CX3CL1) as an amplification circuit of polarized Th1 responses. *J. Clin. Invest.* **107,** 1173–1181.
39. Umehara, H., Bloom, E., Okazaki, T., Domae, N., and Imai, T. (2001) Fractalkine and vascular injury. *Trends Immunol.* **22,** 602–607.
40. Dichmann, S., Herouy, Y., Purlis, D., Rheinen, H., Gebicke-Harter, P., and Norgauer, J. (2001) Fractalkine induces chemotaxis and actin polymerization in human dendritic cells. *Inflamm. Res.* **50,** 529–533.
41. Volin, M. V., Woods, J. M., Amin, M. A., Connors, M. A., Harlow, L. A., and Koch, A. E. (2001) Fractalkine: a novel angiogenic chemokine in rheumatoid arthritis. *Am. J. Pathol.* **159,** 1521–1530.
42. Cockwell, P., Chakravorty, S. J., Girdlestone, J., and Savage, C. O. (2002) Fractalkine expression in human renal inflammation. *J. Pathol.* **196,** 85–90.
43. Boehme, S. A., Lio, F. M., Maciejewski-Lenoir, D., Bacon, K. B., and Conlon, P. J. (2000) The chemokine fractalkine inhibits Fas-mediated cell death of brain microglia. *J. Immunol.* **165,** 397–403.
44. Meucci, O., Fatatis, A., Simen, A. A., and Miller, R. J. (2000) Expression of CX3CR1 chemokine receptors on neurons and their role in neuronal survival. *Proc. Natl. Acad. Sci. USA* **97,** 8075–8080.
45. Harrison, J. K., Jiang, Y., Chen, S., et al. (1998) Role for neuronally derived fractalkine in mediating interactions between neurons and CX3CR1-expressing microglia. *Proc. Natl. Acad. Sci. USA* **95,** 10896–10901.
46. Cook, D. N., Chen, S. C., Sullivan, L. M., et al. (2001) Generation and analysis of mice lacking the chemokine fractalkine. *Mol. Cell. Biol.* **21,** 3159–3165.
47. Bone-Larson, C. L., Simpson, K. J., Colletti, L. M., et al. (2000) The role of chemokines in the immunopathology of the liver. *Immunol. Rev.* **177,** 8–20.
48. Zou, Y. R., Kottmann, A. H., Kuroda, M., Taniuchi, I., and Littman, D. R. (1998) Function of the chemokine receptor CXCR4 in haematopoiesis and in cerebellar development. *Nature* **393,** 595–599.
49. Nagasawa, T., Hirota, S., Tachibana, K., et al. (1996) Defects of B-cell lymphopoiesis and bone-marrow myelopoiesis in mice lacking the CXC chemokine PBSF/SDF-1. *Nature* **382,** 635–638.
50. Rossi, D. L., Hurst, S. D., Xu, Y., et al. (1999) Lungkine, a novel CXC chemokine, specifically expressed by lung bronchoepithelial cells. *J. Immunol.* **162,** 5490–5497.
51. Chen, S. C., Mehrad, B., Deng, J. C., et al. (2001) Impaired pulmonary host defense in mice lacking expression of the CXC chemokine lungkine. *J. Immunol.* **166,** 3362–3368.
52. Neote, K., DiGregorio, D., Mak, J. Y., Horuk, R., and Schall, T. J. (1993) Molecular cloning, functional expression, and signaling characteristics of a C-C chemokine receptor. *Cell* **72,** 415–425.

53. Gao, J. L., Sen, A. I., Kitaura, M., et al. (1996) Identification of a mouse eosinophil receptor for the CC chemokine eotaxin. *Biochem. Biophys. Res. Commun.* **223,** 679–684.
54. Gao, J. L. and Murphy, P. M. (1995) Cloning and differential tissue-specific expression of three mouse beta chemokine receptor-like genes, including the gene for a functional macrophage inflammatory protein-1 alpha receptor. *J. Biol. Chem.* **270,** 17494–17501.
55. Gao, J. L., Kuhns, D. B., Tiffany, H. L., et al. (1993) Structure and functional expression of the human macrophage inflammatory protein 1 alpha/RANTES receptor. *J. Exp. Med.* **177,** 1421–1427.
56. Post, T. W., Bozic, C. R., Rothenberg, M. E., Luster, A. D., Gerard, N., and Gerard, C. (1995) Molecular characterization of two murine eosinophil beta chemokine receptors. *J. Immunol.* **155,** 5299–5305.
57. Blease, K., Mehrad, B., Standiford, T. J., et al. (2000) Airway remodeling is absent in CCR1–/– mice during chronic fungal allergic airway disease. *J. Immunol.* **165,** 1564–1572.
58. Topham, P. S., Csizmadia, V., Soler, D., et al. (1999) Lack of chemokine receptor CCR1 enhances Th1 responses and glomerular injury during nephrotoxic nephritis. *J. Clin. Invest.* **104,** 1549–1557.
59. Gao, J. L., Wynn, T. A., Chang, Y., et al. (1997) Impaired host defense, hematopoiesis, granulomatous inflammation and type 1-type 2 cytokine balance in mice lacking CC chemokine receptor 1. *J. Exp. Med.* **185,** 1959–1968.
60. Shang, X., Qiu, B., Frait, K. A., et al. (2000) Chemokine receptor 1 knockout abrogates natural killer cell recruitment and impairs type-1 cytokines in lymphoid tissue during pulmonary granuloma formation. *Am. J. Pathol.* **157,** 2055–2063.
61. Gao, W., Topham, P. S., King, J. A., et al. (2000) Targeting of the chemokine receptor CCR1 suppresses development of acute and chronic cardiac allograft rejection. *J. Clin. Invest.* **105,** 35–44.
62. Liao, F., Shirakawa, A. K., Foley, J. F., Rabin, R. L., and Farber, J. M. (2002) Human B cells become highly responsive to macrophage-inflammatory protein-3alpha/CC chemokine ligand-20 after cellular activation without changes in CCR6 expression or ligand binding. *J. Immunol.* **168,** 4871–4880.
63. Yamagami, S., Tanaka, H., and Endo, N. (1997) Monocyte chemoattractant protein-2 can exert its effects through the MCP-1 receptor (CC CKR2B). *FEBS Lett.* **400,** 329–332.
64. Garcia-Zepeda, E. A., Combadiere, C., Rothenberg, M. E., et al. (1996) Human monocyte chemoattractant protein (MCP)-4 is a novel CC chemokine with activities on monocytes, eosinophils, and basophils induced in allergic and nonallergic inflammation that signals through the CC chemokine receptors (CCR)-2 and -3. *J. Immunol.* **157,** 5613–5626.
65. Sarafi, M. N., Garcia-Zepeda, E. A., MacLean, J. A., Charo, I. F., and Luster, A. D. (1997) Murine monocyte chemoattractant protein (MCP)-5: a novel CC chemokine that is a structural and functional homologue of human MCP-1. *J. Exp. Med.* **185,** 99–109.
66. Kurihara, T. and Bravo, R. (1996) Cloning and functional expression of mCCR2, a murine receptor for the C-C chemokines JE and FIC. *J. Biol. Chem.* **271,** 11603–11607.
67. Kurihara, T., Warr, G., Loy, J., and Bravo, R. (1997) Defects in macrophage recruitment and host defense in mice lacking the CCR2 chemokine receptor. *J. Exp. Med.* **186,** 1757–1762.
68. Sato, N., Ahuja, S. K., Quinones, M., et al. (2000) CC chemokine receptor (CCR)2 is required for Langerhans cell migration and localization of T helper cell type 1 (Th1)-inducing dendritic cells. Absence of CCR2 shifts the *Leishmania major*-resistant phenotype to a susceptible state dominated by Th2 cytokines, B cell outgrowth, and sustained neutrophilic inflammation. *J. Exp. Med.* **192,** 205–218.
69. Traynor, T. R., Kuziel, W. A., Toews, G. B., and Huffnagle, G. B. (2000) CCR2 expression determines T1 versus T2 polarization during pulmonary *Cryptococcus neoformans* infection. *J. Immunol.* **164,** 2021–2027.
70. Blease, K., Mehrad, B., Standiford, T. J., et al. (2000) Enhanced pulmonary allergic responses to Aspergillus in CCR2–/– mice. *J. Immunol.* **165,** 2603–2611.
71. Kim, Y., Sung, S., Kuziel, W. A., Feldman, S., Fu, S. M., and Rose, C. E. Jr. (2001) Enhanced airway Th2 response after allergen challenge in mice deficient in CC chemokine receptor-2 (CCR2). *J. Immunol.* **166,** 5183–5192.
72. Boring, L., Gosling, J., Chensue, S. W., et al. (1997) Impaired monocyte migration and reduced type 1 (Th1) cytokine responses in C-C chemokine receptor 2 knockout mice. *J. Clin. Invest.* **100,** 2552–2561.

73. Peters, W., Dupuis, M., and Charo, I. F. (2000) A mechanism for the impaired IFN-gamma production in C-C chemokine receptor 2 (CCR2) knockout mice: role of CCR2 in linking the innate and adaptive immune responses. *J. Immunol.* **165,** 7072–7077.
74. Warmington, K. S., Boring, L., Ruth, J. H., et al. (1999) Effect of C-C chemokine receptor 2 (CCR2) knockout on type-2 (schistosomal antigen-elicited) pulmonary granuloma formation: analysis of cellular recruitment and cytokine responses. *Am. J. Pathol.* **154,** 1407–1416.
75. Dawson, T. C., Kuziel, W. A., Osahar, T. A., and Maeda, N. (1999) Absence of CC chemokine receptor-2 reduces atherosclerosis in apolipoprotein E-deficient mice. *Atherosclerosis* **143,** 205–211.
76. Boring, L., Gosling, J., Cleary, M., and Charo, I. F. (1998) Decreased lesion formation in CCR2–/– mice reveals a role for chemokines in the initiation of atherosclerosis [In Process Citation]. *Nature* **394,** 894–897.
77. Fife, B. T., Huffnagle, G. B., Kuziel, W. A., and Karpus, W. J. (2000) CC chemokine receptor 2 is critical for induction of experimental autoimmune encephalomyelitis. *J. Exp. Med.* **192,** 899–905.
78. Izikson, L., Klein, R. S., Charo, I. F., Weiner, H. L., and Luster, A. D. (2000) Resistance to experimental autoimmune encephalomyelitis in mice lacking the CC chemokine receptor (CCR)2. *J. Exp. Med.* **192,** 1075–1080.
79. Bird, J. E., Giancarli, M. R., Kurihara, T., et al. (2000) Increased severity of glomerulonephritis in C-C chemokine receptor 2 knockout mice. *Kidney Int.* **57,** 129–136.
80. Siebert, H., Sachse, A., Kuziel, W. A., Maeda, N., and Bruck, W. (2000) The chemokine receptor CCR2 is involved in macrophage recruitment to the injured peripheral nervous system. *J. Neuroimmunol.* **110,** 177–185.
81. Ma, W., Bryce, P. J., Humbles, A. A., et al. (2002) CCR3 is essential for skin eosinophilia and airway hyperresponsiveness in a murine model of allergic skin inflammation. *J. Clin. Invest.* **109,** 621–628.
82. Humbles, A. A., Lu, B., Friend, D. S., et al. (2002) The murine CCR3 receptor regulates both the role of eosinophils and mast cells in allergen-induced airway inflammation and hyperresponsiveness. *Proc. Natl. Acad. Sci. USA* **99,** 1479–1484.
83. Imai, T., Baba, M., Nishimura, M., Kakizaki, M., Takagi, S., and Yoshie, O. (1997) The T cell directed CC chemokine TARC is a highly specific ligand for CC chemokine receptor 4. *J. Biol. Chem.* **272,** 15036–15042.
84. Imai, T., Chantry, D., Raport, C. J., et al. (1998) Macrophage-derived chemokine is a functional ligand for the CC chemokine receptor 4. *J. Biol. Chem.* **273,** 1764–1768.
85. Power, C. A., Clemetson, J. M., Clemetson, K. J., and Wells, T. N. (1995) Chemokine and chemokine receptor mRNA expression in human platelets. *Cytokine* **7,** 479–482.
86. Chvatchko, Y., Hoogewerf, A. J., Meyer, A., et al. (2000) A key role for CC chemokine receptor 4 in lipopolysaccharide-induced endotoxic shock. *J. Exp. Med.* **191,** 1755–1764.
86a. Schuh, J. M., Power, C. A., Proudfoot, A. E., Kunkel, S. L., Lukacs, N. W., and Hogaboam, C. M. (2002) Airway Hyperresponsiveness, but not airway remodeling, is attenuated during chronic pulmonary allergic responses to Aspergillus in CCR4$^{-/-}$ mice. *FASEB J.* **16,** 1313–1315.
87. Imai, T., Nagira, M., Takagi, S., et al. (1999) Selective recruitment of CCR4-bearing Th2 cells toward antigen-presenting cells by the CC chemokines thymus and activation-regulated chemokine and macrophage-derived chemokine. *Int. Immunol.* **11,** 81–88.
88. Schrum, S., Probst, P., Fleischer, B., and Zipfel, P. F. (1996) Synthesis of the CC-chemokines MIP-1alpha, MIP-1beta, and RANTES is associated with a type 1 immune response. *J. Immunol.* **157,** 3598–3604.
89. Iwasaki, M., Mukai, T., Nakajima, C., et al. (2001) A mandatory role for STAT4 in IL-12 induction of mouse T cell CCR5. *J. Immunol.* **167,** 6877–6883.
90. Alkhatib, G., Combadiere, C., Broder, C. C., et al. (1996) CC CKR5: a RANTES, MIP-1 alpha, MIP-1beta receptor as a fusion cofactor for macrophage-tropic HIV-1. *Science* **272,** 1955–1958.
91. O'Brien, T. R., Winkler, C., Dean, M., et al. (1997) HIV-1 infection in a man homozygous for CCR5 delta 32. *Lancet* **349,** 1219.

92. Picchio, G. R., Gulizia, R. J., and Mosier, D. E. (1997) Chemokine receptor CCR5 genotype influences the kinetics of human immunodeficiency virus type 1 infection in human PBL-SCID mice. *J. Virol.* **71,** 7124–7127.
93. Hall, I. P., Wheatley, A., Christie, G., McDougall, C., Hubbard, R., and Helms, P. J. (1999) Association of CCR5 delta32 with reduced risk of asthma [letter] [see comments]. *Lancet* **354,** 1264–1265.
94. Mitchell, T. J., Walley, A. J., Pease, J. E., et al. (2000) Delta 32 deletion of CCR5 gene and association with asthma or atopy. *Lancet* **356,** 1491–1492.
95. Schuh, J. M., Blease, K., and Hogaboam, C. M. (2002) The role of CC chemokine receptor 5 (CCR5) and RANTES/CCL5 during chronic fungal asthma in mice. *FASEB J.* **16,** 228–230.
96. Zhou, Y., Kurihara, T., Ryseck, R. P., et al. (1998) Impaired macrophage function and enhanced T cell-dependent immune response in mice lacking CCR5, the mouse homologue of the major HIV-1 coreceptor. *J. Immunol.* **160,** 4018–4025.
97. Huffnagle, G. B., McNeil, L. K., McDonald, R. A., et al. (1999) The role of CCR5 in organ-specific and innate immunity to *Cryptococcus neoformans*. *J. Immunol.* **163,** 4642–4646.
98. Aliberti, J., Reis e Sousa, C., Schito, M., et al. (2000) CCR5 provides a signal for microbial induced production of IL-12 by CD8 alpha+ dendritic cells. *Nat. Immunol.* **1,** 83–87.
99. Mazzucchelli, L., Hauser, C., Zgraggen, K., et al. (1996) Differential in situ expression of the genes encoding the chemokines MCP-1 and RANTES in human inflammatory bowel disease. *J. Pathol.* **178,** 201–206.
100. Scheerens, H., Hessel, E., de Waal-Malefyt, R., Leach, M. W., and Rennick, D. (2001) Characterization of chemokines and chemokine receptors in two murine models of inflammatory bowel disease: IL-10–/– mice and Rag-2–/– mice reconstituted with CD4+CD45RBhigh T cells. *Eur. J. Immunol.* **31,** 1465–1474.
101. Agace, W. W., Roberts, A. I., Wu, L., Greineder, C., Ebert, E. C., and Parker, C. M. (2000) Human intestinal lamina propria and intraepithelial lymphocytes express receptors specific for chemokines induced by inflammation. *Eur. J. Immunol.* **30,** 819–826.
102. Andres, P. G., Beck, P. L., Mizoguchi, E., et al. (2000) Mice with a selective deletion of the CC chemokine receptors 5 or 2 are protected from dextran sodium sulfate-mediated colitis: lack of CC chemokine receptor 5 expression results in a NK1.1+ lymphocyte-associated Th2-type immune response in the intestine. *J. Immunol.* **164,** 6303–6312.
103. Krzysiek, R., Lefevre, E. A., Bernard, J., et al. (2000) Regulation of CCR6 chemokine receptor expression and responsiveness to macrophage inflammatory protein-3alpha/CCL20 in human B cells. *Blood* **96,** 2338–2345.
104. Nakayama, T., Fujisawa, R., Yamada, H., et al. (2001) Inducible expression of a CC chemokine liver- and activation-regulated chemokine (LARC)/macrophage inflammatory protein (MIP)-3 alpha/CCL20 by epidermal keratinocytes and its role in atopic dermatitis. *Int. Immunol.* **13,** 95–103.
105. Tanaka, Y., Imai, T., Baba, M., et al. (1999) Selective expression of liver and activation-regulated chemokine (LARC) in intestinal epithelium in mice and humans. *Eur. J. Immunol.* **29,** 633–642.
106. Lukacs, N. W., Prosser, D. M., Wiekowski, M., Lira, S. A., and Cook, D. N. (2001) Requirement for the chemokine receptor CCR6 in allergic pulmonary inflammation. *J. Exp. Med.* **194,** 551–555.
107. Cook, D. N., Prosser, D. M., Forster, R., et al. (2000) CCR6 mediates dendritic cell localization, lymphocyte homeostasis, and immune responses in mucosal tissue. *Immunity* **12,** 495–503.
108. Varona, R., Villares, R., Carramolino, L., et al. (2001) CCR6-deficient mice have impaired leukocyte homeostasis and altered contact hypersensitivity and delayed-type hypersensitivity responses. *J. Clin. Invest.* **107,** R37–R45.
109. Schweickart, V. L., Raport, C. J., Godiska, R., et al. (1994) Cloning of human and mouse EBI1, a lymphoid-specific G-protein-coupled receptor encoded on human chromosome 17q12-q21.2. *Genomics* **23,** 643–650.
110. Burgstahler, R., Kempkes, B., Steube, K., and Lipp, M. (1995) Expression of the chemokine receptor BLR2/EBI1 is specifically transactivated by Epstein-Barr virus nuclear antigen 2. *Biochem. Biophys. Res. Commun.* **215,** 737–743.
111. Sallusto, F., Schaerli, P., Loetscher, P., et al. (1998) Rapid and coordinated switch in chemokine receptor expression during dendritic cell maturation. *Eur. J. Immunol.* **28,** 2760–2769.

112. Forster, R., Schubel, A., Breitfeld, D., et al. (1999) CCR7 coordinates the primary immune response by establishing functional microenvironments in secondary lymphoid organs. *Cell* **99,** 23–33.
113. Saeki, H., Moore, A. M., Brown, M. J., and Hwang, S. T. (1999) Cutting edge: secondary lymphoid-tissue chemokine (SLC) and CC chemokine receptor 7 (CCR7) participate in the emigration pathway of mature dendritic cells from the skin to regional lymph nodes. *J. Immunol.* **162,** 2472–2475.
114. Zingoni, A., Soto, H., Hedrick, J. A., et al. (1998) The chemokine receptor CCR8 is preferentially expressed in Th2 but not Th1 cells. *J. Immunol.* **161,** 547–551.
115. Chensue, S. W., Lukacs, N. W., Yang, T. Y., et al. (2001) Aberrant in vivo T helper type 2 cell response and impaired eosinophil recruitment in CC chemokine receptor 8 knockout mice. *J. Exp. Med.* **193,** 573–584.
116. Uehara, S., Grinberg, A., Farber, J. M., and Love, P. E. (2002) A role for CCR9 in T lymphocyte development and migration. *J. Immunol.* **168,** 2811–2819.
117. Carramolino, L., Zaballos, A., Kremer, L., et al. (2001) Expression of CCR9 beta-chemokine receptor is modulated in thymocyte differentiation and is selectively maintained in CD8(+) T cells from secondary lymphoid organs. *Blood* **97,** 850–857.
118. Zaballos, A., Gutierrez, J., Varona, R., Ardavin, C., and Marquez, G. (1999) Cutting edge: identification of the orphan chemokine receptor GPR-9-6 as CCR9, the receptor for the chemokine TECK. *J. Immunol.* **162,** 5671–5675.
119. Wurbel, M. A., Malissen, M., Guy-Grand, D., et al. (2001) Mice lacking the CCR9 CC-chemokine receptor show a mild impairment of early T- and B-cell development and a reduction in T-cell receptor gammadelta(+) gut intraepithelial lymphocytes. *Blood* **98,** 2626–2632.
120. Gosling, J., Dairaghi, D. J., Wang, Y., et al. (2000) Cutting edge: identification of a novel chemokine receptor that binds dendritic cell- and T cell-active chemokines including ELC, SLC, and TECK. *J. Immunol.* **164,** 2851–2856.
121. Schweickart, V. L., Epp, A., Raport, C. J., and Gray, P. W. (2001) CCR11 is a functional receptor for the monocyte chemoattractant protein family of chemokines. *J. Biol. Chem.* **276,** 856.
122. Murphy, P. M. (2002) International Union of Pharmacology. XXX. Update on chemokine receptor nomenclature. *Pharmacol. Rev.* **54,** 227–229.
123. Horuk, R., Chitnis, C. E., Darbonne, W. C., et al. (1993) A receptor for the malarial parasite *Plasmodium vivax*: the erythrocyte chemokine receptor. *Science* **261,** 1182–1184.
124. Dawson, T. C., Lentsch, A. B., Wang, Z., et al. (2000) Exaggerated response to endotoxin in mice lacking the Duffy antigen/receptor for chemokines (DARC). *Blood* **96,** 1681–1684.
125. Hall, L. R., Diaconu, E., Patel, R., and Pearlman, E. (2001) CXC chemokine receptor 2 but not C-C chemokine receptor 1 expression is essential for neutrophil recruitment to the cornea in helminth-mediated keratitis (river blindness). *J. Immunol.* **166,** 4035–4041.
126. Kielian, T., Barry, B., and Hickey, W. F. (2001) CXC chemokine receptor-2 ligands are required for neutrophil-mediated host defense in experimental brain abscesses. *J. Immunol.* **166,** 4634–4643.
127. Lippert, U., Artuc, M., Grutzkau, A., et al. (1998) Expression and functional activity of the IL-8 receptor type CXCR1 and CXCR2 on human mast cells. *J. Immunol.* **161,** 2600–2608.
128. Heath, H., Qin, S., Rao, P., et al. (1997) Chemokine receptor usage by human eosinophils. The importance of CCR3 demonstrated using an antagonistic monoclonal antibody. *J. Clin. Invest.* **99,** 178–184.
129. Bonecchi, R., Facchetti, F., Dusi, S., et al. (2000) Induction of functional IL-8 receptors by IL-4 and IL-13 in human monocytes. *J. Immunol.* **164,** 3862–3869.
130. Otto, V. I., Stahel, P. F., Rancan, M., et al. (2001) Regulation of chemokines and chemokine receptors after experimental closed head injury. *Neuroreport* **12,** 2059–2064.
131. Devalaraja, R. M., Nanney, L. B., Qian, Q., et al. (2000) Delayed wound healing in CXCR2 knockout mice. *J. Invest. Dermatol.* **115,** 234–244.
132. Addison, C. L., Daniel, T. O., Burdick, M. D., et al. (2000) The CXC chemokine receptor 2, CXCR2, is the putative receptor for ELR+ CXC chemokine-induced angiogenic activity. *J. Immunol.* **165,** 5269–5277.
133. Arenberg, D. A., Kunkel, S. L., Polverini, P. J., Glass, M., Burdick, M. D., and Strieter, R. M. (1996) Inhibition of interleukin-8 reduces tumorigenesis of human non-small cell lung cancer in SCID mice. *J. Clin. Invest.* **97,** 2792–2802.

134. Kitadai, Y., Haruma, K., Sumii, K., et al. (1998) Expression of interleukin-8 correlates with vascularity in human gastric carcinomas. *Am. J. Pathol.* **152,** 93–100.
135. Luan, J., Shattuck-Brandt, R., Haghnegahdar, H., et al. (1997) Mechanism and biological significance of constitutive expression of MGSA/GRO chemokines in malignant melanoma tumor progression. *J. Leukoc. Biol.* **62,** 588–597.
136. Nickoloff, B. J., Mitra, R. S., Varani, J., Dixit, V. M., and Polverini, P. J. (1994) Aberrant production of interleukin-8 and thrombospondin-1 by psoriatic keratinocytes mediates angiogenesis. *Am. J. Pathol.* **144,** 820–828.
137. Keane, M. P., Arenberg, D. A., Lynch, J. P. 3rd, et al. (1997) The CXC chemokines, IL-8 and IP-10, regulate angiogenic activity in idiopathic pulmonary fibrosis. *J. Immunol.* **159,** 1437–1443.
138. Schuh, J. M., Blease, K., and Hogaboam, C. M. (2002) CXCR2 is necessary for the development and persistence of chronic fungal asthma in mice. *J. Immunol.* **168,** 1447–1456.
139. Cacalano, G., Lee, J., Kikly, K., et al. (1994) Neutrophil and B cell expansion in mice that lack the murine IL-8 receptor homolog. *Science* **265,** 682–684.
140. Del Rio, L., Bennouna, S., Salinas, J., and Denkers, E. Y. (2001) CXCR2 deficiency confers impaired neutrophil recruitment and increased susceptibility during *Toxoplasma gondii* infection. *J. Immunol.* **167,** 6503–6509.
141. Goncalves, A. S. and Appelberg, R. (2002) The involvement of the chemokine receptor CXCR2 in neutrophil recruitment in LPS-induced inflammation and in *Mycobacterium avium* infection. *Scand. J. Immunol.* **55,** 585–591.
142. Boisvert, W. A., Santiago, R., Curtiss, L. K., and Terkeltaub, R. A. (1998) A leukocyte homologue of the IL-8 receptor CXCR-2 mediates the accumulation of macrophages in atherosclerotic lesions of LDL receptor-deficient mice. *J. Clin. Invest.* **101,** 353–363.
143. Hancock, W. W., Lu, B., Gao, W., et al. (2000) Requirement of the chemokine receptor CXCR3 for acute allograft rejection. *J. Exp. Med.* **192,** 1515–1520.
144. Rappert, A., Biber, K., Nolte, C., et al. (2002) Secondary lymphoid tissue chemokine (CCL21) activates CXCR3 to trigger a Cl- current and chemotaxis in murine microglia. *J. Immunol.* **168,** 3221–3226.
145. Forster, R., Mattis, A. E., Kremmer, E., Wolf, E., Brem, G., and Lipp, M. (1996) A putative chemokine receptor, BLR1, directs B cell migration to defined lymphoid organs and specific anatomic compartments of the spleen. *Cell* **87,** 1037–1047.
146. Voigt, I., Camacho, S. A., de Boer, B. A., Lipp, M., Forster, R., and Berek, C. (2000) CXCR5-deficient mice develop functional germinal centers in the splenic T cell zone. *Eur. J. Immunol.* **30,** 560–567.
147. Haskell, C. A., Hancock, W. W., Salant, D. J., et al. (2001) Targeted deletion of CX(3)CR1 reveals a role for fractalkine in cardiac allograft rejection. *J. Clin. Invest.* **108,** 679–688.

20

IFN-γ and IFN-γ Receptor Knockout Mice

Dyana Dalton

1. Introduction

Interferon-γ (IFN-γ) was originally characterized as an antiviral compound *(1)*. However, it has a major immunoregulatory role as a key effector cytokine secreted by T-cells during a variety of immune responses. An early review emphasized the pleiotropic and redundant characteristics of T-cell-derived lymphokines *(2)*. Cytokine knockout mice were not yet available to determine the in vivo roles of cytokines. The genetic approach is a powerful method that has been used for decades in lower organisms to determine biologic functions of proteins. The technique of making targeted deletions of genes in mouse embryonic stem cells to produce mutant mice has extended this approach to mammals. Mice with targeted mutations in IFN-γ (IFN-γ knockout) *(3)* and the IFN-γ receptor (IFN-γR knockout) *(4)* have been studied for nearly a decade. There is only one known receptor for IFN-γ *(5)*. Mice lacking IFN-γ and its receptor develop normally and are indistinguishable from wild-type mice—unless they are given an immunologic challenge.

Characterization of the IFN-γ and IFN-γR knockout mice has confirmed pleiotropic activities of IFN-γ. IFN-γ has both effector and regulatory functions. In agreement with the original designation, IFN-γ is required for resistance to some viruses. However, some viral infections are cleared normally in these mice. Furthermore, the lack of IFN-γ attenuates the immunopathology associated with some viral infections. Hence, there is redundancy in the antiviral activities of IFN-γ. IFN α/β may be more important for first-line defense against viral infections *(6)*. However, there are many functions of IFN-γ that are not redundant in vivo. Studies of numerous infectious diseases in IFN-γ and IFN-γR knockout mice show that an essential role of IFN-γ is to protect against a variety of intracellular pathogens (discussed below).

2. IFN-γ and Mycobacterial Infections

A key role of IFN-γ is control of mycobacterial infections. Mycobacteria are intracellular pathogens that colonize the phagosomes of macrophages. Infection of mice with mycobacteria induces the development of Th1 CD4+ T-cell effectors that secrete IFN-γ. A major role of IFN-γ during mycobacterial infection in mice is to activate expression of inducible

From: *Contemporary Immunology: Cytokine Knockouts, 2nd Edition*
Edited by: Giamila Fantuzzi © Humana Press Inc., Totowa, NJ

nitric oxide synthase (iNOS); this enzyme synthesizes reactive nitrogen intermediates (nitric oxide) that control the growth of many, but not all, mycobacterial species (reviewed in ref. *7*). Mice with defects in IFN-γ production or responses are particularly susceptible to mycobacterial infections. This was first shown in the IFN-γ knockout mice *(3)*. Mice lacking IFN-γ were unable to control the growth of the attenuated vaccine strain, *Mycobacterium bovis* [bacille Calmette-Guérin (BCG)]; this resulted in death of the mice. Similarly, BCG grew unrestricted in IFN-γR knockout mice *(8)*.

IFN-γ knockout mice were also found to be highly susceptible to virulent *Mycobacterium tuberculosis (9,10)*. The IFN-γ knockout mice were unable to produce nitric oxide during *M. tuberculosis* infection and thus were unable to restrict the growth of the *M. tuberculosis* bacteria *(9)*. The death of *M. tuberculosis*-infected IFN-γ knockout mice could be delayed, but not prevented, by administration of exogenous IFN-γ either by injections or by an osmotic pump delivery device *(9)*. This suggests that IFN-γ is most effective when locally produced by T-cells, rather than when circulating systemically. It is likely that IFN-γ is secreted, at relatively high concentrations, into the intracellular cleft during cognate T-cell/macrophage interactions *(11,12)*. After aerogenic infection of IFN-γ knockout mice with *M. tuberculosis*, the growth of the organism was uncontrolled; severe immunopathology and necrosis in the lungs resulted in rapid death of the mice *(10)*.

M. tuberculosis uses IFN-γ to evade the adaptive immune response and establish latent infection *(13)*. *M. tuberculosis* usually establishes a persistent infection of the host and does not cause disease unless adaptive immunity fails *(14)*. Thus, the breakdown of latency into uncontrolled infection contributes to death of the host from tuberculosis disease. Latency is accompanied by a metabolic shift in the *M. tuberculosis* organisms. The mycobacterial enzyme isocitrate lyase (ICL), which is essential for fatty acid metabolism, facilitates the persistence of *M. tuberculosis* in activated mouse macrophages *(13)*. This was shown in an elegant study using a mutant tuberculosis strain, Δ*icl*, in which the ICL gene was deleted. The Δ*icl* mutant established persistence in resting macrophages, but not in IFN-γ-activated macrophages. The mutant organism was less virulent and was unable to establish latent infection in wild-type mice. IFN-γ knockout mice are unable to activate their macrophages *(3)*. When the IFN-γ knockout mice were infected with the Δ*icl* mutant, its virulence was restored. Moreover, the Δ*icl* mutant established persistence in IFN-γ knockout mice. Further experiments demonstrated that ICL promotes persistence of mycobacterial infection by enhancing bacterial survival in activated macrophages. This study illustrates the power of using genetic mutations to elucidate biologic mechanisms. The phenotypes of wild-type and mutant *M. tuberculosis* in wild-type and mutant IFN-γ knockout mice revealed a mechanism for how *M. tuberculosis* resists eradication in an immunocompetent host.

The study of mycobacterial infection in IFN-γ and IFN-γ receptor knockout mice has also contributed to the discovery of rare mutations in humans *(15–19)*. The extreme susceptibility of IFN-γ and IFN-γ receptor knockout mice to poorly pathogenic species of *Mycobacterium*, such as BCG, has led to the identification of humans with defects in the IFN-γ receptor *(16,17)* or the interleukin-12 (IL-12) receptor *(18,19)*. Over 3 billion humans worldwide have been vaccinated with BCG *(20)*. In rare instances, BCG-vaccinated children have developed systemic dissemination of the BCG bacteria. The findings that IFN-γ knockout and IFN-γ receptor knockout mice are susceptible to lethal, disseminated infection with BCG prompted clinicians to examine this pathway in children with disseminated BCG or atypical mycobacterial infections. Several types of mutations have been found in the IFN-γ pathway in children with disseminated atypical mycobacterial infections and salmonellosis. A mutation in the IFN-γ receptor led to complete lack of expression of the IFN-γR on lymphocytes; this resulted in unresponsiveness of cells to endogenously produced IFN-γ *(17)*. IFN-γ plus lipopolysaccharide induces the production of tumor necrosis factor-α (TNF-α) in whole blood cells; this was impaired in children with homozygous IFN-γR deficiency. In IFN-γ receptor knockout mice, the CD4+ T-cells produce high levels of IFN-γ, but the macrophages are unable to respond to IFN-γ and produce nitric oxide *(21,22)*. Mutations in the human IL-12 pathway cause impaired production of IFN-γ, increased susceptibility to BCG, *Mycobacterium avium*, and to non-typhi *Salmonella* infections *(18,19)*. Mice that lack IL-12p40 are susceptible to lethal *M. tuberculosis* infection *(23)*.

3. IFN-γ and the Contraction of the Activated CD4+ T-Cell Population

An unexpected result from studies of immune responses in IFN-γ knockout and IFN-γR knockout mice is the critical role that IFN-γ plays in the contraction phase of T-cell responses. When T-cells become activated by antigens during an infection, they proliferate and increase in number. The rapid increase in the effector T-cell population is the expansion phase of a T-cell response. The expansion phase of the T-cell population is followed by a contraction of the T-cell population, in which there is cell death and elimination of the majority of effector cells (reviewed in ref. *24*). The contraction phase often coincides with the clearance of the pathogen; this is especially true for CD8+ T-cell effectors during viral infections. However, intracellular pathogens that induce a Th1 CD4+ T-cell response may persist for months in immunocompetent mice, yet there is a marked contraction of the effector CD4+ T-cell population *(25–27)*. Several studies, discussed below, show that the contraction phase of Th1 CD4+ T-cell responses is impaired without IFN-γ.

A role for IFN-γ in the death of activated T-cells was suspected in the original characterization of the IFN-γ knockout mice *(3)*. Splenocytes from wild-type and IFN-γ knockout mice were stimulated with a T-cell mitogen. Wild-type splenocytes increased in number for 66 h. At this time, the cells stopped proliferating and began to die. In contrast, the death of IFN-γ knockout cells was delayed as the cells continued to proliferate beyond 66 h. The uncontrolled expansion of the IFN-γ knockout cell population could be stopped by addition of exogenous IFN-γ. This suggested that polyclonal T-cell stimulation of IFN-γ knockout cells led to increased expansion and delayed death of T-cells in the cultures. Similarly, IFN-γ knockout spleen cells proliferated more than wild-type in a mixed lymphocyte reaction and developed increased allogeneic cytotoxic T-lymphocyte (CTL) activity compared with wild-type spleen cells.

A similar role for IFN-γ in promoting T-cell death was observed during *M. bovis* (BCG) infection *(25)*. During BCG infection of wild-type mice, CD4+ T-cells expanded into an activated effector T-cell population (enlarged CD4+ T-cells expressing $CD44^{hi}$, $CD62L^{lo}$, and $CD45RB^{lo}$) that peaked in number at 3.5 wk. The splenic CD4+ T-cell effector population then rapidly contracted a week later, despite the persistence of large numbers of BCG organisms in wild-type spleens. The activated CD4+ T-cell population in IFN-γ knockout mice was three times larger than in wild-type mice at 3.5 wk post infection. However, the activated CD4+ T-cell population did not contract in IFN-γ knockout mice. At 8 wk there was necrosis of the spleen in IFN-γ knockout mice, resulting in the nonspecific death of all spleen cells. The uncontrolled growth of BCG in IFN-γ knockout mice probably contributed to greater expansion of the activated CD4+ T-cell population. However, the absence of IFN-γ was a key factor in the failure of the CD4+ T-cell population to contract.

The kinetics of apoptosis of activated CD4+ T-cells was compared in wild-type and IFN-γ knockout mice during BCG infection. After BCG infection, activated CD4+ T-cells in wild-type mice began to increase in number and at the same time to undergo increased apoptosis. Between d 14 and 17 of BCG infection, activated CD4+ T-cells in wild-type mice exhibited a surge of apoptosis from 30 to 50%. This coincided with the appearance of IFN-γ-secreting CD4+ T-cells and control of mycobacterial expansion. Over the next 8 wk BCG-infected wild-type mice maintained a high level of apoptosis of activated effector CD4+ T-cells. However, increased apoptosis did not result in a severe depletion of activated CD4+ T-cells in wild-type mice; the number of activated CD4+ T-cells remained elevated compared with uninfected mice. This finding suggested that a continual replenishment of effector cells (possibly derived from the naive CD4+ T-cells pool) was occurring after the contraction phase. We hypothesized that naive CD4+ T-cells developed into IFN-γ-secreting effectors and then died by apoptosis.

The activated CD4+ T-cell population in BCG-infected IFN-γ knockout mice failed to contract because of impaired apoptosis of these cells. The level of apoptosis of activated CD4+ T-cells did not increase above baseline levels in IFN-γ knockout mice. Activated CD4+CD44^{hi} T-cells of BCG-infected IFN-γ knockout mice expressed significantly lower levels of Fas compared with wild-type CD4+ T-cells. During infection with mycobacteria, in which antigen persists, Fas-dependent activation-induced cell death (AICD) might be essential to promote apoptosis of effector T-cells by repeated antigenic stimulation. Thus, we investigated whether *lpr* mice, which completely lack Fas, also had impaired apoptosis of activated CD4+ T-cells during BCG infection. Interestingly, the activated CD4+ T-cells in *lpr* mice showed the identical kinetics and percentage of apoptosis as the same cells in wild-type mice. Similarly, during *M. tuberculosis* infection, contraction of activated CD4+ CD44^{hi} T-cells in *gld* (Fas ligand mutant) mice was slightly delayed, but occurred to the levels found in wild-type mice *(26)*. Fas/Fas ligand interactions do play a key role in elimination of activated CD4+ T-cells in some models *(28)*. However, Fas/Fas ligand interactions do not appear to play a major role in apoptosis or contraction of the CD4+ T-cell population during two different mycobacterial infections; rather, the data suggest that activated CD4+ T-cell death during mycobacterial infections requires IFN-γ.

During BCG infection, IFN-γ induces apoptosis of activated CD4+ T-cells by a mechanism requiring nitric oxide and macrophages *(25)*. Since activated splenic CD4+ T-cells from BCG-infected IFN-γ knockout mice were not apoptotic ex vivo, exogenous IFN-γ was added to in vitro cultures to induce apoptosis. Pure populations of activated IFN-γ knockout CD4+ T-cells were not directly susceptible to apoptosis upon addition of exogenous IFN-γ. Activated CD4+ T-cells were only susceptible to apoptosis in whole splenocyte cultures. This suggested an indirect effect of IFN-γ on CD4+ T-cells. Cell-depletion experiments and addition of nitric oxide inhibitors indicated that activated macrophages producing nitric oxide were required for IFN-γ-dependent apoptosis.

A recent paper described another mechanism by which IFN-γ limited T-cell expansion and survival in vitro *(29)*. Naive CD4+ T-cells were activated with anti-CD3 and anti-CD28 and then restimulated with anti-CD3. This method mimics repeated antigen stimulation and results in AICD. Thus, wild-type CD4+ T-cells died by apoptosis. However, IFN-γ knockout CD4+ T-cells were resistant to AICD, despite normal expression of Fas and Fas ligand. AICD had been previously shown to be dependent on Fas/Fas ligand interactions *(30,31)*. Further experiments showed that the failure of IFN-γ knockout T-cells to die from AICD was because of reduced expression of caspase 8. Caspase 8 is a critical signal in the apoptosis pathway for T-cells. It remains to be tested whether the failure of IFN-γ-dependent caspase 8 upregulation has a role in contraction of CD4+ T-cells during mycobacterial infection. There may be multiple mechanisms to eliminate potentially dangerous Th1 CD4+ effector cells.

Our hypothesis is that a negative feedback loop eliminates activated Th1 CD4+ T-cells *after* they have performed their effector function of secreting IFN-γ to activate macrophages *(25)*. During BCG infection, IFN-γ-producing Th1 CD4+ effector T-cells activate macrophages to produce nitric oxide. Nitric oxide then controls the proliferation of the mycobacteria. Nitric oxide also triggers apoptotic elimination of the activated CD4+ T-cells that are present in the tissues of BCG-infected mice. The activated CD4+ T effector cells are thereby eliminated after they have accomplished their effector function of secreting IFN-γ. This has two beneficial effects: immunity to BCG is not impaired, and harmful Th1 CD4+ T-cells are eliminated once they have done their job of activating macrophages.

It is likely that the persistence of BCG stimulates continual production of new Th1 CD4+ effectors from the naive CD4+ T-cell pool. Once the naive cells have differentiated into Th1 effectors, their IFN-γ will activate macrophages; the activated macrophages will then trigger apoptosis of the new Th1 effector CD4+ T-cells. This model explains why enhanced apoptosis of splenic CD4+ T-cell effectors occurred for at least 8 wk after BCG infection of wild-type mice. Despite sustained apoptosis of activated CD4+ T-cells in wild-type BCG-infected mice, there were elevated levels of activated CD4+ T-cells throughout BCG infection. Hence, sustained apoptosis of activated CD4+ T-cells did not cause lymphopenia in BCG-infected wild-type mice. There were still large numbers of BCG organisms in the spleens of wild-type mice at 8 wk of BCG infection. The persistent BCG was likely stimulating production of IFN-γ-secreting CD4+ effector T-cells, as well as macrophage nitric oxide, and thus inducing continual apoptosis of activated CD4+ T-cells.

4. The Role of IFN-γ During Infections with Intracellular Pathogens

There is also evidence for a dual role for IFN-γ both in controlling some intracellular pathogens and in eliminating effector CD4+ T-cells during infection. During footpad infection of mice with *Mycobacterium leprae*, there was dramatically increased swelling and inflammation in IFN-γ knockout mice, even though the number of persisting *M. leprae* in IFN-γ knockout mice was only slightly greater than in wild-type mice *(33)*. The histology of the sites of inflammation revealed increased numbers of CD4+ T-cells in IFN-γ knockout mice compared with wild-type mice. There was increased proliferation of IFN-γ knockout cells to *M. leprae* antigens. This suggested that IFN-γ has a role in eliminating CD4+ T-cells during *M. leprae* infection.

Trypanosoma cruzi is a protozoan parasite that may cause lifelong infection of humans. Wild-type mice survived acute infection with *T. cruzi*; however, the parasite was poorly controlled by IFN-γ knockout mice *(34)*. These mice died with severe parasitemia. In wild-type mice, infection with *T. cruzi* causes a period of T-cell unresponsiveness. However, spleen cells from IFN-γ knockout mice proliferated vigorously to a T-cell mitogen. In wild-type mice, *T. cruzi* infection enhanced nitric oxide production and increased expression of Fas on splenocytes, but this was impaired in IFN-γ knockout mice. Apoptosis of splenocytes was also impaired in IFN-γ knockout mice. Addition of IFN-γ to IFN-γ knockout splenocyte cultures induced expression of Fas and production of nitric oxide; this was associated with enhanced apoptosis. Further experiments suggested that IFN-γ regulates apoptosis of splenocytes during *Trypansoma* infection by two independent mechanisms: induction of nitric oxide production and enhancement of Fas/Fas ligand expression. However, the requirement for IFN-γ-dependent induction of Fas on splenocytes was not demonstrated in this model.

Mice lacking IFN-γR are highly susceptible to infection with *Plasmodium yoeli* sporozoites (malaria) *(35)*. In a model of rodent malaria, a role for IFN-γ in elimination of malaria-specific CD4+ effector T-cells was recently demonstrated *(36)*. Malaria-specific Th1 CD4+ T-cell effectors that were transferred to malaria-infected mice were rapidly deleted from the spleen. This resulted in impaired protective immunity to malaria. The authors found that elimination of Fas and TNF-α did not prevent deletion of the protective CD4+ T-cells. However, neutralizing antibodies to IFN-γ did prevent the deletion of the protective CD4+ T-cells. This implicated IFN-γ in mediating the deletion of malarial specific Th1 CD4+ cells.

Superantigens are produced by some bacterial species and cause massive activation of both CD4+ and CD8+ T-cells. Exposure to superantigens can lead to shock and impaired immune responses. CD4+ T-cells from superantigen-treated mice became refractory to restimulation in vitro; this was caused by T-cell death upon restimulation *(37)*. Death was blocked by neutralizing IFN-γ. The suppression of CD4+ T-cells was shown to be dependent on IFN-γ in a mechanism requiring nitric oxide, reactive oxygen intermediates, and myeloid cells.

5. IFN-γ and the Generation of Th1 Memory CD4+ T-cells

A recent study supports the hypothesis that CD4+ Th1 effector cells that secrete IFN-γ are eliminated in vivo *(38)*. IFN-γ-secreting Th1 cells did not develop into memory CD4+ T-cells that persisted in vivo. Naive TCR transgenic CD4+ T-cells were activated under conditions that promoted the development of Th1 cells. This was a heterogeneous population with respect to IFN-γ production. These were sorted into IFN-γ+ and IFN-γ^- populations and then transferred into hosts. The IFN-γ^- CD4+ cells were of the Th1 lineage, since they were T-bet^{hi} and IL-12 receptor^{hi}, IL-4^{lo}, and GATA-3^{lo}. After transfer, the IFN-γ+ CD4+ T-cells rapidly disappeared from the hosts. In contrast, the IFN-γ^- CD4+ T-cells persisted and became resting memory cells. However, these Th1-lineage IFN-γ^- cells were able to secrete IFN-γ after restimulation. This study raises the question of how resting memory Th1 CD4+ T-cells are maintained during infection with intracellular pathogens. If antigen-specific, Th1-lineage, IFN-γ^- cells are generated during an infection, these will eventually encounter antigens from the persisting pathogens. Upon antigen restimulation, the Th1 CD4+ cells will secrete IFN-γ. Secretion of IFN-γ is predicted to induce deletion (apoptosis) of the Th1 CD4+ memory cell. The model predicts that under conditions of continued antigen stimulation, even the IFN-γ^- CD4+ T memory cells would be deleted.

Indeed, serious problems have been encountered in the development of long-lasting vaccines against intracellular pathogens that require CD4 T-cell-mediated immunity. Vaccines against intracellular pathogens may require the continued persistence of live organisms to generate "effector memory" CD4+ T-cells instead of "resting memory" CD4+ T-cells.

The persistence of pathogen would continually stimulate production of new Th1 effectors to replace those lost by apoptosis.

The combined evidence suggests that IFN-γ, via induction of nitric oxide, plays an important role in eliminating effector CD4+ T-cells during Th1 immune responses to persisting pathogens in mice. Since the pathogens persist, there may be continual generation and apoptosis of protective CD4+ T-cells that help control the pathogen by activating macrophages to produce nitric oxide. As long as naive CD4+ T-cells can continue to enter the periphery, Th1 CD4+ cell effectors will continue to be generated. Therefore, we suggest that this mechanism is designed to provide effector Th1 CD4+ cells, while at the same time curtailing the potentially damaging inflammatory response.

6. IFN-γ and the Control of Hematopoiesis

IFN-γ appears to have another role in curbing acute inflammatory responses by suppressing hematopoiesis. Infection of IFN-γ knockout mice with BCG caused unchecked myeloid cell proliferation and massive extramedullary hematopoiesis. *(37)*. Similarly, infection of IFN-γ knockout mice with *M. tuberculosis* results in enhanced inflammation composed of many granulocytes *(27)*. Infection of IFN-γ knockout mice with *Toxoplasma gondii* resulted in a 5- to 10-fold greater recruitment of neutrophils to the peritoneal cavity *(40)*. Moreover, the IFN-γ knockout and IFN-γR knockout mice have large granulocytic infiltrates in the central nervous system (CNS) during experimental autoimmune diseases such as encephalomyelitis and uveitis *(41–43)*. These observations suggest an unexpected role for IFN-γ in the suppression of myeloid cell production and acute inflammatory responses. The mechanism of suppression of myeloid cells by IFN-γ is not yet clear.

7. IFN-γ and Th1 CD4+-Mediated Autoimmune Diseases

Th1 CD4+ T-cell-mediated autoimmune diseases are thought to be driven by the proinflammatory activities of IFN-γ. One such model is experimental autoimmune encephalomyelitis (EAE), a rodent model of the human autoimmune disease multiple sclerosis (MS). EAE is induced in susceptible rodents by immunization with brain and spinal cord antigens emulsified in complete Freund's adjuvant (CFA), thus generating Th1 effector CD4+ T-cells. Since EAE is mediated by activated Th1 CD4+ T-cells *(44)*, IFN-γ was thought to play an exclusively damaging role in development of EAE. Activated CD4+ T-cells can enter the CNS; this allows activated peripheral macrophages to migrate across the normally intact blood-brain barrier. IFN-γ-secreting Th1 CD4+ T-cells, specific for CNS antigens, are thought to activate resident microglia (brain macrophages) and recruit peripheral macrophages that damage oligodendrocytes and the myelin sheath. The activated macrophages secrete nitric oxide, which is toxic for oligodendrocytes. Other proinflammatory effects of IFN-γ are increased expression of MHC class I and II molecules that might facilitate self-antigen presentation in the CNS. IFN-γ has been implicated in induction of the adhesion molecules vascular cell adhesion molecule (VCAM) and intercellular adhesion molecule (ICAM), which might facilitate homing of inflammatory cells to the CNS. Moreover, IFN-γ induces some chemokine molecules that may also attract damaging cells to the CNS. Prior to experiments in IFN-γ and IFN-γ receptor knockout mice, many investigators expected that deletion of the proinflammatory cytokine, IFN-γ, would ameliorate EAE.

Several studies of EAE in IFN-γ or IFN-γ receptor knockout mice have shown that IFN-γ is not required for the induction of EAE. The first study of EAE in IFN-γ knockout mice used B10.PL mice that normally develop severe EAE *(41)*. IFN-γ knockout mice also developed severe disease, and a greater percentage of IFN-γ knockout mice died during EAE. This hinted at a protective role for IFN-γ in EAE. More compelling evidence for a protective role emerged in later studies. 129/Sv and BALB/c mice were found to be highly resistant to EAE unless IFN-γ or its receptor was deleted *(21,45)*. The lack of IFN-γ conferred EAE susceptibility to normally resistant mice. Immunization of mice with a peptide from myelin-oligodendrocyte glycoprotein (MOG) induces a moderate course clinical EAE in C57BL/6 mice. In IFN-γ knockout mice, on the C57BL/6 background, MOG induced a more severe, nonremitting clinical course *(46)*. This was associated with increased numbers of CD4+ T-cells infiltrating the brains and spinal cords of IFN-γ knockout mice.

Remission of EAE in wild-type mice was previously shown to be associated with increased apoptosis of infiltrating mononuclear cells in the CNS *(47,48)*. During EAE there was impaired apoptosis of activated CD4+ T-cells in the CNS and spleens of IFN-γ knockout mice. This was the most likely cause of the increased numbers of CNS-infiltrating CD4+ T-cells in IFN-γ knockout mice with EAE. This was further characterized in vitro. Wild-type CD4+ T-cells from mice with EAE, restimulated with MOG antigen, failed to proliferate and died by apoptosis. In contrast, the IFN-γ knockout CD4+ T-cell population proliferated in response to MOG antigen, and there was significantly less apoptosis. Addition of exogenous IFN-γ induced apoptosis of IFN-γ knockout CD4+ T-cells responding to antigen. Additional support for a role of IFN-γ in promoting apoptosis of activated CD4+ T-cells in the CNS was shown in another study *(49)*. Murine IFN-γ was expressed, from a viral vector, in the cerebrospinal fluid of mice with EAE. This treatment significantly downregulated the severity and duration of EAE. Moreover, remission of EAE in IFN-γ-treated mice was associated with dramatically increased apoptosis of CNS-infiltrating lymphocytes.

The conversion of the resistant 129/Sv to a susceptible strain by deletion of the IFN-γ receptor also suggested that IFN-γ was critical for downregulation of EAE in 129/Sv mice *(21)*. IFN-γR knockout mice and wild-type 129/Sv controls were immunized with MOG. Restimulation of splenocytes with MOG peptide showed that there was little proliferation or IFN-γ production in the resistant wild-type 129/Sv. There was enhanced splenocyte proliferation and enhanced IFN-γ production from the susceptible IFN-γR knockout mice. The authors then adoptively transferrred activated, MOG-stimulated, IFN-γR knockout lymphoid cells into wild-type and IFN-γ receptor knockout mice. Transfer of the IFN-γR knockout cells into IFN-γR knockout recipients led to severe unremitting EAE. However, transfer of IFN-γR knockout cells into wild-type mice produced equally severe disease, but the wild-type recipients fully recovered. These results suggested that IFN-γ was acting indirectly to downregulate EAE. The CD4+ T-cells from IFN-γR knockout mice made extremely high amounts of IFN-γ, yet IFN-γR knockout cells cannot respond to IFN-γ. However, IFN-γR knockout CD4+ T-cell effectors transferred into wild-type recipients were downregulated, inducing remission of disease. This suggested that another cell in the wild-type host may have responded to IFN-γ and downregulated the encephalitogenic effectors.

A later study by the same group implicated nitric oxide production from macrophages in the inhibition of proliferation of MOG-stimulated cells *(22)*. A failure of T-cells to proliferate may be caused by live cells failing to respond to T-cell receptor (TCR) stimulation, or by death of the effector T-cells, or both. Since apoptosis of activated effector cells was not measured, it was not possible to differentiate these possibilities. It was suggested that IFN-γ-driven nitric oxide production from macrophages via the iNOS enzyme downregulated effector cell proliferation, leading to remission of disease. We have found that addition of IFN-γ to spleen and CNS mononuclear cells from IFN-γ knockout mice with EAE stops proliferation and induces apoptosis of effector CD4+ T-cells. IFN-γ-mediated proliferative arrest and apoptosis of effector CD4+ T-cells is blocked by LNIL, a specific inhibitor of inducible nitric oxide synthase *(46)* (Dalton et al., manuscript in preparation). Thus, during EAE, IFN-γ induces nitric oxide production; this stops proliferation and induces apoptosis of CNS-infiltrating cells, thereby inducing remission of disease.

Another role of IFN-γ knockout CD4+ effector cells in promoting inflammation in the CNS may be to attract neutrophils into the CNS. One study showed that IFN-γ knockout mice with EAE expressed higher levels of RNA for macrophage inflammatory protein-2 (MIP-2) and T-cell activation-specific protein-3 (TCA-3), both neutrophil-attracting chemokines *(42)*. There were large numbers of neutrophils in the CNS inflammatory lesions of IFN-γ knockout mice. Since IFN-γ knockout mice with actively induced EAE undergo extramedullary myelopoiesis in the spleen, this suggests a source for the large numbers of neutrophils that migrate to the CNS.

Another model of Th1 CD4+-mediated autoimmunity highlighted the important role of IFN-γ in downregulating autoimmune disease *(50)*. Experimental autoimmune uveitis (EAU) is an organ-specific, autoimmune disease in which there is inflammation and destruction of the neural retina and related tissues. Early administration of IL-12 paradoxically downregulated EAU after induction of the disease. This was associated with high levels of IFN-γ in the serum during IL-12 treatment. IL-12 treatment of mice with EAU led to decreased proliferation of autoantigen-specific lymph node cells. Such mice had significantly decreased numbers of cells in the draining lymph nodes. Additionally, there were increased numbers of apoptotic cells in the lymph nodes of IL-12-treated mice. Neither IFN-γ knockout mice nor iNOS knockout mice were protected from EAU by IL-12 treatment, suggesting that IL-12 induction of IFN-γ and subsequent nitric oxide production were part of the mechanism. It was proposed that IL-12 protected mice from EAU by hyperinduction of IFN-γ. This in turn caused increased nitric oxide production. Nitric oxide then eliminated autoantigen-specific T-cells by apoptosis as they were being primed. The apoptosis induced by IFN-γ and nitric oxide may have been partly regulated by Bcl-2.

8. The Role of IFN-γ in CD8 T-Cell Contraction

IFN-γ also plays a key role in contraction of the CD8 T-cell population (reviewed in ref. *51*). Wild-type mice that are infected with a low dose of lymphocytic choriomeningitis virus (LCMV) develop an expansion of activated CD8 T-cells, which contribute to viral clearance. The IFN-γR knockout mice showed increased levels of viral replication and a delayed clearance of virus *(52)*. The contraction of the CD8 T-cell population in IFN-γR knockout mice was also delayed compared with that of wild-type mice. Moreover, the CD8 T-cells from LCMV-infected IFN-γR knockout mice were resistant to AICD when restimulated in vitro with anti-CD3. In another study, IFN-γ knockout mice were infected with an attenuated strain of *Listeria monocytogenes* that induces protective CD8+ T-cell immunity *(53)*. The clearance of *Listeria* from the spleens of IFN-γ knockout mice was only slightly delayed compared with wild-type mice. However, there was a dramatic impairment of the contraction phase of CD8+ T-cells in IFN-γ knockout mice. In the same study, the investigators also demonstrated that delayed contraction of antigen-specific CD8 T-cells occurred in IFN-γ knockout mice that were infected with LCMV. The mechanism for IFN-γ-mediated contraction of activated CD8 T-cells is not yet clear. IFN-γ may induce apoptosis of activated CD8 T-cells by induction of Fas, or in conjunction with other CD8 T-cell effector molecules such as perforin.

9. The Role of IFN-γ in Viral Infections

The IFN-γ knockout mice are resistant to some viruses and highly susceptible to others. Another class of proteins, IFN-αβ, has antiviral activities early in viral infections; thus, antiviral activity may be a redundant function for IFN-γ. IFN-γ was not required for clearance of influenza virus *(54)*. IFN-γ knockout mice were infected intranasally with a mouse-adapted influenza virus to establish pulmonary infection. At a range of doses, the time to death and minimal lethal dose of influenza virus was identical for IFN-γ knockout and wild-type mice. At the highest doses given, the wild-type mice died slightly faster, ranging from 24 to 48 h. This was suggestive of a role for IFN-γ in viral immunopathology. In another viral infection, neurovirulent Sindbis virus, wild-type mice develop fatal encephalomyelitis that is T-cell-mediated. Clearance of the virus was not impaired in IFN-γ knockout mice *(55)*. However, mice lacking IFN-γ were greatly protected from fatal T-cell-mediated encephalomyelitis. Thus, IFN-γ contributes to viral immunopathology during Sindbis virus infection. As discussed above, the attenuated LCMV Armstrong strain was cleared from IFN-γ knockout mice with slightly delayed kinetics compared with wild-type mice *(52,53)*. However, in other viral infections (vaccinia virus and measles virus encephalitis) IFN-γ knockout or IFN-γR knockout mice were more susceptible than wild-type *(4,56)*.

IFN-γ is important in the resolution of some viral infections in the CNS. For example, a neurotropic strain of mouse hepatitis virus (JHMV) requires both perforin and IFN-γ to control viral replication in the CNS *(57)*. IFN-γ controlled viral replication in myelin-producing oligodendrocytes. The IFN-γ knockout mice had worse clinical symptoms and mortality, despite normal CTL and antibody responses. The viral antigen localized to the oligodendrocytes and was associated with increased infiltration of CD8+ T-cells. A later study of neurotropic JHMV infection demonstrated that perforin-mediated control of CNS viral replication was severely impaired without IFN-γ; this was associated with decreased expression of MHC class I in CNS tissues *(58)*.

10. Conclusions

Characterization of the IFN-γ and IFN-γR knockout mice has provided a wealth of information about IFN-γ. The apparent normality of these mice is only evident when they are kept under conditions of careful animal husbandry. These knockout mice appear to have no defects until they are immunologically challenged. A comparison of the phenotype of the wild-type and IFN-γ-deficient mice after immune challenges has confirmed some ideas of the role of IFN-γ in the immune system. IFN-γ is indeed a pleiotropic cytokine, performing a variety of functions in the immune response. IFN-γ is a proinflammatory cytokine, yet some studies of IFN-γ-deficient mice have implicated IFN-γ as a suppressor of inflammation. Paradoxically, in diseases such as CD4+ T-cell-mediated autoimmunity, IFN-γ appears to be dispensable for initiating inflammation, yet absolutely critical for suppressing inflammation. An unexpected role for IFN-γ is in T-cell homeostasis. The immune system must eliminate the large number of effector T-cells that are generated during an infection, thereby maintaining normal numbers of T-cells. It is most interesting that the contraction of both CD4+ and CD8+ T-cell effectors is critically dependent on the presence of IFN-γ, rather than strictly dependent on the clearance of pathogen.

Acknowledgements

The author acknowledges grant support from The National Multiple Sclerosis Society RG3103A1/1, NIAID R29AI41258-02, NINDS R01NS04335-01, and funds from the Trudeau Institute. The author thanks Mark Gardner for critical review of the manuscript.

References

1. Isaacs, A. and Lindenmann, J. (1957) Virus interference. 1. The interferons. *Proc. R. Soc. Lond. B.* **147,** 258–267.
2. Paul, W. E. (1989) Pleiotropy and redundancy: T cell-derived lymphokines in the immune response. *Cell* **57,** 521–524.
3. Dalton, D. K., Pitts-Meek, S., Keshav, S., Figari, I. S., Bradley, A., and Stewart, T. A. (1993) Multiple defects of immune cell function in mice with disrupted interferon-gamma genes. *Science* **259,** 1739–1742.
4. Huang, S., Hendriks, W., Althage, A., et al. (1993) Immune response in mice that lack the interferon-gamma receptor. *Science* **259,** 1742–1745.
5. Farrar, M. A. and Schreiber, R. D. (1993) The molecular cell biology of interferon-gamma and its receptor. *Annu. Rev. Immunol.* **11,** 571–611.
6. De Maeyer, E. and De Maeyer-Guignard, J. (1998) Type I interferons. *Int. Rev. Immunol.* **17,** 53–73.
7. Cooper, A. M., Adams, L. B., Dalton, D. K., Appelberg, R., and Ehlers, S. (2002) IFN-gamma and NO in mycobacterial disease: new jobs for old hands. *Trends Microbiol.* **10,** 221–6.
8. Kamijo, R., Le, J., Shapiro, D., et al. (1993) Mice that lack the interferon-gamma receptor have profoundly altered responses to infection with Bacillus Calmette-Guérin and subsequent challenge with lipopolysaccharide. *J. Exp. Med.* **178,** 1435–1440.
9. Flynn, J. L., Chan, J., Triebold, K. J., Dalton, D. K., Stewart, T. A., and Bloom, B. R. (1993) An essential role for interferon gamma in resistance to *Mycobacterium tuberculosis* infection. *J. Exp. Med.* **178,** 2249–2254.
10. Cooper, A. M., Dalton, D. K., Stewart, T. A., Griffin, J. P., Russell, D. G., and Orme, I. M. (1993) Disseminated tuberculosis in interferon gamma gene-disrupted mice. *J. Exp. Med.* **178,** 2243–2247.
11. Soong, L., Xu, J. C., Grewal, I. S., et al. (1996) Disruption of CD40-CD40 ligand interactions results in an enhanced susceptibility to *Leishmania amazonensis* infection. *Immunity* **4,** 263–273.
12. Poo, W. J., Conrad, L., and Janeway, C. A. Jr. (1988) Receptor-directed focusing of lymphokine release by helper T cells. *Nature* **332,** 378–380.
13. McKinney, J. D., Honer zu Bentrup, K., Munoz-Elias, E. J., et al. (2000) Persistence of *Mycobacterium tuberculosis* in macrophages and mice requires the glyoxylate shunt enzyme isocitrate lyase. *Nature* **406,** 735–738.
14. Kochi, A. (1991) Government intervention programs in HIV/tuberculous infection. Outline of guidelines for national tuberculosis control programs in view of the HIV epidemic. *Bull. Int. Union Tuberc. Lung Dis.* **66,** 33–36.
15. Jouanguy, E., Doffinger, R., Dupuis, S., Pallier, A., Altare, F., and Casanova, J. L. (1999) IL-12 and IFN-gamma in host defense against mycobacteria and salmonella in mice and men. *Curr. Opin. Immunol.* **11,** 346–351.
16. Jouanguy, E., Altare, F., Lamhamedi, S., et al. (1996) Interferon-gamma-receptor deficiency in an infant with fatal bacille Calmette-Guérin infection. *N. Engl. J. Med.* **335,** 1956–1961.
17. Newport, M. J., Huxley, C. M., Huston, S., et al. (1996) A mutation in the interferon-gamma-receptor gene and susceptibility to mycobacterial infection. *N. Engl. J. Med.* **335,** 1941–1949.

18. Altare, F., Durandy, A., Lammas, D., et al. (1998) Impairment of mycobacterial immunity in human interleukin-12 receptor deficiency. *Science* **280,** 1432–1435.
19. Altare, F., Lammas, D. Revy, P., et al. (1998) Inherited interleukin 12 deficiency in a child with bacille Calmette-Guérin and *Salmonella enteritidis* disseminated infection. *J. Clin. Invest.* **102,** 2035–2040.
20. Bloom, B. R. (1989) Vaccines for the Third World. *Nature* **342,** 115–120.
21. Willenborg, D. O., Fordham, S., Bernard, C. C., Cowden, W. B., and Ramshaw, I. A. (1996) IFN-gamma plays a critical down-regulatory role in the induction and effector phase of myelin oligodendrocyte glycoprotein-induced autoimmune encephalomyelitis. *J. Immunol.* **157,** 3223–3227.
22. Willenborg, D. O., Fordham, S. A., Staykova, M. A., Ramshaw, I. A., and Cowden, W. B. (1999) IFN-gamma is critical to the control of murine autoimmune encephalomyelitis and regulates both in the periphery and in the target tissue: a possible role for nitric oxide. *J. Immunol.* **163,** 5278–5286.
23. Cooper, A. M., Magram, J., Ferrante, J., and Orme, I. M. (1997) Interleukin 12 (IL-12) is crucial to the development of protective immunity in mice intravenously infected with *Mycobacterium tuberculosis*. *J. Exp. Med.* **186,** 39–45.
24. Kaech, S. M., Wherry, E. J., and Ahmed, R. (2002) Effector and memory T-cell differentiation: implications for vaccine development. *Nat. Rev. Immunol.* **2,** 251–262.
25. Dalton, D. K., Haynes, L., Chu, C. Q., Swain, S. L., and Wittmer, S. (2000) Interferon gamma eliminates responding CD4 T cells during mycobacterial infection by inducing apoptosis of activated CD4 T cells. *J. Exp. Med.* **192,** 117–122.
26. Pearl, J. E., Orme, I. M., and Cooper, A. M. (2000) CD95 signaling is not required for the down regulation of cellular responses to systemic *Mycobacterium tuberculosis* infection. *Tuberc. Lung Dis.* **80,** 273–279.
27. Pearl, J. E., Saunders, B., Ehlers, S., Orme, I. M., and Cooper, A. M. (2001) Inflammation and lymphocyte activation during mycobacterial infection in the interferon-gamma-deficient mouse. *Cell Immunol.* **211,** 43–50.
28. Van Parijs, L., Ibraghimov, A., and Abbas, A. K. (1996) The roles of costimulation and Fas in T cell apoptosis and peripheral tolerance. *Immunity* **4,** 321–328.
29. Refaeli, Y., Van Parijs, L., Alexander, S. I., and Abbas, A. K. (2002) Interferon gamma is required for activation-induced death of T lymphocytes. *J. Exp. Med.* **196,** 999–1005.
30. Brunner, T., Mogil, R. J., LaFace, D., et al. (1995) Cell-autonomous Fas (CD95)/Fas-ligand interaction mediates activation-induced apoptosis in T-cell hybridomas. *Nature* **373,** 441–444.
31. Dhein, J., Walczak, H., Baumler, C., Debatin, K. M., and Krammer, P. H. (1995) Autocrine T-cell suicide mediated by APO-1/(Fas/CD95). *Nature* **373,** 438–441.
32. MacMicking, J., Xie, Q. W., and Nathan, C. (1997) Nitric oxide and macrophage function. *Annu. Rev. Immunol.* **15,** 323–350.
33. Adams, L. B., Scollard, D. M., Ray, N. A., et al. (2002) The study of *Mycobacterium leprae* infection in interferon-gamma gene-disrupted mice as a model to explore the immunopathologic spectrum of leprosy. *J. Infect. Dis.* **185(Suppl. 1),** S1–S8.
34. Martins, G. A., Vieira, L. Q., Cunha, F. Q., and Silva, J. S. (1999) Gamma interferon modulates CD95 (Fas) and CD95 ligand (Fas-L) expression and nitric oxide-induced apoptosis during the acute phase of *Trypanosoma cruzi* infection: a possible role in immune response control. *Infect. Immun.* **67,** 3864–3871.
35. Tsuji, M., Miyahira, Y., Nussenzweig, R. S., Aguet, M., Reichel, M., and Zavala, F. (1995) Development of antimalaria immunity in mice lacking IFN-gamma receptor. *J. Immunol.* **154,** 5338–5344.
36. Xu, H., Wipasa, J., Yan, H., et al. (2002) The mechanism and significance of deletion of parasite-specific CD4(+) T cells in malaria infection. *J. Exp. Med.* **195,** 881–892.
37. Cauley, L. S., Miller, E. E., Yen, M., and Swain, S. L. (2000) Superantigen-induced CD4 T cell tolerance mediated by myeloid cells and IFN-gamma. *J. Immunol.* **165,** 6056–6066.
38. Wu, C. Y., Kirman, J. R., Rotte, M. J., et al. (2002) Distinct lineages of T(H)1 cells have differential capacities for memory cell generation in vivo. *Nat. Immunol.* **3,** 852–858.
39. Murray, P. J., Young, R. A., and Daley, G. Q. (1998) Hematopoietic remodeling in interferon-gamma-deficient mice infected with mycobacteria. *Blood* **91,** 2914–2924.

40. Scharton-Kersten, T. M., Wynn, T. A., Denkers, E. Y., et al. (1996) In the absence of endogenous IFN-gamma, mice develop unimpaired IL-12 responses to *Toxoplasma gondii* while failing to control acute infection. *J. Immunol.* **157,** 4045–4054.
41. Ferber, I. A., Brocke, S., Taylor-Edwards, C., et al. (1996) Mice with a disrupted IFN-gamma gene are susceptible to the induction of experimental autoimmune encephalomyelitis (EAE). *J. Immunol.* **156,** 5–7.
42. Tran, E. H., Prince, E. N., and Owens, T. (2000) IFN-gamma shapes immune invasion of the central nervous system via regulation of chemokines. *J. Immunol.* **164,** 2759–2768.
43. Jones, L. S., Rizzo, L. V., Agarwal, R. K., et al. (1997) IFN-gamma-deficient mice develop experimental autoimmune uveitis in the context of a deviant effector response. *J. Immunol.* **158,** 5997–6005.
44. Wekerle, H. (1997) CD4 effector cells in autoimmune diseases of the central nervous system. In: Keane, H. F., ed. *Immunology of the Nervous System.* Oxford University Press, New York, pp. 460–492.
45. Krakowski, M. and Owens, T. (1996) Interferon-gamma confers resistance to experimental allergic encephalomyelitis. *Eur. J. Immunol.* **26,** 1641–1646.
46. Chu, C. Q., Wittmer, S., and Dalton, D. K. (2000) Failure to suppress the expansion of the activated CD4 T cell population in interferon gamma-deficient mice leads to exacerbation of experimental autoimmune encephalomyelitis. *J. Exp. Med.* **192,** 123–128.
47. Tabi, Z., McCombe, P. A., and Pender, M. P. (1995) Antigen-specific down-regulation of myelin basic protein-reactive T cells during spontaneous recovery from experimental autoimmune encephalomyelitis: further evidence of apoptotic deletion of autoreactive T cells in the central nervous system. *Int. Immunol.* **7,** 967–973.
48. Xiao, B. G., Huang, Y. M., Xu, L. Y., Ishikawa, M., and Link, H. (1999) Mechanisms of recovery from experimental allergic encephalomyelitis induced with myelin basic protein peptide 68-86 in Lewis rats: a role for dendritic cells in inducing apoptosis of CD4+ T cells. *J. Neuroimmunol.* **97,** 25–36.
49. Furlan, R., Brambilla, E., Ruffini, F., et al. (2001) Intrathecal delivery of IFN-gamma protects C57BL/6 mice from chronic-progressive experimental autoimmune encephalomyelitis by increasing apoptosis of central nervous system-infiltrating lymphocytes. *J. Immunol.* **167,** 1821–1829.
50. Tarrant, T. K., Silver, P. B., Wahlsten, J. L., et al. (1999) Interleukin 12 protects from a T helper type 1-mediated autoimmune disease, experimental autoimmune uveitis, through a mechanism involving interferon gamma, nitric oxide, and apoptosis. *J. Exp. Med.* **189,** 219–230.
51. Harty, J. T. and Badovinac, V. P. (2002) Influence of effector molecules on the CD8(+) T cell response to infection. *Curr. Opin. Immunol.* **14,** 360–365.
52. Lohman, B. L. and Welsh, R. M. (1998) Apoptotic regulation of T cells and absence of immune deficiency in virus-infected gamma interferon receptor knockout mice. *J. Virol.* **72,** 7815–7821.
53. Badovinac, V. P., Tvinnereim, A. R., and Harty, J. T. (2000) Regulation of antigen-specific CD8+ T cell homeostasis by perforin and interferon-gamma. *Science* **290,** 1354–1358.
54. Graham, M., Dalton, D., Giltinan, D., Braciale, V., Stewart, T., and Braciale, T. (1993) Response to influenza infection in mice with a targeted disruption of the interferon-γ gene. *J. Exp. Med.* **178,** 1725–1732.
55. Rowell, J. F. and Griffin, D. E. (2002) Contribution of T cells to mortality in neurovirulent Sindbis virus encephalomyelitis. *J. Neuroimmunol.* **127,** 106–114.
56. Finke, D., Brinckmann, U. G., ter Meulen, V., and Liebert, U. G. (1995) Gamma interferon is a major mediator of antiviral defense in experimental measles virus-induced encephalitis. *J. Virol.* **69,** 5469–5474.
57. Parra, B., Hinton, D. R., Marten, N. W., et al. (1999) IFN-gamma is required for viral clearance from central nervous system oligodendroglia. *J. Immunol.* **162,** 1641–1647.
58. Bergmann, C., Parra, B., Hinton, D. R., Chandran, R., Morrison, M., and Stohlman, S. A. (2002) Perforin mediated effector function within the CNS requires IFN-γ mediated MHC upregulation. *Viral Immunol.* **14,** 1–18.

21

Macrophage Migration Inhibitory Factor (MIF)-Deficient Mice

Gunter Fingerle-Rowson, Abhay E. Satoskar, and Richard Bucala

Summary

Although first described almost 40 years ago, MIF was not cloned until 1989, and knowledge regarding its biological functions has emerged only recently. From an initial view of MIF as a lymphocyte-derived cytokine, a much broader concept of MIF function has developed that emphasizes the mediator's fundamental activities in cell activation and proliferation. Biochemical and functional interactions between MIF and regulators of cell physiology such as the MAPK (ERK-1/2) pathway, the transcription factors AP-1, and the p53 tumor suppressor have been identified. The recent development of MIF-deficient mice has confirmed the important regulatory role of MIF in inflammatory and autoimmune disease, and these strains will be of great value for continued research in the fields of immunology and tumor biology, as well as other areas.

Key words

carcinogenesis, inflammation, MIF

1. Introduction

In 1966, Barry Bloom and John David independently characterized a protein from the culture supernatants of antigen-stimulated lymphocytes that could act at a distance to inhibit the random movement or migration of phagocytes *(1,2)*. Named macrophage migration inhibitory factor (MIF), this "activity" was reported over the next 20 years to influence macrophage adherence, phagocytosis, and tumoricidal potential *(3–5)*. When human and murine MIFs were cloned in 1989 *(6)* and 1993 *(7)*, respectively, a more detailed understanding of MIF's biologic, biochemic, and biophysical properties began to emerge. The subsequent development of neutralizing MIF-specific antibodies also helped to illuminate the role of this protein in physiology and pathology.

It soon was found that a great variety of cells express MIF, including macrophages, which were long considered to be the primary target of MIF action. Normal tissue expression of MIF includes epithelial and endothelial cells, neurons, hepatocytes, keratinocytes, and different mesenchymal cell types such as hematopoietic cells, osteoblasts, and fibroblasts. Many biologic effects have been associated with MIF action (Table 1).

For historical reasons, the most intensively investigated area of MIF biology has involved immunology. MIF was shown to act as a proinflammatory mediator that regulates the expression of cytokines (TNF-α, IL-1β, IL-2, IL-6, IL-8, IFNγ) *(8–11)*, other inflammatory

From: *Contemporary Immunology: Cytokine Knockouts, 2nd Edition*
Edited by: Giamila Fantuzzi © Humana Press Inc., Totowa, NJ

Table 1
Tissue and Cellular Distribution of Migration Inhibitory Factor and Suggested Biologic Functions

Cell type	Stimuli	Function	Reference
Anterior pituitary	CRF, LPS	Endocrine hormone	*7*
Corticotropic cells		Glucocorticoid antagonist	*50*
Immune system			
Monocytes/macrophages	LPS, TNFα, IFN-γ, glucocorticoids	Proinflammatory mediator Glucocorticoid antagonist	*52*
	TSST- 1, exotoxin A, PPD		*53*
	Malarial pigment (hemozoin)		*55*
T-cells, mast cells	αCD3, PMA/ionomycin		*17*
	PHA		*100*
Eosinophils	PMA, C5a, IL-5		*70*
Adrenal gland			
Cortex: zona glomerulosa, zona fasciculata	LPS	Unknown	*103*
Lung			
Bronchial epithelium	LPS	Unknown	*103*
Alveolar macrophages		Proinflammatory mediator Glucocorticoid antagonist	*9*
Kidney			
Mesangial cells	LPS, PDGF-AB, IFN-γ	Unknown	*60*
Glomerular epithelial/ endothelial cells	LPS		*101*
Tubular epithelial cells	LPS	Unknown	*102*
Liver			
Hepatocytes around central vein	LPS	Unknown	*103*
Kupffer cells		Proinflammatory mediator Glucocorticoid antagonist	
Skin			
Keratinocytes, sebaceous glands, hair follicle, endothelial cells	LPS, croton oil	Unknown	*56,104*
	UV-B		*56,73*
	Acute inflammation		*105*
	Acute inflammation		*106*
Testis			
Leydig cells, seminiferous epithelium		Inhibitor of inhibit Spermatogenesis?	*92,107*
Epididymis			
Epithelial cells		Sperm maturation?	*61*
Prostate			
Epithelial cells		Unknown	*65*
Ovary			
Granulosa cells		Unknown	*108*
Uterus			
Myometrial cells		Unknown	*108*
Pancreas			
Islet b-cells	Glucose	Regulation of insulin secretion	*79*

Table 1 (Continued)

Cell type	Stimuli	Function	Reference
Eye			
Corneal epithelial cells		Regulator of proliferation/ differentiation	*95*
Endothelial cells, lens			*109*
Iris, ciliary epithelium			*110*
Brain			
Neurons in cortex, hypothalamus,	LPS	Proinflammatory mediator	*64*
Cerebellum, glial cells, ependyma			
Peripheral nervous system			
Neurons, Schwann cells	Injury	Nerve regeneration?	*111,112*
Bone			
Osteoblasts, osteoclasts			*113,114*
Fat tissue			
Adipocytes	TNF-α, glucose, insulin	Regulator of glucose homeostasis	*115,116*
Vasculature			
Endothelial cells	LPS	Angiogenesis	*117*
Connective tissue			
Fibroblast		Inhibitor of p53 activity	*18*
		Regulator of carcinogenesis	*118*
		Regulator of transformation	*119,120*
		Stimulator of MAPK	*12*

CRF, corticotropin-releasing factor; IFN-γ, interferon-γ; IL, interleukin; LPS, lipopolysaccharide; PDGF, platelet-derived growth factor; PHA, phytohemagglutin; PMA, phorbol myristate acetate; PPD, purified protein derivative; TNF-α, tumor necrosis factor-α; TSST-1, toxic shock syndrome toxin-1; UV-B, ultraviolet B.

mediators [nitric oxide *(11)*, prostaglandins *(12,13)*, and matrix metalloproteinases *(14–16)*], the proliferation of lymphocytes *(17)*, and the apoptosis of macrophages *(13,18)*. In several animal models of inflammatory disease, MIF was demonstrated to be critically involved in the pathogenesis of sepsis *(7,19)*, acute respiratory distress syndrome (ARDS) *(9,20)*, arthritis *(21–25)*, colitis *(26)*, skin wound healing *(27)*, allograft rejection *(28)*, and glomerulonephritis *(29)*. Observations from the areas of developmental research and tumor biology further illustrated that MIF participates in growth and differentiation processes and directly affects pathways mediated by mitogen-activated protein kinase (MAPK) *(12)*, p53 *(18)*, and $p27^{KIP1}$ *(30)*. The fact that many tumors overexpress MIF *(31–35)* supports the potential clinical importance of this line of research. It has become apparent that the biologic function of MIF, although important in many immunologic pathways, probably resides in more fundamental processes related to cell activation.

2. The MIF Gene

2.1. Genomic Organization

The mouse *mif* gene (NCBI accession no. Z23048) is located on chromosome 10 *(36, 37)*, and the human MIF gene (NCBI accession no. Z23063) lies on chromosome 22q11.2

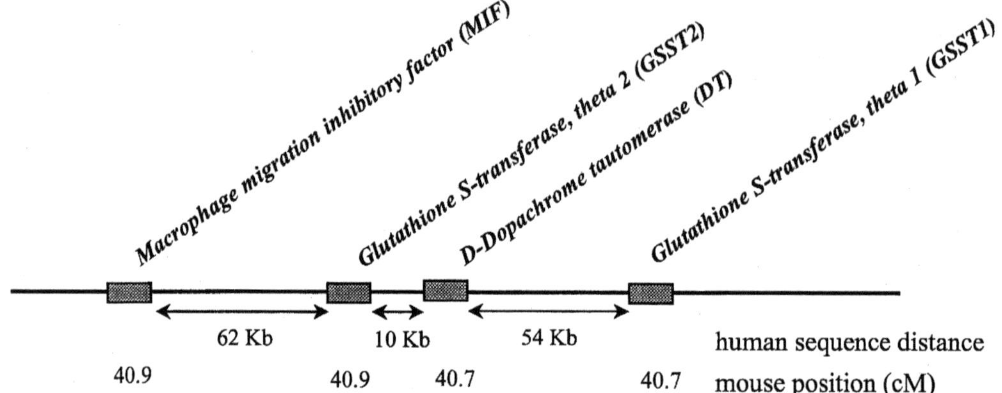

Fig. 1. The MIF/DT-GSST1/2 cluster. The neighboring genes and genomic distances are taken from the sequence of human chromosome 22 as published at www.sanger.ac.uk/HGP/Chr22/Mouse/Maps/hm_genes.shtml. cM, centi Morgan.

(38). Both genes are small (approximately 1,7 kb in size), possess only three exons, and display a similar exon/intron organization. Although the human gene is present in only a single copy in the genome, multiple MIF-related sequences exist within the mouse genome. Nine of these sequences constitute pseudogenes that have been mapped to chromosomes 1, 2, 3, 7, 8, 9, 12, 17, and 19 *(37,39)*. A likely reason for the presence of many pseudogenes is the existence of a retrotransposon of the intracisternal A-particle type (IAP) located less than 3 kb upstream from exon 1. This retrotransposon is conserved among different mouse strains, and although it is believed to be highly mutated and unlikely to be active as a "jumping transposon," it may still have recombinogenic potential *(40)*.

Interestingly, there is another gene, named D-dopachrome tautomerase (DT), that is very similar in structure to MIF (35% identity in protein sequence) *(41)*. Based on the human sequence and the physical map of the mouse, the MIF and the DT genes lie closely apposed to the glutathione-S transferase genes GSST-1 and GSST-2 in a configuration suggesting that the MIF/DT-GSST1/GSST2 cluster might have arisen through a duplication event *(42)* (Fig. 1).

Another interesting feature of MIF is the striking degree of evolutionary conservation that is unsurpassed by any other cytokine. MIF not only has homologs in vertebrates such as the zebrafish, but also in nematodes (*Caenorhabditis elegans*), insects (*Amblyomma americanum*), plants (*Arabidopsis thaliana*), and even protozoa (*Entamoeba histolytica, Trypanosoma cruzi*) *(43)* (G. Fingerle-Rowson, unpublished results). Of note, the recently completed *C. elegans* database reveals the presence of at least five MIF homologs within a single species, suggesting that MIF may be part of a larger protein family *(44)*. Emerging studies also implicate different vector and parasitic MIF homologs in human disease pathogenesis *(45,46)*.

2.2. Gene Expression

Although a systematic analysis of the MIF promoter has not yet been performed, several consensus sequences that may be important in the transcriptional regulation of the human and murine MIF gene have been identified. These include a c-fos motif, an Sp-1 site, a cAMP-

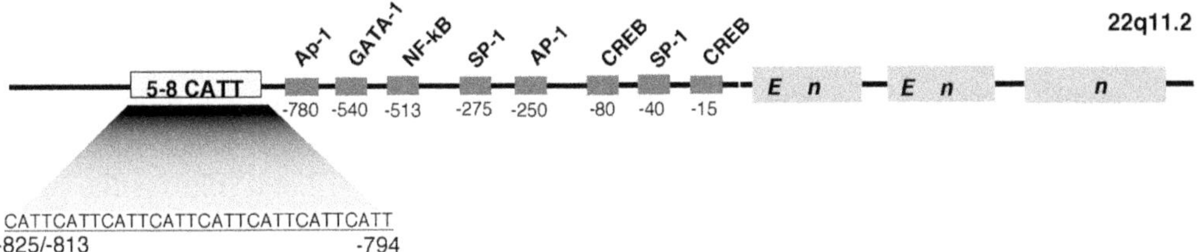

Fig. 2. The human *Mif* gene showing the position of the 5–8 CATT promoter polymorphism and the location of potential transcription factor binding sites.

responsive element (CRE), an activation protein-2 (AP-2) site, a negative glucocorticoid-responsive element (nGRE), a CK-1, and nuclear factor-κB (NF-κB) site *(36)*.

Of importance, two different promoter polymorphisms in human *mif* have been reported and linked to autoimmune disease. The first is a single nucleotide polymorphism (SNP) consisting of a G-to-C transition at position –173 (relative to the transcription start site). In a cohort of U.K. Caucasian patients, the MIF 173*C SNP was shown to be associated with an increased risk of systemic-onset juvenile idiopathic arthritis *(47)*. This G-to-C transition creates a potential AP-4 transcription factor binding site; however, the functional effect of this mutation on MIF gene expression is unknown.

A functionally important tetranucleotide repeat polymorphism (5-, 6-, 7-, 8-CATT) at position –794 of the human *Mif* gene also has been identified (Fig. 2). In model gene reporter assays performed in different cell lines, there is a virtually linear relationship between repeat number and basal and stimulated promoter activity. The presence of the 5-CATT repeat confers low susceptibilty to rheumatoid arthritis and correlates with low disease severity in those patients with rheumatoid arthritis *(48)*. Interestingly, the CATT repeat falls within a Pit-1 transcription factor binding site, rekindling interest in MIF's role as a neuroendocrine mediator *(49,50)* (G. Fingerle-Rowson et al., in press) and in the potential influence of the hypothalamic-pituitary-adrenal axis in immune responsiveness *(51)*.

The *mif* gene appears to be constitutively expressed at a basal level in most cell types; however, its expression can be upregulated by various stimuli. *mif* expression also varies depending on the cellular and tissue context. Stimulants of *mif* expression or MIF production in monocytes/macrophages include bacterial endotoxin [like lipopolysaccharide (LPS)] *(52)* and exotoxins [toxic shock syndrome toxin-1 (TSST-1) and SPEA] *(53)*, purified protein derivative (PPD) *(54)*, malarial pigment *(55)*, tumor necrosis factor-α (TNF-α), interferon-γ (IFN-γ), and glucocorticoid hormones (in low concentrations) *(8)*, ultraviolet (UV)-B in keratinocytes *(56)*, glucose in β-cells of the pancreatic islands *(57)*, corticotropin-releasing factor (CRF) in anterior pituitary cells *(58)*, human choriogonadotropin (hCG) *(59)*, and platelet-derived growth factor (PDGF) in kidney mesangial cells *(60)* (Table 1).

2.3. MIF-Secretion

The gene for MIF does not encode an N-terminal leader sequence that directs protein export *(6,36)*. There is ultrastructural evidence for a vesicular pathway of protein secretion *(50,61)*, but the molecular details of this pathway are unknown. MIF can be detected in serum and bodily fluids such as urine *(62,63)*, cerebrospinal fluid *(64)*, seminal plasma *(65)*, and epididymal *(61)* and follicular fluid *(66)*. The functional importance of extracellular MIF has been documented by many studies. MIF plasma levels are elevated in patients with inflammatory diseases such as sepsis *(19,67–69)*, ARDS *(9,20)*, asthma *(70,71)*, Crohn's disease *(72)*, atopic dermatitis *(73)*, iridocyclitits *(74)*, uveitis *(75)*, and Behçet's disease *(76)*. Locally, high levels of MIF also have been measured in the synovial fluid of patients with rheumatoid arthritis *(23)*. In mouse models of inflammatory disease, recombinant MIF exacerbates the mortality of LPS-induced endotoxemia *(7)* and inhibits the protective effects of glucocorticoids in endotoxemia *(8)* and antigen-induced arthritis *(25)*. Many of these immunopathologic effects were inhibited by the use of MIF-specific monoclonal antibodies.

3. Mechanism of Action

Studies with recombinant MIF and neutralizing anti-MIF antibodies have shown that MIF induces or promotes proinflammatory mediator production. In many cases, this action is linked to the broad, counterregulating action of MIF on glucocorticoid suppression of cellular responses. In the case of activated monocytes/macrophages for instance, MIF promotion of TNF-α production leads to further MIF release, producing a "reentrant" activation pathway that is required for the optimal expression of TNF-α *(52)*. This phenomenon probably explains the self-propagating activation state of cultured macrophages obtained from the alveolar airspaces of ARDS patients, or from the synovia of rheumatoid arthritis patients *(9,23)*. MIF-treated macrophages are more actively phagocytic and better able to destroy intracellular pathogens such as *Leishmania* species *(77,78)*. MIF also promotes the activation of T-cells *(17)* and fibroblasts *(12)*, enhances insulin release from pancreatic β-cells *(79)*, and mediates the long-reported effects of TNF-α on cellular glucose catabolism and lactate production *(80)*.

How does MIF exert its activating effects on cells? Molecular characterization of the cell surface receptor proteins for MIF is under way in our laboratories; however, an examination of the phosphorylated substrates within MIF-stimulated cells has revealed a significant increase in the phosphorylation and activation of the p44/p42 extracellular signal-regulated kinases (ERK-1/2) family of MAP kinase proteins *(12)*. ERK-1/2 are proline-directed, serine/threonine kinases and components of the Ras-Raf-MEK-ERK MAP kinase cascade *(81)*. ERK phosphorylation occurs as early as 30 min after MIF addition but, remarkably, is sustained for a period of at least 24 h. This is surprising because in physiologic processes mediated by Ras protein, ERK-1/2 activation is almost always terminated in less than 90 min. Notable exceptions include transformation by oncogenic *ras* and certain costimulation phenomena mediated by integrin ligation *(82)*. Although ERK-1/2 kinase has been best characterized for its role in growth control, ERK-1/2 also activates several downstream effector proteins that are involved in the inflammatory response, such as transcription factors (*c-myc*, NF-κB, Fos, and Ets), cytoskeletal proteins mediating membrane activation and phagocytosis, and other protein kinases *(81)*. Among these targets, cytoplasmic phospholipase A_2 ($cPLA_2$) is an important component of the inflammatory cascade, and its product, arachidonic acid, is the precursor for the synthesis of prostaglandins and leukotrienes *(83)*. Arachidonic acid activates the *c-jun* N-terminal kinase, which is required for the efficient translation of TNF-α mRNA *(84)*. $cPLA_2$ also is an important target for the antiinflammatory action of glucocortiocids, and subsequent studies showed that MIF could fully "override" glucocorticoid inhibition of $cPLA_2$ activation, providing one point of molecular interaction by which MIF—via sustained ERK-1/2 activation—counterregulates glucocorticoid effects on macrophages *(12)*.

Another target of interaction between MIF and glucocorticoids has been revealed by studies of the NF-κB pathway. NF-κB regulates the expression of over 60 proinflammatory cytokines and cell surface proteins, and it is normally maintained in an inactive state by binding to the cytoplasmic protein IκB. Glucocorticoids mediate an additional spectrum of their antiinflammatory action by increasing IκB expression *(85)*, thereby preventing NF-κB translocation to the nucleus and activating a proinflammatory gene response. Daun and Cannon reported evidence that MIF can enhance NF-κB activity by inhibiting glucocorticoid-induced IκB synthesis *(86)*. MIF also upregulates the expression of Toll-like receptor-4 (TLR-4) *(87)*, which mediates Gram-negative endotoxin (LPS) binding and activation of monocytes/macrophages. This observation suggests a potentially important role for MIF in the early recognition phase of the innate immune response to Gram-negative endotoxin.

MIF also can inhibit p53-dependent apoptosis in cultured tumor cells, which is an activity that was uncovered in a cell-based screen for tumor-promoting genes *(18)*. As discussed further below, macrophages from MIF knockout mice primed with LPS were noted to show decreased viability, which was owing to an increase in macrophage apoptosis, compared with wild-type controls *(13)*. There is accumulating evidence that activation-induced macrophage apoptosis is a normal mechanism for downregulating the innate immune response. This may serve to limit macrophage activation to the actual site of infection or tissue invasion. Prevention of this downregulatory pathway by high MIF expression and/or by the sustained nature of MIF signaling is likely to play an important role in the exaggerated inflammatory response that underlies the pathophysiology of disease states such as ARDS and sepsis.

Kleemann et al. *(30)* recently reported a new, intriguing way by which MIF might work that involves an intercellular mechanism that may bypass the need for a cell surface receptor. The authors showed that MIF binds directly to a cytoplasmic protein, Jab1, which is presumably accessed by MIF translocation across the membrane after endocytosis. This protein usually induces the phosphorylation of c-Jun, a protein involved in inducing cell growth and the activity of AP-1, a transcription factor that activates the expression of various proinflammatory genes. Jab1 also binds to and promotes the degradation of $p27^{Kip1}$, a protein that halts the cell division cycle. The downstream consequences of the direct, physical interaction between MIF and Jab1 suggest a way by which MIF may exert an antiinflammatory spectrum of action. This is incongruent with the known proinflammatory and proproliferative effects of MIF, but it may account for MIF's bell-shaped dose-response profile and the downregulation of responses that occur at high concentrations of MIF. Alternatively, Jab1 may have a role in regulating MIF expression by direct binding to MIF prior to its secretion from cells *(30,88)*.

4. Macrophage MIF-Deficient Mice

4.1. Generation of the MIF Null Mutation

To our knowledge, three laboratories have independently created strains of MIF knockout mice. These strains differ in many features such as the embryonic stem cells employed, the gene targeting strategy, the size of the deletion in the *Mif* locus, and the genetic background of the mouse (Table 2). Bozza et al. *(10)* and Honma et al. *(89)* utilized a traditional *neo* replacement-technique to disrupt the MIF locus, and Fingerle-Rowson *(90,118)* made use of the Cre-loxP-technique. Honma et al. *(89)* replaced only the 3'-end of exon 1 and half of intron 1 by *neo*, whereas Bozza et al. *(10)* replaced a larger portion of the gene that spanned

Table 2
Summary of Different Migration Inhibitory Factor Knockout Strains

	Bozza et al. *(10)*	Honma et al. *(89)*	Fingerle-Rowson *(90)*
Genomic DNA	129/SvJ	129/SvJ	129/SvJ
ES cells	J1 (129/SvJae)	R1 (129/Sv x 129/Sv-CP)F1	Bruce 4 (C57Bl/6)
Targeting strategy	*neo*-replacement	*neo*-replacement	Cre-loxP
Deletion	End of exon-2 to 3'-UTR	End of exon-1 to beginning of intron-1	Promoter + all exons
Genetic background	Mixed (129/SvJae/C57Bl6)	Mixed (129/Sv x 129SvJ/C57Bl6)	Pure (C57/Bl6)
Presence of *neo*	Yes	Yes	No
Option for inducible/ cell-type specific *mif*-targeting	No	No	Yes

ES, embryonic cell.

the end of exon 2 to the 3'-untranslated region. Fingerle-Rowson *(90)* flanked the entire gene (promoter and all three exons) with loxP sites and excised it in vitro with the Cre recombinase. Of note, the generation of a mouse that carries a loxP-flanked *Mif*-allele (MIF^{flox}-mouse) together with the international development of a vast array of tissue-specific, Cre-transgenic mice will enable researchers in the future to generate cell-specific or inducible MIF knockout mice for detailed experimental investigations *(91)* (Fingerle-Rowson et al., in preparation).

4.2. Phenotype of the MIF Knockout Mouse

The first MIF knockout strain was reported in 1999, and the first phenotypic data were obtained on a mixed 129Sv/C57Bl6 background *(10)*. The amount of biologic information that has been generated by the study of MIF knockout mice is still limited, but it is increasing rapidly. We discuss below the results that have been obtained in all three models of MIF deficiency; however, many of these data and observations are incomplete.

4.2.1. Reproduction and Development

MIF expression in the male and female reproductive tract as well as its expression during embryogenesis has suggested that MIF might play a role in the control of fertility, embryonic development, or pregnancy *(61,66,92,93)*. However, all three mouse models of MIF deficiency are fertile and produce normal-sized litters. The reported genotype distribution of the offspring from heterozygous matings varies slightly between the individual groups. On the mixed 129Sv/C57Bl6 background, there was a slightly reduced frequency of MIF$^{-/-}$ males. Bozza et al. *(10)* initially reported a low frequency of MIF$^{-/-}$ offspring (16%); however, this deviation from the expected Mendelian pattern did not hold true with more extensive breeding (J. David, personal communication). On the pure C57Bl/6 background, the inheritance of the MIF knockout allele follows an expected mendelian pattern *(90)*.

MIF knockout mice appear healthy, and no differences in either life span or gross behavior have been observed to date. Histopathologic examination at the tissue level has also

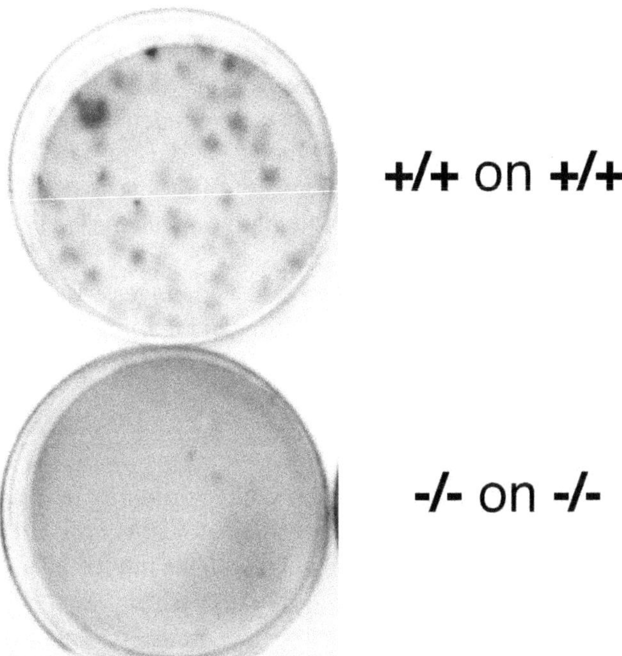

Fig. 3. MIF deficiency and oncogenic transformation in murine embryonic fibroblasts. Using retroviral gene transfer, $MIF^{+/+}$ and $MIF^{-/-}$ MEFs were immortalized by c-myc and subsequently transformed by oncogenic N-ras. For the focus formation assay, 1000 transformed cells were mixed with 300,000 nontransformed primary cells and cultured for 14 d in DMEM/5% FCS. Colonies were stained with Giemsa and photographed at 4× magnification. Although $MIF^{+/+}$-transformed cells form colonies efficiently, MIF deficiency significantly impairs colony formation.

not revealed any abnormalities. Initial studies suggest that hematopoiesis is normal and that T- and B-cell lineages are not affected by the lack of the MIF gene.

4.2.2. In Vitro Studies with MIF-Deficient Embryonic Fibroblasts

MIF was identified as a "delayed early response gene" in NIH/3T3 fibroblasts *(94)*, and its expression has been correlated with tissue development and differentiation *(93,95)*. The increased expression of MIF in several human malignancies and its likely role in the regulation of cell cycle regulatory proteins, such as MAPK, p53, and Jab1/AP-1, prompted Petrenko et al. to study the growth properties of murine embryonic fibroblasts (MEFs) derived from MIF knockout and their wild-type counterparts. Primary MEFs proliferated equally well from both strains, but upon reaching confluency the MIF knockout cells arrested at a 30% lower density than wild-type cells. During the process of immortalization and malignant transformation using various oncogenes such as adenoviral E1A, dominant-negative p53, or c-myc, the decreased growth potential of MIF knockout fibroblasts was much more apparent. Immortalized MIF knockout MEFs proliferated significantly more slowly than wild-type MEFs. Most importantly, MIF knockout MEFs were defective in malignant transformation mediated by oncogenic ras and produced fewer malignant clones in the focus formation assay (Fig. 3). The ability to undergo malignant transformation was clearly dependent on the presence of MIF, as demonstrated by rescue expression of MIF cDNA in knockout cells. In a series of experiments using MIF-deficient mice from the Bozza et al. and the Fingerle-Rowson et al. strains on different genetic backgrounds, Petrenko et al. provided evidence that the transcription factor E2F1 is part of the growth-restraining mechanism in MIF-null fibroblasts. MIF knockout fibroblasts appear to possess a more inhibitory Rb/E2F pathway leading to growth inhibition and resistance to malignant transformation *(95a)*.

Both knockout models generated by Bozza et al. and Fingerle-Rowson et al. yielded cells with clear differences in growth, immortalization, and malignant transformation, demonstrating that this phenotypic property of MIF-deficient fibroblasts is independent of the gene targeting strategy that was employed.

4.2.3. In Vivo Studies and Disease Models

The effect of MIF-deletion in vivo has been studied primarily in models of infection and inflammation, as follows: (1) endo- and exotoxemia, (2) infection with the Gram-negative pathogen *Pseudomonas aeruginosa*, (3) infection with the intracellular parasite *Leishmania major*, (4) infection with the helminth *Taenia crassiceps*, and (5) experimental autoimmune colitis.

4.2.3.1. Endotoxemia Models

LPS (endotoxin) is a potent immunostimulatory and toxic component of the cell wall of Gram-negative bacteria that triggers a strong proinflammatory response from macrophages. LPS interacts with CD14/TLR-4 and in high doses leads to an overwhelming inflammatory response that produces multiorgan failure and death within 1–3 days *(96)*.

All three available MIF knockout mice have been tested with respect to their sensitivity toward LPS. On the mixed 129Sv/C57Bl6 background, Bozza et al. reported that MIF deficiency leads to resistance to the lethal effects of LPS that was associated with a 50% diminution in the production of TNF-α, a key toxic effector cytokine. The production of the other cytokines tested, such as interleukin (IL)-6, IL-10 or IL-12, was unaffected, and the secretion of nitric oxide (NO) was slightly increased *(10)*. These results were entirely expected, given that immunoneutralization of MIF protects mice from endotoxic shock *(7)*. The deficient TNF-α response by macrophages from the Bozza et al. MIF knockout strain has since been replicated by other groups *(13,87)*. It subsequently was found that MIF knockout macrophages express lower levels of TLR-4 mRNA and display slightly lower levels of TLR-4/MD2 on their surface *(87)*. This effect probably contributes to the resistance of these MIF knockout mice to LPS, but it is insufficient to explain their resistance to Gram-positive exotoxins *(10)*, or to infection by intracellular pathogens such as *Plasmodium chabaudii* (J. Xie and R. Bucala, unpublished observations).

Macrophages from MIF knockout mice primed with LPS were also noted to show decreased viability, owing to an increase in macrophage apoptosis, compared with wild-type controls. At the same time, MIF knockout macrophages exhibit a corresponding decrease in their expression of TNF-α, IL-1β, and prostaglandin E_2 (PGE_2). Follow-up experiments established that a significant effect of MIF during LPS priming in vivo was to promote monocyte/macrophage survival and to enhance proinflammatory function by suppressing activation-induced p53-dependent apoptosis *(13)*.

We note that at the present time the concept of MIF as a critical mediator of acute endotoxemia is not without challenge. Honma et al. *(89)* tested their MIF knockout strain for resistance to LPS shock and observed no significant difference between MIF knockout and wild-type littermates. Although data were provided to support the absence of immunoreactive MIF protein in this particular strain of KO mice, the status of MIF transcription was not examined. From the technical perspective of gene deletion, this model may be the product of a "soft" gene targeting approach, and it is difficult at present to conclude if this model is a stringent knockout, or an MIF "knockdown" mouse.

The MIF-deficient mice created on the pure C57Bl/6 background by Cre-loxP recombination are devoid of any residual MIF protein or MIF mRNA. At present, our experiments have failed to show any significant difference in survival or in LPS-elicited cytokine production (TNF-α, IL-6, PGE_2) in these MIF knockout mice compared with C57Bl/6 littermate controls *(90)*. The reason for the differences in LPS sensitivity between these MIF knockout models remains under study, but additional factors such as genetic background and the underlying microbial environment may play a role. These possibilities are supported by the unpublished observation that the MIF knockout mice created by Bozza et al. lose the LPS-resistant phenotype after re-derivation under strict specific pathogen-type (SPF)-free conditions and backcrossing to C57Bl/6 for one generation (A. Billich, personal communication). C57Bl/6 mice are well known to tolerate higher doses of endotoxin than BALB/c or 129/Sv mice *(97)*, but the genes that influence this differential sensitivity to LPS are not yet known. Alternatively, the observation that the MIF knockout mice created by Honma et al. were housed under strict SPF conditions and did not show any endotoxin resistance points to the possibility that microbial colonization may be required to elicit the endotoxin-resistant phenotype. This situation is reminiscent of the IL-2 knockout mouse, which does not develop inflammatory bowel disease when housed under germ-free conditions *(98)*.

Given MIF's clear upstream role as a regulator, rather than an "effector" of innate and acquired immunity, such an influence of background colonization would not be surprising. Future experiments controlling carefully for these variables are needed to unravel these different influences. Such studies could prove to be important in furthering our understanding of human susceptibility to bacterial infection, which is clearly influenced by an interplay of genetic and environmental factors. In fact, recent observations that MIF knockout 129Sv/C57Bl6 mice are resistant to the helminth *Taenia crassiceps*, whereas those on the BALB/c genetic background are susceptible (Rodriguez-Sosa et al., submitted), suggest that the genetic background of the mouse may influence the role of MIF in determining disease outcome in this model.

4.2.3.2. *Leishmania major* Infection

Cutaneous *Leishmania major* infection is a well-established model of parasitic infection that has contributed greatly to the development of the Th1-Th2 paradigm of T-cell regulation. The ability of mice to resolve cutaneous *L. major* infection is associated with a strong Th1 response. Following infection with *L. major*, MIF knockout mice are susceptible to disease and develop significantly larger lesions and greater parasite burdens than wild-type mice *(11)*. This increased susceptibility was not owing to a dysregulation of Th1 and Th2 responses, but rather to a deficiency in the production of NO and superoxide and to an overproduction of IL-6.

4.2.3.3. *Taenia crassiceps* Infection

Cysticercosis is an helminthic infection caused by larvae of the cestode *T. solium* affecting humans and pigs. The development of protective immunity in the experimental model of murine cysticercosis caused by *Taenia crassiceps* is critically dependent on the induction of a Th1-like response. Although MIF knockout mice on the mixed 129Sv/C57Bl6 background are as resistant as wild-type mice to *T. crassiceps*, those on a BALB/c genetic background are highly susceptible to this parasite (Rodriguez-Sosa et al., submitted). Moreover, enhanced susceptibility of MIF knockout BALB/c mice to *T. crassiceps* is not owing to the lack of Th1 development but appears to be associated with impaired TNF-α and NO production from macrophages.

4.2.3.4. Chronic Autoimmune Colitis

Murine models of chronic colitis are valuable systems for analysis of molecules involved in the pathogenesis of autoimmune inflammatory disease, and in many features these models mimic human inflammatory bowel disease. Both activated Th1 cells and antigen-presenting cells are crucial effector cells in the pathogenesis of chronic murine colitis. MIF knockout mice on a mixed 129Sv/C57Bl6 background were protected from both trinitrobenzene sulfonic acid-induced acute colitis and chronic autoimmune colitis in the $CD45RB^{hi}$ T-cell transfer model. Colitis score, end weight, and colonic pathology were markedly ameliorated in the absence of MIF. Through an elegant series of T-cell and bone marrow transfer experiments, de Jong et al. *(26)* were able to show that it was MIF produced by monocytes/macrophages that was the crucial determinant of disease susceptibility.

Acknowledgments

These studies were supported by NIH grants 1RO1-AI42310 and 1R01-AR049610 (to R.B.). We are grateful for our collaboration with Glenn Dranoff and John David (Harvard University, Cambridge, MA), and Klaus Rajewsky and Werner Muller (Institute of Genetics, Cologne University, Germany).

References

1. Bloom, B. R. and Bennett, B. (1966) Mechanism of a reaction in vitro associated with delayed-type hypersensitivity. *Science* **111,** 514–521.
2. David, J. (1966) Delayed hypersensitivity in vitro: its mediation by cell-free substances formed by lymphoid cell-antigen interaction. *Proc. Natl. Acad. Sci. USA* **56,** 72–77.
3. Nathan, C. F., Remold, H. G., and David, J. R. (1973) Characterization of a lymphocyte factor which alters macrophage functions. *J. Exp. Med.* **137,** 275–290.
4. Nathan, C. F., Karnovsky, M. L., and David, J. R. (1971) Alterations of macrophage functions by mediators from lymphocytes. *J. Exp. Med.* **133,** 1356–1376.
5. Churchill, W. H. Jr., Piessens, W. F., Sulis, C. A., and David, J. R. (1975) Macrophages activated as suspension cultures with lymphocyte mediators devoid of antigen become cytotoxic for tumor cells. *J. Immunol.* **115,** 781–786.
6. Weiser, W. Y., Temple, P. A., Witek-Giannotti, J. S., Remold, H. G., Clark, S. C., and David, J. R. (1989) Molecular cloning of a cDNA encoding a human macrophage migration inhibitory factor. *Proc. Natl. Acad. Sci. USA* **86,** 7522–7526.
7. Bernhagen, J., Calandra, T., Mitchell, R. A., et al. (1993) MIF is a pituitary-derived cytokine that potentiates lethal endotoxaemia. *Nature* **365,** 756–759.
8. Calandra, T., Bernhagen, J., Metz, C. N., et al. (1995) MIF as a glucocorticoid-induced modulator of cytokine production. *Nature* **377,** 68–71.

9. Donnelly, S. C., Haslett, C., Reid, P. T., et al. (1977) Regulatory role for macrophage migration inhibitory factor in acute respiratory distress syndrome. *Nat. Med.* **3,** 320–323.
10. Bozza, M., Satoskar, A. R., Lin, G., et al. (1999) Targeted disruption of migration inhibitory factor gene reveals its critical role in sepsis. *J. Exp. Med.* **189,** 341–346.
11. Satoskar, A. R., Bozza, M., Rodriguez, S. M., Lin, G., and David, J. R. (2001) Migration-inhibitory factor gene-deficient mice are susceptible to cutaneous *Leishmania major* infection. *Infect. Immun.* **69,** 906–911.
12. Mitchell, R. A., Metz, C. N., Peng, T., and Bucala, R. (1999) Sustained mitogen-activated protein kinase (MAPK) and cytoplasmic phospholipase A2 activation by macrophage migration inhibitory factor (MIF). Regulatory role in cell proliferation and glucocorticoid action. *J. Biol. Chem.* **274,** 18100–18106.
13. Mitchell, R. A., Liao, H., Chesney, J., et al. (2002) Macrophage migration inhibitory factor (MIF) sustains macrophage proinflammatory function by inhibiting p53: regulatory role in the innate immune response. *Proc. Natl. Acad. Sci. USA* **99,** 345–350.
14. Meyer-Siegler, K. (2000) Macrophage migration inhibitory factor increases MMP-2 activity in DU-145 prostate cells. *Cytokine* **12,** 914–921.
15. Onodera, S., Kaneda, K., Mizue, Y., Koyama, Y., Fujinaga, M., and Nishihira, J. (2000) Macrophage migration inhibitory factor up-regulates expression of matrix metalloproteinases in synovial fibroblasts of rheumatoid arthritis. *J. Biol. Chem.* **275,** 444–450.
16. Onodera, S., Nishihira, J., Iwabuchi, K., et al. (2002) Macrophage migration inhibitory factor up-regulates matrix metalloproteinase-9 and -13 in rat osteoblasts. Relevance to intracellular signaling pathways. *J. Biol. Chem.* **277,** 7865–7874.
17. Bacher, M., Metz, C. N., Calandra, T., et al. (1996) An essential regulatory role for macrophage migration inhibitory factor in T-cell activation. *Proc. Natl. Acad. Sci. USA* **93,** 7849–7854.
18. Hudson, J. D., Shoaibi, M. A., Maestro, R., Carnero, A., Hannon, G. J., and Beach, D. H. (1999) A proinflammatory cytokine inhibits p53 tumor suppressor activity. *J. Exp. Med.* **190,** 1375–1382.
19. Calandra, T., Echtenacher, B., Roy, D. L., et al. (2000) Protection from septic shock by neutralization of macrophage migration inhibitory factor. *Nat. Med.* **6,** 164–170.
20. Guo, Y. and Xie, C. (2002) [The pathogenic role of macrophage migration inhibitory factor in acute respiratory distress syndrome]. *Zhonghua Jie He He Hu Xi Za Zhi* **25,** 337–340.
21. Mikulowska, A., Metz, C. N., Bucala, R., and Holmdahl, R. (1997) Macrophage migration inhibitory factor is involved in the pathogenesis of collagen type II-induced arthritis in mice. *J. Immunol.* **158,** 5514–5517.
22. Leech, M., Metz, C., Santos, L., et al. (1998) Involvement of macrophage migration inhibitory factor in the evolution of rat adjuvant arthritis. *Arthritis Rheum.* **41,** 910–917.
23. Leech, M., Metz, C., Hall, P., et al. (1999) Macrophage migration inhibitory factor in rheumatoid arthritis: evidence of proinflammatory function and regulation by glucocorticoids. *Arthritis Rheum.* **42,** 1601–1608.
24. Leech, M., Metz, C., Bucala, R., and Morand, E. F. (2000) Regulation of macrophage migration inhibitory factor by endogenous glucocorticoids in rat adjuvant-induced arthritis. *Arthritis Rheum.* **43,** 827–833.
25. Santos, L., Hall, P., Metz, C., Bucala, R., and Morand, E. F. (2001) Role of macrophage migration inhibitory factor (MIF) in murine antigen-induced arthritis: interaction with glucocorticoids. *Clin. Exp. Immunol.* **123,** 309–314.
26. de Jong, Y. P., Abadia-Molina, A. C., Satoskar, A. R., et al. (2001) Development of chronic colitis is dependent on the cytokine MIF. *Nat. Immunol.* **2,** 1061–1066.
27. Abe, R., Shimizu, T., Ohkawara, A., and Nishihira, J. (2000) Enhancement of macrophage migration inhibitory factor (MIF) expression in injured epidermis and cultured fibroblasts. *Biochim. Biophys. Acta* **1500,** 1–9.
28. Hou, G., Valujskikh, A., Bayer, J., Stavitsky, A. B., Metz, C., and Heeger, P. S. (2001) In vivo blockade of macrophage migration inhibitory factor prevents skin graft destruction after indirect allorecognition. *Transplantation* **72,** 1890–1897.
29. Lan, H. Y., Bacher, M., Yang, N., et al. (1997) The pathogenic role of macrophage migration inhibitory factor in immunologically induced kidney disease in the rat. *J. Exp. Med.* **185,** 1455–1465.

30. Kleemann, R., Hausser, A., Geiger, G., et al. (2000) Intracellular action of the cytokine MIF to modulate AP-1 activity and the cell cycle through Jab1. *Nature* **408,** 211–216.
31. Markert, J. M., Fuller, C. M., Gillespie, G. Y., et al. (2001) Differential gene expression profiling in human brain tumors. *Physiol. Genomics* **5,** 21–33.
32. Meyer-Siegler, K. and Hudson, P. B. (1996) Enhanced expression of macrophage migration inhibitory factor in prostatic adenocarcinoma metastases. *Urology* **48,** 448–452.
33. Meyer-Siegler, K. (2000) Increased stability of macrophage migration inhibitory factor (MIF) in DU-145 prostate cancer cells. *J. Interferon Cytokine Res.* **20,** 769–778.
34. del Vecchio, M. T., Tripodi, S. A., Arcuri, F., et al. (2000) Macrophage migration inhibitory factor in prostatic adenocarcinoma: correlation with tumor grading and combination endocrine treatment-related changes. *Prostate* **45,** 51–57.
35. Karan, D., Kelly, D. L., Rizzino, A., Lin, M. F., and Batra, S. K. (2002) Expression profile of differentially-regulated genes during progression of androgen-independent growth in human prostate cancer cells. *Carcinogenesis* **23,** 967–975.
36. Mitchell, R., Bacher, M., Bernhagen, J., Pushkarskaya, T., Seldin, M. F., and Bucala, R. (1995) Cloning and characterization of the gene for mouse macrophage migration inhibitory factor (MIF). *J. Immunol.* **154,** 3863–3870.
37. Bozza, M., Kolakowski, L. F., Jenkins, N. A., et al. (1995) Structural characterization and chromosomal location of the mouse macrophage migration inhibitory factor gene and pseudogenes. *Genomics* **27,** 412–419.
38. Budarf, M., McDonald, T., Sellinger, B., Kozak, C., Graham, C., and Wistow, G. (1997) Localization of the human gene for macrophage migration inhibitory factor (MIF) to chromosome 22q11.2. *Genomics* **39,** 235–236.
39. Kozak, C. A., Adamson, M. C., Buckler, C. E., Segovia, L., Paralkar, V., and Wistow, G. (1995) Genomic cloning of mouse MIF (macrophage inhibitory factor) and genetic mapping of the human and mouse expressed gene and nine mouse pseudogenes. *Genomics* **27,** 405–411.
40. Kobayashi, S., Yoshida, K., Ohshima, T., et al. (1998) DNA sequence motifs are associated with aberrant homologous recombination in the mouse macrophage migration inhibitory factor (Mif) locus. *Gene* **215,** 85–92.
41. Nishihira, J., Fujinaga, M., Kuriyama, T., et al. (1998) Molecular cloning of human D-dopachrome tautomerase cDNA: N-terminal proline is essential for enzyme activation. *Biochem. Biophys. Res. Commun.* **243,** 538–544.
42. Coggan, M., Whitbread, L., Whittington, A., and Board, P. (1998) Structure and organization of the human theta-class glutathione S-transferase and D-dopachrome tautomerase gene complex. *Biochem. J.* 334 (Pt 3)**,** 617–623.
43. Swope, M. D. and Lolis, E. (1999) Macrophage migration inhibitory factor: cytokine, hormone, or enzyme? *Rev. Physiol. Biochem. Pharmacol.* **139,** 1–32.
44. Marson, A. L., Tarr, D. E., and Scott, A. L. (2001) Macrophage migration inhibitory factor (mif) transcription is significantly elevated in *Caenorhabditis elegans* dauer larvae. *Gene* **278,** 53–62.
45. Jaworski, D. C., Jasinskas, A., Metz, C. N., Bucala, R., and Barbour, A. G. (2001) Identification and characterization of a homologue of the pro-inflammatory cytokine macrophage migration inhibitory factor in the tick, *Amblyomma americanum. Insect Mol. Biol.* **10,** 323–331.
46. Pastrana, D. V., Raghavan, N., FitzGerald, P., et al. (1998) Filarial nematode parasites secrete a homologue of the human cytokine macrophage migration inhibitory factor. *Infect. Immun.* **66,** 5955–5963.
47. Donn, R. P., Shelley, E., Ollier, W. E., and Thomson, W. (2001) A novel 5'-flanking region polymorphism of macrophage migration inhibitory factor is associated with systemic-onset juvenile idiopathic arthritis. *Arthritis Rheum.* **44,** 1782–1785.
48. Baugh, J. A., Chitnis, S., Donnelly, S. C., et al. (2002) A functional promoter polymorphism in the macrophage migration inhibitory factor (MIF) gene associated with disease severity in rheumatoid arthritis. *Genes Immun.* **3,** 170–176.
49. Bernhagen, J., Calandra, T., Cerami, A., and Bucala, R. (1994) Macrophage migration inhibitory factor is a neuroendocrine mediator of endotoxaemia. *Trends Microbiol.* **2,** 198–201.

50. Nishino, T., Bernhagen, J., Shiiki, H., Calandra, T., Dohi, K., and Bucala, R. (1995) Localization of macrophage migration inhibitory factor (MIF) to secretory granules within the corticotrophic and thyrotrophic cells of the pituitary gland. *Mol. Med.* **1,** 781–788.
51. Tonelli, L., Webster, J. I., Rapp, K. L., and Sternberg, E. (2001) Neuroendocrine responses regulating susceptibility and resistance to autoimmune/inflammatory disease in inbred rat strains. *Immunol. Rev.* **184,** 203–211.
52. Calandra, T., Bernhagen, J., Mitchell, R. A., and Bucala, R. (1994) The macrophage is an important and previously unrecognized source of macrophage migration inhibitory factor. *J. Exp. Med.* **179,** 1895–1902.
53. Calandra, T., Spiegel, L. A., Metz, C. N., and Bucala, R. (1998) Macrophage migration inhibitory factor is a critical mediator of the activation of immune cells by exotoxins of Gram-positive bacteria. *Proc. Natl. Acad. Sci. USA* **95,** 11383–11388.
54. Bernhagen, J., Bacher, M., Calandra, T., et al. (1996) An essential role for macrophage migration inhibitory factor in the tuberculin delayed-type hypersensitivity reaction. *J. Exp. Med.* **183,** 277–282.
55. Martiney, J. A., Sherry, B., Metz, C. N., et al. (2000) Macrophage migration inhibitory factor release by macrophages after ingestion of *Plasmodium chabaudi*-infected erythrocytes: possible role in the pathogenesis of malarial anemia. *Infect. Immun.* **68,** 2259–2267.
56. Shimizu, T., Abe, R., Ohkawara, A., and Nishihira, J. (1999) Ultraviolet B radiation upregulates the production of macrophage migration inhibitory factor (MIF) in human epidermal keratinocytes. *J. Invest. Dermatol.* **112,** 210–215.
57. Plaisance, V., Thompson, N., Niederhauser, G., et al. (2002) The mif gene is transcriptionally regulated by glucose in insulin-secreting cells. *Biochem. Biophys. Res. Commun.* **295,** 174–181.
58. Waeber, G., Thompson, N., Chautard, T., et al. (1998) Transcriptional activation of the macrophage migration-inhibitory factor gene by the corticotropin-releasing factor is mediated by the cyclic adenosine 3',5'-monophosphate responsive element-binding protein CREB in pituitary cells. *Mol. Endocrinol.* **12,** 698–705.
59. Wada, S., Kudo, T., Kudo, M., et al. (1999) Induction of macrophage migration inhibitory factor in human ovary by human chorionic gonadotrophin. *Hum. Reprod.* **14,** 395–399.
60. Tesch, G. H., Nikolic-Paterson, D. J., Metz, C. N., et al. (1998) Rat mesangial cells express macrophage migration inhibitory factor in vitro and in vivo. *J. Am. Soc. Nephrol.* **9,** 417–424.
61. Eickhoff, R., Wilhelm, B., Renneberg, H., et al. (2001) Purification and characterization of macrophage migration inhibitory factor as a secretory protein from rat epididymis: evidences for alternative release and transfer to spermatozoa. *Mol. Med.* **7,** 27–35.
62. Brown, F. G., Nikolic-Paterson, D. J., Chadban, S. J., et al. (2001) Urine macrophage migration inhibitory factor concentrations as a diagnostic tool in human renal allograft rejection. *Transplantation* **71,** 1777–1783.
63. Brown, F. G., Nikolic-Paterson, D. J., Hill, P. A., et al. (2002) Urine macrophage migration inhibitory factor reflects the severity of renal injury in human glomerulonephritis. *J. Am. Soc. Nephrol.* **13(Suppl. 1),** S7–S13.
64. Bacher, M., Meinhardt, A., Lan, H. Y., et al. (1998) MIF expression in the rat brain: implications for neuronal function. *Mol. Med.* **4,** 217–230.
65. Frenette, G., Tremblay, R. R., Dube, J. Y., Lazure, C., and Lemay, M. (1998) High concentrations of the macrophage migration inhibitory factor in human seminal plasma and prostatic tissues. *Arch. Androl.* **41,** 185–193.
66. Wada, S., Fujimoto, S., Mizue, Y., and Nishihira, J. (1997) Macrophage migration inhibitory factor in the human ovary: presence in the follicular fluids and production by granulosa cells. *Biochem. Mol. Biol. Int.* **41,** 805–814.
67. Joshi, P. C., Poole, G. V., Sachdev, V., Zhou, X., and Jones, Q. (2000) Trauma patients with positive cultures have higher levels of circulating macrophage migration inhibitory factor (MIF). *Res. Commun. Mol. Pathol. Pharmacol.* **107,** 13–20.
68. Gando, S., Nishihira, J., Kobayashi, S., Morimoto, Y., Nanzaki, S., and Kemmotsu, O. (2001) Macrophage migration inhibitory factor is a critical mediator of systemic inflammatory response syndrome. *Intensive Care Med.* **27,** 1187–1193.

69. Lehmann, L. E., Novender, U., Schroeder, S., et al. (2001) Plasma levels of macrophage migration inhibitory factor are elevated in patients with severe sepsis. *Intensive Care Med.* **27,** 1412–1415.
70. Rossi, A. G., Haslett, C., Hirani, N., et al. (1998) Human circulating eosinophils secrete macrophage migration inhibitory factor (MIF). Potential role in asthma. *J. Clin. Invest.* **101,** 2869–2874.
71. Yamaguchi, E., Nishihira, J., Shimizu, T., et al. (2000) Macrophage migration inhibitory factor (MIF) in bronchial asthma. *Clin. Exp. Allergy* **30,** 1244–1249.
72. de Jong, Y. P., Abadia-Molina, A. C., Satoskar, A. R., et al. (2001) Development of chronic colitis is dependent on the cytokine MIF. *Nat. Immunol.* **2,** 1061–1066.
73. Shimizu, T., Abe, R., Ohkawara, A., Mizue, Y., and Nishihira, J. (1997) Macrophage migration inhibitory factor is an essential immunoregulatory cytokine in atopic dermatitis. *Biochem. Biophys. Res. Commun.* **240,** 173–178.
74. Kitaichi, N., Kotake, S., Mizue, Y., Matsuda, H., Onoe, K., and Nishihira, J. (2000) Increase of macrophage migration inhibitory factor in sera of patients with iridocyclitis. *Br. J. Ophthalmol.* **84,** 1423–1425.
75. Kitaichi, N., Kotake, S., Sasamoto, Y., et al. (1999) Prominent increase of macrophage migration inhibitory factor in the sera of patients with uveitis. *Invest. Ophthalmol. Vis. Sci.* **40,** 247–250.
76. Niino, M., Ogata, A., Kikuchi, S., Tashiro, K., and Nishihira, J. (2000) Macrophage migration inhibitory factor in the cerebrospinal fluid of patients with conventional and optic-spinal forms of multiple sclerosis and neuro-Behçet's disease. *J. Neurol. Sci.* **179,** 127–131.
77. Onodera, S., Suzuki, K., Matsuno, T., Kaneda, K., Takagi, M., and Nishihira, J. (1997) Macrophage migration inhibitory factor induces phagocytosis of foreign particles by macrophages in autocrine and paracrine fashion. *Immunology* **92,** 131–137.
78. Juttner, S., Bernhagen, J., Metz, C. N., Rollinghoff, M., Bucala, R., and Gessner, A. (1998) Migration inhibitory factor induces killing of *Leishmania major* by macrophages: dependence on reactive nitrogen intermediates and endogenous TNF-alpha. *J. Immunol.* **161,** 2383–2390.
79. Waeber, G., Calandra, T., Roduit, R., et al. (1997) Insulin secretion is regulated by the glucose-dependent production of islet beta cell macrophage migration inhibitory factor. *Proc. Natl. Acad. Sci. USA* **94,** 4782–4787.
80. Benigni, F., Atsumi, T., Calandra, T., et al. (2000) The proinflammatory mediator macrophage migration inhibitory factor induces glucose catabolism in muscle. *J. Clin. Invest.* **106,** 1291–1300.
81. Vojtek, A. B. and Der, C. J. (1998) Increasing complexity of the Ras signaling pathway. *J. Biol. Chem.* **273,** 19925–19928.
82. Roovers, K., Davey, G., Zhu, X., Bottazzi, M. E., and Assoian, R. K. (1999) Alpha5beta1 integrin controls cyclin D1 expression by sustaining mitogen-activated protein kinase activity in growth factor-treated cells. *Mol. Biol. Cell.* **10,** 3197–3204.
83. Murakami, M., Nakatani, Y., Atsumi, G., Inoue, K., and Kudo, I. (1997) Regulatory functions of phospholipase A2. *Crit. Rev. Immunol.* **17,** 225–283.
84. Joyce, D. A., Gimblett, G., and Steer, J. H. (2001) Targets of glucocorticoid action on TNF-alpha release by macrophages. *Inflamm. Res.* **50,** 337–340.
85. Scheinman, R. I., Cogswell, P. C., Lofquist, A. K., and Baldwin, A. S. Jr. (1995) Role of transcriptional activation of I kappa B alpha in mediation of immunosuppression by glucocorticoids. *Science* **270,** 283–286.
86. Daun, J. M. and Cannon, J. G. (2000) Macrophage migration inhibitory factor antagonizes hydrocortisone-induced increases in cytosolic IkappaBalpha. *Am. J. Physiol. Regul. Integr. Comp. Physiol.* **279,** R1043–R1049.
87. Roger, T., David, J., Glauser, M. P., and Calandra, T. (2001) MIF regulates innate immune responses through modulation of Toll-like receptor 4. *Nature* **414,** 920–924.
88. Bucala, R. (2000) A most interesting factor. *Nature* **408,** 146–147.
89. Honma, N., Koseki, H., Akasaka, T., et al. (2000) Deficiency of the macrophage migration inhibitory factor gene has no significant effect on endotoxaemia. *Immunology* **100,** 84–90.
90. Fingerle-Rowson, G. (2001) A genetic approach to the biologic function of macrophage migration inhibitory factor (MIF). The Picower Institute for Medical Research, Manhasset, NY. Thesis/ Dissertation.
91. Rajewsky, K., Gu, H., Kuhn, R., et al. (1996) Conditional gene targeting. *J. Clin. Invest.* **98,** 600–603.

92. Meinhardt, A., Bacher, M., McFarlane, J. R., et al. (1996) Macrophage migration inhibitory factor production by Leydig cells: evidence for a role in the regulation of testicular function. *Endocrinology* **137,** 5090–5095.
93. Kobayashi, S., Satomura, K., Levsky, J. M., et al. (1999) Expression pattern of macrophage migration inhibitory factor during embryogenesis. *Mech. Dev.* **84,** 153–156.
94. Lanahan, A., Williams, J. B., Sanders, L. K., and Nathans, D. (1992) Growth factor-induced delayed early response genes. *Mol. Cell. Biol.* **12,** 3919–3929.
95. Wistow, G. J., Shaughnessy, M. P., Lee, D. C., Hodin, J., and Zelenka, P. S. (1993) A macrophage migration inhibitory factor is expressed in the differentiating cells of the eye lens. *Proc. Natl. Acad. Sci. USA* **90,** 1272–1275.
95a. Petrenko, O., Fingerle-Rowson, G., Peng, T., Mitchell, R. A., and Metz, C. N. (2003) Macrophage Migration Inhibitory Factor deficiency is associated with altered cell growth and reduced susceptibility to Ras-mediated transformation. *J. Biol. Chem.* **278,** 11078–11085.
96. Karima, R., Matsumoto, S., Higashi, H., and Matsushima, K. (1999) The molecular pathogenesis of endotoxic shock and organ failure. *Mol. Med. Today* **5,** 123–132.
97. Galanos, C. and Freudenberg, M. A. (1993) Mechanisms of endotoxin shock and endotoxin hypersensitivity. *Immunobiology* **187,** 346–356.
98. Sadlack, B., Merz, H., Schorle, H., Schimpl, A., Feller, A. C., and Horak, I. (1993) Ulcerative colitis-like disease in mice with a disrupted interleukin-2 gene. *Cell* **75,** 253–261.
99. Morales-Montor, J., Baig, S., Kabbani, A., and Damian, R. T. (2002) Do interleukin-6 and macrophage-migration inhibitory factor play a role during sex-associated susceptibility in murine cysticercosis? *Parasitol. Res.* **88,** 901–904.
100. Chen, H., Centola, M., Altschul, S. F., and Metzger, H. (1998) Characterization of gene expression in resting and activated mast cells. *J. Exp. Med.* **188,** 1657–1668.
101. Lan, H. Y., Mu, W., Yang, N., et al. (1996) De Novo renal expression of macrophage migration inhibitory factor during the development of rat crescentic glomerulonephritis. *Am. J. Pathol.* **149,** 1119–1127.
102. Imamura, K., Nishihira, J., Suzuki, M., et al. (1996) Identification and immunohistochemical localization of macrophage migration inhibitory factor in human kidney. *Biochem. Mol. Biol. Int.* **40,** 1233–1242.
103. Bacher, M., Meinhardt, A., Lan, H. Y., et al. (1997) Migration inhibitory factor expression in experimentally induced endotoxemia. *Am. J. Pathol.* **150,** 235–246.
104. Shimizu, T., Ohkawara, A., Nishihira, J., and Sakamoto, W. (1996) Identification of macrophage migration inhibitory factor (MIF) in human skin and its immmunohistochemical localization. *FEBS Lett.* **381,** 199–202.
105. Gomez, R. S., Diepgen, T. L., Neumann, C., and Sorg, C. (1990) Detection of migration inhibitory factor (MIF) by a monoclonal antibody in the microvasculature of inflamed skin. *Arch. Dermatol. Res.* **282,** 374–378.
106. Goebeler, M., Gutwald, J., Roth, J., and Sorg, C. (1991) The severity of irritant contact dermatitis in various strains of mice correlates with endothelial expression of migration inhibitory factor (MIF). *Arch. Dermatol. Res.* **283,** 246–250.
107. Meinhardt, A., Bacher, M., Metz, C., et al. (1998) Local regulation of macrophage subsets in the adult rat testis: examination of the roles of the seminiferous tubules, testosterone, and macrophage-migration inhibitory factor. *Biol. Reprod.* **59,** 371–378.
108. Suzuki, H., Kanagawa, H., and Nishihira, J. (1996) Evidence for the presence of macrophage migration inhibitory factor in murine reproductive organs and early embryos. *Immunol. Lett.* **51,** 141–147.
109. Matsuda, A., Kotake, S., Tagawa, Y., Matsuda, H., and Nishihira, J. (1996) Detection and immunolocalization of macrophage migration inhibitory factor in rat iris and ciliary epithelium. *Immunol. Lett.* **53,** 1–5.
110. Matsuda, A., Tagawa, Y., Matsuda, H., and Nishihira, J. (1996) Identification and immunohistochemical localization of macrophage migration inhibitory factor in human cornea. *FEBS Lett.* **385,** 225–228.
111. Nishio, Y., Minami, A., Kato, H., Kaneda, K., and Nishihira, J. (1999) Identification of macrophage migration inhibitory factor (MIF) in rat peripheral nerves: its possible involvement in nerve regeneration. *Biochim. Biophys. Acta* **1453,** 74–82.

112. Nishio, Y., Nishihira, J., Ishibashi, T., Kato, H., and Minami, A. (2002) Role of macrophage migration inhibitory factor (MIF) in peripheral nerve regeneration: anti-MIF antibody induces delay of nerve regeneration and the apoptosis of schwann cells. *Mol. Med.* **8,** 509–520.
113. Onodera, S., Suzuki, K., Matsuno, T., Kaneda, K., Kuriyama, T., and Nishihira, J. (1996) Identification of macrophage migration inhibitory factor in murine neonatal calvariae and osteoblasts. *Immunology* **89,** 430–435.
114. Onodera, S., Suzuki, K., Kaneda, K., Fujinaga, M., and Nishihira, J. (1999) Growth factor-induced expression of macrophage migration inhibitory factor in osteoblasts: relevance to the plasminogen activator system. *Semin. Thromb. Hemost.* **25,** 563–568.
115. Sakaue, S., Nishihira, J., Hirokawa, J., et al. (1999) Regulation of macrophage migration inhibitory factor (MIF) expression by glucose and insulin in adipocytes in vitro. *Mol. Med.* **5,** 361–371.
116. Hirokawa, J., Sakaue, S., Furuya, Y., et al. (1998) Tumor necrosis factor-alpha regulates the gene expression of macrophage migration inhibitory factor through tyrosine kinase-dependent pathway in 3T3-L1 adipocytes. *J. Biochem. (Tokyo)* **123,** 733–739.
117. Chesney, J., Metz, C., Bacher, M., Peng, T., Meinhardt, A., and Bucala, R. (1999) An essential role for macrophage migration inhibitory factor (MIF) in angiogenesis and the growth of a murine lymphoma. *Mol. Med.* **5,** 181–191.
118. Fingerle-Rowson, G., Petrenko, O., Metz, C., et al. (2003) The p53-dependent effects of macrophage migration inhibitory factor revealed by gene targeting, *submitted.*
119. Liao, H., Bucala, R., and Mitchell, R. (2003) Adhesion-dependent signaling by macrophage migration inhibitory factor (MIF). *J. Biol. Chem.* **278,** 76–81.

22

Osteopontin, a Surprisingly Flexible Cytokine

Functions Revealed from Osteopontin Knockout Mice

Susan R. Rittling, Anthony W. O'Regan, and Jeffrey S. Berman

Summary

In many ways, osteopontin is an atypical cytokine. From its unusual, flexible structure to its participation in a variety of different systems, the protein almost defies categorization. It clearly meets the criteria for a cytokine *(1)*, and has multiple effects on the immune system. Yet it also regulates mineralization, and is an important component and regulator of normal and abnormal calcified tissues and structures. In addition, it regulates fibrosis in various pathologies, but whether this activity relates to its function as a cytokine is still an open question. Thus the flexibility of the protein structurally is mirrored in its functional flexibility. Osteopontin is a multitasking protein, and since many of its functions have been best defined through analysis of the OPN-knockout mouse, this volume is a most appropriate venue in which to review these functions. Here we review the role of OPN in a number of systems in which it participates, including bone, the immune system, renal and cardiovascular physiology, and tumorigenesis and metastasis, with especial emphasis on studies utilizing the OPN knockout mice. Furthermore, we consider the idea that many of the functions of OPN are mediated by its ability to regulate cellular recruitment.

Key words

osteopontin, cytokine, macrophages, bone, migration, fibrosis, mineralization, integrin, SIBLING, osteoclast, kidney, cardiovascular, tumorigenesis

1. Osteopontin Structure

The primary structure of OPN is unusual. The secreted protein is 298 amino acids in the human and 278 in the mouse and is highly and variably posttranslationally modified. Of the 278 amino acids in the mouse protein, 22% are serine or threonine, and the protein is highly acidic, with a pI of 4.18. There are no disulfide bonds in the molecule. Analysis of posttranslationally modified OPN by nuclear magnetic resonance (NMR) reveals that there is little secondary structure and that the protein has a flexible conformation in solution *(2)*. It has been suggested that this conformation may be stabilized through interaction of OPN with a number of binding partners, including complement factor H *(3)*. There are two splice variants of the human mRNA but as yet no indication that these variants differ functionally.

Posttranslational modifications of OPN are clearly important in its function, but the details of this issue are just now becoming understood. The protein is highly and variably phosphorylated and O-glycosylated; although the protein has been thought to be subject to N-glycosylation *(2)*, other studies fail to confirm this *(4,5)*. The protein from bone can be fractionated according to phosphorylation status: the most highly and the least phosphorylated fractions are known as OPN-1 and OPN-2, respectively *(6)*. Functionally, these isoforms can

From: *Contemporary Immunology: Cytokine Knockouts, 2nd Edition*
Edited by: Giamila Fantuzzi

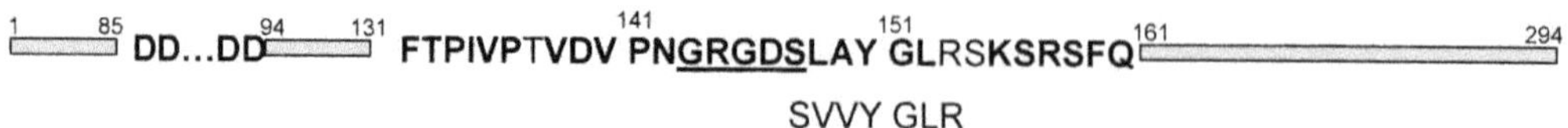

Fig. 1. Cartoon of mouse OPN structure. Sequences discussed are indicated by the one-letter amino acid code. DD...DD represents the poly-aspartate sequence. The central loop containing the GRGDS sequence (underlined), the thrombin cleavage site, and Thr 137 (both in non-bold type) are indicated. The sequence of the human $\alpha_9\beta_1$ binding site is shown below.

be distinguished by some cell types but not others, indicating that different OPN receptors may differentially recognize the various phosphorylated forms of the protein *(7)*, (C. Farach-Carson, personal communication). Additionally, there are hints that the glycosylation state of the protein may regulate function *(8)*. The protein is a substrate for several proteases including thrombin and matrix metalloproteinases (MMP-3 and MMP-7) *(9)*. The cleaved forms of OPN have been reported to have either increased *(9,10)* or decreased *(11)* activities in vitro depending on the assay and cell type used. These differing results may result from different OPN-receptor interactions, as discussed below.

2. Osteopontin Receptors

OPN binds to several different integrins, most notably those of the α_v class [$\alpha_v\beta_3$, $\alpha_v\beta_5$, and $\alpha_v\beta_1$, *(12–14)*], but interaction of OPN with a series of β_1-containing integrins has been more recently reported, including $\alpha_9\beta_1$ *(15,16)*, $\alpha_5\beta_1$ *(17)*, $\alpha_4\beta_1$ *(18)*, and $\alpha_4\beta_7$ *(19)*. The ability of OPN to mediate cell attachment through the $\alpha_v\beta_5$ and $\alpha_v\beta_1$ integrins has recently been questioned, however *(20)*. In addition, interaction of OPN with a non-integrin cell surface receptor, CD44, has been described *(21)*. CD44, although transcribed from a single copy gene, exists in a variety of forms generated by differential splicing, and the presence of the v6 and/or the v7 exons appears to be required for interaction with OPN *(21,22)*. The nature of the interaction of OPN with CD44 is not well understood: it has been suggested that OPN may not interact directly with CD44, rather that the appropriate form(s) of CD44 interact with β_1-containing integrins bound to OPN, but this point is controversial *(22–24)*.

The α_v-containing integrins most likely interact with OPN through the RGD sequence and can mediate cell adhesion to OPN *(25)*. The β_1-interacting sequences have been studied extensively recently: the SVVYGLR (of human OPN) has been shown to be the binding site for the $\alpha_9\beta_1$ integrin *(16)*, as well as $\alpha_4\beta_7$ *(19)*; an additional sequence that binds the $\alpha_4\beta_1$ integrin has been described at amino acids 131–143 in human OPN, although this sequence is apparently missing from mouse OPN *(26)*. The SVVYGLR sequence is contiguous with the RGD sequence (Fig. 1) and the thrombin cleavage site. The SVVYGLR sequence is cryptic *(15)* and is only active when OPN is cleaved by thrombin at the RS sequence just downstream of this sequence (Fig. 1) This has been shown in the case of the $\alpha_4\beta_7$ interaction to be owing to a requirement for an acidic residue at the COOH-terminal end of this sequence: this negative charge can be supplied by the free COO^- moiety in the thrombin-cleaved molecule *(19)*. In a proB cell line, OPN has been shown to prevent apoptosis via an interaction that involves CD44 *(24)*. Thr137 and Ser147 are required for this interaction, and their mutation to alanine results in dominant negative forms of OPN. In bovine milk OPN, Thr137 is glycosylated *(27)*, suggesting a functional role for this modification in this system. A poly-aspartate sequence in the NH_2-terminal half of the molecule functions in OPN binding to hydroxyapatite.

CD44 is variably expressed on lymphocytes, and its variant forms are expressed on many metastatic cells *(28)*. It is intriguing that several aspects of the biology of the CD44 variants, particularly those containing v6/v7, parallel that of OPN. Expression of the CD44 v6 exon or of OPN is associated with acquisition of a metastatic phenotype, as well as with activation of lymphocytes (reviewed in ref. *28*). Mice in which theCD44 v6/v7 exons are specifically deleted fail to develop pathology in experimental colitis: this pathology involves a Th1 autoimmune response *(29)*, and this resistance to pathology is strikingly similar to that seen in autoimmune models in OPN-deficient mice *(30–32)*.

3. Osteopontin Localization and Function

By *in situ* hybridization, OPN mRNA has been identified in a wide variety of tissues throughout the body—a recurrent theme is its appearance in epithelial cells, particularly at epithelial surfaces *(33)*. This observation is consistent with the protein's accumulation in a variety of bodily fluids, including blood, bile, saliva, cerebrospinal fluid, and urine (see below). The protein is made at high levels in the lactating mammary gland *(34)*, and it has been isolated from human and bovine milk *(4,18)*. In addition, it is present in high levels in bone and is induced by a variety of stimuli in a series of cell types, including inflammatory cells such as lymphocytes and macrophages (reviewed in ref. *35*). Unlike many interleukins, OPN is expressed at relatively high levels in many cell types and is readily detectable by immunohistochemistry.

Owing to the presence of OPN in the mineralized matrix of bone, together with its integrin binding properties, OPN achieved a reputation as a component of the extracellular matrix. Although this is certainly the case in bone, OPN is clearly a soluble protein in tumors *(36)* and probably in most soft tissues as well. This consideration has important implications for the function of the protein, as a major in vitro activity of the protein is mediating adhesion of cells to surfaces via its binding to a series of adhesive receptors. This adhesive activity is unlikely therefore to be relevant to its function in soft tissues, although stimulation of migration, which can be mediated through the same adhesive receptors, is undoubtedly a key function of OPN *(12,37)*. Other functions of the protein in vitro are less well defined and include inhibition of apoptosis *(24,38,39)* and regulation of cytokine production *(30,40)*.

Mice with a disrupted OPN gene are viable and fertile and show no evidence of abnormality under typical laboratory animal care conditions *(41,42)*. They have a normal growth rate, and the litter size is normal. Although OPN may be a member of a gene family [the SIBLING family *(2)*, which apparently diverged from a common ancestor based on structural similarity at the level of organization of the gene], there is no evidence that the closest member of this family, BSP, is misexpressed in OPN-deficient mice *(41,43)*. These observations are consistent with a role for the protein primarily in pathologic situations. Accordingly, as described in detail in the following sections, the OPN knockout mice have dramatic phenotypes in a series of different pathologic conditions.

4. Osteopontin in Bone

One of the earliest descriptions of OPN was as a major noncollagenous protein of bone *(44)*. When the protein was isolated from bone and subsequently cloned, its high affinity for hydroxyapatite and the presence of the RGD sequence led to the suggestion of the name osteopontin to reflect a function of the protein as a bridge linking various bone cells to the mineralized matrix of bone *(45)*. OPN is made by a variety of bone cells, including osteoblasts and osteoclasts, and accumulates in the mineralized matrix, particularly at sites previously occupied by bone cells, cement lines, and lamina limitantes *(46)*. In vitro experiments have demonstrated that OPN acts to inhibit crystal formation from supersaturated hydroxyapatite solutions *(47)*, and, indeed, the OPN-deficient mice have hypermineralized bones that show increased crystal size *(48)*.

Noda and colleagues have used the OPN knockout mice to demonstrate elegantly the critical role OPN plays in bone. Using a variety of models, this group showed that bone resorption in pathologic situations is severely inhibited in the absence of osteopontin *(49–52)*. For instance, in the mouse, there is significant bone resorption that occurs in the first 2 wk following ovariectomy, a model for postmenopausal osteoporosis in women. OPN-deficient mice are completely protected from this bone loss *(49)*. Similarly, OPN-deficient mice are protected from bone loss following immobilization, in experiments in which mice are prevented from using their hind legs for 2 wk *(52,53)*. This situation is particularly applicable to persons restricted to bed rest or astronauts exposed to microgravity. Bone resorption is a critical aspect of normal bone growth, and although it at first appeared that bone structure in the OPN-deficient mice was normal *(41)*, subsequent analyses indicate slightly increased bone density in the absence of OPN *(49,52,54)*.

Bone resorption is mediated by osteoclasts, multinucleated cells that differentiate from the same hematopoietic precursors as macrophages *(55)*. These cells form a tight seal against the bone and secrete protons and proteases into the enclosed space, thus dissolving the mineralized matrix, in a pattern of interconnected pits. Osteoclasts express high amounts of the $\alpha_v\beta_3$ integrin, which is critical for bone resorption *(56)*. It is clear from the in vivo studies that OPN has a major role in osteoclast function. Experiments with osteoclasts in vitro show that OPN-deficient osteoclasts are defective in bone resorption owing to impaired mobility in addition to reduced resorption, as evidenced by reduced pit depth *(54,57)*. OPN is required for osteoclast function both as a soluble molecule and as a component of bone. Soluble OPN added to OPN-deficient osteoclasts can only partially correct the defect in bone resorption, restoring osteoclast motility but not pit depth *(54)*. This observation indicates that OPN in the bone, either endogenous or secreted into the resorption space by osteoclasts, has an important role in bone resorption. Osteoclast differentiation is also impaired in the absence of OPN: OPN-deficient osteoclasts have on average fewer nuclei *(57)*, and this reduced cell size is associated with impaired resorptive activity. Whether the altered crystal structure of the OPN-deficient bones also plays a role in the bone resorption defect is still unknown. The observation that OPN-deficient cells show impaired migration is not unique to osteoclasts. Both fibroblasts and macrophages from OPN-deficient mice show a similar reduction in migration *(57,58)*. Since integrins are critically involved in migration *(59)*, these observations are consistent with a critical interaction between OPN and various integrins in mediating migration, although in the case of macrophages, migration in response to only a subset of chemokines depends on OPN *(60)*. An intracellular interaction between OPN and CD44 has been suggested as mediating these effects of OPN on migration *(58)*.

5. Osteopontin in Inflammation and Immunity

Two seminal observations formed the basis of the now well-described role for OPN in immune responses. First, OPN was independently identified and cloned from T-cells as early T-cell activation gene 1 (Eta-1) by Patarca et al. (reviewed in refs. *61* and *62*). OPN was found to be the most abundant early T-cell transcript in activated T-cells. It was further demonstrated that early expression of OPN was required for resistance to infection with *Rickettsia tsutsugamushi* in mice and that the OPN gene mapped to the rickettsial resistance locus. Later, using differential display, Nau et al. *(63)* demonstrated that OPN was the most prominent transcript expressed by macrophages after mycobacterial infection compared with infection with other bacteria. These results suggested that OPN was an abundantly expressed early protein in immune responses.

Subsequently it has been shown that OPN is indeed expressed by a variety of inflammatory cells including macrophages, dendritic cells, T-cells, and natural killer (NK) cells *(62)*. Extensive in vitro data have demonstrated that macrophages and T-cells adhere to OPN and that OPN is chemotactic for macrophages, dendritic cells, and T-cells *(40,62,64)*. Indeed, a recent study in mice demonstrated that OPN could both drive interleukin-12 (IL-12) and inhibit IL-10 expression by macrophages *(30)*. Interestingly phosphorylation of OPN was required for its effect on IL-12 but not IL-10. In view of Th1/Th2 cytokine cross-inhibition and self-amplification, these data indicate that OPN should induce a profound polarization of the immune response toward the Th1 pole. Collectively these studies suggest that OPN may regulate cellular recruitment to and early Th1/Th2 cytokine expression at sites of inflammation. The availability of OPN knockout mice has provided in vivo evidence to support these in vitro studies, as described below.

5.1. Cellular Recruitment: Macrophages

Several, although not all, studies have demonstrated deficient inflammatory cell recruitment in OPN-deficient mice. Although Liaw et al. *(42)* showed that macrophage recruitment was normal to sites of cutaneous wound repair, studies in kidney, lung, and skin models of inflammation have shown that macrophage accumulation was markedly reduced *(30,65–68)*. In the absence of OPN expression, granulomatous inflammation in both the lung (in response to eggs of *Schistosoma mansoni*) *(65)* and skin (in response to polyvinyl pyrrolidone) *(30)* was associated with a dramatic reduction in macrophage numbers. The models of granulomatous inflammation studied reflect both a foreign body and hypersensitivity response suggesting that defective cellular recruitment is not an antigen-dependent phenomenon. Interestingly, although Nau et al. *(69)* showed defective control of mycobacterial growth in OPN-deficient mice, these authors could not demonstrate abnormal macrophage recruitment to peritoneum or to sites of mycobacterial accumulation in vivo.

In several models of renal injury such as obstructive uropathy *(68)* and cyclosporin A nephropathy *(70)*, macrophage accumulation in OPN-deficient animals was also decreased and associated with reduced transforming growth factor-β (TGF-β) expression, fibrosis, arteriolopathy, and epithelial cell apoptosis. In contrast, although OPN is expressed in Goodpasture's nephritis in humans, deficient OPN expression had no impact on the initiation or progression of experimental antiglomerular basement membrane nephritis *(71)*. Finally, a recent study of antibody-mediated inflammatory arthritis showed that OPN knockout mice developed less inflammation and swelling as well as less chondrocyte apoptosis *(72)*. It was suggested that these findings represented distinct functions of OPN on cellular recruitment and chrondrocyte survival and together contributed to a dramatic decrease in the severity of inflammatory arthritis. These studies suggest that although OPN does appear to regulate macrophage accumulation in vivo, its effects are organ- and insult-specific.

The mechanism of defective macrophage accumulation in OPN-deficient mice is unclear. Based on extensive in vitro data, it is likely to reflect aberrant macrophage migration. OPN has direct chemotactic effects on a variety of inflammatory cells and thus may be the major macrophage chemoattractant expressed in certain immune responses such as granulomatous inflammation. Although this explanation is plausible, the dramatic decrease in macrophage accumulation and the fact that numerous additional macrophage-monocyte chemoattractants are present during granuloma formation raise the possibility that OPN may regulate intrinsic migratory mechanisms central to macrophage chemotaxis in vivo. Interestingly Giachelli et al. *(73)* have shown that the chemotactic response to fMLP in rat skin can be inhibited by pretreatment with anti-OPN antibodies. Similarly, Zohar et al. *(58)* have shown that OPN-deficient macrophages demonstrate reduced in vitro migration to fMLP. This group also demonstrated that intracellular OPN colocalizes with CD44 and the actin binding protein ezrin at the leading intracellular edge of migrating cells. This suggests that an intracellular form of OPN functions to regulate the cytoskeletal apparatus of migrating cells. Other studies have shown that OPN regulates the expression of several MMPs including MMP-1, -2, and -9 *(74–76)*. Failure to traverse matrix and endothelial boundaries efficiently because of impaired MMP expression represents another potential mechanism for failure of macrophage migration in OPN-deficient animals.

Increased macrophage apoptosis could also account for reduced accumulation of macrophages at sites of inflammation. In fact, OPN has been shown to be a survival factor for vascular smooth muscle cells *(77)*, endothelial cells *(78)*, and hematopoietic cells *(79)*. Although OPN may form cell-matrix interactions that protect cells from *anoikis* (anchorage-dependent apoptosis), soluble OPN has also been shown to provide survival signals to endothelial cells *(78)*, and OPN is required for the antiapoptotic effects of IL-3 and granulocyte/macrophage colony-stimulating factor (GM-CSF) on a murine pro-B-cell line *(79)*. Despite these data, no studies have shown increased macrophage apoptosis in OPN-deficient cells or animals. In schistosome-induced granulomatous inflammation in the lung, we have found no difference in macrophage apoptosis in OPN-deficient compared with $OPN^{+/+}$ animals (A. O'Regan, unpublished observations). Thus at present there is no evidence that the effects of OPN on macrophage accumulation in vivo is due to altered macrophage survival.

5.2. Cellular Recruitment: Dendritic Cells and B-Cells

A recent study demonstrated that OPN-deficient mice also showed defective migration of dendritic cells to regional lymph nodes following a cutaneous antigenic challenge *(80)*. The profound defect in dendritic cell migration could potentially result in defective antigen presentation and impaired downstream antigen-specific immune responses. It is unclear whether such a mechanism could account for the defective killing of mycobacteria despite seemingly normal inflammatory cell accumulation.

Despite convincing effects of OPN deficiency on macrophage and dendritic cell migration, transgenic mice overexpressing OPN develop a B-cell peritonitis *(81)*. Accumulating B-cells were predominantly of the B1 type, and there was an associated expression of anti-double-stranded DNA autoantibodies. No increase in T-cells or macrophages was seen in the peritoneum. Phenotypic differences in other organs in these mice were not described. The effects of OPN overexpression are similar to the B-cell proliferation seen in *lpr/lpr* mice. These mice develop a lymphoproliferative disease at adulthood, with an increase in

B1-lymphocytes, polyclonal B-cell activation with elevated immunoglobulin levels, and autoimmune renal disease. OPN has been implicated as the driving force behind the B-cell proliferation *(61,82,83)*, and a recent study showed that OPN-deficient mice bred onto the *lpr/lpr* background had delayed B-cell proliferation and production of autoantibodies, whereas the late lymphoproliferation and renal disease was unaltered *(84)*. In vitro, OPN can stimulate CD40L expression on T-cells *(40)*: a similar effect of the protein in vivo on T-cells could mediate effects on B-cell proliferation and function.

5.3. Th1 Cytokine Responses in Infection and Autoimmunity

Ashkar et al. *(30)* reported a dramatic defect in Th1 responses in OPN-deficient mice. When challenged with prototypical Th1 infection such as *Listeria* and herpes simplex virus (HSV)-1, OPN-deficient mice failed to mount a protective Th1 response and consequently developed more severe infection with increased mortality. The Th1-mediated autoimmune HSV-1 keratitis was also attenuated in the absence of OPN. Cytokine expression studies suggested that this phenotype reflected not only reduced interferon-γ (IFN-γ) and IL-12 expression but also increased IL-10 expression. It is still unclear whether abnormalities in cellular recruitment also accounted for some of the phenotypic consequences in this model.

Nau et al. *(69)* demonstrated that OPN-deficient animals were more susceptible to infection with *Mycobacterium bovis* (bacille Calmette-Guérin; BCG). In this model, mice were infected by intraperitoneal injection; OPN-deficient animals demonstrated an increased bacterial burden, although the numbers of organisms declined by 12 wk, indicating eventual control of infection. Peritoneal macrophages from knockout animals were deficient in their ability to control mycobacterial growth in vitro, although in this study there was no decrease in knockout macrophage production of IFN-γ in response to mycobacterial antigens, nor was there a decrease in production of nitric oxide. In this study no defect was found in the numbers of macrophages or other cells recruited to the peritoneum in response to thioglycollate or to mycobacteria. The exact defect in mycobacterial control in OPN knockout animals has not been delineated.

In contrast to these results, a recent study demonstrated that deficiency in OPN did not influence the numbers of spirochetes in tissues from *Borrelia burgdorferi*-infected mice or the level of arthritis or the outcome *(85)*. OPN maps to a locus implicated in mouse strain-specific susceptibility to *B. burgdorferi*, but these studies suggest that OPN is not part of the host defense against *Borrelia*.

Two recent studies have evaluated experimental models of multiple sclerosis in OPN-deficient mice *(31,86)*. Experimental allergic encephalomyelitis (EAE) is a Th1-dependent model in which mice are challenged with the central nervous system (CNS) antigen myelin basic protein to simulate multiple sclerosis. In two independent studies virtually identical results were found in which OPN-deficient mice were protected from EAE disease. Knockout animals exhibited significantly less morbidity and virtually absent mortality from the disease. This phenotype was associated with impaired Th1 cytokine production with reduced expression of IFN-γ and tumor necrosis factor (TNF)-α mRNA in the brains of OPN-deficient challenged mice. Similarly, CD4-positive T-cells stimulated ex vivo with the antigen used to induce CNS disease produced less IFN-γ, TNF-α, and IL-2, along with increased amounts of IL-10. Again, it is unclear whether defective cellular recruitment accounted for any of these changes, as only one of the two studies reported reduced CNS inflammation in OPN-deficient mice.

6. Osteopontin and Renal Function

Osteopontin mRNA is expressed in kidney at levels as high as any other tissue; paradoxically, however, the protein is difficult to detect in this tissue *(87)*. This observation implies that OPN made in the kidney is quantitatively secreted, predominantly into the urine. OPN has long been recognized as an inhibitor of kidney stone formation *(88,89)* and is incorporated into calcium oxalate stones *(90)*. Correspondingly, urinary stones form readily in OPN-deficient mice fed the calcium oxalate precursor ethylene glycol, whereas wild-type, OPN-expressing mice are protected from stone formation *(70)*.

OPN is clearly also an important regulator of pathology in a variety of other models of renal pathology. In a wide variety of different models of renal damage in rats and mice (reviewed in ref. *66*), OPN is upregulated, and a neutralizing antibody to OPN has been shown to suppress the appearance of pathologic changes *(67)*, which frequently involve macrophage infiltration and fibrosis *(91,92)*. When ischemia is induced in mouse kidneys by ureteral ligation, OPN-deficient mice have less macrophage infiltration, TGF-β expression, and reduced cell death in the affected kidney than in wild-type mice, although the extent of disease is similar in mice of both genotypes *(68)*. Similarly, in chronic renal failure, functional analysis reveals no difference between wild-type and OPN-deficient mice. There is, however, strikingly reduced macrophage infiltration and fibrosis, with significantly less immunoreactive collagens I and IV (V.P. Percy, personal communication). Renal damage induced by cyclosporin treatment is also ameliorated in OPN-deficient mice, which show reduced pathology, macrophage infiltration, and fibrosis *(93)*. In ischemia induced by ligation of the renal artery, on the other hand, mice deficient for OPN show a more progressive acute disease, in a manner consistent with increased nitric oxide production in the absence of OPN *(94)*. Indeed, in macrophages and kidney proximal tubular epithelial cells, OPN suppresses nitric oxide production *(95,96)*, and OPN expression is inhibited by NO in what may be a regulatory feedback loop *(97,98)*.

7. Vascular and Cardiac Effects of Osteopontin

Ectopic calcification results in pathology in a variety of situations, most notably in the cardiovascular system, but also in such diverse conditions as breast cancer, granulomatous inflammation, and dental plaques *(99)*. The association of OPN with various forms of calcified matrices and its ability in vitro to inhibit mineralization *(47,100)* suggest that the protein may play a role in ectopic calcification in vivo. In vascular smooth muscle cells in culture, OPN inhibits calcification *(101)*: phosphorylation of the protein is a strict requirement for this activity *(102)*. Indeed, Giachelli and Steitz *(103)* demonstrated an important role for OPN in calcification in vivo. When implanted in mice, glutaraldehyde-fixed porcine aortic valves undergo calcification in wild-type mice: in the absence of OPN, this calcification is increased by five- to eightfold, consistent with a role of OPN as an inhibitor of calcification *(103)*. This effect can be ameliorated by injection of OPN into the OPN-deficient mice and may be mediated through carbonic anhydrase II *(103)*. This role of OPN in vascular calcification was further confirmed by using mice deficient for matrix Gla protein. These mice develop spontaneous vascular calcification *(104)*, as early as 2 wk after birth, and OPN localizes to these sites of calcification. When these mice were crossed to the osteopontin knockout mice, doubly deficient mice developed significantly more severe calcification and died earlier than their wild-type littermates *(105)*. The mechanism of these effects of OPN probably includes the protein's ability to inhibit mineralization but may involve additional signaling functions of the molecule as well.

Mice deficient for OPN confirm striking roles for the protein in the cardiovascular system. OPN is made in a variety of vascular cell types, particularly during pathogenesis, including macrophages and their derivatives foam cells, smooth muscle cells, and myocytes, as well as endothelial cells and cardiac fibroblasts *(106)*, (reviewed in ref. *107*). In a murine model of myocardial remodeling following infarction, several aspects of the disease are altered in the OPN-deficient mice, including increased left ventricular dilation and myocyte length *(108)*. Intriguingly, collagen deposition in the damaged region of the heart was entirely absent in the OPN-deficient animals, as measured at the levels of both protein and mRNA *(108)*, possibly resulting from increased MMP activity (K. Singh, personal communication). In experimentally induced hypertension, OPN expression in the aorta is increased (F. Alameddine et al., manuscript in preparation), and the protein is present in the adventitial, medial, and intimal layers *(107)*. In OPN-deficient mice, vascular hypertrophy was dramatically reduced, such that thickening of the vessel wall was significantly lessened. In wild-type mice, vessel wall thickening in response to hypertension was accompanied by macrophage infiltration into all layers of the vessel wall: this infiltration was strikingly absent in the OPN-deficient mice (F. Alameddine et al., manuscript in preparation). Thus, in this model, OPN mediates intimal thickening and macrophage recruitment into the aorta in response to mechanical strain.

8. Osteopontin in Tumorigenesis and Metastasis

The first description of OPN was as a transformation- associated protein *(109)*: OPN is upregulated in a variety of different tumor models in mice *(66)* and is increasingly being suggested as a tumor marker in human cancer *(110–114)*. It is clear that OPN acts to accelerate tumor growth in several models: OPN-overexpressing cells grow more rapidly as tumors and/or show increased metastasis *(115,116)*, and transformed cells expressing antisense RNA for OPN are less transformed and/or tumorigenic than their control transfected counterparts *(117–119)*. Similarly, *ras*-transformed embryonic fibroblast cells from OPN-deficient mice form tumors and metastases more slowly than their wild-type counterparts *(120)*.

Analysis of tumorigenesis in the OPN knockout mice, however, has revealed complex roles for the protein in tumorigenesis and metastasis, and this complexity may reflect differing effects of host and tumor-produced OPN on tumor growth and metastasis. In various models, tumor development has been found to be altered in OPN-deficient mice, but in unexpected ways: tumor growth is accelerated in sarcomas *(121)*; unchanged in primary mammary tumorigenesis *(43)*; and suppressed in a model of melanoma metastasis *(122)* in OPN-deficient mice compared with wild-type. Although differences in the function of the protein in different tumor types may represent one possibility for these differences, an alternative explanation for these divergent results may be differing effects of host and tumor protein. Although OPN expression in tumor cells themselves clearly enhances tumor growth *(120)*, host expression of the protein may act to suppress tumor development through stimulation of the type 1 immune response *(30)* and/or effects on macrophage function *(121)*. Which of these effects predominate in any single tumor type remains unclear.

9. Conclusions

Clearly, the biology of osteopontin is complex, evidenced by the diversity of systems that are affected and the apparent multiplicity of actions of the protein. A few overriding themes, however, have emerged from the last decade of work on the protein. A main feature of the protein is its ability to affect cell migration, both in vivo and in vitro, and this function may underlie many of its actions in vivo. A second, and probably independent, function of OPN is as a regulator of mineralization, both in bone and in soft tissues. Do these two functions of the protein account for its key role in regulating the immune response and bone resorption and in supporting the fibrotic response in multiple pathologies? Are other reported activities of the protein, such as its ability to regulate cytokine and nitric oxide production, independent of these two well-characterized functions? And if so, how did a protein of such seemingly simple structure evolve this complex set of activities? These are critical questions for the field that will probably be addressed in the near future. The OPN knockout mice have been a key tool in understanding the important role the protein plays in vivo and in beginning to understand its mechanism of action. In vitro systems for studying the function of OPN on the cellular and molecular level and understanding the role, if any, of its posttranslational modifications will be critical for further understanding of how this important cytokines regulates biologic processes.

References

1. WHO-IUIS (1991) Nomenclature for secreted regulatory proteins of the immune system (interleukins). WHO-IUIS Nomenclature Subcommittee on Interleukin Designation. *Bull. World Health Organ* **69,** 483–486.
2. Fisher, L. W., Torchia, D. A., Fohr, B., Young, M. F., and Fedarko, N. S. (2001) Flexible structures of SIBLING proteins, bone sialoprotein, and osteopontin. *Biochem. Biophys. Res. Commun.* **280,** 460–465.
3. Fedarko, N. S., Fohr, B., Robey, P. G., Young, M. F., and Fisher, L. W. (2000) Factor H binding to bone sialoprotein and osteopontin enables tumor cell evasion of complement-mediated attack. *J. Biol. Chem.* **275,** 16666–16672.
4. Sørensen, E. S., Hojrup, P., and Petersen, T. E. (1995) Post-translational modification of bovine osteopontin: identification of twenty-eight phosphorylation and three O-glycosylation sites. *Protein Sci.* **4,** 2040–2049.
5. Neame, P. J. and Butler, W. T. (1996) Posttranslational modification in rat bone osteopontin. *Connect. Tissue Res.* **35,** 145–150.
6. Safran, J. B., Butler, W. T., and Farach-Carson, M. C. (1998) Modulation of osteopontin post-translational state by 1,25-$(OH)_2$-vitamin D_3. Dependence on Ca^{2+} influx. *J. Biol. Chem.* **273,** 29935–29941.
7. Razzouk, S., Brunn, J. C., Qin, C., Tye, C. E., Goldberg, H. A., and Butler, W. T. (2002) Osteopontin posttranslational modifications, possibly phosphorylation, are required for in vitro bone resorption but not osteoclast adhesion. *Bone* **30,** 40–47.
8. D'Alonzo, R. C., Kowalski, A. J., Denhardt, D. T., Nickols, G. A., and Partridge, N. C. (2002) Regulation of collagenase-3 and osteocalcin gene expression by collagen and osteopontin in differentiating MC3T3-E1 Cells. *J. Biol. Chem.* **277,** 24788–24798.
9. Agnihotri, R., Crawford, H. C., Haro, H., Matrisian, L. M., Havrda, M. C., and Liaw, L. (2001) Osteopontin, a novel substrate for matrix metalloproteinase-3 (stromelysin-1) and matrix metalloproteinase-7 (matrilysin). *J. Biol. Chem.* **276,** 28261–28267.
10. Senger, D. R. and Perruzzi, C. A. (1996) Cell migration promoted by a potent GRGDS-containing thrombin-cleavage fragment of osteopontin. *Biochim. Biophys. Acta* **1314,** 13–24.
11. Xuan, J. W., Hota, C., and Chambers, A. F. (1994) Recombinant GST-human osteopontin fusion protein is functional in RGD-dependent cell adhesion. *J. Cell Biochem.* **54,** 247–255.

12. Liaw, L., Skinner, M. P., Raines, E. W., et al. (1995) The adhesive and migratory effects of osteopontin are mediated via distinct cell surface integrins: role of $\alpha_v\beta_3$ in smooth muscle migration to osteopontin *in vitro*. *J. Clin. Invest.* **95,** 713–724.
13. Hu, D. D., Hoyer, J. R., and Smith, J. W. (1995) Calcium suppresses cell adhesion to osteopontin by attenuating binding affinity for integrin $\alpha_v\beta_3$. *J. Biol. Chem.* **270,** 9917–9925.
14. Hu, D. D., Lin, E. C., Kovach, N. L., Hoyer, J. R., and Smith, J. W. (1995) A biochemical characterization of the binding of osteopontin to integrins $\alpha_v\beta_1$ and $\alpha_v\beta_5$. *J. Biol. Chem.* **270,** 26232–26238.
15. Smith, L. L., Cheung, H. K., Ling, L. E., et al. (1998) Osteopontin N-terminal domain contains a cryptic adhesive sequence recognized by $\alpha_9\beta_1$ integrin. *J. Biol. Chem.* **271,** 28485–28491.
16. Yokosaki, Y., Matsuura, N., Sasaki, T., et al. (1999) The integrin alpha(9)beta(1) binds to a novel recognition sequence (SVVYGLR) in the thrombin-cleaved amino-terminal fragment of osteopontin. *J. Biol. Chem.* **274,** 36328–36334.
17. Denda, S., Reichardt, L. F., and Müller, U. (1998) Identification of osteopontin as a novel ligand for the integrin $\alpha_8\beta_1$ and potential roles for this integrin-ligand interaction in kidney morphogenesis. *Mol. Biol. Cell* **9,** 1425–1435.
18. Bayless, K. A., Meininger, G. A., Scholtz, J. M., and Davis, G. E. (1998) Osteopontin is a ligand for the $\alpha_4\beta_1$ integrin. *J. Cell Sci.* **111,** 1165–1174.
19. Green, P. M., Ludbrook, S. B., Miller, D. D., Horgan, C. M., and Barry, S. T. (2001) Structural elements of the osteopontin SVVYGLR motif important for the interaction with alpha(4) integrins. *FEBS Lett.* **503,** 75–79.
20. Caltabiano, S., Hum, W. T., Attwell, G. J., et al. (1999) The integrin specificity of human recombinant osteopontin. *Biochem. Pharmacol.* **58,** 1567–1578.
21. Weber, G. F., Ashkar, S., Glimcher, M. J., and Cantor, H. (1996) Receptor-ligand interaction between CD44 and osteopontin (ETA-1). *Science* **271,** 509–512.
22. Katagiri, Y. U., Sleeman, J., Fujii, H., et al. (1999) CD44 variants but not CD44s cooperate with beta1-containing integrins to permit cells to bind to osteopontin independently of arginine-glycine-aspartic acid, thereby stimulating cell motility and chemotaxis. *Cancer Res.* **59,** 219–226.
23. Smith, L. L., Greenfield, B. W., Aruffo, A., and Giachelli, C. M. (1999) CD44 is not an adhesive receptor for osteopontin. *J. Cell Biochem.* **73,** 20–30.
24. Lin, Y. H. and Yang-Yen, H. F. (2001) The osteopontin-CD44 survival signal involves activation of the phosphatidylinositol-3-kinase/Akt signaling pathway. *J. Biol. Chem.* **276,** 46024–46030.
25. Xuan, J. W., Hota, C., Shigeyama, Y., D'Errico, J. A., Somerman, M. J., and Chambers, A. F. (1995) Site-directed mutagenesis of the arginine-glycine-aspartic acid sequence in osteopontin destroys cell adhesion and migration functions. *J. Cell Biochem.* **57,** 680–690.
26. Bayless, K. J. and Davis, G. E. (2001) Identification of dual $\alpha_4\beta_1$ integrin binding sites within a 38 amino acid domain in the N-terminal thrombin fragment of human osteopontin. *J. Biol. Chem.* **276,** 13483–13489.
27. Sørensen, E. S., Hojrup, P., and Petersen, T. E. (1995) Post-translational modification of bovine osteopontin: identification of twenty-eight phosphorylation and three O-glycosylation sites. *Protein Sci.* **4,** 2040–2049.
28. Naot, D., Sionov, R. V., and Ish-Shalom, D. (1997) CD44: structure, function, and association with the malignant process. *Adv. Cancer Res.* **71,** 241–319.
29. Wittig, B. M., Johansson, B., Zoller, M., Schwarzler, C., and Gunthert, U. (2000) Abrogation of experimental colitis correlates with increased apoptosis in mice deficient for CD44 variant exon 7 (CD44v7). *J. Exp. Med.* **191,** 2053–2064.
30. Ashkar, S., Weber, G. F., Panoutsakopoulou, V., et al. (2000) Eta-1 (osteopontin): an early component of type-1 (cell-mediated) immunity. *Science* **287,** 860–864.
31. Chabas, D., Baranzini, S. E., Mitchell, D., et al. (2001) The influence of the proinflammatory cytokine, osteopontin, on autoimmune demyelinating disease. *Science* **294,** 1731–1735.
32. Yumoto, K., Ishijima, M., Rittling, S. R., et al.(2001) Osteopontin-deficiency supresses joint swelling, chondrocyte apoptosis and joint destruction in antibody-induced rheumatoid arthritis model. *J. Bone Min. Res.* **16,** S450.
33. Brown, L. F., Berse, B., Van De Water, L., et al. (1992) Expression and distribution of osteopontin in human tissues: widespread association with luminal epithelial surfaces. *Mol. Biol. Cell* **3,** 1169–1180.

34. Rittling, S. R. and Novick, K. W. (1997) Osteopontin expression in mammary gland development and tumorigenesis. *Cell Growth Differ.* **8,** 1061–1069.
35. Denhardt, D. T. and Noda, M. (1998) Osteopontin expression and function: role in bone remodeling. *J. Cell Biochem.* **S30/31,** 92–102.
36. Rittling, S. R., Chen, Y., Feng, F., and Wu, Y. (2002) Tumor-derived osteopontin is soluble, not matrix associated. *J. Biol. Chem.* **277,** 9175–9182.
37. Zohar, R., Cheifetz, S., McCulloch, C. A., and Sodek, J. (1998) Analysis of intracellular osteopontin as a marker of osteoblastic cell differentiation and mesenchymal cell migration. *Eur. J. Oral Sci.* **106(Suppl. 1),** 401–407.
38. Scatena, M., Almeida, M., Chaisson, M. L., Fausto, N., Nicosia, R. F., and Giachelli, C. M. (1998) NF-κB mediates $\alpha_v\beta_3$ integrin-induced endothelial cell survival. *J. Cell Biol.* **141,** 1083–1093.
39. Malyankar, U. M., Scatena, M., Suchland, K. L., Yun, T. J., Clark, E. A., and Giachelli, C. M. (2000) Osteoprotegerin is an αvβ3-induced, NF-κB-dependent survival factor for endothelial cells. *J. Biol. Chem.* **275,** 20959–20962.
40. O'Regan, A. W., Hayden, J. M., and Berman, J. S. (2000) Osteopontin augments CD3-mediated interferon-gamma and CD40 ligand expression by T cells, which results in IL-12 production from peripheral blood mononuclear cells. *J. Leukoc. Biol.* **68,** 495–502.
41. Rittling, S. R., Matsumoto, H. N., McKee, M. D., et al. (1998) Mice lacking osteopontin show normal development and bone structure but display altered osteoclast formation *in vitro*. *J. Bone Min. Res.* **13,** 1101–1111.
42. Liaw, L., Birk, D. E., Ballas, C. B., Whitsitt, J. S., Davidson, J. M., and Hogan, B. L. M. (1998) Altered wound healing in mice lacking a functional osteopontin gene (spp1). *J. Clin. Invest.* **101,** 1468–1478.
43. Feng, F. and Rittling, S. R. (2000) Mammary tumorigenesis is normal in the absence of osteopontin. *Breast Cancer Res. Treat.* **63,** 71–79.
44. Heinegard, D. and Oldberg, A. (1989) Structure and biology of cartilage and bone matrix noncollagenous macromolecules. *FASEB J.* **3,** 2042–2051.
45. Reinholt, F. P., Hultenby, K., Oldberg, A., and Heinegard, D. (1990) Osteopontin—a possible anchor of osteoclasts to bone. *Proc. Natl. Acad. Sci. USA* **87,** 4473–4475.
46. McKee, M. D., Farach-Carson, M. C., Butler, W. T., Hauschka, P. V., and Nanci, A. (1993) Ultrastructural immunolocalization of noncollagenous (osteopontin and osteocalcin)and plasma (albumin and a_2HS-glycoprotein) in rat bone. *J. Bone Miner. Res.* **8,** 485–496.
47. Hunter, G. K., Hauschka, P. V., Poole, A. R., Rosenberg, L. C., and Goldberg, H. A. (1996) Nucleation and inhibition of hydroxyapatite formation by mineralized tissue proteins. *Biochem. J.* **317,** 59–64.
48. Boskey, A. L., Spevak, L., Paschalis, E., Doty, S. B., and McKee, M. D. (2002) Osteopontin deficiency increases mineral content and mineral crystallinity in mouse bone. *Calcif. Tissue Int.* **71,** 145–154.
49. Yoshitake, H., Rittling, S. R., Denhardt, D. T., and Noda, M. (1999) Osteopontin-deficient mice are resistant to ovariectomy-induced bone resorption . *Proc. Natl. Acad. Sci. USA* **96,** 8156–8160.
50. Asou, Y., Rittling, S. R., Yoshitake, H., et al. (2001) Osteopontin facilitates angiogenesis, accumulation of osteoclasts, and resorption in ectopic bone. *Endocrinology* **142,** 1325–1332.
51. Ihara, H., Denhardt, D. T., Furuya, K., et al. (2001) Parathyroid hormone-induced bone resorption does not occur in the absence of osteopontin. *J. Biol. Chem.* **276,** 13065–13071.
52. Ishijima, M., Rittling, S. R., Yamashita, T., et al. (2001) Enhancement of osteoclastic bone resorption and suppression of osteoblastic bone formation in response to reduced mechanical stress do not occur in the absence of osteopontin. *J. Exp. Med.* **193,** 399–404.
53. Ishijima, M., Tsuji, K., Rittling, S. R., et al. (2002) Resistance to unloading-induced three-dimensional bone loss in osteopontin-deficient mice. *J. Bone Miner. Res.* **17,** 661–667.
54. Chellaiah, M., Kizer, N., Biswas, R., et al. (2003) Osteopontin deficiency produces osteoclast dysfunction due to reduced CD44 surface expression. *Mol. Biol. Cell.* **14,** 173–189.
55. Väänänen, K. (1996) Osteoclast function: biology and mechanism. In: Bilezikian, J. P., Raisz, L. G., and Rodan, G. A., eds. *Principles of Bone Biology*. Academic Press, San Diego, pp. 103–114.
56. McHugh, K. P., Hodivala-Dilke, K., Zheng, M. H., et al. (2000) Mice lacking beta3 integrins are osteosclerotic because of dysfunctional osteoclasts. *J. Clin. Invest.* **105,** 433–440.

57. Suzuki, K., Zhu, B., Rittling, S. R., et al. (2002) Colocalization of intracellular osteopontin with CD44 is associated with migration, cell fusion, and resorption in osteoclasts. *J. Bone Miner. Res.* **17,** 1486–1497.
58. Zohar, R., Suzuki, N., Suzuki, K., et al. (2000) Intracellular osteopontin is an integral component of the CD44-ERM complex involved in cell migration. *J. Cell Physiol.* **184,** 118–130.
59. Keely, P., Parise, L., and Juliano, R. (1998) Integrins and GTPases in tumour cell growth, motility and invasion. *Trends Cell Biol.* **8,** 101–106.
60. Zhu, B., Suzuki, K., Goldberg, H. A., et al. (2002) Association of intracellular osteopontin with CD44: impaired migration and osteoclast formation in osteopontin- and CD44-null peritoneal macrophages, *submitted.*
61. Weber, G. F. and Cantor, H. (1996) The immunology of Eta-1/osteopontin. *Cytokine Growth Factor Rev.* **7,** 241–248.
62. O'Regan, A. and Berman, J. S. (2000) Osteopontin: a key cytokine in cell-mediated and granulomatous inflammation. *Int. J. Exp. Pathol.* **81,** 373–390.
63. Nau, G. J., Guilfoile, P., Chupp, G. L., et al. (1997) A chemoattractant cytokine associated with granulomas in tuberculosis and silicosis. *Proc. Natl. Acad. Sci. USA* **94,** 6414–6419.
64. Wu, Y., Tewari, M., Cui, S., and Rubin, R. (1996) Activation of the insulin-like growth factor-I receptor inhibits tumor necrosis factor-induced cell death. *J. Cell Physiol.* **168,** 499–509.
65. O'Regan, A. W., Hayden, J. M., Body, S., et al. (2001) Abnormal pulmonary granuloma formation in osteopontin-deficient mice. *Am. J. Respir. Crit. Care Med.* **164,** 2243–2247.
66. Rittling, S. R. and Denhardt, D. T. (1999) Osteopontin (OPN) function in pathology: lessons from OPN-deficient mice. *Exp. Nephrol.* **7,** 103–113.
67. Yu, X. Q., Nikolic-Paterson, D. J., Mu, W., et al. (1998) A functional role for osteopontin in experimental crescentic glomerulonephritis in the rat. *Proc. Assoc. Am. Phys.* **110,** 50–64.
68. Ophascharoensuk, V., Giachelli, C. M., Gordon, K., et al. (1999) Obstructive uropathy in the mouse: role of osteopontin in interstitial fibrosis and apoptosis. *Kidney Int.* **56,** 571–580.
69. Nau, G. J., Liaw, L., Chupp, G. L., Berman, J. S., Hogan, B. L., and Young, R. A. (1999) Attenuated host resistance against *Mycobacterium bovis* BCG infection in mice lacking osteopontin. *Infect. Immun.* **67,** 4223–4230.
70. Wesson, J. A., Johnson, R. J., Mazzali, M., et al. (2003) Osteopontin is a critical inhibitor of calcium oxalate crystal formation and retention in renal tubules. *J. Am. Soc. Nephrol.* **14,** 139–147.
71. Bonvini, J. M., Schatzmann, U., Beck-Schimmer, B., et al. (2000) Lack of in vivo function of osteopontin in experimental anti-GBM nephritis. *J. Am. Soc. Nephrol.* **11,** 1647–1655.
72. Yumoto, K., Ishijima, M., Rittling, S. R., et al. (2002) Osteopontin deficiency protects joints against destruction in anti-type II collagen antibody-induced arthritis in mice. *Proc. Natl. Acad. Sci. USA* **99,** 4556–4561.
73. Giachelli, C. M., Lombardi, D., Johnson, R. J., Murry, C. E., and Almeida, M. (1998) Evidence for a role of osteopontin in macrophage infiltration in response to pathological stimuli *in vivo. Am. J. Pathol.* **152,** 353–358.
74. Nemir, M., Bhattacharyya, D., Li, X., Singh, K., Mukherjee, A. B., and Mukherjee, B. B. (2000) Targeted inhibition of osteopontin expression in the mammary gland causes abnormal morphogenesis and lactation deficiency. *J. Biol. Chem.* **275,** 969–976.
75. Philip, S., Bulbule, A., and Kundu, G. C. (2001) Osteopontin stimulates tumor growth and activation of pro-matrix metalloproteinase-2 through NF-κB mediated induction of membrane type 1-matrix metalloproteinase in murine melanoma cells. *J. Biol. Chem.* **276,** 44926–44935.
76. Bendeck, M. P., Irvin, C., Reidy, M., et al. (2000) Smooth muscle cell matrix metalloproteinase production is stimulated via alpha(v)beta(3) integrin. *Arterioscler. Thromb. Vasc. Biol.* **20,** 1467–1472.
77. Cowan, K. N., Jones, P. L., and Rabinovitch, M. (2000) Elastase and matrix metalloproteinase inhibitors induce regression, and tenascin-C antisense prevents progression, of vascular disease. *J. Clin. Invest.* **105,** 21–34.
78. Khan, S. A., Lopez-Chua, C. A., Zhang, J., Fisher, L. W., Sorensen, E. S., and Denhardt, D. T. (2002) Soluble osteopontin inhibits apoptosis of adherent endothelial cells deprived of growth factors *J. Cell Biochem.* **85,** 728–736.

79. Lin, Y. H., Huang, C. J., Chao, J. R., et al. (2000) Coupling of osteopontin and its cell surface receptor CD44 to the cell survival response elicited by interleukin-3 or granulocyte-macrophage colony-stimulating factor. *Mol. Cell Biol.* **20,** 2734–2742.
80. Weiss, J. M., Renkl, A. C., Maier, C. S., et al. (2001) Osteopontin is involved in the initiation of cutaneous contact hypersensitivity by inducing Langerhans and dendritic cell migration to lymph nodes. *J. Exp. Med.* **194,** 1219–1229.
81. Iizuka, J., Katagiri, Y., Tada, N., et al. (1998) Introduction of an osteopontin gene confers the increase in B1 cell population and the production of anti-DNA autoantibodies. *Lab. Invest.* **78,** 1523–1533.
82. Lampe, M. A., Patarca, R., Iregui, M. V., and Cantor, H. (1991) Polyclonal B-cell activation by the Eta-1 cytokine and the development of autoimmune disease. *J. Immunol.* **147,** 2902–2906.
83. Patarca, R., Wei, F., Singh, P., Morasso, M., and Cantor, H. (1990) Dysregulated expresion of the T cell cytokine ETA-1 in CD4-8- lymphocytes during development of murine autoimmune disease. *J. Exp. Med.* **172,** 1177–1183.
84. Adler, B., Ashkar, S., Cantor, H., and Weber, G. F. (2001) Costimulation by extracellular matrix proteins determines the response to TCR ligation. *Cell Immunol.* **210,** 30–40.
85. Potter, M. R., Rittling, S. R., Denhardt, D. T., et al. (2002) Role of osteopontin in murine Lyme arthritis and host defense against *Borrelia burgdorferi. Infect. Immun.* **70,** 1372–1381.
86. Jansson, M., Panoutsakopoulou, V., Baker, J., Klein, L., and Cantor, H. (2002) Cutting edge: attenuated experimental autoimmune encephalomyelitis in eta-1/osteopontin-deficient mice. *J. Immunol.* **168,** 2096–2099.
87. Rittling, S. R. and Feng, F. (1998) Detection of mouse osteopontin by western blotting. *Biochem. Biophys. Res. Commun.* **250,** 287–292.
88. Shiraga, H., Min, W., VanDusen, W. J., et al. (1992) Inhibition of calcium oxalate crystal growth *in vitro* by uropontin, a new member of the aspartic-acid rich protein superfamily. *Proc. Natl. Acad. Sci. USA* **89,** 426–430.
89. Worcester, E. M., Blumenthal, S. S., Beshensky, A. M., and Lewand, D. L. (1992) The calcium oxalate crystal growth inhibitor protein produced by mouse kidney cortical cells in culture is osteopontin. *J. Bone Miner. Res.* **7,** 1029–1036.
90. McKee, M. D., Nanci, A., and Khan, S. R. (1995) Ultrastructural immunodetection of osteopontin and osteocalcin as major matrix components of renal calculi. *J. Bone Miner. Res.* **10,** 1913–1929.
91. Hudkins, K. L., Giachelli, C. M., Eitner, F., Couser, W. G., Johnson, R. J., and Alpers, C. E. (2000) Osteopontin expression in human crescentic glomerulonephritis. *Kidney Int.* **57,** 105–116.
92. Pichler, R., Giachelli, C. M., Lombardi, D., et al. (1994) Tubulointerstitial disease in glomerulonephritis. Potential role of osteopontin. *Am. J. Pathol.* **144,** 915–926.
93. Mazzali, M., Hughes, J., Dantas, M., et al. (2002) Effects of cyclosporine in osteopontin null mice. *Kidney Int.* **62,** 78–85.
94. Noiri, E., Dickman, K., Miller, F., et al. (1999) Reduced tolerance to acute renal ischemia in mice with a targeted disruption of the osteopontin gene. *Kidney Int.* **56,** 74–82.
95. Hwang, S. M., Lopez, C. A., Heck, D. E., et al. (1994) Osteopontin inhibits induction of nitric oxide synthase gene expression by inflammatory mediators in mouse kidney epithelial cells. *J. Biol. Chem.* **269,** 711–715.
96. Rollo, E. E., Laskin, D. L., and Denhardt, D. T. (1996) Osteopontin inhibits nitric oxide production and cytotoxicity by activated RAW 264.7 macrophages. *J. Leukoc. Biol.* **60,** 397–404.
97. Guo, H., Cai, C. Q., Schroeder, R. A., and Kuo, P. C. (2001) Osteopontin is a negative feedback regulator of nitric oxide synthesis in murine macrophages. *J. Immunol.* **166,** 1079–1086.
98. Wuthrich, R. P., Fan, X., Ritthaler, T., et al. (1998) Enhanced osteopontin expression and macrophage infiltration in MRL-Fas(lpr) mice with lupus nephritis. *Autoimmunity* **28,** 139–150.
99. Giachelli, C. M. (2001) Ectopic calcification: new concepts in cellular regulation. *Z. Kardiol.* **90(Suppl. 3),** 31–37.
100. Boskey, A. L., Maresca, M., Ullrich, W., Doty, S. B., Butler, W. T., and Prince, C. W. (1993) Osteopontin-hydroxyapatite interactions *in vitro*: inhibition of hydroxyapatite formation and growth in a gelatin gel. *Bone Miner.* **22,** 147–159.

101. Wada, T., McKee, M. D., Steitz, S., and Giachelli, C. M. (1999) Calcification of vascular smooth muscle cell cultures: inhibition by osteopontin. *Circ. Res.* **84,** 166–178.
102. Jono, S., Peinado, C., and Giachelli, C. M. (2000) Phosphorylation of osteopontin is required for inhibition of vascular smooth muscle cell calcification. *J. Biol. Chem.* **275,** 20197–20203.
103. Steitz, S. A., Speer, M. Y., McKee, M. D., et al. (2002) Osteopontin inhibits mineral deposition and promotes regression of ectopic calcification. *Am. J. Pathol.* **161,** 2035–2046.
104. Luo, G., Ducy, P., McKee, M. D., et al. (1997) Spontaneous calcification of arteries and cartilage in mice lacking matrix GLA protein. *Nature* **386,** 78–81.
105. Speer, M. Y., McKee, M. D., Guldberg, R. E., et al. (2002) Osteopontin, an inducible inhibitor of vascular calcification in matrix Gla protein-deificent mice. *J. Exp. Med.* **196,** 1047–1055.
106. Singh, K., Balligand, J. L., Fischer, T. A., Smith, T. W., and Kelly, R. A. (1995) Glucocorticoids increase osteopontin expression in cardiac myocytes and microvascular endothelial cells. Role in regulation of inducible nitric oxide synthase. *J. Biol. Chem.* **270,** 28471–28478.
107. Giachelli, C. M., Schwartz, S. M., and Liaw, L. (1995) Molecular and cellular biology of osteopontin. *Trends Cardiovasc. Med.* **5,** 88–95.
108. Trueblood, N. A., Xie, Z., Communal, C., et al. (2001) Exaggerated left ventricular dilation and reduced collagen deposition after myocardial infarction in mice lacking osteopontin. *Circ. Res.* **88,** 1080–1087.
109. Senger, D. R., Perruzzi, C. A., Gracey, C. F., Papadopoulous, A., and Tenen, D. G. (1988) Secreted phospohoproteins associated with neoplastic transformation: close homology with plasma proteins cleaved during blood coagulation. *Cancer Res.* **48,** 5770–5774.
110. Tuck, A. B., O'Malley, F. P., Singhal, H., et al. (1998) Osteopontin expression in a group of lymph node negative breast cancer patients. *Int. J. Cancer* **79,** 502–508.
111. Agrawal, D., Chen, T., Irby, R., et al. (2002) Osteopontin identified as lead marker of colon cancer progression, using pooled sample expression profiling. *J. Natl. Cancer Inst.* **94,** 513–521.
112. Kim, J. H., Skates, S. J., Uede, T., et al. (2002) Osteopontin as a potential diagnostic biomarker for ovarian cancer. *JAMA* **287,** 1671–1679.
113. Bellahcène, A. and Castronovo, V. (1995) Increased expression of osteonectin and osteopontin, two bone matrix proteins, in human breast cancer. *Am. J. Pathol.* **146,** 95–100.
114. Rudland, P. S., Platt-Higgins, A., El Tanani, M., et al. (2002) Prognostic significance of the metastasis-associated protein osteopontin in human breast cancer. *Cancer Res.* **62,** 3417–3427.
115. Oates, A. J., Barraclough, R., and Rudland, P. S. (1997) The role of osteopontin in tumorigenesis and metastasis. *Invasion Metastasis* **17,** 1–15.
116. Morris, V. L., Tuck, A. B., Wilson, S. M., Percy, D., and Chambers, A. F. (1993) Tumor progression and metastasis in murine D2 hyperplastic alveolar nodule mammary tumor cell lines. *Clin. Exp. Metastasis* **11,** 103–112.
117. Su, L., Mukherjee, A. B., and Mukherjee, B. B. (1995) Expression of antisense osteopontin mRNA inhibits tumor promoter-induced neoplastic transformation of mouse JB6 epidermal cells. *Oncogene* **10,** 2163–2169.
118. Gardner, H. A. R., Berse, B., and Senger, D. R. (1994) Specific reduction in osteopontin synthesis by antisense RNA inhibits the tumorigenicity of transformed Rat1 fibroblasts. *Oncogene* **9,** 2321–2326.
119. Behrend, E. I., Craig, A. M., Wilson, S. M., Denhardt, D. T., and Chambers, A. F. (1994) Reduced malignancy of ras-transformed NIH 3T3 cells expressing antisense osteopontin RNA. *Cancer Res.* **54,** 832–837.
120. Wu, Y. M., Denhardt, D. T., and Rittling, S. R. (2000) Osteopontin is required for full expression of the transformed phenotype by the ras oncogene. *Br. J. Cancer* **83,** 156–163.
121. Crawford, H. C., Matrisian, L. M., and Liaw, L. (1998) Distinct roles of osteopontin in host defense activity and tumor survival during squamous cell carcinoma progression in vivo. *Cancer Res.* **58,** 5206–5215.
122. Nemoto, H., Rittling, S. R., Yoshitake, H., et al. (2001) Osteopontin deficiency reduces experimental tumor cell metastasis to bone and soft tissues. *J. Bone Miner. Res.* **16,** 652–659.

23

RANKL, RANK, and OPG

Young-Yun Kong and Josef M. Penninger

Summary

Tumor necrosis factor (TNF) and TNF receptor (R) family proteins play important roles in the control of cell death, proliferation, autoimmunity, the function of immune cells, or the organogenesis of lymphoid organs. Recently, novel members of this large family have been identified that couple immunity with other organ systems such as bone morphogenesis and mammary gland formation in pregnancy. The TNF-family molecule receptor activator of nuclear factor κB ligand (RANKL) [osteoprotegerin (OPGL), TNF-related activation-induced cytokine (TRANCE) osteoclast differentiation factor (ODF)], its receptor RANK, and the decoy receptor osteoprotegerin (OPG) are essential for the development and activation of osteoclasts and are key regulators of bone remodeling. Intriguingly, RANKL/RANK interactions also regulate T-cell/dendritic cell communications, dendritic cell survival, and lymph node formation. T-cell-derived RANKL can mediate bone loss in arthritis and periodontal disease. Moreover, RANKL and RANK are expressed in mammary gland epithelial cells, where they control the development of a lactating mammary gland during pregnancy required for the propagation of mammalian species. RANKL can also induce angiogenesis, and inflammatory cytokines can trigger the expression of RANKL, RANK, and OPG in vascular endothelial cells. Modulation of these systems provides us with a unique opportunity to design novel therapeutics to inhibit bone loss in osteoporosis, arthritis, periodontal disease, and cancer metastasis.

1. RANKL: Identification of the Critical Osteoclast Differentiation Factor

The receptor activator of nuclear factor κB ligand (RANKL)/tumor necrosis factor-related activation-induced cytokine (TRANCE)/osteoclast differentiation factor (ODF) was cloned simultaneously by four independent groups *(1–4)*. The *rankl* gene encodes a tumor necrosis factor (TNF) superfamily molecule of 316 amino acids (38 kDa), and three RANKL subunits assemble to form the functional trimeric molecule. Trimeric RANKL is initially made as a membrane-anchored molecule and can be subsequently released from the cell surface as soluble homotrimeric molecules following proteolytic cleavage by the metalloprotease-disintegrin TNF-α convertase (TACE) *(5)*. It remains to be seen whether TACE is indeed the critical protease required for the release of RANKL from the cell surface. Although slight functional differences may exist, both soluble and membrane-bound RANKL can function as potent agonistic ligands for osteoclastogenesis in vitro *(2,5,6)*. However, other studies have suggested that membrane-bound RANKL may work more efficiently than soluble RANKL *(7)*. The crystal structure of RANKL revealed that it associates as a homotrimer with four unique surface loops that distinguish it from other TNF cytokines. Mutagenesis of selected residues in these loops modulates RANK activation, suggesting that structural

From: *Contemporary Immunology: Cytokine Knockouts, 2nd Edition*
Edited by: Giamila Fantuzzi © Humana Press Inc., Totowa, NJ

Table 1
Molecules that Regulate RANKL and OPG Levels

	RANKL	OPG
Hormones		
Vitamin D_3	Increased	Increased
PTH	Increased	Decreased
PTHrP	Increased	Decreased
Estradiol	No change	Increased
Cytokines		
TNF-α	Increased	Increased
IL-1	Increased	Increased
IL-6	Increased	n.t.
IL-11	Increased	n.t.
IL-17	Increased	n.t.
Growth factors		
TGF-β	Decreased	Increased
BMP-2	n.t.	Increased
Others		
Prostaglandin E_2	Increased	Decreased
Glucocorticoid	Increased	Decreased
CD40L	Increased	n.t.

BMP-2, bone morphogenetic protein-2; n.t., not tested; PTH, parathyroid hormone; PTHrP, PTH-related peptide; TGF-β, transforming growth factor-β; TNF-α, tumor necrosis factor-α.

determinants of RANKL-RANK interactions can be selectively targeted to block RANKL/RANK function *(8,9)*.

RANKL is strongly expressed in osteoblast/stromal cells, primitive mesenchymal cells surrounding the cartilaginous anlagen, and hypertrophied chondrocytes. RANKL mRNA has also been observed in prehypotrophic and hypertrophic chondrocytes at d 15 of embryogenesis and in extraskeletal tissues such as the brain, heart, kidneys, skeletal muscle, and skin throughout mouse development *(10)*. RANKL expression can be upregulated by bone-resorbing factors such as glucocorticoids, vitamin D_3, interleukin-1 (IL-1), IL-6, IL-11, IL-17, TNF-α, prostaglandin E_2 (PGE_2), parathyroid hormone (PTH), and others (Table 1) *(4)*. Using in vitro culture systems, it has been shown that RANKL can both activate mature osteoclasts and mediate osteoclastogenesis in the presence of colony-stimulating factor-1 (CSF-1) *(4)*. *rankl*$^{-/-}$ mice display severe osteopetrosis, stunted growth, and a defect in tooth eruption owing to a complete absence of osteoclasts. Importantly, osteoblast cell lines derived from *rankl*$^{-/-}$ mice do not support osteoclast formation, indicating that the defect in osteoclastogenesis observed in *rankl*$^{-/-}$ mice is owing to an intrinsic defect in osteoblastic stroma. However, these mice contain hematopoietic precursors that can differentiate into phenotypically and functionally mature osteoclasts in vitro in the presence of recombinant RANKL and CSF-1.

Whereas *csf-1* mutant *op/op* mice display a developmental arrest in both monocyte/macrophage and osteoclast lineages, *rankl*$^{-/-}$ mice display normal monocyte/macrophage dif-

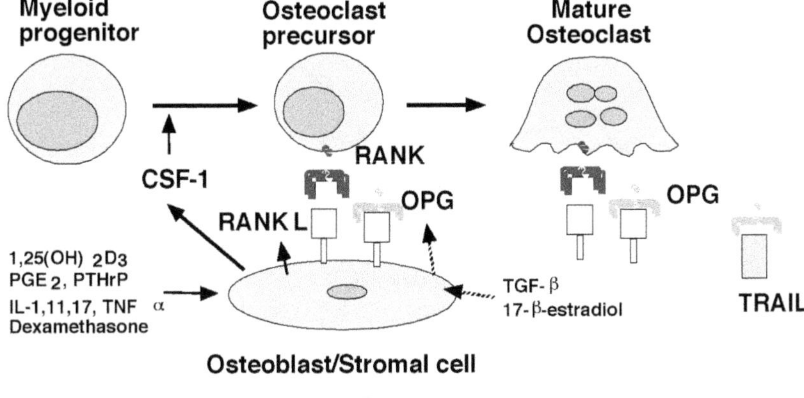

Figure 1

ferentiation and normal differentiation of dendritic cells (DCs). The osteoclast defect in *csf-1* mutant *op/op* mice is not absolute, and older *op/op* mice do have, albeit only a few, osteoclasts. Moreover, the defect in *op/op* mice can be reversed by transgenic overexpression of Bcl-2 in the osteoclast/monocyte lineage, indicating that CSF-1 expression is not essential for osteoclast development *(11)*. Thus, RANKL is a specific and essential differentiation factor for osteoclast precursors and an activation factor for mature osteoclasts (Fig. 1).

2. RANK: Identification of the Receptor for RANKL

The receptor for RANKL is RANK (receptor activator of NF-κB; also known as TRANCE-R, or TNFRSF11A), a member of the TNF receptor superfamily. RANK is expressed as a transmembrane heterotrimer on the surface of hematopoietic osteoclast progenitors, mature osteoclasts, chondrocytes, and mammary gland epithelial cells *(1,12)*. In vitro ligation of RANK with RANKL results in osteoclastogenesis from progenitor cells and the activation of mature osteoclasts *(12–14)*. Mice with a genetic mutation of RANK are phenocopies of *rankl*$^{-/-}$ mice and have a complete block in osteoclast development that can be restored by reintroduction of RANK into bone marrow progenitor cells *(15,16)*. The osteopetrosis observed in these mice can be reversed by transplantation of bone marrow cells from *rag1*$^{-/-}$ mice, indicating that *rank*$^{-/-}$ mice have an intrinsic defect in the differentiation of hematopoietic osteoclast progenitor cells *(16)*. Thus, the interaction between RANKL expressed by stromal cells/osteoblasts and its receptor RANK expressed on osteoclast precursors is essential for osteoclastogenesis (Fig. 1).

In human familial expansile osteolysis, a rare autosomal dominant bone disorder characterized by focal areas of increased bone remodeling *(17)*, a heterozygous insertion mutation in exon 1 of RANK has been noted that appears to increase RANK-mediated NF-κB activation and thus might be causal for the disease. These genetic results in humans and mutant mice established the absolute dependency of osteoclast differentiation and activation of mature osteoclasts on the expression of RANKL and RANK.

2.1. RANK Signaling

When RANK on osteoclasts is activated, it sends signals into the cells through adapter proteins (Fig. 2). RANK contains 383 amino acids in its intracellular domain (residues 234–

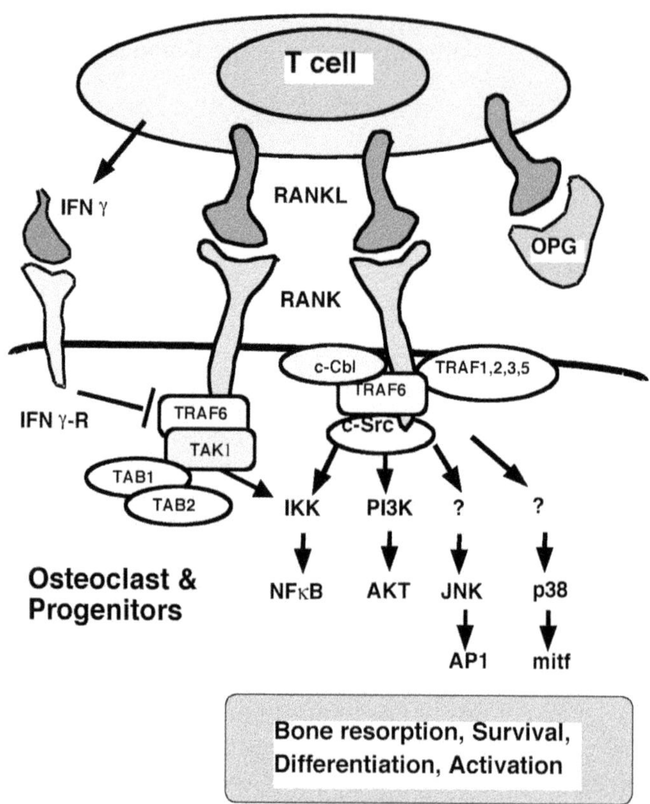

Figure 2

616), which contains three putative binding domains (termed I, II, and III) for TNF receptor-associated factors (TRAFs) *(18)*. RANK interacts with TRAFs 1, 2, 3, 5, and 6 both in vitro and in cells *(19)*. Mapping of the structural requirements for TRAF/RANK interaction revealed multiple TRAF binding sites clustered in two distinct domains in the RANK cytoplasmic tail. These TRAF binding domains were shown to be functionally important for the RANK-dependent induction of NF-κB and c-Jun NH_2-terminal kinase (JNK) activities. In particular, TRAF-6 interacts with membrane-proximal determinants distinct from those binding TRAFs 1, 2, 3, and 5. When this membrane-proximal TRAF-6 interaction domain was deleted, RANK-mediated NF-κB signaling was completely inhibited, whereas JNK activation was only partially inhibited *(18–21)*, suggesting that interaction with TRAF-6 is necessary for NF-κB activation but not essential for activation of the JNK pathway. Indeed, mice lacking TRAF-6 have bone phenotypes similar to that of *rankl*$^{-/-}$ and *rank*$^{-/-}$ mice owing to a partial block in osteoclastogenesis and defective activation of mature osteoclasts *(22–24)*. It should be noted that TRAF-6 mutant mice still have detectable numbers of TRAP+ osteoclasts *(23)*, whereas NF-κB1/NF-κB2 double mutant mice lack all TRAP+ osteoclasts *(25,26)*. Thus, TRAF-6 is a critical factor involved in the activation of mature osteoclasts, but other TRAFs (and possibly other molecules) appear to be able to partially substitute for the loss of TRAF-6 during osteoclast development. In line with these data, osteoclastogenesis can be initiated in *rank*$^{-/-}$ mice by transfer of mutant RANK that lacks the TRAF-6 binding site *(16)*.

RANKL activates the TAK-1 MEKK kinase through TRAF-6 and TAB-2. Dominant negative forms of TAK-1 and TAB-2 inhibit NF-κB activation induced by RANKL, and TAK-1 is activated in response to RANKL stimulation, suggesting that the formation of the TRAF-6/TAB-2-/TAK-1 complex is involved in the RANK signaling pathway leading to NF-κB activation *(27)*. Interestingly, I-κB kinase (IKK) activation by TRAF-6 requires two intermediary factors, TRAF-6-regulated IKK activator-1 (TRIKA-1) and TRIKA-2 *(28)*. TRIKA is a dimeric ubiquitin-conjugating enzyme complex that catalyzes the formation of a lysine-linked polyubiquitin chain that mediates IKK activation. TRIKA is composed of TAK-1, TAB-1, and TAB-2, and the TAK-1 kinase complex activates IKK in a manner that depends on TRAF-6 and Ubc-Uev1A *(29)*. This kinase complex can also phosphorylate MKK-6, which acts upstream of the p38 mitogen-activated protein (MAP) kinase pathway *(29)*. In response to RANKL stimulation, p38 MAP kinase phosphorylates the microphthalmia transcription factor (Mitf), which regulates osteoclast target genes like TRAP, cathepsin K, and E-cadherin by binding to a 7-bp conserved sequence TCANGTA found in the promoter regions of these genes. Mitf (*mi*) mutant osteoclast precursors cannot fuse to form multinuclear cells, lack a ruffled border, express low levels of TRAP and cathepsin K, and cannot efficiently resorb bone *(30)*. Moreover, RANKL induces transcription of Fosl1 in a c-fos-dependent manner, establishing a link between RANK signaling and the expression of activation protein-1 (AP-1) proteins in osteoclast differentiation *(31)*.

RANKL also activates the antiapoptotic serine/threonine kinase Akt/PKB through a signaling complex involving c-Src and TRAF-6 *(32)*. c-Src and TRAF-6 interact with each other and with RANK following receptor engagement, and a deficiency in c-Src or the addition of Src family kinase inhibitors blocks RANKL-mediated Akt/PKB activation in osteoclasts. TRAF-6, in turn, enhances the kinase activity of c-Src leading to tyrosine phosphorylation of downstream signaling molecules such as c-Cbl *(32)*. Moreover, RANK can recruit TRAF-6, Cbl family scaffolding proteins, and the phospholipid kinase PI3K in a ligand- and Src-dependent manner. RANKL-mediated Akt/PKB activation is defective in *cbl-b*$^{-/-}$ DCs *(33)*. These findings implicate Cbl family proteins not only as negative regulators of signaling, but also as positive modulators of TNFR superfamily signaling. Moreover, these data provided the evidence of crosstalk between TRAF proteins and Src family kinases. In addition, it should be noted that inhibition of p38 kinases using SB203580 and overexpression of dominant negative p38α or MKK-6 inhibit RANKL-induced differentiation of the osteoclast-like cell line RAW264 *(34)*. The in vivo role of JNKs in osteoclast development and function needs to be established.

3. Osteoprotegerin: Protector of the Bone

Osteoprotegerin [OPG, "protector of the bone"; also known as osteoclastogenesis inhibitory factor (OCIF)] is a secreted protein with homology to members of the TNF receptor family *(2,4,35,36)*. The *opg* gene encodes a 44-kDa protein that is posttranslationally modified to a 55-kDa molecule through N-linked glycosylation. Although OPG is a member of the TNFR family, whose members normally assemble as molecular trimers, OPG is secreted as a 110-kDa homodimer. OPG functions as a soluble decoy receptor to RANKL and competes with RANK for RANKL binding. Consequently, OPG is an effective inhibitor of osteoclast maturation and activation in vitro and in vivo (Fig. 1) *(2,35)*. High systemic levels of OPG in OPG transgenic mice cause osteopetrosis with normal tooth eruption and bone elongation, and these levels also inhibit the development and activity of endosteal, but not periosteal, osteoclasts *(35)*. OPG-deficient mice display severe osteoporosis associated with a high incidence of fractures *(37,38)*. Thus, the level of bone mass correlates with the levels of OPG in mice.

Expression of OPG in the ST2 stromal cell line and in human bone marrow stromal cells is downregulated by bone-resorbing factors such as vitamin D_3 [1,25$(OH)_2D_3$), prostaglandin E_2 (PGE_2), or glucocorticoids and is upregulated by Ca^{2+} ions and transforming growth factor-β (TGF-β) *(36,39,40)*. OPG is also expressed in follicular DCs (identified as FDCR-1) and is upregulated following CD40 ligation in these DCs *(41)*. In addition to osteoporosis, some but not all OPG mutant mice develop calcification of their large arteries *(37)*, and RANKL and RANK transcripts are detected in the calcified arteries of $OPG^{-/-}$ mice *(42)*. Transgenic OPG delivered from midgestation through adulthood does prevent the formation of arterial calcification in *opg*$^{-/-}$ mice by blocking a process resembling osteoclastogenesis *(42)*. These data indicate that the OPG/RANKL/RANK pathway may play an important role in both pathologic and physiologic calcification processes. Such findings may also explain the observed high clinical incidence of vascular calcification in the osteoporotic patient population *(43)*. Since women with osteoporosis have an increased incidence of strokes *(44,45)*, OPG, RANKL, and RANK may play, similar to the CD40 and CD40L system *(46)*, a role in the pathogenesis of atherosclerosis, strokes, or heart attacks via a yet unknown regulation of endothelial cells.

4. The Role of RANKL, RANK, and OPG in Bone Remodeling

All genetic and functional experiments by many different groups indicate that the balance between RANKL-RANK signaling and the levels of biologically active OPG regulate development and activation of osteoclasts and bone metabolism (Figs. 1 and 2). Intriguingly, all factors that inhibit or enhance bone resorption via osteoclasts act via regulation of RANKL-RANK and/or OPG. Thus, it appears that the complex system of osteoclast-regulated bone remodeling is critically controlled by these three molecules. However, although RANKL is also expressed in many other tissues than the bone and osteoclast development is restricted to the bone microenvironment, another factor may exist that acts in concert with RANKL/RANK to confer tissue specificity. It has recently been shown in vitro that TNF-α and IL-1 can apparently induce the development of TRAP+ osteoclasts in the absence of RANK/RANKL. However, in our own genetic experiments using RANK-deficient osteoclast progenitors, TNF-α as well as interleukin-1 (IL-1)-dependent osteoclastogenesis are strictly dependent on RANK expression. Thus, whereas TNF-α and IL-1 appear to potentiate the development of osteoclasts *(47)*, presumably via activation of common second messenger systems such as NF-κB activation, both of these molecules rely on the expression of RANKL/RANK. It should also be noted that mutations of TNF-α, TNFRI, or TNFRII do not cause any alterations in bone metabolism or osteoclast development/activation in vivo. Intriguingly, TNF-α-TNFRp55 might play a physiologic role in old-age osteoporosis acting upstream of RANKL since ovarectomy-induced bone loss appears to depend on T-cell-derived TNF-α production *(48,49)*.

In addition to the association between RANKL and OPG, OPG can also bind to the TNF-family molecule TNF-related apoptosis-inducing ligand (TRAIL) at low stoichiometry (approx. 10,000 times less binding to TRAIL than to RANKL) *(50)*. OPG-Fc binds TRAIL with an affinity of 3.0 n*M*, which is slightly weaker than the interaction of TRID-Fc or DR5-Fc with TRAIL. Functionally, high doses of OPG inhibit TRAIL-induced apoptosis of

Jurkat cells, and TRAIL can block the antiosteoclastogenic activity of OPG *(50)*. These data suggest potential crossregulatory mechanisms by OPG and TRAIL. However, it is still not known whether OPG-TRAIL interactions have any functional relevance in vivo. Importantly, OPG expression is induced by estrogen in cell lines and in vivo *(51,52)*, which might explain postmenopausal osteoporosis in women, that is, reduced ovarian function leads to reduced estrogen levels and hence reduced OPG levels, which release RANKL from the inhibition by the decoy receptor. Injection of OPG into ovariectomized female rats blocks bone loss and osteoporosis normally associated with the loss of ovarian function *(35)*. Thus, OPG and/or modulation of RANKL-RANK function via small molecules are promising avenues to prevent postmenopausal osteoporosis. In essence, OPG appears to function in bone loss similar to insulin in diabetes: injection of OPG prevents osteoclast activation and osteopenia in essentially every model system of osteoclast-mediated bone loss.

5. The Role of RANKL and OPG in Cancer-Induced Bone Destruction

It has long been recognized that many epithelial cancers such as breast, prostate, or colon cancers have the ability to invade and grow as metastases in bone *(53)*. Most of them form osteolytic lesions, and most studies indicate that cancer-induced bone destruction is mediated by the osteoclast. A recent study demonstrated that breast and colon cancers regulate RANKL expression of stromal osteoblasts, which leads to osteoclast activation, and that OPG inhibits this activation *(54)*. Furthermore, massive bone destruction is a prominent feature of multiple myeloma and adult T-cell leukemias. Multiple myeloma is a B-cell neoplasm characterized by clonal expansion of plasma cells, and it either induces RANKL expression on stromal osteoblasts or myeloma B-cells express RANKL on the surface that leads directly to osteoclast activation *(55,56)*. In a murine model of human myeloma, both OPG and RANK-Fc administration prevents myeloma-induced bone destruction and inhibits myeloma progression *(57)*, suggesting that the RANKL/RANK/OPG system may play a critical role in development of osteolytic bone diseases and that targeting this system may have therapeutic potential.

The most common symptom of bone cancer is pain. This pain is constant, increases with time, and occurs in patients with primary bone cancer and in patients with cancer that has metastasized to bone from distinct sites such as the breast, colon, and lung *(58)*. Bone cancer pain is commonly associated with cancer-induced bone destruction owing to osteoclast activation. In a murine model of bone cancer, cancer-induced osteoclastogenesis and bone destruction were prevented by treatment of OPG. In addition, treatment of OPG substantially diminished pain-related behaviors and prevented the neurochemical reorganization of the spinal cord seen in mice with bone cancer pain *(59)*, indicating that excessive cancer-induced bone destruction is involved in the generation of bone cancer pain. Thus, OPG may provide an effective treatment for cancer-induced bone destruction and pain in humans.

6. RANKL and RANK in the Immune System

RANKL (TRANCE) was independently cloned by two groups as a molecule expressed on the surface of activated T-cells *(1,3,60)*. Both soluble and membrane-bound RANKL is produced by activated CD4+ and CD8+ T-cells *(6,60)*. RANKL is also expressed in lymph nodes, spleen, thymus, intestinal lymphoid patches *(2)*, and immature CD4–/CD8– thymocytes *(1)*. RANKL expression in T-cells is induced by antigen receptor engagement and is regulated by calcineurin, extracellular signal-regulated kinase (ERK)-1/ERK-2, and protein kinase C (PKC)-regulated signaling pathways *(6,60)*. RANK is expressed on the surface of DCs, mature T-cells, and hematopoietic precursors; RANKL-RANK interactions can induce cluster formation, Bcl-XL expression, survival, CD40 expression, and IL-12 production in DCs *(1,60,61)*. In addition, OPG was found in a screen to identify novel genes expressed in follicular DCs. OPG can be found on the cell surface of DCs, probably by capturing soluble OPG at the cell membrane via binding of a hyalurinic acid binding region present in OPG *(41)*. Thus, like the interactions between CD40-L and CD40, or CD28 and CD80/CD86, the binding of RANKL to RANK can regulate DC functions, T-cell activation, and T-cell-DC communication in vitro *(1,3)*. Moreover, OPG may modulate this interaction.

7. Lymph Node Organogenesis

During the initial analyses of *rankl*$^{-/-}$ and later of *rank* mutant mice, a completely unexpected phenotype became evident: *rankl*$^{-/-}$ and *rank*$^{-/-}$ mice displayed complete absence of all lymph nodes *(15,16,62)*. Recent studies of mice deficient for lymphotoxin-α (LT-α) *(63,64)*, LT-β *(65,66)*, TNFR1 (TNFRp55) *(67)*, LT-β receptor (LT-βR) *(68,69)*, or Id2 *(70)* have revealed important roles for each of these molecules in the development and organization of secondary lymphoid tissues. For example, TNF-α activation of the TNFR1 is required for the formation of splenic B-lymphocyte follicles, follicular dendritic networks, and germinal center formation *(67,71)*. Mice with disrupted LT-α, LT-β, or LT-βR genes lack lymph nodes, Peyer's patches, and follicular DCs; such mice also show altered splenic architecture *(64–66,68)*. Thus, it was assumed that lymph node organogenesis and the development of Peyer's patches are always genetically linked. Surprisingly, *rankl*$^{-/-}$ and *rank*$^{-/-}$ mice lack all lymph nodes but display intact splenic architecture and develop Peyer's patches normally, suggesting that RANKL and RANK have a specific and essential role in lymph node organogenesis. Importantly, RANKL disruption provided the first evidence that development of lymph nodes and Peyer's patches can be genetically uncoupled.

The concerted activity of several cell lineages including fibroblasts, macrophages, reticular cells, and endothelial cells is required for the morphogenesis of primordial lymph nodes *(72)*. These primordial lymph nodes are subsequently seeded by T- and B-cells and CD4+/CD3–/LTβ+ cells that differentiate into natural killer (NK) cells, antigen-presenting cells, and follicular cells to form mature compact nodes *(73)*. *In situ* hybridization of normal lymph nodes has shown that RANKL- and RANK-expressing cells are present in lymph nodes, located mainly in the cortical areas adjacent to subcapsular sinuses *(35)*. The identity of these cells has yet to be determined. Since RANK and RANKL are also expressed in the spleen and Peyer's patches, restricted RANKL-RANK expression cannot account for the selective lack of lymph nodes. Moreover, because defective homing of *rankl*$^{-/-}$ lymphocytes was excluded as the cause of defective lymph node formation and normal bone marrow cells cannot rescue the lymph node defect in *rankl*$^{-/-}$ mice in chimeric transfer experiments, we speculated that RANKL may act as a growth and/or survival factor on a lymph node-organizing cell during embryonic development *(62)*.

Recently it has been shown that the defective lymph node development in *rankl*$^{-/-}$ mice correlates with a significant reduction in LT-αβ+/α4β7+/CD45+/CD4+/CD3– cells and their failure to form clusters in rudimentary mesenteric lymph node oncogene *(74)*. Transgenic RANKL-mediated restoration of lymph node development required LT-αβ expression on CD45+/CD4+/CD3– cells as lymph node formation could not be induced in *LT-α*$^{-/-}$ mice.

The authors proposed that both RANKL and LT-αβ regulate the colonization and cluster formation by CD45+/CD4+/CD3− cells during lymph node organogenesis *(74)*.

Similar to *rankl*$^{-/-}$ and *rank*$^{-/-}$ mice, TNFR1$^{-/-}$ mice exhibit retained but small Peyer's patches *(67,71)*, which suggests that both TNFR1 and RANKL may have a potential, albeit not essential, role in the formation of Peyer's patches. We have recently generated *rankl-tnfr1* double knockout mice, and these mice completely lack Peyer's patches in the small intestine without further affecting the defects in splenic architecture observed in *tnfr1* single mutant mice (Y. Kong and J. M. Penninger, unpublished data). Thus, RANKL is essential for lymph node formation and cooperates with the TNFR1 in the formation of Peyer's patches. The exact cellular and molecular mechanisms of RANKL-RANK-regulated lymph node morphogenesis and the linkage between lymph node and Peyer's patch formation need to be tested.

8. RANKL/RANK and Dendritic Cells

Similar to the CD40L/CD40 system, interactions between RANKL expressed on activated T-cells and RANK expressed on DCs can mediate DC survival via Bcl-XL induction and upregulation of the costimulatory molecule CD40 on DCs *(1,3,61)*. Recently it has also been shown that RANKL activates the antiapoptotic serine/threonine kinase Akt/protein kinase B (PKB) through a signaling complex involving TRAF-6 and c-Src on mature DCs and osteoclasts *(32)*. In addition to Akt/PKB activation, NF-κB and ERK are activated by RANKL. Because NK-κB, ERK, and Akt/PKB promote cell survival by inhibiting apoptosis-inducing pathways, activation of these antiapoptotic molecules seems to be at least partially responsible for the RANKL-mediated DC survival. In addition to these in vitro studies, it has been shown that treatment of antigen-pulsed mature DCs with soluble RANKL in vitro enhances the number and persistence of antigen-presenting DCs in the draining lymph nodes in vivo *(61)*. Furthermore, RANKL treatment increased antigen-specific primary T-cell responses. Interestingly, significant memory responses were observed only in mice injected with RANKL-treated DCs *(61)*. The increase in primary and memory T-cell responses following vaccination with RANKL-treated DCs could be caused by enhanced/altered cytokine production such as expression of IL-12 and/or an increased number of antigen-pulsed DCs.

Both CD40L and RANKL have functional similarity, are expressed on activated T-cells, and enhance the activation and survival of DCs *(1,3)*. However, in contrast to CD40L/CD40, RANKL/RANK signaling does not alter the expression of cell surface molecules such as MHC class II, CD80, CD86, and CD54. Whereas CD40L is primarily expressed on activated CD4+ T-cells, RANKL is expressed on activated CD4+ and CD8+ T-cells *(6,75)*. Moreover, the maximal level of RANKL following the initial T-cell activation event occurs at 48 h, and high levels of RANKL expression are sustained until 96 h, whereas CD40L is rapidly expressed and downregulated *(76)*. Thus, CD40L-CD40 interactions may primarily control the initial priming stage, whereas RANKL-RANK may act at later times than does CD40L during the immune response. For example, CD40L is essential for the T-cell-dependent B-cell responses such as germinal center formation, affinity maturation, and class switching *(77,78)*. By contrast, in *rankl*$^{-/-}$ mice, germinal center formation, Ig class switching, and the production of neutralizing antiviral antibodies are not overtly affected, and all the B-cell defects could be explained by the absence of lymph nodes (Y.-Y. Kong and J. M. Penninger, unpublished data).

Inhibition of RANKL in vivo using a soluble RANK-Fc molecule does not block the priming of LCMV-specific T-cells, but it does impair proliferation of CD4+ T-cells to an LCMV-antigen at later time points after infection *(79)*. This impaired CD4+ T-cell response in RANK-Fc-treated mice was especially apparent in the absence of CD40 expression. Thus, at later stages of the immune response, RANKL can regulate CD40L-independent activation of CD4+ T-helper cells *(79)*. These observations suggest that although CD40L and RANKL have functional similarity and may cooperate, RANKL and CD40-L may also have fundamentally different functions in the control of immune responses: CD40L regulates T/B responses, and RANKL appears to have a role in memory T-cell responses.

Only activated T-cells, but not resting T-cells, express RANKL, which promotes DC survival *(3)*. DCs reside in tissues as immature cells and are specialized to capture and process antigens that lead to maturation of DCs in response to inflammatory stimuli. Mature DCs that have captured antigens migrate to T-cell zones of secondary lymphoid organs by afferent lymphatics in order to present antigen to antigen-specific T-cells. The T-cell areas of secondary lymphoid organs represent the microenvironment that allows interactions among DCs, T-cells, and B-cells to initiate adaptive immune responses (reviewed in ref. *80*). Antigen-bearing DCs are in direct contact with naive antigen-specific T-cells within the T-cell areas of lymph nodes, and after interaction with T-cells these DCs are eliminated rapidly *(81)*. Activated T-cells induce apoptosis of DCs by producing the TNF-family molecules TRAIL, FasL, and TNF-α. Accumulation and prolonged survival of DCs were reported in patients with human autoimmune lymphoproliferative syndrome type II. These patients have a caspase-10 mutation that rendered DCs resistant to TRAIL-induced cell death *(82)*. Thus, it appears that mature DCs have short life spans and that mature DCs presenting antigens to T-cells must be effectively eliminated to avoid excessive immune responses. The life span of DCs may be an important checkpoint to control for the induction of tolerance, priming, and chronic inflammation *(83)*.

Since both TRAIL and RANKL are produced by activated T-cells, the balance between RANKL and TRAIL may also influence DC survival *(84–86)*. Both RANKL and TRAIL can bind to OPG *(50)*, and OPG is made by DCs *(41)*, which suggests that these factors might control the fate of DCs. Based on these studies, various groups are currently trying to control the DC fate via RANKL-RANK and OPG to modulate in vivo DC survival and to enhance the efficiency of DC-based vaccinations for antitumor therapy or the treatment of autoimmune diseases. In the final analyses of all the published genetic and functional studies on RANKL, RANK, and OPG, it appears that although these molecules can influence some aspects of lymphocyte and DC functions, none of these molecules plays an essential function in T-cells, B-cells, or DCs that cannot be compensated for by other molecules such as CD40L/CD40.

Thus, the essential and true functions of RANKL/RANK in the immune system and communication between DCs and T-cells need to be elucidated. Intriguingly, a recent study suggested that TRANCE-RANK interactions may be important for the development of regulatory T-cells in mice *(87)*, suggesting that TRANCE-RANK signals constitute a third pathway (along with CD28-B7 and CD154-CD40) that is critical for the generation of regulatory CD4+/CD25+ T-cell responses. CD4+/CD25+ Treg cells prevent β-cell destruction following localized inflammation in the islets of Langerhans. These Treg cells accumulate preferentially in the pancreatic lymph nodes (PLNs) and islets but not other lymph nodes or spleen. PLN-derived Treg cells are needed to prevent diabetes development, and their capacity to regulate appears to depend on RANKL-RANK signaling. Indeed, blockade of this pathway results in decreased frequency of CD4+/CD25+ Treg cells in the PLN, resulting in intraislet differentiation of CD8+ T-cells into cytotoxic lymphocytes (CTLs) and rapid progression to diabetes. Moreover, since expression of these molecules can be controlled by sex hormones *(51,88)*, we speculate that this system may control gender-specific differences in immunity and could be involved in the higher incidence of autoimmune diseases like arthritis in women.

9. Lymphocyte Differentiation

Two principal genetic checkpoints regulate thymocyte differentiation. The first checkpoint, at the CD44–/CD25+ stage of development, depends on the expression of the pre-T-cell receptor (TCR) on CD4–/CD8– thymocyte precursors, which regulates expansion of these precursor cells. The second checkpoint regulates progression from CD4+/CD8+ immature to mature CD4+ or CD8+ thymocytes and correlates with positive thymocyte selection. Various mutations that arrest thymocyte development at the stage of pre-TCR expression have been reported *(89)*. All these mutations either affect the pre-TCR complex directly or affect signaling molecules thought to be downstream of the pre-TCR. RANKL expression has been detected on CD4–CD8– early thymocyte precursors *(1)*. RANKL-deficient mice showed the block in the progression of CD4–/CD8–/CD44–/CD25+ precursors to CD4–/CD8–/CD44–/CD25– thymocytes. This developmental defect does not reside in the thymic environment but is intrinsic to bone marrow-derived cells *(62)*. These data suggested that the TNF-family cytokine RANKL is important for the progression of CD25+/CD44– precursors to CD25–/CD44– thymocytes at the stage of pre-TCR expression.

However, thymuses of newborn *rankl*$^{-/-}$ mice and differentiation of *rankl*$^{-/-}$ thymocytes in fetal thymic organ cultures appear normal, and the defects of thymocyte development in *rankl*$^{-/-}$ mice are only apparent at around 2 wk of age, a phenotype reminiscent of thymic defects in mice lacking the proapoptotic bcl-2 family molecule bim *(90)*. Age-dependent interactions between RANKL-expressing thymocyte precursors and as yet unknown thymic stromal cells expressing RANK could contribute to early thymocyte development and thymocyte expansion, whereas later stages appear to be RANKL independent. However, although RANK mRNA can be found in the thymus using *in situ* hybridization *(62)*, *rank*$^{-/-}$ mice do not display any obvious defects in thymocyte maturation *(15,16)*. This difference in thymocyte differentiation is the only discernable distinction between *rankl* and *rank* mutant mice, and it suggests that RANKL might act on another, as yet unidentified, receptor during early thymocyte development. Additional work in the future should provide evidence of whether RANKL and RANK indeed play a role in thymocyte development in a cell-autonomous fashion. For example, since RANKL and OPG expression can be controlled by sex hormones, it would be interesting to test whether the thymocyte differentiation defects observed in *rankl*$^{-/-}$, but not *rank*$^{-/-}$ mice, are dependent on sex hormone levels, a scenario that could explain age-related differences. For instance, estrogen deficiency results in enhanced expression of Smoothened of the Hedgehog signaling in the thymus and affects thymocyte development *(91)*.

In addition to T-cells, *rankl* and *rank* knockout mice have reduced numbers of mature B220+/IgD+ and B220+/IgM+ B-cells in the spleen and lymph nodes and slightly disorganized B-cell areas in primary splenic follicles *(12,15,62)*. Since *rankl* and *rank*-null mice have no bone marrow cavities, the reduced cellularity of B-cells could be owing to an altered microenvironment or to changes in the composition of stromal cells outside the bone marrow cavity that affect B-cell differentiation. For example, *rankl*$^{-/-}$ mice form an ectopically organized extramedullary hematopoietic tissue localized at the outer surfaces of vertebral bodies *(62)*. This tissue exhibits morphologic and phenotypic features characteristic of hematopoiesis and proliferating precursor cells. Whether these hematopoietic islands in *rankl*$^{-/-}$ mice represent a defect in the homing of precursors during the switch from hepatic to bone marrow hematopoiesis, or is an event secondary to osteopetrosis that interferes with the seeding of bone marrow cavities, remains to be determined.

In fetal liver cell chimeras, RANKL regulates early B-cell differentiation from the B220+/CD43+/CD25– pro-B-cell to the B220+/CD43–/CD25+ pre-B-cell stage of development, which indicates that the TNF-family cytokine RANKL is indeed a regulator of early B lymphocyte development *(62)*. Recent evidence on *opg* mutant mouse strain confirms the notion that the interplay of RANKL-RANK and the molecular decoy receptor OPG may regulate the development and possibly the function of B-lymphocytes *(92)*. Ex vivo, *opg*$^{-/-}$ pro-B-cells have enhanced proliferation to IL-7, and type 1 transitional B-cells accumulate in the spleens of *opg*$^{-/-}$ mice. Thus, loss of OPG may control B-cell maturation. Moreover, it should be noted that OPG is a CD40-regulated gene in B-cells and DCs *(92)* and that PGE_2 treatment can increase the amount of RANKL messenger RNA in B220+ B-cells in an estrogen-dependent manner *(93)*. Activated B-cells expressed many osteoclastogenic factors including RANKL, TNF-α, IL-6, macrophage inflammatory protein-1 (MIP-1), and macrophage chemoattractant protein-3 (MCP-3) and induced osteoclast differentiation in the presence of M-CSF *(94)*. Whether RANKL acts as a survival factor required for early B- and T-cell development or whether RANKL directly affects antigen receptor-driven lymphocyte maturation remains to be seen.

10. Osteoimmunology

Since RANKL is made by T-cells and B-cells following antigen-receptor stimulation, T- and B-cell-derived RANKL can regulate the development and activation of osteoclasts, that is, activated lymphocytes can modulate bone turnover via RANKL. In an in vitro cell culture system, activated T-cells directly trigger osteoclastogenesis via RANKL *(6)*. Importantly, systemic activation of T-cells in vivo leads to a RANKL-dependent increase in osteoclastogenesis followed by bone loss. All in vitro and in vivo effects of T-cells on osteoclasts could be blocked by the administration of the decoy receptor OPG *(6)*. Moreover, in a recent elegant study it has been shown that transgenic overexpression of RANKL in T-cells restores osteoclastogenesis in a *rankl*$^{-/-}$ background and partially restores normal bone marrow cavities *(95)*. These data showed that systemic activation of T-cells leads to bone loss, indicating that, through their production of RANKL, T-cells are crucial mediators of bone loss in vivo. The results also provided a novel paradigm for T-cells and possibly B-cells as regulators of bone physiology.

Because mutant mice that lack T-cells and B-cells still have normal bone cavities and tooth eruption, T-cells are probably not required for normal bone homeostasis *(62)*. However, chronic systemic T- and B-cell activation such as in autoimmune diseases, viral infections, or local inflammation within the bone owing to metastasis, infections, and fractures, or joint inflammation in arthritis all probably attract T-cells that then actively participate in bone remodeling via production of RANKL. Moreover, glucocorticoids, which are used to treat autoimmune diseases and allergic disorders, strongly induce RANKL expression and decrease OPG *(4,96)*. Thus, in certain diseases such as asthma, primary activation of T-cells together with immunosuppressive treatment may in fact exacerbate osteopenia via synergistic activation of RANKL expression on T-cells. Intriguingly, it has recently been shown that ovariectomy-induced bone loss in wild-type mice but not in T-cell-deficient nude mice, which was restored by adoptive transfer of wild-type T-cells. Moreover, this effect appears to depend on TNF-α-TNFRp55 interactions that act presumably upstream of RANKL *(49)*. Upregulation of TNF-producing T-cells in the bone marrow appears to be a key mechanism by which estrogen deficiency induces bone loss in vivo *(49)*. If these observations hold true in humans, it is possible that T-cells are the principal cells that contribute to bone loss in old age.

These findings provide a molecular explanation for bone loss associated with diseases having immune system involvement, such as adult and childhood leukemias, cancer metastasis, autoimmunity, and various viral infections. Inhibition of RANKL function via OPG or a related molecule may therefore prevent bone destruction in multiple diseases.

11. A Molecular Scenario of T-Cell-Regulated Bone Loss

Reduced bone mineral densities can also be seen in many human diseases such as adult and childhood leukemia *(97)*, chronic infections such as hepatitis C or HIV *(98–100)*, autoimmune disorders such as diabetes mellitus *(101)* and lupus erythematosus *(102)*, allergic diseases such as asthma *(103)*, lytic bone metastases in multiple cancers such as breast cancer *(104)*, and of course arthritis *(105)*. These osteopenic disorders can cause irreversible crippling, thereby severely disrupting the lives of significant numbers of patients. For example, many patients with lupus require hip replacement surgery, and essentially all children who survive leukemia experience severe bone loss and growth retardation. In North America and Europe, 1 in 100 people develop rheumatoid arthritis (RA) and 1 in 10 people develop osteoarthritis. In particular, bone loss represents a major unsolved problem in RA, and skeletal complications of RA consist of focal bone erosions and periarticular osteoporosis at sites of active inflammation, as well as generalized bone loss with reduced bone mass *(106)*. In most of these osteopenic disorders, disease pathogenesis correlates with the activation of T-cells (Fig. 3).

In inflammatory or autoimmune disease states, activated T-cells produce RANKL and proinflammatory cytokines such as TNF-α, IL-1, or IL-11, all of which can induce RANKL expression in osteoblasts and bone marrow stromal cells *(107)*. Thus, it appears that T-cells promote bone resorption directly via RANKL expression and indirectly via expression of proinflammatory cytokines that mediate RANKL expression in non-T-cells (Fig. 3). These results are in line with the findings that T-cells and non-T-cell populations express RANKL in arthritic joints. Bone resorption induced by local injection of IL-1β or TNF-α over the calvaria of mice can be blocked by concurrent systemic injection of OPG, which indicates that RANKL is the mediator of the bone-damaging effects of TNF-α and IL1-β in vivo *(108)*. Although inhibition of TNF-α and IL-1 using soluble receptor antagonists to some extent prevents inflammation and bone loss in arthritis *(109–111)*, inhibition of RANKL function via OPG might therefore prevent bone destruction and cartilage damage in arthritis irrespective of the initial trigger.

Inhibition of RANKL via OPG has no effect on inflammation but completely prevents bone loss and protects cartilage in a rat model of adjuvant arthritis *(6)*. Genetic ablation of RANKL also protects from bone loss and partially protects from cartilage damage but does

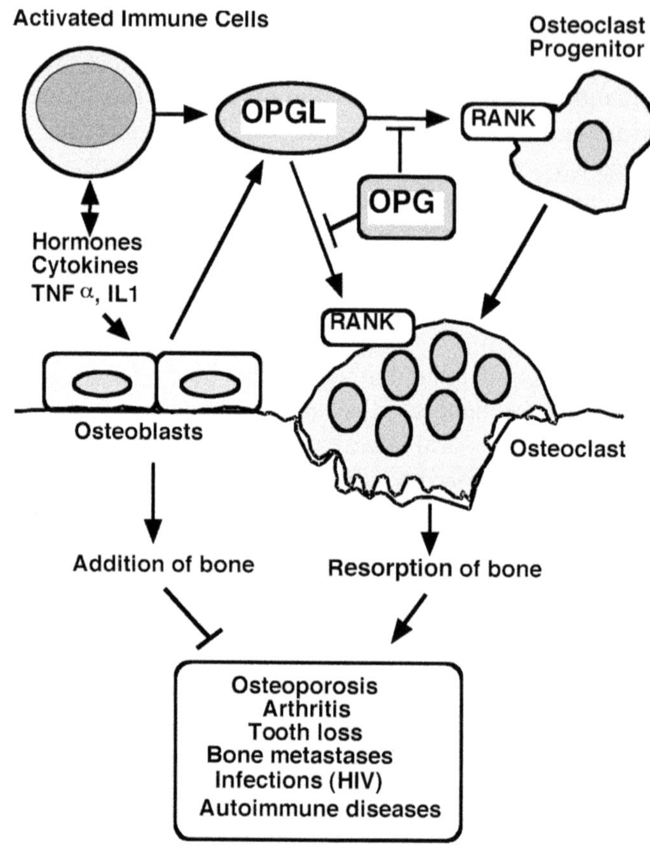

Figure 3

not prevent inflammation, in an antibody-mediated model of arthritis using the K/BxN serum transfer model *(112)*. RANK, RANKL, and OPG expression have been recently observed in normal cartilage *(66)*. However, the functional relevance of RANKL-RANK expression in chondrocytes is still not known *(113)*.

Moreover, inhibition of RANKL via OPG prevents bone loss and has a beneficial effect on cartilage destruction without affecting inflammation in a TNF-α-induced arthritis model, indicating that TNF-α-triggered joint destruction is critically dependent on RANKL expression *(114)*. It has also been recently suggested that the RANKL-RANK system plays an important role for osteoclastogenesis in both local and systemic osteolytic lesions in autoimmune type II collagen-induced arthritis in mice *(115)*. Thus, in all animal models of arthritis studied so far, the RANKL/RANK system is the trigger of bone loss and crippling, making OPG the prime drug candidate for therapeutic intervention in different forms of arthritis. In addition, T-cell-derived RANKL contributes to alveolar bone resorption and tooth loss in an animal model that mimics human periodontal disease. The alveolar bone resorption around the teeth can be inhibited with OPG *(116)*.

Short-term activation of T-cells normally does not result in any detectable bone loss, not even in some chronic T-cell and TNF-α-mediated diseases such as ankylosis spondylitis *(117)*. Moreover, T-cells are working constantly to fight off the universe of foreign particles in which we live, so, at any point in time, some T-cells are activated *(118)*. What is it that prevents these T-cells from causing extensive bone loss every time we have an infection? A crucial counterregulatory mechanism, by which activated T-cells can inhibit the RANKL-induced maturation and activation of osteoclasts, has been recently discovered (Fig. 2) *(119)*. It turns out that interferon (IFN)-γ blocks RANKL-induced osteoclast differentiation in vitro. Moreover, *IFN-γ receptor* knockout mice develop more bone destruction in inflammatory arthritis than do normal mice. Mechanistically, IFN-γ can activate the ubiquitin-proteasome pathway within the osteoclasts, resulting in the degradation of TRAF-6. Thus, it appears that IFN-γ can prevent uncontrolled bone loss during inflammatory T-cell responses.

Moreover, T-cell-derived IL-12 alone, and IL-12 in synergy with IL-18, inhibits osteoclast formation in vitro *(120)*, and IL-4 can abrogate osteoclastogenesis through STAT-6-dependent inhibition of NF-κB signaling and blockade of the JNK, p38, and ERK MAP kinase pathways *(121,122)*. Thus, multiple T-cell-derived cytokines appear to be able to interfere with RANK signaling and therefore with osteoclastogenesis and osteoclast functions. In addition to these regulatory mechanisms, autoregulatory mechanisms appear to exist. For instance, it has been reported that RANKL induces IFN-β gene expression in osteoclast precursors and that IFN-β inhibits the osteoclast differentiation by interfering with the RANKL-induced expression of c-fos, which is the essential transcription factor for osteoclast formation *(123)*. These new findings on the regulation of RANKL-induced osteoclast differentiation provide novel insights on the molecular control of osteoclast activation and bone turnover.

In the future it will be interesting to determine the mechanisms that control the balance between T-cell-mediated bone loss and inhibition of osteoclastogenesis. Nonetheless it has become clear now that inhibition of RANKL-mediated activation of RANK via OPG or a related molecule ameliorates many osteopenic conditions. RANKL inhibition appears to be the most rational and advisable strategy to prevent bone destruction in multiple diseases, to possibly eradicate major human diseases such as osteoporosis, to curtail crippling, and to limit tooth loss, diseases that affect millions of people.

12. Bone Loss, Mammary Gland Formation, and Mammalian Evolution

The expression of RANKL and OPG is regulated by multiple hormones and cytokines shown to affect the development and activation of osteoclasts, including 25-dihydroxyvitamin D_3, IL-1, IL-11, PGE_2, calcitonin, and TNF-α *(124)*. Intriguingly, expression of RANKL and OPG is also strongly influenced by the female sex hormones progesterone and estrogen and by hormones involved in reproduction and lactation such as prolactin and parathyroid hormone-related peptide (PTHrP) *(125)*. Reduction of ovarian function following menopause in women and ovariectomy in animal models result in osteoporosis and fractures, conditions that can be completely reversed at least in animals by treatment with OPG *(35)*. However, the evolutionary and functional rationale for RANKL/OPG regulation by reproductive hormones and the prevalence of hormonally regulated and gender-biased osteoporosis in older females were not known.

In mammals, sex and pregnancy hormones control mammary gland morphogenesis and formation of a lactating mammary gland. Mammary gland morphogenesis proceeds in distinct steps, beginning with a fetal mammary anlage that undergoes ductal elongation and branching *(126)*. During pregnancy, increased ductal side branching and development of lobuloalveolar structures result from the expansion and proliferation of ductal and alveolar epithelium *(127)*. Formation of a lactating mammary gland provides essential nourishment to mammalian newborns in the form of milk. Calcium is an important component of milk, and the main source of calcium for a newborn mammal is its mother's breast milk *(128)*. Calcium transport from mothers to the fetus and neonates is a vital process to preserve species. Deficits in maternal calcium transfer or calcium handling in the offspring have severe consequences for newborns, ranging from rickets to heart and brain defects *(129)*. Mothers meet the increased requirements for calcium during pregnancy and lactation by doubling their intestinal calcium absorption and demineralizing their skeletons via activation of bone-resorbing osteoclasts *(130)*.

Surprisingly, our mice lacking RANKL or its receptor RANK fail to form lobuloalveolar mammary gland structures during pregnancy and show a complete block in the formation of a lactating mammary gland, leading to the death of newborn pups *(88)*. RANKL expression in mammary epithelial cells is induced by pregnancy hormones, whereas RANK is constitutively expressed on these cells. Transplantation and local RANKL-rescue experiments in *rankl*$^{-/-}$ and *rank*$^{-/-}$ pregnant females showed that RANKL acts directly on RANK-expressing mammary epithelial cells. The effects of RANKL are autonomous to epithelial cells. The mammary gland defect in female *rankl*$^{-/-}$ mice is characterized by enhanced apoptosis and by failures in proliferation and Akt/PKB activation in lobuloalveolar buds that can be reversed by recombinant RANKL treatment *(88)*. Thus, RANKL and RANK, the master regulators of skeletal calcium release, are essential for the formation of the lactating mammary gland, the organ required for transmission of maternal calcium to neonates in mammalian species. Importantly, these data provided a novel function for TNF and TNFR-family proteins and a new paradigm in the formation of a lactating mammary gland.

In phylogenetic evolution, the formation of lactating mammary glands is a relatively recent event, occurring when the first mammals appeared about 200 million years ago. Thus, mammals took a gene product that is the master regulator of bone metabolism and calcium turnover in the whole organism and subverted it to stimulation of mammary gland development during pregnancy. Intriguingly, genetic and functional models have shown that osteoclast-regulated bone remodeling is under the control of powerful sex and pregnancy hormones *(124)*. When estrogen production falls, such as occurs in ovarectomy models in animals or in postmenopausal women, induction of OPG is decreased, allowing uncontrolled demineralization of bone by RANKL-stimulated osteoclasts *(35)*. Osteoporosis is strongly associated with increased morbidity and premature death in older women. The evolutionary question then arises of why has the RANKL/RANK/OPG system, a key regulator of a structural organ such as the skeleton, come under the regulatory umbrella of reproductive hormones? Our results provided an unexpected molecular and evolutionary explanation for gender bias and the high incidence of osteoporosis in females. The strong bias toward bone loss in postmenopausal women may be because the RANKL/RANK/OPG system is essential for reproduction and the survival of mammalian offspring.

In contrast to the synergy between CSF-1 and RANKL in osteoclastogenesis, CSF-1 appears to act independently of RANKL/RANK during mammary gland formation. Unlike *rankl*$^{-/-}$ and *rank*$^{-/-}$ mice, *csf-1* mutant mice show increased lobuloalveolar development of mammary epithelium during pregnancy and ovarian defects *(131)*. Thus, it appears that RANKL/RANK has a specific and unique role in mammary gland development that is regulated by pregnancy hormones. Mice deficient for the *stat5a*, *cyclin D1*, or *prolactin receptor* genes have defects in mammary gland development similar to those observed in *rankl*$^{-/-}$

and *rank*$^{-/-}$ females *(126,132,133)*, which suggests that RANKL/RANK, Cyclin D1, Stat5a, and/or prolactin might cooperate to stimulate lobuloalveolar development. The exact functional and genetic relationships among RANKL/RANK and pregnancy hormones, signaling molecules, and cell cycle regulatory molecules await elucidation.

Interestingly, kinase-defective IKK-α mutant mice display a severe lactation defect owing to impaired proliferation of mammary epithelial cells *(134)*. IKK-α activity is required for NF-κB activation in mammary gland epithelial cells in response to RANKL, which leads to cyclin D1 induction. Overexpression of a Cyclin D1 transgene in mammary tissue rescues the defects in kinase-defective IKK-α mutant mice, indicating that IKK-α/NF-κB/Cyclin D1 are critical intermediates in RANK signaling pathway leading to proliferation of mammary epithelial cells. In addition, OPGL induces β-casein transcription through the CCAAT/enhancer binding protein (C/EBPβ) *(135)*. In both HC11 cell lines and primary mammary epithelial cells, RANKL stimulation triggers rapid nuclear translocation of C/EBP-β, which is critical for the expression of the β-casein gene. Mutation of C/EBP-β binding sites in the β-casein gene promoter completely abrogated RANKL-induced β-casein promoter activity. By contrast, RANKL stimulation does not result in STAT-5 phosphorylation. In vivo immunohistochemistry studies further demonstrated defective nuclear translocation of C/EBP-β, but normal STAT-5 activation, in OPGL-deficient mice *(135)*. These data show that RANKL is a critical activator of β-casein gene expression via the transcription factor C/EBP-β, providing new insights into the understanding of the molecular events involved in milk protein gene expression.

These data have another intriguing implication. Both RANKL and RANK are required for lymph node organogenesis, and RANKL expressed on T-cells provides activation and survival signals to DCs. DCs, which express OPG, are specialized antigen-presenting cells that initiate and integrate immune responses. Like calcium uptake, immune responses must be modified during pregnancy so that a mother does not reject her allogeneic fetus, although the same mother can still reject an allogeneic skin transplant. Other examples of immune system alterations include the observed amelioration of clinical symptoms of multiple sclerosis during pregnancy and the onset of severe T-cell-regulated food allergies in some pregnant women *(136,137)*. Thus, pregnancy is associated with alterations to the immune system that do not impair the general response to infections but lead to selective immunologic adjustments *(136)*. Moreover, like osteoporosis, the development of autoimmunity shows a gender bias, and various sex/pregnancy hormones such as estrogen and prolactin influence the function and development of various lymphocyte populations *(138,139)*. TRANCE-RANK interactions are crucial to the development of regulatory responses *(87)*. Since RANKL, RANK, and OPG provide a genetic interface among the immune system, bone remodeling, and formation of a lactating mammary gland, this system is an intriguing starting point to address these questions at the genetic level.

13. RANKL as a New Angiogenic Factor?

Angiogenesis is a fundamental step in a variety of physiologic and pathologic conditions including wound healing, embryonic development, chronic inflammation, and tumor growth *(140)*. The angiogenic process is tightly controlled by a wide variety of positive and negative regulators, which are composed of growth factors, cytokines, lipid metabolites, or cryptic fragments of hemostatic proteins. Many of these factors were initially characterized in other biologic activities. A recent study suggested that RANKL possesses angiogenic activity *(141)*. RANKL stimulates DNA synthesis, chemotactic motility, and capillary-like tube formation in primary cultured human umbilical vein endothelial cells. Both Matrigel plug assay in mice and chick chorioallantoic membrane assays revealed that RANKL potently induces neovascularization in vivo. Angiogenic activity of RANKL is mediated through the Src-PLC-FAK signaling cascade upon receptor engagement in endothelial cells, suggesting a role of RANKL in neovasculogenesis under physiologic and pathologic conditions.

Vascular endothelial cells in bone are thought to have significant roles in pathologic bone resorption such as bone metastasis and hypercalcemia because this resorption is often seen where blood vessels are abundant *(142)*. TGF-β is abundantly stored in bone matrix and is released and activated during bone resorption. Interestingly, TGF-β upregulates the expression of RANKL in bone marrow-derived endothelial cells and in primary vascular endothelial cells but not in osteoblasts *(143)*. Further analysis revealed that protein kinase A and p38 signaling pathways are involved in TGF-β-induced RANKL expression by stimulating transcription factors that bind to the cAMP-responsive element (CRE)-like domains. These findings suggest that TGF-β stimulates osteoclastogenesis and angiogenesis by promoting RANKL expression in endothelial cells under pathologic conditions. Since the expression levels of RANKL, RANK, and OPG in vascular endothelial cells are regulated by inflammatory cytokines, cytokine-activated endothelial cells may contribute to inflammatory-mediated bone loss, vessel calcification, and angiogenesis *(144)*. It remains to be seen whether these effects of RANKL on angiogenesis in in vitro assays have any physiologic significance.

14. Conclusions

RANKL, its receptor RANK, and the decoy receptor OPG are the key regulators for osteoclast development and the activation of mature osteoclasts. Surprisingly, the same molecules that regulate osteoclastogenesis were identified as key factors in early lymphocyte differentiation and the development of lymph nodes. In the immune system, RANKL is produced by activated T- and B-cells and acts as a potent survival factor of DCs. The understanding and manipulation of DC fate by RANKL/RANK provides a new avenue for antitumor vaccination and the treatment of autoimmune diseases. RANKL produced by activated T-cells and B-cells can directly induce osteoclastogenesis. Systemic or local activation of T-cells triggers bone loss via expression of RANKL. These findings provide the molecular explanation for bone loss associated with diseases having immune system involvement, such as adult and childhood leukemias, autoimmunity, and various viral infections. Moreover, T-cells have been recently implicated as important regulatory cells in old-age osteoporosis. Inhibition of RANKL function via OPG or a related molecule might therefore ameliorate many osteopenic conditions and prevent the bone destruction and cartilage damage that ultimately cause crippling in arthritis. Moreover, RANKL and RANK, the master regulators of skeletal calcium release, are essential for the morphogenesis of a lactating mammary gland, which provides an evolutionary rationale for hormonal regulation of osteoporosis.

Acknowledgments

J.M.P. holds a Canadian Research Chair in Cell Biology and is supported by the Premier's Research Excellence Award of Canada and The Institute for Molecular Biotechnology of the Austrian Academy of Sciences. Y.Y. Kong is supported by a Vascular System Research grant from KOSEF and the Molecular Medicine Research Group Program (M1-0106-01-0001) from the Ministry of Science and Technology. We thank all the members of our laboratories for vital contributions and discussion.

References

1. Anderson, D. M., Maroskovsky, E., Billingsley, W. L., et al. (1997) A homologue of the TNF receptor and its ligand enhance T-cell growth and dendritic-cell function. *Nature* **390,** 175–179.
2. Lacey, D. L., Timms, E., Tan, H. L., et al. (1998) Osteoprotegerin ligand is a cytokine that regulates osteoclast differentiation and activation. *Cell* **93,** 165–176.
3. Wong, B. R., Josien, R. Lee, S. Y., et al. (1997) TRANCE (tumor necrosis factor [TNF]-related activation-induced cytokine), a new TNF family member predominantly expressed in T cells, is a dendritic cell-specific survival factor. *J. Exp. Med.* **186,** 2075–2080.
4. Yasuda, H., Shima, N., Nakagawa, N., et al. (1998) Osteoclast differentiation factor is a ligand for osteoprotegerin/osteoclastogenesis-inhibitory factor and is identical to TRANCE/RANKL. *Proc. Natl. Acad. Sci. USA* **95,** 3597–3602.
5. Lum, L., Wong, B. R., Josien, R., et al. (1999) Evidence for a role of a tumor necrosis factor-alpha (TNF-alpha)-converting enzyme-like protease in shedding of TRANCE, a TNF family member involved in osteoclastogenesis and dendritic cell survival. *J. Biol. Chem.* **274,** 13613–13618.
6. Kong, Y. Y., Feige, U., Sarosi, I., et al. (1999) Activated T cells regulate bone loss and joint destruction in adjuvant arthritis through osteoprotegerin ligand. *Nature* **402,** 304–309.
7. Nakashima, T., Kobayashi, Y., Yamasaki, S., et al. (2000) Protein expression and functional difference of membrane-bound and soluble receptor activator of NF-kappaB ligand: modulation of the expression by osteotropic factors and cytokines. *Biochem. Biophys. Res. Commun.* **275,** 768–775.
8. Lam, J., Nelson, C. A., Ross, F. P., Teitelbaum, S. L., and Fremont, D. L. (2001) Crystal structure of the TRANCE/RANKL cytokine reveals determinants of receptor-ligand specificity. *J. Clin. Invest.* **108,** 971–979.
9. Ito, S., Wakabayashi, K., Obukata, O., Hayashi, S., Okada, F., and Hata, T. (2002) Crystal structure of the extracellular domain of mouse RANK ligand at 2.2-A resolution. *J. Biol. Chem.* **277,** 6631–6636.
10. Kartsogiannis, V., Zhou, H., Horwood, N. J., et al. (1999) Localization of RANKL (receptor activator of NF kappa B ligand) mRNA and protein in skeletal and extraskeletal tissues. *Bone* **25,** 525–534.
11. Lagasse, E. and Weissman, I. L. (1997) Enforced expression of Bcl-2 in monocytes rescues macrophages and partially reverses osteopetrosis in op/op mice. *Cell* **89,** 1021–1031.
12. Hsu, H., Lacey, D. L., Dunstan, C. R., et al. (1999) Tumor necrosis factor receptor family member RANK mediates osteoclast differentiation and activation induced by osteoprotegerin ligand. *Proc. Natl. Acad. Sci. USA* **96,** 3540–3545.
13. Burgess, T. L., Qian, Y., Kaufman, S., et al. (1999) The ligand for osteoprotegerin (OPGL) directly activates mature osteoclasts. *J. Cell. Biol.* **145,** 527–538.
14. Nakagawa, N., Kinosaki, M., Yamaguchi, K. et al. (1998) RANK is the essential signaling receptor for osteoclast differentiation factor in osteoclastogenesis. *Biochem. Biophys. Res. Commun.* **253,** 395–400.
15. Dougall, W. C., Glaccum, M., Charrier, K., et al. (1999) RANK is essential for osteoclast and lymph node development. *Genes Dev.* **13,** 2412–2424.
16. Li, J., Sarosi, I., Yan, X. Q., et al. (2000) RANK is the intrinsic hematopoietic cell surface receptor that controls osteoclastogenesis and regulation of bone mass and calcium metabolism. *Proc. Natl. Acad. Sci. USA* **97,** 1566–1571.
17. Hughes, A. E., Ralston, S. H., Marken, J., et al. (2000) Mutations in TNFRSF11A, affecting the signal peptide of RANK, cause familial expansile osteolysis. *Nat. Genet.* **24,** 45–48.
18. Darnay, B. G., Haridas, V., Ni, J., Moore, P. A., and Aggarwal, B. B. (1998) Characterization of the intracellular domain of receptor activator of NF-kappaB (RANK). Interaction with tumor necrosis factor receptor-associated factors and activation of NF-kappaB and c-Jun N-terminal kinase. *J. Biol. Chem.* **273,** 20551–20555.

19. Galibert, L., Tometsko, M. E., Anderson, D. M., Cosman, D., and Dougall, W. C. (1998) The involvement of multiple tumor necrosis factor receptor (TNFR)-associated factors in the signaling mechanisms of receptor activator of NF-kappaB, a member of the TNFR superfamily. *J. Biol. Chem.* **273,** 34120–34127.
20. Lee, Z. H., Kwack, K., Kimm, K. K., Lee, S. H., and Kim, H. H. (2000) Activation of c-Jun N-terminal kinase and activator protein 1 by receptor activator of nuclear factor kappaB. *Mol. Pharmacol.* **58,** 1536–1545.
21. Wong, B. R., Josien R., Lee, S. Y., Vologodskaia, M., Steinman, R. M., and Choi, Y. (1998) The TRAF family of signal transducers mediates NF-kappaB activation by the TRANCE receptor. *J. Biol. Chem.* **273,** 28355–28359.
22. Kobayashi, N., Kadono, Y., Naito, A., et al. (2001) Segregation of TRAF6-mediated signaling pathways clarifies its role in osteoclastogenesis. *EMBO J.* **20,** 1271–1280.
23. Lomaga, M. A., Yeh, W. C., Sarosi, I., et al. (1999) TRAF6 deficiency results in osteopetrosis and defective interleukin-1, CD40, and LPS signaling. *Genes Dev.* **13,** 1015–1024.
24. Naito, A., Azuma, S., Tanaka, S., et al. (1999) Severe osteopetrosis, defective interleukin-1 signalling and lymph node organogenesis in TRAF6-deficient mice. *Genes Cells* **4,** 353–362.
25. Franzoso, G., Carlson, L., Xing, L., et al. (1997) Requirement for NF-kappaB in osteoclast and B-cell development. *Genes Dev.* **11,** 3482–3496.
26. Iotsova, V., Caamano, J., Loy, J., Yang, Y., Lewin, A., and Bravo, R. (1997) Osteopetrosis in mice lacking NF-kappaB1 and NF-kappaB2. *Nat. Med.* **3,** 1285–1289.
27. Mizukami, J., Takaesu, G., Akatsuka, H., et al. (2002) Receptor activator of NF-kappaB ligand (RANKL) activates TAK1 mitogen-activated protein kinase kinase kinase through a signaling complex containing RANK, TAB2, and TRAF6. *Mol. Cell. Biol.* **22,** 992–1000.
28. Deng, L., Wang, C., Spencer, E. et al. (2000) Activation of the IkappaB kinase complex by TRAF6 requires a dimeric ubiquitin-conjugating enzyme complex and a unique polyubiquitin chain. *Cell* **103,** 351–361.
29. Wang, C., Deng, L., Hong, M., Akkaraju, G. R., Inoue, J., and Chen, Z. J. (2001) TAK1 is a ubiquitin-dependent kinase of MKK and IKK. *Nature* **412,** 346–351.
30. Mansky, K. C., Sankar, U., Han, J., and Ostrowski, M. C. (2002) Microphthalmia transcription factor is a target of the p38 MAPK pathway in response to receptor activator of NF-kappa B ligand signaling. *J. Biol. Chem.* **277,** 11077–11083.
31. Matsuo, K., Owens, J. M., Tonko, M., Elliott, C., Chambers, T. J., and Wagner, E. F. (2000) Fosl1 is a transcriptional target of c-Fos during osteoclast differentiation. *Nat. Genet.* **24,** 184–187.
32. Wong, B. R., Besser, D., Kim, N., et al. (1999) TRANCE, a TNF family member, activates Akt/PKB through a signaling complex involving TRAF6 and c-Src. *Mol. Cell* **4,** 1041–1049.
33. Arron, J. R., Vologodskaia, M., Wong, B. R., et al. (2001) A positive regulatory role for Cbl family proteins in tumor necrosis factor-related activation-induced cytokine (trance) and CD40L-mediated Akt activation. *J. Biol. Chem.* **276,** 30011–30017.
34. Matsumoto, M., Sudo, T., Saito, T., Osada, H., and Tsujimoto, M. (2000) Involvement of p38 mitogen-activated protein kinase signaling pathway in osteoclastogenesis mediated by receptor activator of NF-kappa B ligand (RANKL). *J. Biol. Chem.* **275,** 31155–31161.
35. Simonet, W. S., Lacey, D. L., Dunstan, C. R., et al. (1997) Osteoprotegerin: a novel secreted protein involved in the regulation of bone density. *Cell* **89,** 309–319.
36. Yasuda, H., Shima, N., Nakagawa, N., et al. (1998) Identity of osteoclastogenesis inhibitory factor (OCIF) and osteoprotegerin (OPG): a mechanism by which OPG/OCIF inhibits osteoclastogenesis in vitro. *Endocrinology* **139,** 1329–1337.
37. Bucay, N., Sarosi, I., Dunstan, C. R., et al. (1998) Osteoprotegerin-deficient mice develop early onset osteoporosis and arterial calcification. *Genes Dev.* **12,** 1260–1268.
38. Mizuno, A., Murakami, A., Nakagawa, N., et al. (1998) Structure of the mouse osteoclastogenesis inhibitory factor (OCIF) gene and its expression in embryogenesis. *Gene* **215,** 339–343.
39. Brandstrom, H., Jonsson, K. B., Ohlsson, C., Vidal, O., Ljunghall, S., and Ljunggren, O. (1998) Regulation of osteoprotegerin mRNA levels by prostaglandin E2 in human bone marrow stroma cells. *Biochem. Biophys. Res. Commun.* **247,** 338–341.

40. Brandstrom, H., Jonsson, K. K., Vidal, O., Ljunghall, S., Ohlsson, C., and Ljunggren, O. (1998) Tumor necrosis factor-alpha and -beta upregulate the levels of osteoprotegerin mRNA in human osteosarcoma MG-63 cells. *Biochem. Biophys. Res. Commun.* **248,** 454–457.
41. Yun, T. J., Chaudhary, P. M., Shu, G. L., et al. (1998) OPG/FDCR-1, a TNF receptor family member, is expressed in lymphoid cells and is up-regulated by ligating CD40. *J. Immunol.* **161,** 6113–6121.
42. Min, H., Morony, S., Sarosi, I., et al. (2000) Osteoprotegerin reverses osteoporosis by inhibiting endosteal osteoclasts and prevents vascular calcification by blocking a process resembling osteoclastogenesis. *J. Exp. Med.* **192,** 463–474.
43. Parhami, F. and Demer, L. L. (1997) Arterial calcification in face of osteoporosis in ageing: can we blame oxidized lipids? *Curr. Opin. Lipidol.* **8,** 312–314.
44. Walker-Bone, K., Dennison, E., and Cooper, C. (2001) Epidemiology of osteoporosis. *Rheum. Dis. Clin. North Am.* **27,** 1–18.
45. Jorgensen, L., Engstad, T., and Jacobsen, B. K. (2001) Bone mineral density in acute stroke patients: low bone mineral density may predict first stroke in women. *Stroke* **32,** 47–51.
46. Mach, F., Schonbeck, U., Sukhova, G. K., Atkinson, E., and Libby, P. (1998) Reduction of atherosclerosis in mice by inhibition of CD40 signalling. *Nature* **394,** 200–203.
47. Zhang, Y. H., Heulsmann, A., Tondravi, M. M., Mukherjee, A., and Abu-Amer, Y. (2001) Tumor necrosis factor-alpha (TNF) stimulates RANKL-induced osteoclastogenesis via coupling of TNF type 1 receptor and RANK signaling pathways. *J. Biol. Chem.* **276,** 563–568.
48. Cenci, S., Weitizmann, M. N., Roggia, C., et al. (2000) Estrogen deficiency induces bone loss by enhancing T-cell production of TNF-alpha. *J. Clin. Invest.* **106,** 1229–1237.
49. Roggia, C., Gao, Y., Cenci, S., et al. (2001) Up-regulation of TNF-producing T cells in the bone marrow: a key mechanism by which estrogen deficiency induces bone loss in vivo. *Proc. Natl. Acad. Sci. USA* **98,** 13960–13965.
50. Emery, J. G., McDonnell, P., Burke, M. B., et al. (1998) Osteoprotegerin is a receptor for the cytotoxic ligand TRAIL. *J. Biol. Chem.* **273,** 14363–14367.
51. Hofbauer, L. C., Khosla, S., Dunstan, C. R., Lacey, D. L., Spelsberg, T. C., and Riggs, B. L. (1999) Estrogen stimulates gene expression and protein production of osteoprotegerin in human osteoblastic cells. *Endocrinology* **140,** 4367–4370.
52. Saika, M., Inoue, D., Kido, S., and Matsumoto, T. (2001) 17beta-estradiol stimulates expression of osteoprotegerin by a mouse stromal cell line, ST-2, via estrogen receptor-alpha. *Endocrinology* **142,** 2205–2212.
53. Mundy, G. R. (1997) Mechanisms of bone metastasis. *Cancer* **80(8 Suppl.),** 1546–1556.
54. Thomas, R. J., Guise, T. A., Yin, J. J., Elliott, J., Horwood, N. J., Martin, T. J., and Gillespie, M. T. (1999) Breast cancer cells interact with osteoblasts to support osteoclast formation. *Endocrinology* **140,** 4451–4458.
55. Croucher, P. I., Shipman, C. M., Lippitt, J., et al. (2001) Osteoprotegerin inhibits the development of osteolytic bone disease in multiple myeloma. *Blood* **98,** 3534–3540.
56. Nosaka, K., Miyamoto, T., Sakai, T., Mitsuya, H., Suda, T., and Matsuoka, M. (2002) Mechanism of hypercalcemia in adult T-cell leukemia: overexpression of receptor activator of nuclear factor kappaB ligand on adult T-cell leukemia cells. *Blood* **99,** 634–640.
57. Pearse, R. N., Sordillo, E. M., Yaccoby, S., et al. (2001) Multiple myeloma disrupts the TRANCE/osteoprotegerin cytokine axis to trigger bone destruction and promote tumor progression. *Proc. Natl. Acad. Sci. USA* **98,** 11581–11586.
58. Thompson, S. W. and Tonge, D. (2000) Bone cancer gain without the pain. *Nat. Med.* **6,** 504–505.
59. Honore, P., Luger, N. M., Sabino, M. A., et al. (2000) Osteoprotegerin blocks bone cancer-induced skeletal destruction, skeletal pain and pain-related neurochemical reorganization of the spinal cord. *Nat. Med.* **6,** 521–528.
60. Wong, B. R., Rho, J., Arron, J., et al. (1997) TRANCE is a novel ligand of the tumor necrosis factor receptor family that activates c-Jun N-terminal kinase in T cells. *J. Biol. Chem.* **272,** 25190–25194.

61. Josien, R., Li, H. L., Ingulli, E., et al. (2000) TRANCE, a tumor necrosis factor family member, enhances the longevity and adjuvant properties of dendritic cells in vivo. *J. Exp. Med.* **191,** 495–502.
62. Kong, Y. Y., Yoshida, H., Sarosi, I., et al. (1999) OPGL is a key regulator of osteoclastogenesis, lymphocyte development and lymph-node organogenesis. *Nature* **397,** 315–323.
63. Rennert, P. D., Browning, J. L., and Hochman, P. S. (1997) Selective disruption of lymphotoxin ligands reveals a novel set of mucosal lymph nodes and unique effects on lymph node cellular organization. *Int. Immunol.* **9,** 1627–1639.
64. De Togni, P., Goellner, J., Ruddle, N. H., et al. (1994) Abnormal development of peripheral lymphoid organs in mice deficient in lymphotoxin. *Science* **264,** 703–707.
65. Koni, P. A., Saca, R., Lawton, P., Browning, J. L., Ruddle, N. H., and Flavell, R. A. (1997) Distinct roles in lymphoid organogenesis for lymphotoxins alpha and beta revealed in lymphotoxin beta-deficient mice. *Immunity* **6,** 491–500.
66. Alimzhanov, M. B., Kuprash, D. V., Kosco-Vilbois, M. H., et al. (1997) Abnormal development of secondary lymphoid tissues in lymphotoxin beta-deficient mice. *Proc. Natl. Acad. Sci. USA* **94,** 9302–9307.
67. Matsumoto, M., Fu, Y. X., Molina, H., et al. (1996) Role of lymphotoxin and the type I TNF receptor in the formation of germinal centers. *Science* **271,** 1289–1291.
68. Rennert, P. D., James, D., Mackay, F., Browning, J. L., and Hochman, P. S. (1998) Lymph node genesis is induced by signaling through the lymphotoxin beta receptor. *Immunity* **9,** 71–79.
69. Futterer, A., Mink, K., Luz, A., Kosco-Vilbois, M. H., and Pfeffer, K. (1998) The lymphotoxin beta receptor controls organogenesis and affinity maturation in peripheral lymphoid tissues. *Immunity* **9,** 59–70.
70. Yokota, Y., Mansouri, A., Mori, S., et al. (1999) Development of peripheral lymphoid organs and natural killer cells depends on the helix-loop-helix inhibitor Id2. *Nature* **397,** 702–706.
71. Pasparakis, M., Alexopoulou, L., Grell, M., Pfizenmaier, K., Bluethmann, H., Kollias, G. (1997) Peyer's patch organogenesis is intact yet formation of B lymphocyte follicles is defective in peripheral lymphoid organs of mice deficient for tumor necrosis factor and its 55-kDa receptor. *Proc. Natl. Acad. Sci. USA* **94,** 6319–6323.
72. Fu, Y. X. and Chaplin, D. D. (1999) Development and maturation of secondary lymphoid tissues. *Annu. Rev. Immunol.* **17**, 399–433.
73. Mebius, R. E., Rennert, P., and Weissman, I. L. (1997) Developing lymph nodes collect CD4+ CD3- LTbeta+ cells that can differentiate to APC, NK cells, and follicular cells but not T or B cells. *Immunity* **7,** 493–504.
74. Kim, D., Mebius, R. E., MacMicking, J. D., et al. (2000) Regulation of peripheral lymph node genesis by the tumor necrosis factor family member TRANCE. *J. Exp. Med.* **192,** 1467–1478.
75. Josien, R., Wong, B. R., Li, H. L., Steinman, R. M., and Choi, Y. (1999) TRANCE, a TNF family member, is differentially expressed on T cell subsets and induces cytokine production in dendritic cells. *J. Immunol.* **162,** 2562–2568.
76. Roy, M., Waldschmidt, T., Aruffo, A., Ledbetter, J. A., and Noelle, R. J. (1993) The regulation of the expression of gp39, the CD40 ligand, on normal and cloned CD4+ T cells. *J. Immunol.* **151,** 2497–2510.
77. Kawabe, T., Naka, T., Yoshida K., et al. (1994) The immune responses in CD40-deficient mice: impaired immunoglobulin class switching and germinal center formation. *Immunity* **1,** 167–178.
78. Xu, J., Foy, T. M., Laman, J. D., et al. (1994) Mice deficient for the CD40 ligand. *Immunity* **1,** 423–431.
79. Bachmann, M. F., Wong, B. R., Josien, R., Steinman, R. M., Oxenius, A., and Choi, Y. (1999) TRANCE, a tumor necrosis factor family member critical for CD40 ligand-independent T helper cell activation. *J. Exp. Med.* **189,** 1025–1031.
80. Banchereau, J. and Steinman, R. M. (1998) Dendritic cells and the control of immunity. *Nature* **392,** 245–252.
81. Ingulli, E., Mondino, A., Khoruts, A., and Jenkins, M. K. (1997) In vivo detection of dendritic cell antigen presentation to CD4(+) T cells. *J. Exp. Med.* **185,** 2133–2141.
82. Wang, J., Zheng, L., Lobito, A., et al. (1999) Inherited human Caspase 10 mutations underlie defective lymphocyte and dendritic cell apoptosis in autoimmune lymphoproliferative syndrome type II. *Cell* **98,** 47–58.

83. Sauter, B., Albert, M. L., Francisco, L., Larsson, M., Somersan, S., and Bhardwaj, N. (2000) Consequences of cell death: exposure to necrotic tumor cells, but not primary tissue cells or apoptotic cells, induces the maturation of immunostimulatory dendritic cells. *J. Exp. Med.* **191,** 423–434.
84. Kayagaki, N., Yamaguchi, N., Nakayama, M., et al. (1999) Involvement of TNF-related apoptosis-inducing ligand in human CD4+ T cell-mediated cytotoxicity. *J. Immunol.* **162,** 2639–2647.
85. Martinez-Lorenzo, M. J., Anel, A., Gamen, S., et al. (1999) Activated human T cells release bioactive Fas ligand and APO2 ligand in microvesicles. *J. Immunol.* **163,** 1274–1281.
86. Thomas, W. D. and Hersey, P. (1998) TNF-related apoptosis-inducing ligand (TRAIL) induces apoptosis in Fas ligand-resistant melanoma cells and mediates CD4 T cell killing of target cells. *J. Immunol.* **161,** 2195–2200.
87. Green, E. A., Choi, Y., and Flavell, R. A. (2002) Pancreatic lymph node-derived CD4(+)CD25(+) Treg cells: highly potent regulators of diabetes that require TRANCE-RANK signals. *Immunity* **16,** 183–191.
88. Fata, J. E., Kong, Y. Y., Li, J., et al. (2000) The osteoclast differentiation factor osteoprotegerin-ligand is essential for mammary gland development. *Cell* **103,** 41–50.
89. von Boehmer, H. and Fehling, H. J. (1997) Structure and function of the pre-T cell receptor. *Annu. Rev. Immunol.* **15,** 433–452.
90. Bouillet, P., Metcalf, D., Huang, D. C., et al. (1999) Proapoptotic Bcl-2 relative Bim required for certain apoptotic responses, leukocyte homeostasis, and to preclude autoimmunity. *Science* **286,** 1735–1738.
91. Li, C. L., Toda, K., Saibara, T., et al. (2002) Estrogen deficiency results in enhanced expression of Smoothened of the Hedgehog signaling in the thymus and affects thymocyte development. *Int. Immunopharmacol.* **2,** 823–833.
92. Yun, T. J., Tallquist, M. D., Aicher, A., et al. (2001) Osteoprotegerin, a crucial regulator of bone metabolism, also regulates B cell development and function. *J. Immunol. 166,* 1482–1491.
93. Kanematsu, M., Ato, T., Takai, H., Watanabe, K., Ikeda, K., and Yamada, Y. (2000) Prostaglandin E2 induces expression of receptor activator of nuclear factor-kappa B ligand/osteoprotegrin ligand on pre-B cells: implications for accelerated osteoclastogenesis in estrogen deficiency. *J. Bone Miner. Res.* **15,** 1321–1329.
94. Choi, Y., Woo, K. M., Ko, S. H., et al. (2001) Osteoclastogenesis is enhanced by activated B cells but suppressed by activated CD8(+) T cells. *Eur. J. Immunol.* **31,** 2179–2188.
95. Kim, N., Odgren, P. R., Kim, D. K., Marks, S. C. Jr., and Choi, Y. (2000) Diverse roles of the tumor necrosis factor family member TRANCE in skeletal physiology revealed by TRANCE deficiency and partial rescue by a lymphocyte-expressed TRANCE transgene. *Proc. Natl. Acad. Sci. USA* **97,** 10905–10910.
96. Vidal, N. O., Brandstrom, H., Jonsson, K. B., and Ohlsson, C. (1998) Osteoprotegerin mRNA is expressed in primary human osteoblast-like cells: down-regulation by glucocorticoids. *J. Endocrinol.* **159,** 191–195.
97. Oliveri, M. B., Mautalen, C. A., Rodriguez Fuchs, C. A., and Romanelli, M. C. (1991) Vertebral compression fractures at the onset of acute lymphoblastic leukemia in a child. *Henry Ford Hosp. Med. J.* **39,** 45–48.
98. Stellon, A. J., Davies, A., Compston, J., and Williams, R. (1985) Bone loss in autoimmune chronic active hepatitis on maintenance corticosteroid therapy. *Gastroenterology* **89,** 1078–1083.
99. Jain, R. G. and Lenhard, J. M. (2002) Select HIV protease inhibitors alter bone and fat metabolism ex vivo. *J. Biol. Chem.* **277,** 19247–19250.
100. Ueland, T., Bollerslev, J., Godang, K., Muller, F., Froland, S. S., and Aukrust, P. (2001) Increased serum osteoprotegerin in disorders characterized by persistent immune activation or glucocorticoid excess—possible role in bone homeostasis. *Eur. J. Endocrinol.* **145,** 685–690.
101. Piepkorn, B., Kann, P., Forst, T., Andreas, J., Pfutzner, A., and Beyer, J. (1997) Bone mineral density and bone metabolism in diabetes mellitus. *Horm. Metab. Res.* **29,** 584–591.
102. Seitz, M. and Hunstein, W. (1985) Enhanced prostanoid release from monocytes of patients with rheumatoid arthritis and active systemic lupus erythematosus. *Ann. Rheum. Dis.* **44,** 438–445.
103. Ebeling, P. R., Erbas, B., Hopper, J. L., Wark, J. D., and Rubinfeld, A. R. (1998) Bone mineral density and bone turnover in asthmatics treated with long-term inhaled or oral glucocorticoids. *J. Bone Miner. Res.* **13,** 1283–1289.

104. Coleman, R. E. (1998) How can we improve the treatment of bone metastases further? *Curr. Opin. Oncol.* **10(Suppl. 1),** p. S7–S13.
105. Feldmann, M., Brennan, F. M., and Maini, R. N. (1996) Role of cytokines in rheumatoid arthritis. *Annu. Rev. Immunol.* **14,** 397–440.
106. Romas, E., Gillespie, M. T., and Martin, T. J. (2002) Involvement of receptor activator of NFkappaB ligand and tumor necrosis factor-alpha in bone destruction in rheumatoid arthritis. *Bone* **30,** 340–346.
107. Hofbauer, L. C., Lacey, D. L., Dunstan, C. R., Spelsberg, T. C., Riggs, B. L., and Khosla, S. (1999) Interleukin-1beta and tumor necrosis factor-alpha, but not interleukin-6, stimulate osteoprotegerin ligand gene expression in human osteoblastic cells. *Bone* **25,** 255–259.
108. Morony, S., Capparelli, C., Lee, R., et al. (1999) A chimeric form of osteoprotegerin inhibits hypercalcemia and bone resorption induced by IL-1beta, TNF-alpha, PTH, PTHrP, and 1, 25(OH)2D3. *J. Bone Miner. Res.* **14,** 1478–1485.
109. Williams, R. O., Feldmann, M., and Maini, R. N. (2000) Cartilage destruction and bone erosion in arthritis: the role of tumour necrosis factor alpha. *Ann. Rheum. Dis.* **59(Suppl. 1),** i75–i80.
110. Fye, K. H. (1999) New treatments for rheumatoid arthritis. Available and upcoming slow-acting antirheumatic drugs. *Postgrad. Med.* **106,** 82–85, 88–90, 92.
111. Graninger, W. B. and Smolen, J. S. (2001) One-year inhibition of tumor necrosis factor-alpha: a major success or a larger puzzle? *Curr. Opin. Rheumatol.* **13,** 209–213.
112. Pettit, A. R., Ji, H., von Stechow, D., et al. (2001) TRANCE/RANKL knockout mice are protected from bone erosion in a serum transfer model of arthritis. *Am. J. Pathol.* **159,** 1689–1699.
113. Komuro, H., Olee, T., Kuhn, K., et al. (2001) The osteoprotegerin/receptor activator of nuclear factor kappaB/receptor activator of nuclear factor kappaB ligand system in cartilage. *Arthritis Rheum.* **44,** 2768–2776.
114. Redlich, K., Hayer, S., Maier, A., et al. (2002) Tumor necrosis factor alpha-mediated joint destruction is inhibited by targeting osteoclasts with osteoprotegerin. *Arthritis Rheum.* **46,** 785–792.
115. Mori, H., Kitazawa, R., Mizuki, S., Nose, M., Maeda, S., and Kitazawa, S. (2002) RANK ligand, RANK, and OPG expression in type II collagen-induced arthritis mouse. *Histochem. Cell Biol.* **117,** 283–292.
116. Teng, Y. T., Nguyen, H., Gao, X., et al. (2000) Functional human T-cell immunity and osteoprotegerin ligand control alveolar bone destruction in periodontal infection. *J. Clin. Invest.* **106,** R59–R67.
117. Brandt, J., Haibel, H., Comely, D., et al. (2000) Successful treatment of active ankylosing spondylitis with the anti-tumor necrosis factor alpha monoclonal antibody infliximab. *Arthritis Rheum.* **43,** 1346–1352.
118. Arron, J. R. and Choi, Y. (2000) Bone versus immune system. *Nature* **408,** 535–536.
119. Takayanagi, H., Ogasawara, K., Hida, S., et al. (2000) T-cell-mediated regulation of osteoclastogenesis by signalling cross-talk between RANKL and IFN-gamma. *Nature* **408,** 600–605.
120. Horwood, N. J., Elliott, J., Martin, T. J., and Gillespie, M. T. (2001) IL-12 alone and in synergy with IL-18 inhibits osteoclast formation in vitro. *J. Immunol.* **166,** 4915–4921.
121. Abu-Amer, Y. (2001) IL-4 abrogates osteoclastogenesis through STAT6-dependent inhibition of NF-kappaB. *J. Clin. Invest.* **107,** 1375–1385.
122. Bendixen, A. C., Shevde, N. K., Dienger, K. M., Willson, T. M., Funk, C. D., and Pike, J. W. (2001) IL-4 inhibits osteoclast formation through a direct action on osteoclast precursors via peroxisome proliferator-activated receptor gamma 1. *Proc. Natl. Acad. Sci. USA* **98,** 2443–2448.
123. Takayanagi, H., Kim, S., Matsuo, K., et al. (2002) RANKL maintains bone homeostasis through c-Fos-dependent induction of interferon-beta. *Nature* **416,** 744–749.
124. Ross, F. P. (2000) RANKing the importance of measles virus in Paget's disease. *J. Clin. Invest.* **105,** 555–558.
125. Karsenty, G. (1999) The genetic transformation of bone biology. *Genes Dev.* **13,** 3037–3051.
126. Robinson, G. W., Karpf, A. B., and Kratochwil, K. (1999) Regulation of mammary gland development by tissue interaction. *J. Mammary Gland Biol. Neoplasia* **4,** 9–19.
127. Robinson, G. W., Hennighausen, L., and Johnson, P. F. (2000) Side-branching in the mammary gland: the progesterone-Wnt connection. *Genes Dev.* **14,** 889–894.

128. Kovacs, C. S. and Kronenberg, H. M. (1997) Maternal-fetal calcium and bone metabolism during pregnancy, puerperium, and lactation. *Endocr. Rev.* **18,** 832–872.
129. Pereira, G. R. and Zucker, A. H. (1986) Nutritional deficiencies in the neonate. *Clin. Perinatol.* **13,** 175–189.
130. Cross, N. A., Hillman, L. S., Allen, S. H., Krause, G. F., and Vieira, N. E. (1995) Calcium homeostasis and bone metabolism during pregnancy, lactation, and postweaning: a longitudinal study. *Am. J. Clin. Nutr.* **61,** 514–523.
131. Pollard, J. W. and Hennighausen, L. (1994) Colony stimulating factor 1 is required for mammary gland development during pregnancy. *Proc. Natl. Acad. Sci. USA* **91,** 9312–9316.
132. Brisken, C., Kaur, S., Chavarria, T. E., et al. (1999) Prolactin controls mammary gland development via direct and indirect mechanisms. *Dev. Biol.* **210,** 96–106.
133. Fantl, V., Edwards, P. A., Steel, J. H., Vonderhaar, B. K., and Dickson, C. (1999) Impaired mammary gland development in Cyl-1(-/-) mice during pregnancy and lactation is epithelial cell autonomous. *Dev. Biol.* **212,** 1–11.
134. Cao, Y., Bonizzi, B., Seagroves, T. N., et al. (2001) IKKalpha provides an essential link between RANK signaling and cyclin D1 expression during mammary gland development. *Cell* **107,** 763–775.
135. Kim, H. J., Yoon, M. J., Lee, J., Penninger, J. M., and Kong, Y. Y. (2002) Osteoprotegerin ligand induces beta-casein gene expression through the transcription factor CCAAT/enhancer-binding protein beta. *J. Biol. Chem.* **277,** 5339–5344.
136. Buyon, J. P. (1998) The effects of pregnancy on autoimmune diseases. *J. Leukoc. Biol.* **63,** 281–287.
137. Whitacre, C. C., Reingold, S. C., and O'Looney, P. A. (1999) A gender gap in autoimmunity. *Science* **283,** 1277–1278.
138. Ahmed, S. A., Hissong, B. D., Verthelyi, D., Donner, K., Becker, K., and Karpuzoglu-Sahin, E. (1999) Gender and risk of autoimmune diseases: possible role of estrogenic compounds. *Environ. Health Perspect.* **107(Suppl. 5),** 681–686.
139. Rider, V. and Abdou, N. I. (2001) Gender differences in autoimmunity: molecular basis for estrogen effects in systemic lupus erythematosus. *Int. Immunopharmacol.* **1,** 1009–1024.
140. Risau, W. (1997) Mechanisms of angiogenesis. *Nature* **386,** 671–674.
141. Kim, Y. M., Kim, Y. M., Lee, Y. M., et al. (2002) TNF-related activation-induced cytokine (TRANCE) induces angiogenesis through the activation of Src and phospholipase C (PLC) in human endothelial cells. *J. Biol. Chem.* **277,** 6799–6805.
142. Gerber, H. P., Vu, T. H., Ryan, A. M., Kowalski, J., Werb, Z., and Ferrara, N. (1999) VEGF couples hypertrophic cartilage remodeling, ossification and angiogenesis during endochondral bone formation. *Nat. Med.* **5,** 623–628.
143. Ishida, A., Fujita, N., Kitazawa, R., and Tsuruo, T. (2002) Transforming growth factor-beta induces expression of receptor activator of NF-kappa B ligand in vascular endothelial cells derived from bone. *J. Biol. Chem.* **277,** 26217–26224.
144. Collin-Osdoby, P., Rothe, L., Anderson, F., Nelson, M., Maloney, W., and Osdoby, P. (2001) Receptor activator of NF-kappa B and osteoprotegerin expression by human microvascular endothelial cells, regulation by inflammatory cytokines, and role in human osteoclastogenesis. *J. Biol. Chem.* **276,** 20659–20672.

24

Targeting the TGF-β Pathway In Vivo

Defining Complex Roles for TGF-β Signaling in Immune Function, Wound Healing, and Carcinogenesis

Lawrence Wolfraim, Mizuko Mamura, Anita Roberts, and John J. Letterio

1. Introduction

Transforming growth factor-β1 (TGF-β1) is a 25-kDa homodimeric peptide and the prototype in a family of structurally related but functionally distinct regulatory proteins. These TGF-β isoforms (TGF-β1, -β2, and -β3 in mammals) bear some structural relationship to a much larger family of peptide signaling molecules, with over 45 known members in this superfamily. The high degree of similarity that exists at the structural level among the isoforms of these growth factors is also accompanied by a significant overlap in function, as defined by many in vitro model systems. Moreover, the signaling pathway is not strictly linear in that there is extensive crosstalk with components of other signaling cascades (Fig. 1), with the TGF-βs typically influencing the manner in which cells interpret other signals in their environment. The evolution of more sophisticated functional genomics approaches has been instrumental in generating unique perspectives into the mechanisms governing the activity of the members of the TGF-β family. The studies outlined in this review serve to demonstrate how these models are more clearly defining the function of this pathway in immune homeostasis, wound healing, and carcinogenesis.

2. Models Targeting the TGF-β Pathway Define Its Important Role in Leukocyte Development and Function

Prior to gene targeting studies in mice, it was difficult to understand clearly the relevance of the complex and often contradictory effects of TGF-β on cells that make up the immune system. This cytokine has been implicated in regulating production and response to both pro- and antiinflammatory cytokines *(1–6)*, free radical production by macrophages *(7)*, the expression of adhesion molecules *(8)*, lymphocyte activation, proliferation, and effector function *(9–13)*, immunoglobulin production *(14,15)*, T-regulatory cell development and function *(16–19)*, and much more (reviewed in refs. *20* and *21*). Although the short survival of the *Tgf-β1*$^{-/-}$ mouse may have limited the use of this model to some extent *(22,23)*, numerous investigators are continuing the pursuit of novel phenotypes in this system and are demonstrating the importance of probing such models to uncover defects linked

From: *Contemporary Immunology: Cytokine Knockouts, 2nd Edition*
Edited by: Giamila Fantuzzi © Humana Press Inc., Totowa, NJ

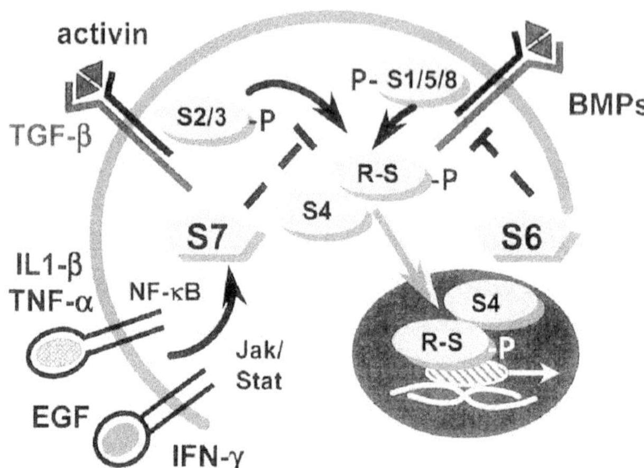

Fig. 1. The signaling pathways for the transforming growth factor-β (TGF-β) family members involve the ligand-induced activation of receptor heterotetramers composed of two type I and two type II receptors. These phosphorylate a class of receptor-activated Smad proteins (R-S), which may distinguish between superfamily ligands (2/3 for TGF-βs/activin; 1/5/8 for BMPs). There are inhibitory Smads (6 and 7) that competitively inhibit the phosphorylation of the receptor-activated Smads. Other cytokines and growth factors are known to modulate TGF-β responses. This cross-talk occurs at multiple levels, including the induction of the inhibitory Smad7 by proinflammatory cytokines such as tumor necrosis factor-α (TNF-α) and interferon-γ (IFN-γ), growth factors such as epidermal growth factor (EGF). IL-1-β, interleukin-1β; NF-κB, nuclear factor-κB.

to disrupted gene expression *(24)*. In addition, newer models directly targeting this pathway in specific leukocyte lineages are confirming many of the conclusions drawn from the *Tgf-β1*$^{-/-}$ mouse by generating phenocopies of this model (Fig. 2).

The mechanisms leading to the aggressive inflammatory syndrome of the *Tgf-β1*$^{-/-}$ mouse have not been clearly defined, but they may reflect the loss of important effects of TGF-β1 on cytokine production or T-cell differentiation (Th1/Th2 balance) *(21,25,26)*. Recent studies have implicated TGF-β and the receptor-activated Smad3 in regulating the expression and activity of key transcription factors involved in T-cell differentiation, *T-bet (26)* and *GATA3 (27,28)*. *Tgf-β1*$^{-/-}$ splenic T-cells activated in vitro and assayed for production of cytokines produce elevated Th2-type cytokines, including interleukin-4 (IL-4), IL-5, and IL-10, and it has been reported that *Tgf-β1*$^{-/-}$ mice have a 30-fold increase in serum IgE levels relative to littermate controls *(29)*. The balance between Th1 and Th2 subsets in *Tgf-β1*$^{-/-}$ mice has also been examined in a study of oral tolerance in this model *(30)*. The mechanisms mediating induction of lymphocyte anergy and tolerance to specific antigens are generally of interest because of their potential in the suppression of various pathologies associated with autoimmune disease *(31,32)*. The concept that tolerance induction at low doses of antigen might be mediated by TGF-β was tested by measuring the response to ovalbumin of lymphocytes isolated from *Tgf-β1*$^{-/-}$ mice, following oral administration of either low or high doses of the antigen for 3 d. The significant suppression of lymphocyte responsiveness detected in *Tgf-β1*$^{-/-}$ mice following both low and high doses of antigen suggests that this cytokine may not be required for induction of oral tolerance. Although enhanced expression of other isoforms of TGF-β is generally not observed

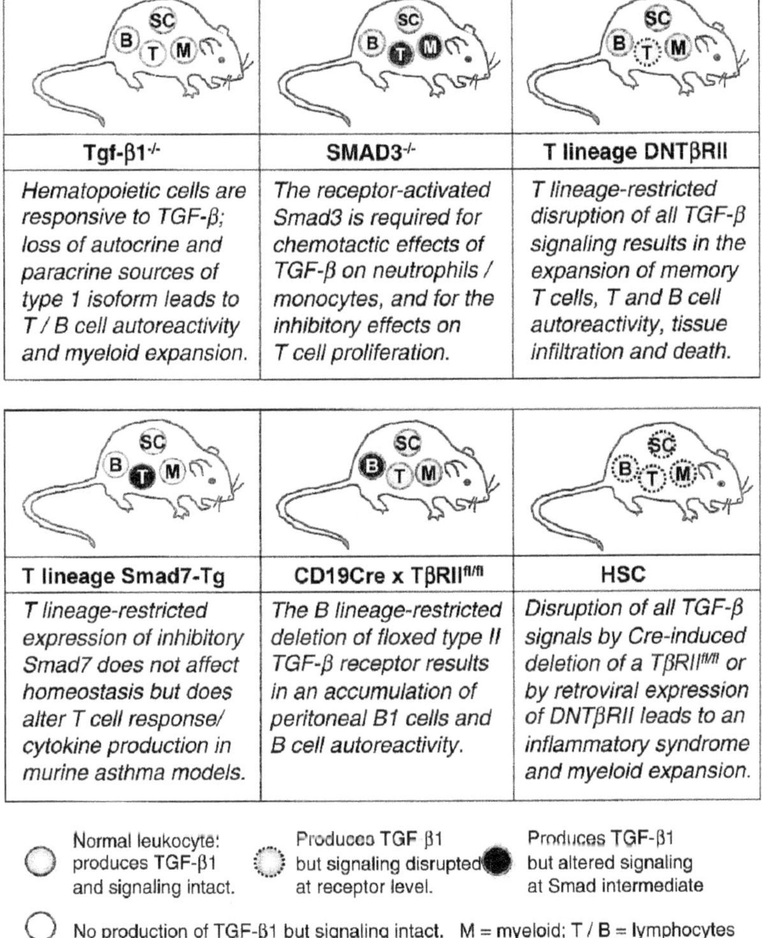

Fig. 2. Several distinct approaches have been taken to disrupt the transforming growth factor-β (TGF-β) pathway in mice. These range from global disruption of gene expression to overexpression of dominant-negative acting forms of TGF-β receptors. In many of these models, alterations in immune and hematopoietic function are prominent phenotypes.

in lymphocytes of *Tgf-β1*$^{-/-}$ mice, the possibility that local production of TGF-β2 or TGF-β3 may play a role in either of these models has not been directly addressed. Regardless, it is clear that other immunomodulators may be sufficient in the absence of the expression of TGF-β1 *(33)*.

Additional studies utilizing *Tgf-β1*$^{+/-}$ mice are demonstrating the existence of relevant gene dosage effects for this isoform with respect to T-cell differentiation and immune function in general. Serum and tissue levels of TGF-β1 protein are significantly reduced in *Tgf-β1*$^{+/-}$ mice, well beyond the 50% reduction that might be predicted by a strict gene dosage effect *(34)*. In an elegant study designed to assess the role of immune cell production of TGF-β1 in transplant arteriosclerosis, the development of intimal thickening was assessed in cardiac allografts placed into *Tgf-β1*$^{+/-}$ mice relative to that found in allografts of wild-type recipients *(35)*. Previous studies in this model system have delineated both the detrimental effects of Th1 subsets to graft survival and the ability of exogenous TGF-β1 to promote and extend graft survival. *Tgf-β1*$^{+/-}$ allograft recipients developed significantly more concentric intimal thickening and luminal occlusion. Intragraft cytokine expression analyses showed that *Tgf-β1*$^{+/-}$ recipients had elevated levels of signal transducer and activator of infection (STAT4), interferon-γ (IFN-γ), and IL-2, consistent with skewing toward a Th1 response, along with unaltered or reduced expression of indicators of Th2 type responses including STAT6, IL-4, and IL-10. The results not only highlight the role of immune sources of TGF-β1 in graft survival and in the attenuation of Th1 responses but also suggest the existence of significant gene dose effects for TGF-β1. This observation illustrates the utility of studies involving TGF-β1 heterozygotes and indicates that compromised polymorphic variants, should they exist for this isoform, might be linked to human susceptibility to specific disease complications.

TGF-β has also been implicated as a factor involved in the development and effector function of regulatory T-cells *(19)*, suggesting that either the loss or altered function of a population of regulatory cells might be a mechanism involved in the pathogenesis of the syndrome of the *Tgf-β1*$^{-/-}$ mouse. One such class of suppressor T-cells is characterized by their expression of CD4 and CD25 and by their ability to potently suppress the proliferation of CD25– T-cells in vitro and in vivo. The mechanisms by which these cells suppress autoimmune diseases in vivo are complex and not entirely clear. However, in vitro, these cells seem to require direct contact with their targets, as their activity has almost invariably been refractory to inhibition by addition of neutralizing anti-cytokine antibodies. The one notable exception has been TGF-β. In some laboratories, suppression of T-cell proliferation by a population of cells defined by CD4+/CD25+ coexpression has been reversible by the addition of high concentrations of an anti-TGF-β neutralizing antibody *(36)*. This controversy has recently been addressed using genetically engineered murine models that either lack expression of TGF-β1 or that, via mutation of the signaling pathway, have T-cells that do not respond to TGF-β. In these studies, *Tgf-β1*$^{-/-}$ T-cells clearly exhibit suppressor function that is indistinguishable from wild-type *(18)*. In addition, when responder T-cells are TGF-β-resistant (i.e., isolated either from mice expressing a dominant-negative TGF-β type II receptor or from Smad3$^{-/-}$ mice), the amount to which they are suppressed by CD4+/CD25+ is equal to that of the wild type. So one might concede that the use of these genetic models provides the most accurate information regarding the role of TGF-β in the function of this class of suppressors. In addition, although there is also in vitro evidence that exogenously added TGF-β can enhance the generation of CD4+/CD25+ T-cells, these cells are present in normal numbers in the *Tgf-β1*$^{-/-}$ mouse. It appears that *Tgf-β1*$^{-/-}$ CD4+/CD25+ T-cells can also function as suppressors in vivo. In adoptive transfer studies using *Tgf-β1*$^{-/-}$ mice as donors and *Tgf-β1*$^{+/+}$/Rag2$^{-/-}$ recipients, the depletion of CD25+ T-cells from whole spleen prior to transfer accelerates the progression of autoimmune manifestations of the the *Tgf-β1*$^{-/-}$ mouse (our unpublished observations). It is interesting to note that this occurs in a background in which there are normal serum and tissue levels of TGF-β1 in the recipients, further supporting the notion that the suppressor activity of these regulatory T-cells is TGF-β1-independent (or at the very least, independent of autocrine production of TGF-β1 by the CD4+/CD25+ T-cells).

Another important aspect of leukocyte biology that is regulated by TGF-β is the proliferation and differentiation of the uncommitted stem cell precursors and of myeloid progenitors. TGF-β is known to regulate the response of progenitors to stem cell factor (SCF) and to suppress expression of the SCF receptor c-kit, to inhibit cell cycle progression in committed progenitors, and to suppress in vitro colony formation in cytokine-supplemented suspension cultures *(37–40)*. Several initial observations made in the *Tgf-β1*$^{-/-}$ mouse suggested that these were significant roles for the endogenous ligand, including the presence of increased numbers of circulating granulocytes, monocytes, and platelets *(22,23)*. Many of these findings could be attributed to chronic exposure to proinflammatory cytokines, which are elevated in *Tgf-β1*$^{-/-}$ mice in immune-competent strains. The persistence of these abnormalities when the *Tgf-β1*$^{-/-}$ genotype is crossed into immune-deficient backgrounds suggests they are the direct result of a loss of the effects of TGF-β1 on hematopoietic precursors *(41)*. Beyond these initial observations, several new studies of isolated populations of cells from the *Tgf-β1*$^{-/-}$ mouse have also implicated autocrine production of TGF-β1 in regulation of hematopoietic progenitors.

Hematopoietic stem cell (HSC) lines derived from marrow of adult *Tgf-β1*$^{-/-}$ mice exhibit enhanced colony-forming efficiency in response to combinations of IL-3, IL-6, and granulocyte colony-stimulating factor (G-CSF), as well as spontaneous differentiation of progenitors into megakaryoctyes (unpublished observations). These findings have been corroborated by a new model system in which the TGF-β pathway is disrupted in hematopoietic progenitors transduced in vitro with a retroviral vector expressing a dominant negative-acting TGF-β type II receptor (TβRII) in a bicistronic vector with green-fluorescent protein (GFP) *(42)*. In mice reconstituted with the transduced HSCs, the bone marrow retains greater than 95% GFP+ cells at 6 mo, and ultimately the mice develop a severe myeloid hyperplasia and anemia. These mice also demonstrate a skewing of T-cells to a memory phenotype, but the myeloid expansion is the most dramatic phenotype and is responsible for their demise. In a similar model involving a Cre-recombinase-mediated deletion of a floxed TβRII allele, mice reconstituted *with TβRII*$^{-/-}$ HSCs go on to develop the aggressive autoimmune manifestations typical of the *Tgf-β1*$^{-/-}$, but no increase in proliferation or number of individual myeloid elements was described *(43)*. Ultimately, comparisons of the outcomes in models taking these distinct approaches will help to clarify the principle activities of TGF-β in the early HSCs and in their committed progenitors.

There are also models in which the T-cell-specific expression of a transgene that encodes a dominant-negative receptor (TβRII) or an inhibitory Smad (Smad7) *(44,45)* has again demonstrated the importance of the TGF-βs in controlling normal differentiation and function in lymphoid tissue. Expression of a kinase-defective TβRII in T-cells under the control of the CD2 promoter results in a progressive lymphoproliferative process characterized by diffuse vasculitis and expansion of CD8+ T-cells in the peripheral lymphoid tissue *(46)*. These T-cells uniformly exhibit a memory phenotype and in some develop abnormal ploidy and evolve into a leukemia-like syndrome that is responsible for early mortality within 3–4 mo of age. The outcome of this model supports observations made in studies of human lymphoid malignancies, in which mutations and loss of cell surface expression of TGF-β receptors occur in both T- and B-lymphoid tumors. By contrast, transgenic mice expressing a dominant negative TβRII under the control of a CD4 promoter (lacking the CD8 silencer) go on to develop an autoimmune process *(47)*. These mice survive beyond 5 mo of age and display many overlapping features with the *Tgf-β1*$^{-/-}$ mice, including perivascular infiltration of mononuclear cells in many organs, circulating autoantibodies, and immune complex deposition in renal glomeruli. The authors of this study also demonstrate that most T-lymphocytes in older CD4-dnTβRII mice spontaneously differentiate into type 1 or type 2 cytokine-secreting cells, with all CD8+ T-cells capable of producing IFN-γ and CD4+ T-cells secreting IFN-γ and/or IL-4 in vitro.

The results demonstrate the importance of TGF-β in maintaining tolerance in T-cells and, moreover, that maintenance of B-cell tolerance to self-antigens is dependent on normal TGF-β signaling in T-cells. In more recent studies, this model has been utilized to demonstrate the impact of T-cell suppression by TGF-β by showing an enhanced cytotoxic T-lymphocyte (CTL)-mediated eradication of tumors *(48)* and a more vigorous Th1 response to the intracellular parasite, *Leishmania major*, when T-cells are refractory to TGF-β *(26)*. Overall, the strategy of expression of a kinase-defective TβRII has been highly successful in unveiling the functions of this pathway in many tissues and physiologic processes *(49)*. The two studies highlighted here also demonstrate the impact of subtle differences in approach, as the choice of two distinct promoters, although restricted to the same lineage, may result in somewhat different phenotypes. Although the popularity of this transgenic approach may ultimately be diminished by the increasing availability of Cre-recombinase models involving tissue-specific conditional mutagenesis, these studies suggest that strategies aiming to inhibit TGF-β signaling in vivo may be clinically useful and that efforts to develop such an approach should continue.

Several studies have focused on the distributions and differentiated functions of mature leukocytes in the *Tgf-β1*$^{-/-}$ mouse, including dendritic cells and platelets. The epidermal dendritic cells, or Langerhans cells (LCs), are presumed to differentiate from a bone marrow-derived myeloid progenitor. In vitro studies of human LC development demonstrated a requirement for TGF-β1 in defined, serum-free conditions *(50,51)*. Analysis of the LC population of the *Tgf-β1*$^{-/-}$ mouse demonstrated their absence in the epidermis *(52)* but also showed that bone marrow progenitors from the *Tgf-β1*$^{-/-}$ mouse can efficiently reconstitute normal LC numbers in the epidermis of lethally irradiated, Ly5-disparate, wild-type recipients *(53)*. Moreover, in a "reverse" set of experiments, Thorbecke and colleagues showed that transfer of marrow progenitors from a *Tgf-β1*$^{+/-}$ SCID mouse is able to reconstitute epidermal LC in both γ-irradiated and -unirradiated *Tgf-β1*$^{-/-}$ SCID recipients *(54)*. In addition, migration of LC into the *Tgf-β1*$^{-/-}$ SCID epidermis could also be accomplished by local (but not systemic) delivery of either recombinant TGF-β1 or TGF-β2 in the epidermis. These data clearly demonstrate a role for both autocrine and paracrine sources of TGF-β in the normal differentiation or migration of LCs to the epidermis and suggest that local availability and activation of the cytokine are essential steps in regulating the activity of this cytokine. Lastly, recent studies of platelets isolated from *Tgf-β1*$^{-/-}$ mice have shown that they are defective in aggregation and that exogenous TGF-β1 can restore this function *(55)*. This result not only highlights the role of TGF-β in the differentiated functions of cells within the myeloid lineage but also indicates the presence of cellular response pathways triggered by extracellular TGF-β1 that do not require gene induction.

Thus, in summary, several different approaches have been utilized to disrupt the TGF-β pathway in mice, both globally and in a leukocyte-specific manner, from ligand to signaling intermediate. Several important conclusions can be drawn from this work. First, there are many similarities in phenotype between models involving a disruption in the expression of the type 1 isoform of TGF-β and disruption of signaling at the receptor level in T-cells. These results suggest that the autocrine production of TGF-β1 is in some manner contributing in a critical way to the homeostatic regulation of this population. A second point to be made is that disruption of a receptor-activated Smad3 and overexpression of the inhibitory Smad7 have yielded different phenotypes, each distinct from the ligand knockout and from models in which signaling is disrupted at the level of the receptor. Moreover, newer models in which the activity of the ligand is neutralized (by transgenic expression of soluble F_C receptors) lack an overt phenotype and suggest that either the autocrine function of the TGF-βs or a tight regulation of their activation and/or production may be critical in the way these cytokines work *(56)*. Thus, one can obviously see that the signaling mechanisms involved in mediating the effects of TGF-β1 on T-cells and other immune cells are complex and will require different approaches to define them clearly, including conditional deletion of other intermediates specifically in T-cells. Lastly, although the mechanisms that underlie the extensive inflammatory syndrome of the *Tgf-β1*$^{-/-}$ mouse may remain unresolved, carefully designed studies, including the use of *Tgf-β1*$^{+/-}$ mice and a variety of adoptive transfer models, have proven useful in answering specific questions regarding the role of TGF-β1 in governing specific immune responses.

3. New Insights into Tissue Repair Based on Knockouts of TGF-β1 and Smad3

The healing of a cutaneous wound involves a temporally defined series of events in which many different cell types participate within the context of a defined tissue architecture *(57)*. Processes include (1) the migration and proliferation of keratinocytes to reestablish the cutaneous barrier; (2) the influx of inflammatory cells, which not only produce other growth factors and cytokines involved in repair but also phagocytose bacteria and other debris in the wound bed; (3) the formation of new blood vessels (angiogenesis); and (4) the recruitment of fibroblasts to deposit and remodel the extracellular matrix to give the wound strength. Not only are all these cellular processes regulated by TGF-β, but TGF-β1 is also a key cytokine released from the α-granules of platelets that contributes to the fibrin clot formed after wounding *(58)*.

It was shown almost 20 years ago that TGF-β had profound effects on the formation of granulation tissue. Injection of TGF-β into Hunt-Schilling wire mesh chambers resulted in the formation of new blood vessels and the deposition of collagen by fibroblasts that invaded the surrounding connective tissue *(59)*. Subsequent studies involving the injection of TGF-β subcutaneously into newborn mice again demonstrated the ability of this growth factor to stimulate formation of granulation tissue, even in the absence of wounding *(60)*. These studies clearly demonstrated that exogenous TGF-β could, either directly or indirectly, stimulate recruitment of inflammatory cells, the production of extracellular matrix and the formation of new blood vessels. Subsequently, many studies involving the topical application of exogenous TGF-β directly to the wound at the time of wounding showed that it could enhance the response in models of impaired healing including those in diabetic animals, aged animals, or animals treated with chemotherapy *(58)*.

Although clearly demonstrating that ectopic TGF-β might have therapeutic activity if applied to wounds, these studies did not address the effects of endogenous TGF-β as it might be activated from the platelet releasate, or produced by cells constituting the granulation tissue and including especially fibroblasts and macrophages. This has now been addressed using mice in which either the ligand, TGF-β1 *(22)*, or one of its key signaling intermediates, Smad3 *(61)*, have been knocked out, and the results have been somewhat surprising. Given that mice lacking the TGF-β1 gene have no TGF-β in their platelets, nor can any of the cells involved in the repair process express TGF-β1, it was expected that wound repair would be retarded or severely compromised. Indeed, studies of healing of cutaneous wounds made in 10-d-old *Tgf-β1*$^{-/-}$ mice showed reduced formation of granulation tissue, vascularity, and collagen deposition *(62)*. These wounds, which were covered with an occlusive dressing also showed reduced epithelization, but interpretation was confounded by the severe inflammatory and wasting phenotype of the mice. Other studies in *Tgf-β1*$^{-/-}$ mice wounded at 30 d of age and maintained on rapamycin to suppress the inflammatory phenotype showed strongly accelerated epithelial covering of wounds, again with reduced amounts of granulation tissue *(63)*. This positive effect on reepithelization was confirmed in *Tgf-β1*$^{-/-}$ mice on a background lacking the cyclin-dependent kinase inhibitor, p21^{Cip1}, in which many of the effects of the *Tgf-β1*$^{-/-}$ phenotype are suppressed *(63)*.

In contrast to these results, large excisional wounds made in *Tgf-β1*$^{-/-}$ mice lacking T- and B-lymphocytes (*Tgf-β1*$^{-/-}$/*Scid*$^{-/-}$) and covered with an occlusive dressing showed an unexpected delay in all phases of wound healing including closure, influx of inflammatory cells, proliferation, and maturation compared with *Tgf-β1*$^{+/+}$/*Scid*$^{-/-}$ mice *(64)*. These results have been interpreted to suggest that lymphocytes and TGF-β1 might play an early, redundant role in initiating wound healing and, further, that altered expression patterns of the other TGF-β isoforms, TGF-β2 and TGF-β3, may also contribute.

Targeted disruption of the TGF-β-activin signaling intermediate Smad3 has provided yet another opportunity to examine the role of this particular pathway in wound healing. Signals from TGF-β receptors are transduced through many downstream pathways including those of the mitogen-activated protein kinase (MAPK) family, phosphatidylinositol 3-kinase (PI3K), and the Smad pathway *(65)*. The latter involves Smad2 and Smad3, each of which are phosphorylated directly by TGF-β and activin receptors, but which clearly have distinct gene targets *(66)*. Study of the healing of cutaneous wounds made in *SMAD3*$^{Exon8-/-}$ mice suggests that the Smad3 pathway is key in mediating effects of TGF-β in tissue repair. There is a strong overlap with features of wound healing in the *Tgf-β1*$^{-/-}$ mice, yet the effects are more dramatic in *SMAD3*$^{Exon8-/-}$ mice since signaling of *all* isoforms of TGF-β as well as activin is restricted by loss of this pathway. Most prominent are the striking acceleration of epithelialization and the reduction of the influx of inflammatory cells *(67)*. This latter effect is probably based on the observation that Smad3 is required for chemotaxis of neutrophils *(61)* and macrophages *(67)* to TGF-β. We have shown that chemotaxis of keratinocytes and fibroblasts to TGF-β is also impaired by loss of Smad3, the latter underlying the reduced numbers of myofibroblasts found in the wound bed *(68)*. Wound strength is reduced in *SMAD3*$^{Exon8-/-}$ mice *(68)*, probably as a result of the reduced levels of TGF-β in the wound bed, the resultant reduced cellularity, and the decreased production of matrix proteins, such as the interstitial collagens, which are Smad3-dependent (Fig. 3) *(69)*. An interesting therapeutic opportunity arises from these studies in that induction of expression of some matrix proteins by TGF-β, particularly fibronection, has been shown to be independent of the Smad pathway *(70)*. Thus the use of a putative inhibitor of Smad3 signaling together with TGF-β may present a particularly efficacious approach to enhancing both epithelialization and matrix deposition in wounds *(71)*.

In summary, although exogenous TGF-β has beneficial effects when applied topically to a wound, endogenous TGF-β inhibits reepithelialization of cutaneous wounds but is required to recruit inflammatory cells and fibroblasts into the wound bed and to promote vigorous deposition of matrix proteins, which impart strength to the wound. Understanding these distinct effects of TGF-β on the different cellular components involved in wound healing should aid in the rational design of new approaches to treatment of chronic wounds.

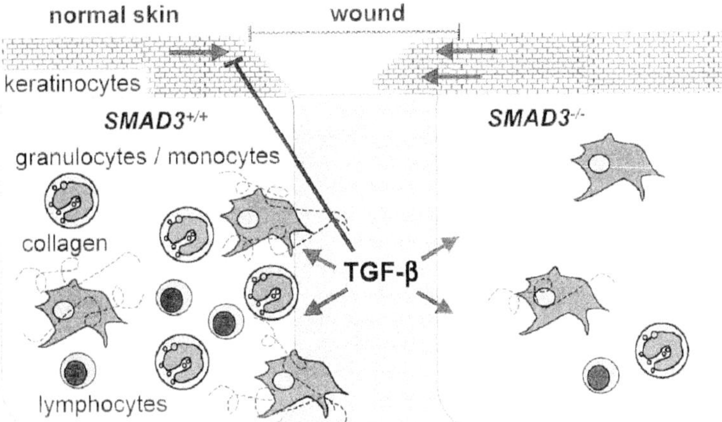

Fig. 3. In the normal sequence of wound repair and tissue regeneration, transforming growth factor-β (TGF-β) released from platelets at the site of a wound will stimulate the chemotaxis of immune cells (monocytes, granulocytes, lymphocytes) and fibroblasts that participate in the resolution of the injury. It also is important for the induction of collagen but is inhibitory to reepithelialization. Studies in the *Smad3*$^{-/-}$ mouse have demonstrated that these events are all dependent on Smad3 expression and have suggested the potential therapeutic benefit of inhibitors of Smad3 in preventing fibrosis and in accelerating reepithelialization of wounds.

4. Carcinogenesis: Lessons Learned from Mice Deficient for TGF-β or Components of the TGF-β Signaling Pathway

The roles played by TGF-β in carcinogenesis are complex (Fig. 4). During the earliest stages, TGF-β acts principally as a tumor suppressor. However, during later stages of malignant progression, production of bioactive TGF-β by the tumor cell is common and can aid tumor growth and metastasis through its immunosuppressive properties and proangiogenic effects. By this time, most tumors have become refractory to the growth-inhibitory effects of the cytokine, often through mechanisms involving the downregulation of expression of TGF-β receptors at the cell surface.

Although disruption of the *Tgf-β1* gene in mice is compatible with only limited survival beyond the neonatal period, this model has still proved useful in examining the role of this ligand in the process of carcinogenesis. Indeed, studies in *Tgf-β1*$^{+/-}$ mice have demonstrated that homozygous deletion of *Tgf-β1* is not required to confer increased risk of tumorigenesis. *Tgf-β1*$^{+/-}$ mice are grossly indistinguishable from their wild-type littermates but show enhanced tumorigenesis following treatment with chemical carcinogens *(34)*. After 9 mo of study, mice heterozygous for the null *Tgf-β1* allele presented with larger tumors, increased multiplicity of tumors, and more tumors exhibiting malignant features. Whereas mRNA levels in the heterozygous mice were roughly 50% those seen in wild-type mice, levels of TGF-β1 protein were much lower than would be predicted from a simple gene dosage relationship. Levels of TGF-β1 protein in *Tgf-β1*$^{+/-}$ mice were only 11% of normal in serum and 30% of normal in liver. Levels of TGF-β2 and TGF-β3 were not significantly changed in *Tgf-β1*$^{+/-}$ mice and are therefore unlikely to compensate for reduced levels of TGF-β1. Classical tumor suppressor genes typically exhibit loss of hetero-

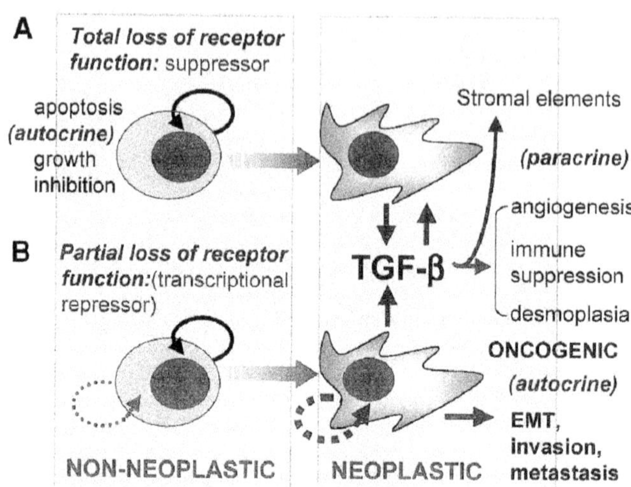

Fig. 4. The transforming growth factor-β (TGF-β) pathway exhibits both tumor-suppressor and tumor-promoting properties, displaying a complex mode of activity in the process of tumorigenesis. In most normal, nonneoplastic tissues, TGF-β can suppress the proliferation of most cell lineages and often induces apoptosis. In transformed cells, total loss of TGF-β receptor expression eliminates these responses in the tumor cell, which often also acquires the capacity to express TGF-β and thereby stimulate events such as matrix production, angiogenesis, and immune suppression, all of which promote tumor progression. If the loss of a TGF-β response is only partial, there may be more prominent effects on differentiation, as is the case with v-*ras*-transformed epithelial cells, in which the apoptotic effects of TGF-β are lost, while the ability to promote epithelial-to-mesenchymal transition (EMT) is observed.

zygosity (LOH) such that the remaining wild-type allele is lost. Interestingly, tumors from *Tgf-β1*$^{+/-}$ mice did not show loss of the remaining wild-type *Tgf-β1* allele, and in fact both TGF-β1 mRNA and protein were clearly detectable in all tumors. Moreover, immunohistochemical analysis of tumors reveals that TGF-β1 protein was even upregulated beyond the expression found in adjacent normal tissue. TGF-β1 is thereby the prototype in a novel class of tumor suppressor genes that show true haploid insufficiency in their ability to protect against tumorigenesis.

The persistent expression of TGF-β1 from the remaining wild-type allele in this model reflects the complex dual role of TGF-β1 in tumorigenesis and supports the notion that this factor exhibits a pro-oncogenic role at later stages of tumorigenesis, at a time when the malignant cell has escaped the growth-suppressive effects of this cytokine. The authors of this study proposed that if the effective threshold dose is lower for oncogenic than for tumor suppressor activities, any additional proliferative advantage gained by the tumor through loss of the remaining wild-type allele in a *Tgf-β1*$^{+/-}$ mouse would be offset by the generation of a less permissive stroma. This idea would be consistent with the results of xenograph experiments using v-*ras*^{Ha}-initiated kerationcytes described earlier in which *Tgf-β1*$^{-/-}$ stroma is less effective in supporting tumor growth *(72)*. In this elegant series of experiments using a skin grafting model system, Glick and colleagues *(73)* showed that autocrine and paracrine TGF-β1 have opposing effects on tumor cell proliferation. Keratinocytes with a targeted deletion of the *Tgf-β1* gene were initiated in vitro using oncogenic v-*ras*^{Ha}, grafted onto athymic mice, in combination with either wild-type or *Tgf-β1*$^{-/-}$ dermal fibroblasts as stroma, and assessed for their tumorigenic properties. Sixty percent of grafts using *Tgf-β1*$^{-/-}$ keratinocytes rapidly progressed to multifocal squamous cell carcinomas. The remainder formed dysplastic papillomas. The multifocal nature of these lesions indicated that malignant conversion was occurring independently in multiple cells throughout the tumor. None of the grafts using wild-type, initiated keratinocytes produced squamous cell carcinoma but instead formed benign, well-differentiated papillomas.

These studies suggest that loss of autocrine TGF-β1 increases the rate and incidence of premalignant progression and malignant conversion. Interestingly, malignant progression was not associated with loss of responsiveness to TGF-β1. The tumor cell labeling index was higher in grafts using initiated *Tgf-β1*$^{-/-}$ keratinocytes than in those using initiated wild-type or *Tgf-β1*$^{+/-}$ cells when grafted onto wild-type fibroblasts. In contrast, the labeling index of all tumors was diminished when *Tgf-β1*$^{-/-}$ fibroblasts were used to form the stroma. Therefore, whereas autocrine TGF-β1 suppresses malignant conversion, paracrine TGF-β1 from stromal fibroblasts enhances tumor cell proliferation, without influencing conversion. The authors demonstrate that whereas normal *Tgf-β1*$^{-/-}$ keratinocytes sequester paracrine TGF-β1 from the stroma and are growth-suppressed, tumor cells, regardless of genotype, do not sequester paracrine TGF-β1 and are consequently not growth-suppressed. Thus, paracrine sources of TGF-β1 cannot suppress the effect (malignant conversion) of genotypic loss of autocrine TGF-β1. This is probably not because of lesions in the TGF-β1 signaling pathway, as cells cultured from these tumors respond to exogenous TGF-β1. These studies elegantly illustrate that the influence of TGF-β1 in carcinogenesis differs depending on the particular compartment in which the ligand is expressed and that there are distinct roles for autocrine versus paracrine TGF-β.

Another approach that has proved successful in uncovering tumor suppressor activity of the type 1 isoform involves the intercross of the *Tgf-β1*$^{-/-}$ mouse with immune deficient strains. Re-deriving the *Tgf-β1*$^{-/-}$ mice onto a *Rag2*$^{-/-}$ mixed strain (129S6 × CF-1) background, which lacks both B- and T-cells, extended the survival of these mice into adulthood *(74)*. In the original report of this model, the *Tgf-β1*$^{+/+}$/*Rag2*$^{-/-}$ mice develop an inflammation-associated hyperplasia of the cecum and colon soon after weaning that does not progress to frank carcinoma. Crypt organization is unaltered. However, *Tgf-β1*$^{-/-}$/*Rag2*$^{-/-}$ mice developed severe hyperplasia that progressed to multiple adenomas and nonmetastatic carcinomas of the cecum and colon by 5 mo of age with 100% penetrance. Adenomatous growth was associated with a profound expansion of the mucosal layer and moderate loss of mucosal architecture. Carcinomas exhibited significant loss of mucosal architecture, stratification of the crypt epithelium, and nuclear atypia.

This study also demonstrated a clear gene dosage effect of TGF-β1 in that there is an inverse correlation between *Tgf-β1* gene dosage and the frequency of transition of hyperplasia to adenoma and carcinoma. Only 20% of *Tgf-β1*$^{+/+}$/*Rag2*$^{-/-}$ mice developed carcinoma, whereas malignant conversion was present in 43% of the *Tgf-β1*$^{+/-}$/*Rag2*$^{-/-}$ mice, a rate intermediate between wild-type and *Tgf-β1*$^{-/-}$ mice. Surprisingly, there was no difference in either the rates of proliferation or cell death among the different genotypes, suggesting that the initiation of dysplasia in *Tgf-β1*$^{-/-}$/*Rag2*$^{-/-}$ mice is owing to an event distinct from excessive cell proliferation. In addition, no differences in inflammation, microsatellite instability, or cellular distribution of β-catenin were found. These results suggest that TGF-β1 suppresses intestinal carcinogenesis in these mice by maintaining mucosal architecture after cell proliferation has been initiated, rather than through effects on epithelial cell proliferation, granulocyte-mediated inflammation, or genetic stability.

On the contrary, there is evidence to suggest that autocrine expression of TGF-β1 is important for maintaining genomic stability, including data from studies involving keratinocyte cell lines derived from *Tgf-β1*$^{-/-}$ mice. In this in vitro model, TGF-β1 suppresses genomic instability associated with gene amplification in response to treatment with the drug *N*-phosphonoacetyl-L-aspartate (PALA) *(75)*. PALA, which mediates G1 growth arrest in wild-type cells, does not trigger arrest in *Tgf-β1*$^{-/-}$ keratinocytes, in spite of the presence of functional p53. Exogenous TGF-β1 suppressed gene amplification in cultures of *Tgf-β1*$^{-/-}$ keratinocytes at doses that did not lead to growth arrest. This ability to suppress genomic instability was independent of pRb or p53 status or G1 growth arrest but was dependent on the presence of an intact TβRII.

In contrast to the results of targeting the individual isoforms of TGF-β, global deletion of TβRII uniformly results in a more severe embryonic phenotype, with lethality in all homozygous null embryos at d 10.5 of gestation *(76)*. Death is the result of defective yolk sac hematopoiesis and vasculogenesis. Mice that are heterozygous for the null allele (*TβRII*$^{+/-}$) are viable and, similar to the *Tgf-β1*$^{+/-}$ mice, have been assessed for their susceptibility to tumorigenesis. There is no increase in the incidence of spontaneous tumorigenesis in *TβRII*$^{+/-}$ mice. However, *TβRII*$^{+/-}$ mice exhibit an enhanced susceptibility to hepatocellular carcinomas following treatment with the chemical carcinogen diethylnitrosamine (DEN) *(77)*. Animals treated with a single initiating dose of the drug at 15 d of age show a significantly increased incidence of neoplastic lesions in the liver compared with wild-type littermates without evidence of metastatic disease. *TβRII*$^{+/-}$ hepatocytes displayed a reduced sensitivity to exogenous TGF-β1 and a mild increase in the proliferation index as assessed by bromodeoxyuridine incorporation. Exposure to carcinogen may have resulted in the loss of the remaining wild-type allele, although this possibility was not directly examined in this study. However, the finding of positive immunohistochemical staining for TβRII in *TβRII*$^{+/-}$ tumors suggests that the retained allele is not silenced. Therefore, a reduction in gene dosage for either the type 1 TGF-β isoform or for a key component of the signaling complex results in an increased susceptibility to tumorigenesis, and each serves as an example of a haploinsufficient tumor suppressor. The relevance of these observations in mice is suggested by the demonstration that loss of expression of the TGF-β type II receptor occurs in pancreatic cancer, colon cancer associated with microsatellite instability, gastric cancers, and gliomas. However, TβRII appears to behave more like a classic tumor suppressor in humans in that LOH is frequently observed in these tumors.

Mutations in genes encoding distal components of the signaling pathway have also been associated with human cancer. Mutations in the *SMAD4* (DPC4) gene are associated with pancreatic and colorectal cancer in humans. Loss of heterozygosity and mutations in the *SMAD4* gene have been reported in invasive and metastatic carcinomas *(78)*. A subset of juvenile polyposis patients has been reported to harbor germline mutations in the *SMAD4* gene *(79,80)*. In mice, homozygous deletion of *SMAD4* is embryonic lethal. *SMAD4*$^{+/-}$ mice are viable and fertile and have been used in tumorigenesis studies. *SMAD4*$^{+/-}$ mice spontaneously developed multiple gastric polyps beyond 1 yr of age *(81)*. According to this study, LOH at the *SMAD4* locus was one of the earliest events in polyp formation, perhaps the triggering event for the formation of both gastric and duodenal polyps. Interestingly, neither *SMAD4*$^{+/-}$ mice nor compound heterozygous mice (*smad4*$^{+/-}$/*Apc*^{D716}) develop pancreatic tumors—a surprising finding given that *SMAD4* is homozygously inactivated in roughly 50% of pancreatic cancers in humans *(82)*. The authors of this study did not look at susceptibility to chemically induced tumors. The gastric and duodenal polyps that developed in these mice were similar in morphology to human juvenile polyps. One obvious difference, the greater relative latency in the mouse model, may indicate the need for other cooperating oncogenic events in the mouse.

In humans, *SMAD2*, like *SMAD4*, is located on chromosome 18q21, a region that is frequently altered in a number of tumors including pancreatic, colorectal, breast, and head and neck carcinomas *(83)*. Mice that lack Smad2 die around embryonic d 8.5 (E8.5) as a result of a failure to undergo egg cylinder elongation, gastrulation, and mesoderm induction *(84)*. The embryonic lethality of a *SMAD2* deletion has precluded a study of the role it may play in suppression of tumorigenesis in vivo. *SMAD2*$^{+/-}$ mice are phenotypically normal and exhibit growth rates and litter sizes comparable to those of their wild-type littermates. In one study in which these mice were followed during a 9-mo study period, the *SMAD2* heterozygotes did not show an accelerated rate of spontaneous tumorigenesis. No chemical mutagenesis studies have been reported thus far.

The other receptor-activated Smad in the TGF-β pathway, Smad3, has been targeted in three distinct mouse models *(61,85,86)*. Of these, only one group *(85)* has reported an enhanced development of tumors. In this report, mice that were homozygous for the *SMAD3* null allele spontaneously developed metastatic colorectal adenocarcinomas beyond 18 mo of age. Multiple lesions were found exclusively in the large intestine and were deeply invasive. The penetrance of this phenotype was 100% on an inbred SvEv129 background but declined to 30% on a mixed background of Sv127 × BL/6. These tumors continue to express adenomatous polyposis coli (APC), suggesting that inactivation of the β-catenin/APC pathway is not a prerequisite for the development of these tumors. Lymph nodes were reportedly frequently enlarged and showed evidence of infiltration by carcinoma. However, in a more recent study that combined this particular *SMAD3* deletion with a disruption of the cdk inhibitor, p27^{Kip1}, there was no evidence for metastasis, and loss of either one or both alleles of p27^{Kip1} had no effect on the frequency or spectrum of tumors in the *SMAD3*$^{-/-}$ mice *(87)*. Neither of these studies described analysis for LOH at the remaining *SMAD3* allele.

To date, no mutations in *SMAD3* have been reported in human colorectal tumors. In addition, the absence of true colorectal cancers in the two additional *SMAD3*$^{-/-}$ models developed independently with distinct constructs calls into question the validity of this earlier study. It is noteworthy that in the study by Zhu et al. *(85)*, the gene targeting strategy employed results in the generation of a truncated 77-amino acid peptide. Although the authors of this study made some attempt to rule out the possibility that this peptide had residual Smad activity, it remains possible that this null allele may be hypomorphic or neomorphic *(88)*. Recent evidence suggests that infection of mice with the gut pathogen *Helicobacter pylori* leads to the development of gastric adenocarcinomas in mice in which the TGF-β signaling pathway has been disrupted through expression of a dominant negative TβRII receptor (dnTβRII) *(89)*. The inflammation that ensues following infection may tip the balance toward malignant progression in the absence of TGF-β signaling. Although the precise role of this gut pathogen in gastric carcinogenesis remains a topic of active debate, it is worth noting that the World Health Organization International Agency for Research on Cancer (WHO-IARC) defines *H. pylori* infection as a class I carcinogen *(89)*. If the mice generated by Zhu et al. were infected with the common murine pathogen *H. hepaticus*, whereas the other two colonies of mice were *Helicobacter*-negative, this could explain why the former mice developed colon adenocarcimonas. This hypothesis is currently being tested in our laboratory using *Smad3*-deficient mice, rederived onto a pure SvEv129 background and infected with *H. pylori*.

In summary, evidence from studies using mice deficient for *Tgf-β1* and various components of the TGF-β signaling pathway indicate that a disruption at various levels of this signaling pathway can increase the risk of tumorigenesis. At least two of the components of this pathway, the TGF-β1 ligand and the type II receptor, exhibit true haploinsufficiency as tumor suppressors.

5. Conclusions

The studies presented in this review, involving murine models with altered TGF-β expression/signaling, are raising new questions regarding the role of these peptide signaling molecules in processes such as wound healing and the immune response. Given the vast array of overlapping activities that has been demonstrated for the TGF-β family ligands, the application of these more modern in vivo tests of function has proved valuable for determining the essential functions of the TGF-βs and their signaling pathway in normal physiology and disease pathogenesis. These models have helped to define the specific and nonredundant activities of the individual isoforms in the context of the environments in which cells respond to them in vivo. Newer strategies involving conditional or inducible disruption of gene expression will be needed to overcome the global embryonic lethality associated with disruption of most TGF-β pathway intermediates. The major goal for continuing these studies should be to learn how to apply these soluble signaling peptides (or their antagonists) to modulate hematopoietic and immune function in settings in which defects in these processes underlie disease pathogenesis and to define how such agents might augment wound repair and tissue regeneration and enhance therapeutic attempts at immune-mediated eradication of tumors.

References

1. Barral-Netto, M., Barral, A., Brownell, C. E., et al. (1992) Transforming growth factor-beta in leishmanial infection: a parasite escape mechanism. *Science* **257,** 545–548.
2. Strober, W., Kelsall, B., Fuss, I., et al. (1997) Reciprocal IFN-gamma and TGF-β responses regulate the occurrence of mucosal inflammation. *Immunol. Today* **18,** 61–64.
3. Tang, J., Nuccie, B. L., Ritterman, I., Liesveld, J. L., Abboud, C. N., and Ryan, D. H. (1997) TGF-β down-regulates stromal IL-7 secretion and inhibits proliferation of human B cell precursors. *J. Immunol.* **159,** 117–125.
4. Espevik, T., Waage, A., Faxvaag, A., and Shalaby, M. R. (1990) Regulation of interleukin-2 and interleukin-6 production from T cells: involvement of interleukin-1 beta and transforming growth factor-beta. *Cell Immunol.* **126,** 47–56.
5. Fargeas, C., Wu, C. Y., Nakajima, T., Cox, D., Nutman, T., and Delespesse, G. (1992) Differential effect of transforming growth factor beta on the synthesis of Th1- and Th2-like lymphokines by human T lymphocytes. *Eur. J. Immunol.* **22,** 2173–2176.
6. Wahl, S. M. (1992) Transforming growth factor beta (TGF-β) in inflammation: a cause and a cure. *J. Clin. Immunol.* **12,** 61–74.
7. Bogdan, C. and Nathan, C. (1993) Modulation of macrophage function by transforming growth factor beta, interleukin-4, and interleukin-10. *Ann. NY Acad. Sci.* **685,** 713–739.

8. Riedl, E., Stockl, J., Majdic, O., et al. (2000) Functional involvement of E-cadherin in TGF-beta 1-induced cell cluster formation of in vitro developing human Langerhans-type dendritic cells. *J. Immunol.* **165,** 1381–1386.
9. Kehrl, J. H., Wakefield, L. M., Roberts, A. B., et al. (1986) Production of transforming growth factor beta by human T lymphocytes and its potential role in the regulation of T cell growth. *J. Exp. Med.* **163,** 1037–1050.
10. Swain, S. L., Huston, G., Tonkonogy, S., and Weinberg, A. (1991) Transforming growth factor-beta and IL-4 cause helper T cell precursors to develop into distinct effector helper cells that differ in lymphokine secretion pattern and cell surface phenotype. *J. Immunol.* **147,** 2991–3000.
11. Ahuja, S. S., Paliogianni, F., Yamada, H., Balow, J. E., and Boumpas, D. T. (1993) Effect of transforming growth factor-beta on early and late activation events in human T cells. *J. Immunol.* **150,** 3109–3118.
12. Cerwenka, A., Bevec, D., Majdic, O., Knapp, W., and Holter, W. (1994) TGF-β 1 is a potent inducer of human effector T cells. *J. Immunol.* **153,** 4367–4377.
13. Cerwenka, A., Kovar, H., Majdic, O., and Holter, W. (1996) Fas- and activation-induced apoptosis are reduced in human T cells preactivated in the presence of TGF-β1. *J. Immunol.* **156,** 459–464.
14. Kehrl, J. H., Roberts, A. B., Wakefield, L. M., et al. (1986) Transforming growth factor beta is an important immunomodulatory protein for human B lymphocytes. *J. Immunol.* **137,** 3855–3860.
15. Coffman, R. L., Lebman, D. A., and Shrader, B. (1989) Transforming growth factor beta specifcally enhances IgA production by lipopolysaccharide-stimulated murine B lymphocytes. *J. Exp. Med.* **170,** 1039–1044.
16. Annunziato, F., Comi, L., Liotta, F., et al. (2002) Phenotype, localization, and mechanism of suppression of $CD4^+CD25^+$ human thymocytes. *J. Exp. Med.* **196,** 379–387.
17. Yamagiwa, S., Gray, J. D., Hashimoto, S., and Horwitz, D. A. (2001) A role for TGF-β in the generation and expansion of $CD4^+$ $CD25^+$ regulatory T cells from human peripheral blood. *J. Immunol.* **166,** 7282–7289.
18. Piccirillo, C. A., Letterio, J. J., Thornton, A. M., et al. (2002) CD4(+)CD25(+) Regulatory T cells can mediate suppressor function in the absence of transforming growth factor beta1 production and responsiveness. *J. Exp. Med.* **196,** 237–246.
19. Shevach, E. M. (2002) CD4+ CD25+ suppressor T cells: more questions than answers. *Nat. Rev. Immunol.* **2,** 389–400.
20. Letterio, J. J. and Roberts, A. B. (1998) Regulation of immune responses by TGF-β. *Annu. Rev. Immunol.* **16,** 137–161.
21. Gorelik, L. and Flavell, R. A. (2002) Transforming growth factor-β in T-cell biology. *Nat. Immunol. Rev.* **2,** 46–53.
22. Kulkarni, A. B, Huh, C. G., Becker, D., et al. (1993) Transforming growth factor beta 1 null mutation in mice causes excessive inflammatory response and early death. *Proc. Natl. Acad. Sci. USA* **90,** 770–774.
23. Shull, M. M., Ormsby, I., Kier, A. B., et al. (1992) Targeted disruption of the mouse transforming growth factor-beta 1 gene results in multifocal inflammatory disease. *Nature* **359,** 693–699.
24. Doetschman, T. (1999) Interpretation of phenotype in genetically engineered mice. *Lab. Anim. Sci.* **49,** 137–143.
25. Blokzijl, A., ten Dijke, P., and Ibanez, C. (2002) Physical and functional interaction between GATA-3 and Smad3 allows TGF-β regulation of GATA target genes. *Curr. Biol.* **12,** 35–45.
26. Gorelik, L., Constant, S., and Flavell, R. A. (2002) Mechanism of transforming growth factor-β-induced inhibition of T helper type 1 differentiation. *J. Exp. Med.* **195,** 1499–1505.
27. Gorelik, L., Fields, P. E., and Flavell, R. A. (2000) Cutting edge: TGF-β inhibits Th type 2 development through inhibition of GATA-3 expression. *J. Immunol.* **165,** 4773–4777.
28. Heath, V. L., Murphy, E. E., Crain, C., Tomlinson, M. G., and O'Garra, A. (2000) TGF-β1 down-regulates Th2 development and results in decreased IL-4-induced STAT6 activation and GATA-3 expression. *Eur. J. Immunol.* **30,** 2639–2649.
29. van Ginkel, F. W., Wahl, S. M., Kearney, J. F., et al. (1999) Partial IgA-deficiency with increased Th2-type cytokines in TGF-beta 1 knockout mice. *J. Immunol.* **163,** 1951–1957.
30. Barone, K. S., Tolarova, D. D., Ormsby, I., Doetschman, T., and Michael, J. G. (1998) Induction of oral tolerance in TGF-beta 1 null mice. *J. Immunol.* **161,** 154–160.

31. Fukaura, H., Kent, S. C., Pietrusewicz, M. J., Khoury, S. J., Weiner, H. L., and Hafler, D. A. (1996) Induction of circulating myelin basic protein and proteolipid protein-specific transforming growth factor-beta1-secreting Th3 T cells by oral administration of myelin in multiple sclerosis patients. *J. Clin. Invest.* **98,** 70–77.
32. Chen, Y., Kuchroo, V. K., Inobe, J., Hafler, D. A., and Weiner, H. L. (1994) Regulatory T cell clones induced by oral tolerance: suppression of autoimmune encephalomyelitis. *Science* **265,** 1237–1240.
33. Rizzo, L. V., Morawetz, R. A., Miller-Rivero, N. E., et al. (1999) IL-4 and IL-10 are both required for the induction of oral tolerance. *J. Immunol.* **162,** 2613–2622.
34. Tang, B., Bottinger, E. P., Jakowlew, S. B., et al. (1998) Transforming growth factor-beta1 is a new form of tumor suppressor with true haploid insufficiency. *Nat. Med.* **4,** 802–807.
35. Koglin, J., Glysing-Jensen, T., Raisanen-Sokolowski, A., and Russell, M. E. (1998) Immune sources of transforming growth factor-beta1 reduce transplant arteriosclerosis: insight derived from a knockout mouse model. *Circ. Res.* **83,** 652–660.
36. Nakamura, K., Kitani, A., and Strober, W. (2001). Cell contact-dependent immunosuppression by CD4+ CD25+ regulatory T cells is mediated by cell surface-bound transforming growth factor beta. *J. Exp. Med.* **194,** 629–644.
37. Fortunel, N., Hatzfeld, J., Kisselev, S., et al. (2000). Release from quiescence of primitive human hematopoietic stem/progenitor cells by blocking their cell-surface TGF-β type II receptor in a short-term in vitro assay. *Stem Cells* **18,** 102–111.
38. Fortunel, N. O., Hatzfeld, A., and Hatzfeld, J. A. (2000). Transforming growth factor-β: pleiotropic role in the regulation of hematopoiesis. *Blood* **96,** 2022–2036.
39. Keller, J. R., McNiece, I. K., Sill, K. T., et al. (1990) Transforming growth factor β directly regulates primitive murine hematopoietic cell proliferation. *Blood* **75,** 596–602.
40. Soma, T., Yu, J. M., and Dunbar, C. E. (1996) Maintenance of murine long-term repopulating stem cells in ex vivo culture is affected by modulation of transforming growth factor-β but not macrophage inflammatory protein-1α activities. *Blood* **87,** 4561–4567.
41. Letterio, J. J., Geiser, A. G., Kulkarni, A. B., et al. (1996) Autoimmunity associated with TGF-β1-deficiency in mice is dependent on MHC class II antigen expression. *J. Clin. Invest.* **98,** 2109–2119.
42. Shah, A. H., Tabayoyong, W. B., Kimm, S. Y., Kim, S. J., Van Parijs, L., and Lee, C. (2002) Reconstitution of lethally irradiated adult mice with dominant negative TGF-beta type II receptor-transduced bone marrow leads to myeloid expansion and inflammatory disease. *J. Immunol.* **169,** 3485–3491.
43. Leveen, P., Larsson, J., Ehinger, M., et al. (2002) Induced disruption of the transforming growth factor beta type II receptor gene in mice causes a lethal inflammatory disorder that is transplantable. *Blood* **100,** 560–568.
44. Kanamaru, Y., Nakao, A., Mamura, M., et al. (2001) Blockade of TGF-beta signaling in T cells prevents the development of experimental glomerulonephritis. *J. Immunol.* **166,** 2818–2823.
45. Nakao, A., Miike, S., Hatano, M., et al. (2000) Blockade of transforming growth factor beta/Smad signaling in T cells by overexpression of Smad7 enhances antigen-induced airway inflammation and airway reactivity. *J. Exp. Med.* **192,** 151–158.
46. Lucas, P. J., Kim, S. J., Melby, S. J., and Gress, R. E. (2000) Disruption of T cell homeostasis in mice expressing a T cell-specific dominant negative transforming growth factor beta II receptor. *J. Exp. Med.* **191,** 1187–1196.
47. Gorelik, L. and Flavell, R. A. (2000). Abrogation of TGF-β signaling in T cells leads to spontaneous T cell differentiation and autoimmune disease. *Immunity* **12,** 171–181.
48. Gorelik, L. and Flavell, R. A. (2001) Immune-mediated eradication of tumors through the blockade of transforming growth factor-beta signaling in T cells. *Nat. Med.* **7,** 1118–1122.
49. Bottinger, E. P., Letterio, J. J., and Roberts, A. B. (1997) Biology of TGF-beta in knockout and transgenic mouse models. *Kidney Int.* **51,** 1355–1360.
50. Strobl, H., Riedl, E., Scheinecker, C., et al. (1996) TGF-β 1 promotes in vitro development of dendritic cells from CD34C hemopoietic progenitors. *J. Immunol.* **157,** 1499–1507.
51. Riedl, E., Strobl, H., Majdic, O., and Knapp, W. (1997) TGF-β 1 promotes in vitro generation of dendritic cells by protecting progenitor cells from apoptosis. *J. Immunol.* **158,** 1591–1597.

52. Borkowski, T. A., Letterio, J. J., Farr, A. G., and Udey, M. C. (1996) A role for endogenous transforming growth factor beta 1 in Langerhans cell biology: the skin of transforming growth factor beta 1 null mice is devoid of epidermal Langerhans cells. *J. Exp. Med.* **184,** 2417–2422.
53. Borkowski, T. A., Letterio, J. J., Mackall, C. L., et al. (1997) A role for TGF-β1 in Langerhans cell biology: further characterization of the epidermal Langerhans cell defect in TGF-β1 null mice. *J. Clin. Invest.* **100,** 575–581.
54. Thomas, R. M., Belsito, D. V., Huang, C., et al. (2001) Appearance of Langerhans cells in the epidermis of TGF-β1(-/-) SCID mice: paracrine and autocrine effects of transforming growth factor-beta 1 and -beta2. *J. Invest. Dermatol.* **117,** 1574–1580.
55. Hoying, J. B., Yin, M., Diebold, R., Ormsby, I., Becker, A., and Doetschman, T. (1999) Transforming growth factor beta1 enhances platelet aggregation through a non-transcriptional effect on the fibrinogen receptor. *J. Biol. Chem.* **274,** 31008–31013.
56. Yang, Y. A., Dukhanina, O., Tang, B., et al. (2002) Lifetime exposure to a soluble TGF-beta antagonist protects mice against metastasis without adverse side effects. *J. Clin. Invest.* **109,** 1607–1615.
57. Singer, A. J. and Clark, R. A. (1999) Cutaneous wound healing. *N. Engl. J. Med.* **341,** 738–746.
58. Roberts, A. B. (1995) Transforming growth factor-beta: activity and efficacy in animal models of wound healing. *Wound Rep. Reg.* **3,** 408–418.
59. Sporn, M. B., Roberts, A. B., Shull, J. H., Smith, J. M., Ward, J. M., and Sodek, J. (1983) Polypeptide transforming growth factors isolated from bovine sources and used for wound healing in vivo. *Science* **219,** 1329–1331.
60. Roberts, A. B., Sporn, M. B., Assoian, R. K., et al. (1986) Transforming growth factor type beta: rapid induction of fibrosis and angiogenesis in vivo and stimulation of collagen formation in vitro. *Proc. Natl. Acad. Sci. USA* **83,** 4167–4171.
61. Yang, X., Letterio, J. J., Lechleider, R. J., et al. (1999) Targeted disruption of SMAD3 results in impaired mucosal immunity and diminished T cell responsiveness to TGF-beta. *EMBO J.* **18,** 1280–1291.
62. Brown, R. L., Ormsby, I., Doetschman, T. C., and Greenhalgh, D.G. (1995) Wound healing in the transforming growth factor-β1-deficient mouse. *Wound Rep. Reg.* **3,** 25–36.
63. Koch, R. M., Roche, N. S., Parks, W. T., Ashcroft, G. S., Letterio, J. J., and Roberts, A. B. (2000) Incisional wound healing in transforming growth factor-beta1 null mice. *Wound Repair Regen.* **8,** 179–191.
64. Crowe, M. J., Doetschman, T., and Greenhalgh, D. G. (2000) Delayed wound healing in immunodeficient TGF-beta 1 knockout mice. *J. Invest. Dermatol.* **115,** 3–11.
65. Wakefield, L. M. and Roberts, A. B. (2002) TGF-beta signaling: positive and negative effects on tumorigenesis. *Curr. Opin. Genet. Dev.* **12,** 22–29.
66. Piek, E., Ju, W. J., Heyer, J., et al. (2001) Functional characterization of transforming growth factor beta signaling in Smad2- and Smad3-deficient fibroblasts. *J. Biol. Chem.* **276,** 19945–19953.
67. Ashcroft, G. S., Yang, X., Glick, A. B., et al. (1999) Mice lacking Smad3 show accelerated wound healing and an impaired local inflammatory response. *Nat. Cell Biol.* **1,** 260–266.
68. Arabshahi, A., Major, C. D., Aburime, E. E., et al. (2002) Interference with TGF-β/activin signaling results in accelerated healing of wounds compromised by irradiation. Submitted.
69. Verrecchia, F., Chu, M. L., and Mauviel, A. (2001) Identification of novel TGF-beta/Smad gene targets in dermal fibroblasts using a combined cDNA microarray/promoter transactivation approach. *J. Biol. Chem.* **276,** 17058–17062.
70. Hocevar, B. A., Brown, T. L., and Howe, P. H. (1999) TGF-beta induces fibronectin synthesis through a c-Jun N-terminal kinase-dependent, Smad4-independent pathway. *EMBO J.* **18,** 1345–1356.
71. Ashcroft, G. S. and Roberts, A. B. (2000) Loss of Smad3 modulates wound healing. *Cytokine Growth Factor Rev.* **11,** 125–131.
72. Glick, A. B., Kulkarni, A. B., Tennenbaum, T., et al. (1993) Loss of expression of transforming growth factor beta in skin and skin tumors is associated with hyperproliferation and a high risk for malignant conversion. *Proc. Natl. Acad. Sci. USA* **90,** 6076–6080.
73. Glick, A. B., Lee, M. M., Darwiche, N., Kulkarni, A. B., Karlsson, S., and Yuspa, S. H. (1994) Targeted deletion of the TGF-beta 1 gene causes rapid progression to squamous cell carcinoma. *Genes Dev.* **8,** 2429–2440.

74. Engle, S. J., Haying, J. B., Boivin, G. P., Ormsby, I., Gartside, P. S., and Doetschman, T. (1999) Transforming growth factor beta1 suppresses nonmetastatic colon cancer at an early stage of tumorigenesis. *Cancer Res.* **59,** 3379–3386.
75. Glick, A. B., Weinberg, W. C., Wu, I. H., Quan, W., and Yuspa, S. H. (1996) Transforming growth factor beta 1 suppresses genomic instability independent of a G1 arrest, p53, and Rb. *Cancer Res.* **56,** 3645–3650.
76. Oshima, M., Oshima, H., and Taketo, M. M. (1996) TGF-beta receptor type II deficiency results in defects of yolk sac hematopoiesis and vasculogenesis. *Dev. Biol.* **179,** 297–302.
77. Im, Y. H., Kim, H. T., Kim, I. Y., et al. (2001) Heterozygous mice for the transforming growth factor-beta type II receptor gene have increased susceptibility to hepatocellular carcinogenesis. *Cancer Res.* **61,** 6665–6668.
78. Miyaki, M., Iijima, T., Konishi, M., et al. (1999) Higher frequency of Smad4 gene mutation in human colorectal cancer with distant metastasis. *Oncogene* **18,** 3098–3103.
79. Howe, J. R., Roth, S., Ringold, J. C., et al. (1998) Mutations in the SMAD4/DPC4 gene in juvenile polyposis. *Science* **280,** 1086–1088.
80. Friedl, W., Kruse, R., Uhlhaas, S., et al. (1999) Frequent 4-bp deletion in exon 9 of the SMAD4/ MADH4 gene in familial juvenile polyposis patients. *Genes Chromosomes Cancer* **25,** 403–406.
81. Taketo, M. M. and Takaku, K. (2000) Gastro-intestinal tumorigenesis in Smad4 mutant mice. *Cytokine Growth Factor Rev.* **11,** 147–157.
82. Hahn, S. A., Schutte, M., Hoque, A. T. M. S., et al. (1996) DPC4, a candidate tumor suppressor gene at human chromosome 18q21.1. *Science* **271,** 350–353.
83. Hata, A., Shi, Y., and Massague, J. (1998) TGF-beta signaling and cancer: structural and functional consequences of mutations in Smads. *Mol. Med. Today* **4,** 257–262.
84. Weinstein, M., Yang, X., Li, C., Xu, X., Gotay, J., and Deng, C. X. (1998) Failure of egg cylinder elongation and mesoderm induction in mouse embryos lacking the tumor suppressor smad2. *Proc. Natl. Acad. Sci. USA* **95,** 9378–9383.
85. Zhu, Y., Richardson, J. A., Parada, L. F., and Graff, J. M. (1998) Smad3 mutant mice develop metastatic colorectal cancer. *Cell* **94,** 703–714.
86. Datto, M. B., Frederick, J. P., Pan, L., Barton, A. J., Zhuang, Y., and Wang, X. F. (1999) Targeted disruption of Smad3 reveals an essential role in transforming growth factor beta-mediated signal transduction. *Mol. Cell Biol.* **19,** 2495–2504.
87. Philipp-Staheli, J., Kim, K.-H., Payne, S. R., et al. (2002) Pathway-specific tumor suppression: reduction of p27 accelerates gastrointestinal tumorigenesis in *Apc* mutant mice, but not in *Smad3* mutant mice. *Cancer Cell* **1,** 355–368.
88. Weinstein, M., Yang, X., and Deng, C. (2000) Functions of mammalian Smad genes as revealed by targeted gene disruption in mice. *Cytokine Growth Factor Rev.* **11,** 49–58.
89. Hahm, K. B., Lee, K. M., Kim, Y. B., et al. (2002) Conditional loss of TGF-beta signalling leads to increased susceptibility to gastrointestinal carcinogenesis in mice. *Aliment. Pharmacol. Ther.* **16(Suppl. 2),** 115–127.

25

Physiologic Roles of Members of the TNF and TNF Receptor Families as Revealed by Knockout Models

Sergei A. Nedospasov, Sergei I. Grivennikov, and Dmitry V. Kuprash

Summary

Members of the tumor necrosis factor (TNF) and TNF receptor (TNFR) families mediate many important functions in the mammalian organism. Ligand-receptor interactions result in signals promoting cell activation, proliferation, inhibition or death. Advances in gene targeting technology continue to uncover biological functions of these molecules in vivo. The review discusses the current state of the field with specific emphasis on the role of TNF and TNFR family members in host defense and their contrasting roles in cancer development and progression. Other features, such as defects in lymphopoiesis, lymphoid organogenesis, and epidermal development are also briefly reviewed.

Key words

TNF, lymphotoxin, cytokines, immunity, host defense, cancer

1. Introduction

Tumor necrosis factor (TNF or TNF-α), the founding member of the TNF ligand superfamily, was discovered because of its antitumor activity in an animal model *(1)*. As subsequent studies have shown, this antitumor effect of TNF was not because of a direct and specific action on tumor cells, but was rather a consequence of several pleiotropic activities of this cytokine, in particular its stimulatory effects on vascular endothelium *(2)*. Lymphotoxin (LT), the closest TNF relative [as proved by later molecular studies *(3)*], was initially discovered as a cytotoxic factor produced by lymphocytes *(4)* and was related to the phenomenon of delayed hypersensitivity *(5)*. However, later studies, based on experiments performed on knockout mice, revealed that the main biologic function of LT is mediated by its membrane-bound form, not its soluble form, and this function was linked to the generation and maintenance of secondary lymphoid tissues, rather than to cytotoxicity *(6)*.

These two examples serve to illustrate the long and winding road from the initial description of biologic activity of many cytokines, through the stages of biochemical purification, then through often painstaking molecular characterization of a distinct gene and gene product, and finally to the resultant opportunity to characterize its function properly in vivo. In this regard, knockout models have provided an extraordinarily powerful method to address the physiologic role of a cytokine activity in the context of the whole animal.

From: *Contemporary Immunology: Cytokine Knockouts, 2nd Edition*
Edited by: Giamila Fantuzzi © Humana Press Inc., Totowa, NJ

Studies of cytokine gene knockout mice, including those reviewed in this chapter, often identified unexpected and surprising biologic features of the cytokines, not anticipated on the basis of prior in vitro studies. Conversely, some activities identified in vitro turned out to be nonessential or minimally important in vivo, perhaps because of redundancy in function. It is important to emphasize that genes and gene products may have unique, redundant, or complementary functions. In case of redundancy, phenotype of a mouse deficient in a single gene may not necessarily reveal all physiologically relevant features.

TNF and lymphotoxin genes (including the second subunit of LT, called LT-β, which is encoded by a separate gene) belonged initially to a small family, which later grew into a super-family of TNF-related cytokines. As with many other cytokines, the most consistent classification is based on homologies between receptor molecules and similarities in postreceptor events. Based on receptor homologies, two ligand-receptors pairs were quickly recognized and added to the initial members by the early 1990s: Fas (Apo-1) and CD40 and their respective ligands, FasL and CD40L *(7)*. Several additional members of the TNF family were identified as ligands for orphan TNF receptors, rather than through direct homology with TNF and LT cytokines. In 1993, a biotech representative announced at a cytokine conference that proprietary human expression databases predicted the existence of an additional 10 members of the TNF and about 15 members of the TNF receptor (R) families. This stunning information proved to be correct, and during the next 10 years the number of currently known ligands and receptors rose to 18 and 27, respectively (see http://www.gene.ucl.ac.uk/nomenclature/genefamily/tnftop.html for one of the nomenclatures for TNFSFs and TNFRSFs)

The first three engineered knockouts of the TNF and TNFR family included TNFRI *(8,9)*, LT-α *(10,11)*, and TNF *(12–14)* and produced a big surprise: LT deficiency was linked to both irreversible and reversible defects in lymphoid tissues, whereas TNF deficiency proved that TNF was a critical host defense molecule and also contributed to the maintenance of lymphoid organ architecture.

To date, mice deficient in 14 different TNF receptor family members have been reported, as well as mice with natural or engineered deficiencies in 13 TNF ligand proteins. The phenotypic characterization of many of these mice is incomplete and ongoing. Perhaps surprisingly, none of the reported knockouts is embryonic lethal, suggesting the absence of a unique indispensable function associated with any single TNF family ligand or receptor. Additional functions mediated by receptors of the TNFR family may be revealed in mice with multiple knockouts of ligands, receptors, or their combination (depending on chromosomal localization).

Additionally, several cytokine and cytokine receptor genes from these families have been inactivated conditionally, allowing investigators to address distinct contributions of various cell types as well as to bypass the effects of the knockout on embryonic development. Recent advances in knockout technology also allowed the generation of several *knockin* mice, which represent analogs of limited site-directed mutagenesis in vivo. Yet additional modality can be provided by reactivatable knockout of the genes, as exemplified by TNFRI knockout mice in which dysfunction can be restored (G. Kollias, personal communication).

Phenotypes of selected knockout mice are reviewed below with specific emphasis on the role of TNF family members in the genesis of complex cellular microenvironment, host defense, and pro- and antitumorigenic functions.

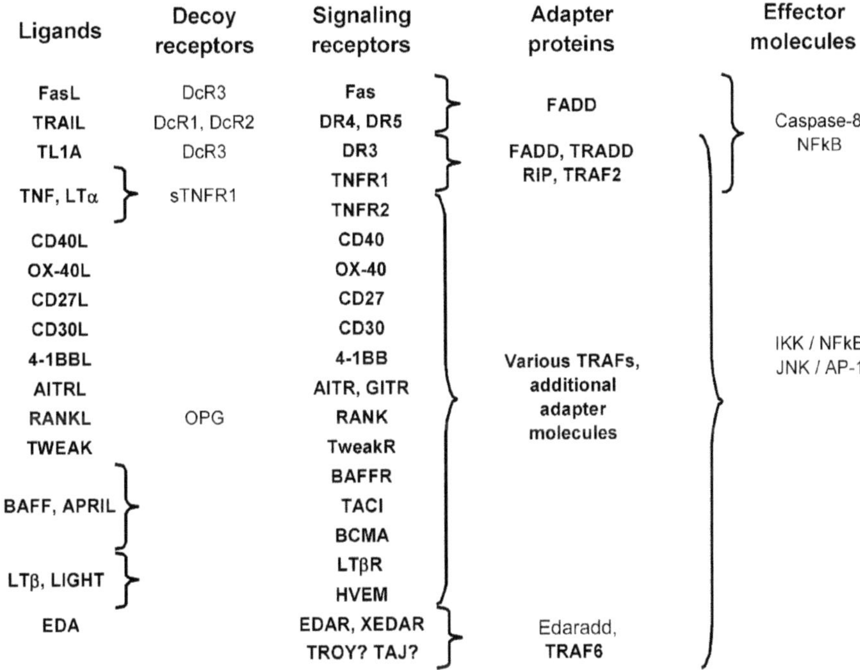

Fig. 1. The growing complexity of ligands, receptors, and adaptor molecules for the TNF/TNFR superfamily. The latest addition is Edaradd (*crinkled*), an adaptor molecule for ectodysplasin receptors and their recently identified homologs expressed in epidermal appendixes. The link between TROY, TAJ, and EDAR has been suggested based on structural homology only. See Table 1 for the abbreviations of TNF/TNFR common names. Other abbreviations: AP1, activating protein-1; DR, death receptor; FADD, Fas-associated death domain; IKK, IkappaB kinase; JNK, c-Jun NH(2)-terminal kinase; NFkB, nuclear factor kappaB; RIP, receptor interacting protein; TRADD, TNF receptor-associated death domain protein; TRAF, TNF receptor-associated factor.

2. Paradigms for the Signaling Pathways

Ligand-receptor interactions of TNF superfamily members transmit several types of intracellular signals, most notably leading to transcriptional activation or to cell death. Knockout technology has significantly contributed to our understanding of these seemingly opposite signal transduction pathways (Figs. 1 and 2).

The receptor signaling characteristic of the TNFR family involves several types of intracellular adaptor molecules that through homotypic and heterotypic aggregations activate one of the following pathways. The activating pathway involves TNF-associated factors (TRAFs), RIP, and mitogen-activated protein kinases (MAPKs) and acts through the IKK complex and nuclear factor-κB (NF-κB) or through c-Jun-N-terminal kinase (JNK) and activation protein-1 (AP-1) *(15)* (Fig. 1). Intracellular proapoptotic pathways induced by extracellular signals and mediated by FADD and are very similar for the entire group of death domain-containing receptors, a subfamily of the TNFR superfamily, and in this case Fas (Apo-1) may serve as a reference model for FADD/caspase-8-dependent pathways *(16)*.

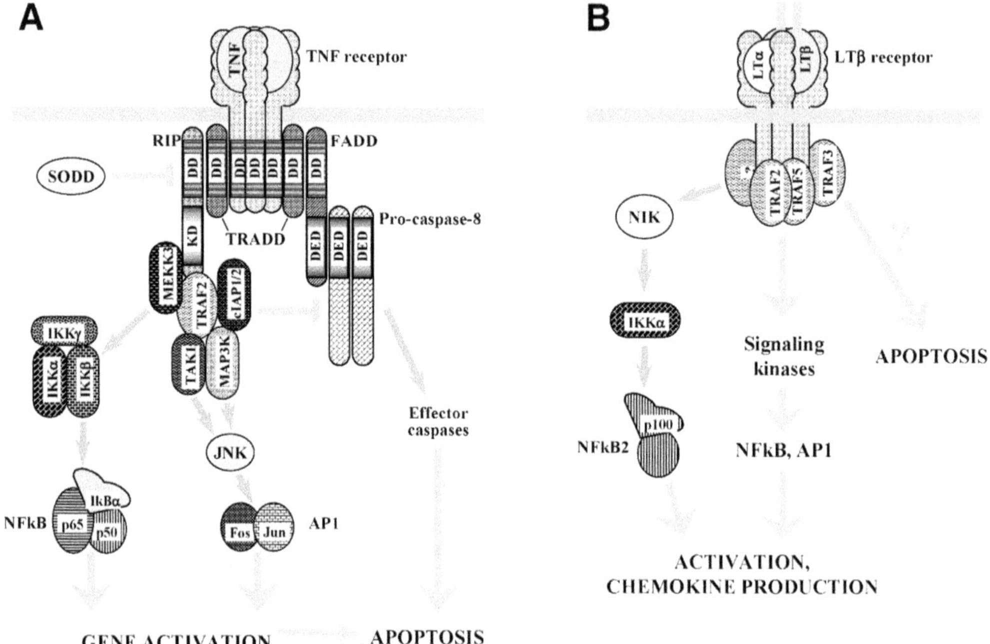

Fig. 2. Examples of tumor necrosis factor/tumor necrosis factor receptor (TNF/TNFR) superfamily signaling. (**A**) TNFRI pathways as an example of DD-containing receptor signaling. (**B**) LTβR pathways as an example of a non-DD receptor signaling. Note the alternative NF-κB activation pathway through NIK and IKK-α. DD, death domain, DED, death effector domain, SODD, silencer of death domain, TRAF, TNF receptor-associated factor, NIK, NF-κB inducing kinase. Abbreviations: cIAP, cellular inhibitor of apoptosis protein; DED, death effector domain; MAPK, mitogen-activated protein kinase; ERK, extracellular signal-regulated kinase; MEKK, MAPK/ERK kinase kinase; NIK, NF-kappaB inducing kinase; SODD, silencer of death domain; TAK1, transforming growth factor-beta-activated kinase-1. See Fig. 1 for additional abbreviations.

Pathways involving TNF and TNFR families are characterized by promiscuity in ligand-receptor relations: a given cytokine can interact with more than one receptor, and each receptor may bind more than one cytokine. The situation becomes even more complex at the level of intracellular signaling, where several pathways converge on the same receptor adaptor molecules or on the same downstream signaling molecules regulating activation or cell death.

It is conceivable that some of the current signaling schemes, both extracellular and intracellular, await further corrections and modifications, especially if the paradigm of heteromeric cytokines, first discovered for the LT-βR ligand LT-α_1LT-β_2 and recently shown to be true for BAFF and APRIL *(17)*, will be extended to other family members.

The recently described phenotype of NF-κB-inducing kinase (NIK) knockout mice and NIK-deficient cells *(18)*, together with earlier studies linking mutation in NIK to the *aly/aly* phenotype *(19)*, helped to define an alternative NF-κB pathway *(20,21)* in LT-βR signaling *(22)*. The alternative pathway is also downstream of CD40 and BAFF-R *(23,24)* but not of TNFRI (Fig. 2).

3. Genomics, Evolution, and Redundancy

Adaptive immunity emerged owing to acquisition of a recombination system involved in T-cell receptor (TCR) and Ig gene rearrangements, and it was proposed that TNF and TNF receptor genes evolved around that time *(7)*. It is interesting that some of the downstream signaling components of both the activating arm (such as RIP and IKK proteins) and the proapoptotic arm (FADD, caspases) evolved much earlier and have been utilized by Toll receptor pathways for innate immunity functions *(25)*. Recent finding of a TNF-like gene, *Eidar*, in *Drosophila (26)* implies that the TNF-TNFR pathway is more ancient than was previously thought. The current three-arm signaling (consisting of JNK, IKK/NF-κB, and FADD/caspase arms; *see* Fig. 2) emerged later in evolution by addition of some of the downstream components of the Toll pathway to the JNK pathway.

Several loci in the human and mouse genome contain clusters of genes belonging to the TNF ligand and TNF receptor families, the best studied being the compact segment inside the class III region of both human and mouse MHC, which contains the TNF, LT-α, and LT-β genes *(7)*. Genes coding for receptors are even more clustered than those coding for their ligands. For example, eight TNFR-like genes are located at 1p36 in humans (mouse chromosome 4), and three genes are clustered at 12p13 (mouse chromosome 6), including two principal receptors of the TNF/LT signaling discussed in this chapter in some detail: TNFRI and LT-βR (Fig. 2). Thorough analysis of the evolution of TNF and TNFR superfamilies awaits complete sequencing of a larger number of diverse mammalian genomes.

Knockout technology at times reveals physiologically essential, but redundant functions that are not observed in single knockout mice. To this end, several multiple knockout models for TNF and TNFR families have been already generated and evaluated. For example, simultaneous disruption of TNFRI and LT-βR is not easy owing to a genetic link between these receptors on chromosome 4. However, these two pathways could be simultaneously inactivated by crossing the TNFRI knockout with the LT-β knockout mouse *(27)*. Comparison of such TNFR/LT-β double knockout mice with TNF/LT-β double knockout mice *(28)* suggested the existence of an additional role of LT-α signaling via TNFRI in the genesis of several types of lymph nodes. Similarly, a LIGHT/LT-β double knockout mouse was recently generated and revealed a limited role of LIGHT-LT-βR interaction in the formation of mesenterial lymph nodes *(29)*. The triple TNF/LT-α/LT-β knockout mouse *(30)* provided additional insight into the redundancy in signaling by two principal receptors of this subfamily: TNFRI and LT-βR (Fig. 1). Another double knockout, FasL/TNF, revealed that in the absence of Fas signaling TNF is an important mediator of lymphoproliferative syndromes caused by Fas *(31)*.

4. Physiologic Roles of Individual TNF Family Cytokines and Receptors Revealed by Knockout Mice

As exemplified by the best studied cytokine of this family, TNF, other TNF-like ligands may be pleiotropic and exhibit a variety of downstream functions, depending on the type of the cell, and on physiologic context. The most important function of many of these cytokines and receptors is to deliver signals necessary for genesis of multicellular structures, such as lymphoid organs and granulomas, with specific reference to reversible tissue remodeling. Recent discoveries of ectodysplasin ligand-receptor systems *(32)* and of an adaptor molecule, Edaradd (*crinkled*) specific for this pathway, also established the role of TNF and TNFR-like molecules in morphogenesis and embryogenesis outside of the immune system. Another function common to several of these cytokines and receptors is delivery of costimulatory or inhibitory signals to T-cells from antigen-presenting cells (APCs), such as dendritic cells (DCs) or B-cells, or from T-cells to B-cells.

Table 1 surveys the phenotypes of knockout mice with ablation of single members of the TNF or TNFR family.

4.1. Role in Host Defense

Host defense relies on the recruitment of inflammatory immune cells to the sites of infection, induction of adaptive immunity, localizing the infection by containment, and finally on feedback inhibition of the inflammatory response and restoration of normal tissue homeostasis. This sequence of events prevents or minimizes the replication of the infectious agent in the host and then prevents negative consequences of persistent inflammatory reaction and tissue damage by turning off the inflammatory response. Several TNF family members and their corresponding receptors contribute to these host defense functions (summarized in Table 2).

4.1.1. TNF/TNFRI/TNFRII

The role of TNF and its receptors in host defense against pathogens has been studied extensively and is well documented. In the pre-knockout era, Vassalli's group used blocking antibodies to demonstrate that locally produced TNF is important for the resistance of mice to mycobacterial infection and for granuloma formation *(91)*. This fundamental finding was fully confirmed in knockout and transgenic mice *(93,122)*. Similarly, transgenic mice expressing high levels of soluble TNFRI (which can inhibit TNF and partly LT-α) were highly susceptible to *Listeria*, *Leishmania*, *Corynebacterium*, and mycobacterial infections *(101,122,123)*. Soluble TNFRI expressed in adenoviral vectors increased susceptibility to *Mycobacterium tuberculosis (124)*. Finally, targeted disruption of either the TNF or TNFRI genes resulted in impaired granuloma formation in both the mycobacterial and the listerial models, clearly confirming that this ligand-receptor combination is indispensable for the control of intracellular bacterial infections *(8,12,39,93,125–127)*. In addition, the susceptible phenotype was characterized by lack of macrophage activation, failure to upregulate inducible nitric oxide synthase (iNOS) and adhesion molecules *(128)*, disorganized infiltration of T-cells, and excessive recruitment of neutrophils to the infected organs and to areas of tissue necrosis. Experiments with bone marrow-transplanted radiation chimeras proved that for effective host defense TNF must be expressed by radiosensitive hematopoietic cells. TNF-deficient mice *(95,129)* and TNFRI null mice *(130)* are susceptible to leishmaniasis and show both increased mortality after subcutaneous challenge and increased parasitic burden. In this model TNF is necessary for granuloma development and for the control of inflammation in infected organs *(129)*. Other studies implicated TNF and TNFRI in the resistance to tularemia *(131)* and *Trypanosoma brucei (132)*.

An interesting feature of TNF was discovered during evaluation of challenge with heat-killed *Corynebacterium parvum (13,133)*, as TNF was found to play not only a proinflammatory, but also an antiinflammatory role by suppressing interferon-γ (IFN-γ)-induced interleukin-12 (IL-12) production. The disruption of this pathway by TNF ablation resulted in uncontrolled inflammation leading to death *(133)*.

These experiments, therefore, illuminated a critical role of TNF in promoting the reversible development of multicellular structures—granulomas—that are critical for containment and elimination of infection. The role of TNF in granuloma formation cannot be compensated for by excessive IFN-γ and IL-12 production.

TNF is clearly implicated in both human and murine malaria. In the murine brain-stage malaria model induced by *Plasmodium berghei*, TNF and TNFRII appear to play a detrimental role in the upregulation of adhesion molecules and breakdown of the blood-brain barrier *(98,122)*. However, it was reported recently that locally upregulated LT-α is uniquely responsible for the major symptoms of brain-stage malaria *(105)* (*see* next section).

The contribution of TNF in promoting resistance against pathogens occurs in part via its membrane-associated form *(134)*. Transgenic mice were generated in which the expression of noncleavable transmembrane TNF occurred on either TNF-deficient *(102)* or TNF/LT-α double-deficient background *(103)*. Analysis of bacille Calmette-Guérin (BCG) infection in such mice revealed that membrane-associated TNF provided at least partial resistance against this pathogen. The mice had significantly lower bacterial load, less tissue necrosis, and comparatively well-defined granulomas compared with knockout animals without transmembrane TNF. These granulomas were smaller in size and in number than in wild-type controls *(103)*. Transmembrane TNF was found to be sufficient for the mediation of liver damage and apoptosis in an experimental hepatitis model *(102)*. However, all the above results await verification in a better defined system, such as a knockin of transmembrane TNF [*(43)* and G. Kollias, personal communication] rather than a transgene.

4.1.2. LT-α

LT-α plays an important role in the development of secondary lymphoid organs by forming a membrane complex with LT-β (mostly on lymphocytes) and signaling through the LT-βR expressed on stromal cells. Additionally, the LT-α homotrimer on its own can signal through TNF receptors, as was shown by recent transgenic studies *(135–137)*. Until recently, every defect in host defense described for the LT-α knockout appeared to be secondary to structural defects in lymphoid organs owing to inactivation of LT-βR signaling. However, two recent reports imply a distinct role of locally produced soluble LT-α homotrimer in granuloma formation during the course of pulmonary tuberculosis *(104)* and in promotion of the brain-stage malaria via intercellular adhesion molecule (ICAM) upregulation and lymphocyte infiltration *(105)*.

Soluble LT-α_3 signaling through TNFRI may partially compensate for the absence of TNF in vivo, and, indeed, TNF/LT-α double knockout mice showed a total lack of recruitment of neutrophils and rapid death in response to systemic candidiasis *(138)*, as opposed to single TNF knockout mice. TNF/LT-α double knockout mice also were more susceptible to *Staphylococcus aureus* infection than single TNF knockout *(97)*.

4.1.3. LT/LT-βR

Disruption of the LT/LT-βR pathway (achieved in either LT-β, LT-α, or LT-βR single knockouts) leads to severe defects in the development and maintenance of secondary lymphoid organs and to a deficient immune response in general. Even so, disruption of LT-βR signaling in mice produces only a limited effect in infectious models. Using LT-β-Ig fusion protein, Lucas and colleagues *(139)* have found that LT-βR is important for both proper granuloma formation and iNOS activation during BCG infection. LT-β signaling appears to be necessary for the clearance of *Listeria monocytogenes (108)*.

Table 1
Overview of the Reported Knockout Phenotypes (TNF and TNFR Families)

Ligand and receptor	Phenotypic features of mouse null mutant	References
TNF TNFRI	Deficient GC formation, disrupted primary B-cell follicles, and absence of mature FDC; partially defective MZ; defective PPs; resistant to LPS + D-Gal shock; multiple host defense abnormalities[a] (deficiency in granuloma development); deregulated Ig class switching and inflammatory responses; resistant to skin carcinogenesis; partial resistance to EAE	*8,9,12,13,33–38*
TNFRII	Grossly normal, decreased sensitivity to TNF, some host defense abnormalities[a]	*39–42*
Transmembrane TNF	Reduced or absent GCs and FDCs in spleen; resistance to LPS + D-Gal shock; partial host defense abnormalities[a]	*43*
LT-α[b] LT-β LT-βR[c]	Absence of PPs and either peripheral (LT-β) or all (LT-α, LT-βR) LNs; defective segregation of B- and T-cells within the white pulp of the spleen; absence of MZ, GCs and FDCs; impaired antibody affinity maturation and Ig switch; defective recruitment of NK cells and DCs; defective response to various infections[a]	*10,11,27,28, 44–48*
LT-β in B cells	Normal PP and all LNs; partial disruption of MZ; lack of GCs, residual FDCs (dependent on LT-β produced by T-cells); impaired antibody responses	*47*
CD40L CD40	Decreased IgM and no GCs in response to thymus-dependent antigens; low or absent serum IgG, IgA, and IgE; defective CD8+ CTL memory cells; impaired inflammatory responses; increased occurrence of opportunistic infections and neoplasms[a]	*49–51*; reviewed in *52*
FasL Fas	Excessive lymphoproliferation resulting from accumulation of CD4/CD8 lymphocytes; excessive immune response in immune-privileged sites; late B-cell lymphomas; resistant to diabetes on NOD background; autoimmune syndromes[a]	*31,53–58*
Ox40L Ox40	Defects in APC function; impaired contact hyper-sensitivity response and DC-dependent T-cell responses; impaired Th2 response. In asthma model: diminished lung inflammation, eosinophilia, and mucus production, attenuated airway hyperreactivity; resistant to EAE	*59–62*
CD30L CD30	Normal negative selection (contrary to initial report); CD30-deficient autoreactive CD8+ T-cells are highly autoaggressive	*63–65*
CD27L CD27	Impaired T-cell memory	*66*
BAFF BAFF-R	Loss of follicular and marginal zone B-lymphocytes but normal B1-cells; B-cell arrest at T1 stage. Strongly reduced total and antigen-specific serum Ig; absence or inhibition of GC formation	*67–70*; reviewed in *71*
APRIL BCMA	APRIL- and BCMA-deficient mice are grossly normal; TACI knockout mice show impaired	*72–75*

Table 1 (Continued)

Ligand and receptor	Phenotypic features of mouse null mutant	References
TACI	T-cell-dependent antibody responses; TACI$^{-/-}$ B-cells hyperproliferate and produce increased amounts of nonspecific immunoglobulins in vitro.	
4-1BBL 4-1BB	4-1BBL knockout mouse: slightly weaker CTL response to influenza virus, but normal general CTL response, IgG and IgM production 4-1BB knockout mouse: enhanced T-cell proliferation in response to mitogens or anti-CD3; diminished T-cell responses; resistant to EAE	*76,77*
LIGHT[d]	Normal spleen microarchitecture; less frequent mesenterial LNs in LIGHT/LT-β compared with LT-β knockout mouse; defective CD8 response; prolonged skin graft survival in LIGHT/CD28 double knockout mouse	*29,78*
RANK RANKL OPG[e]	Low body weight, teeth eruption, extramedullary hematopoiesis in liver and spleen; absence of all LNs; decreased thymic cellularity and thymus size; fewer B-cells in spleen; reduced cytokine production and response to DC stimulation by T-cells; block of T-cell differentiation at the stage of CD4–/CD8–/CD44–/CD25+ precursors	*79–81*
TRAIL DR5[f]	Defects in NK cells: cytotoxic function and tumor surveillance; defective thymocyte accelerated autoimmune diseases	*82–84,84a*
GITR GITRL[f]	Grossly normal; T-cells are hypersensitive to activation-induced cell death and show enhanced proliferation in response to anti-CD3	*85*
Ectodysplasin Edar Xedar[f]	Ectodysplasin: *tabby* mutation in mice, X-linked hypohydrotic ectodermal dysplasia (EDA): defects in teeth, hair, skin, and sweat gland Edar: *downless* mutation in mice, EDA	*86–89*
NGFR	Grossly normal; long-lasting increase in the number of basal forebrain cholinergic neurons; no defects in immune system reported	*90*

[a]See also Table 2.

[b]LT-α can also signal via TNFRI. Sole genetic inactivation of LT-α → TNFRI pathway is not possible because of the involvement of LT-α in LT-βR signaling and of TNFRI in TNF signaling.

[c]Both transmembrane LT and LIGHT can signal via LT-βR.

[d]LIGHT can bind at least two distinct receptors: HVEM and LT-βR. An HVEM knockout mouse has not been reported yet.

[e]Decoy receptor.

[f]No knockout or natural mutation reported.

APC, antigen-presenting cell; APRIL, a proliferation-inducing ligand; 4-1BBL, 4-1BB(CD137) ligand; BCMA, B cell maturation antigen; CTL, cytotoxic T-lymhocyte; D-Gal, D-galactosamine; EAE, experimental autoimmune encephalomyelitis; FDC, follicular dendritic cell; GC, germinal center; GITR, glucocorticoid-induced tumor necrosis factor receptor; GITRL, GITR ligand; HVEM, herpes virus entry mediator; LIGHT, *H*omologous to Lymphotoxins, *I*nducible expression, competes with HSV *G*lycoprotein D for *H*VEM, a receptor expressed on *T*-lymhocytes; LN, lymph node; LPS, lipopolysaccharide; LT, lymphotoxin; MZ, marginal zone; NFGR, nerve growth factor receptor; NK, natural killer (cell); NOD, nonobese diabetic; PP, Peyer's patches; RANK, receptor activator of nuclear factor-kappaB; RANKL, RANK ligand; TACI, transmembrane activator and CAML interactor; TRAIL, TNF-related activation-induced cytokine; OPG, osteoprotegrin.

Table 2
Host Defense: Phenotypes of Selected TNF and TNFR Family Knockout Mice

Ligand and receptor	Host defense phenotype of knockout mice	Infectious agents and references
TNF TNFRI	Susceptibility to bacterial pathogens, certain parasites, and viruses; resistance to TNF-mediated toxicity such as LPS + D-Gal shock and several types of septic shock during infections	*Listeria, Candida,* BCG, *M. tuberculosis (8,12,91–94), Leishmania (95), M. avium (96), St. aureus (97), Plasmodium (42,98–100), Corynebacterium parvum (101), hepatitis (102)*
TNFRII	Susceptibility to brain-stage malaria, partial susceptibility to *M. tuberculosis*	*41,42*
Transmembrane TNF	Transgene on TNF/LT-deficient background confers partial resistance to BCG infection	*103*
LT-β LT-α LT-βR	Impaired immunity to certain bacteria, parasites, and viruses	Tested in LT-α knockout mice: *M. tuberculosis (104), malaria (105),* LCMV *(106),* MCMV *(107)* Tested in LT-β knockout mice: *Listeria (108)* LCMV (LT-βR) *(109)*
CD40L CD40	Impaired adaptive immunity to a wide range of pathogens, especially viruses, owing to defective costimulation	Leishmania *(110–112),* malaria *(113),* viruses *(114–116)*
OX40L Ox40	Increased resistance to *Leishmania*	*60*
FasL Fas	Failure to control early stage of some intracellular infections owing to reduced apoptosis of infected cells	*Pseudomonas aeruginosa (117,118), Helicobacter pylori (119), Listeria (120), S. aureus (121)*

BCG, bacille Calmette-Guérin (*M. bovis*); LCMV, lymphocytic choriomeningitis virus; MCMV, murine cytomegalovirus. For other abbreviations, see footnote to Table 1.

LT-β knockout mice are more susceptible to lymphocytic choriomeningitis virus (LCMV) infection because of the failure to mount a functional antibody response *(109)*. LT-α/LT-β-LT-βR interactions are also implicated in propagation of prion diseases, presumably because of their role in the development and maintenance of follicular dendritic cells (FDCs) *(140,141)*.

4.1.4. Fas/FasL

The main feature of the Fas/FasL system in resistance to infections is the ability to induce apoptosis of infected cells, thus limiting the area of infection and eliminating the pathogen together with the infected cell. FasL may be upregulated by some types of immune cells in response to lipopolysaccharides, which may reflect the role of FasL-Fas interaction at early stages of host defense against bacterial pathogens *(121)*. Both *lpr* and *gld* mice are unable to induce lung cell apoptosis during *Pseudomonas aeruginosa* infection and are subject to fatal sepsis *(118)*. Interestingly, bone marrow transfer experiments between wild-type and *gld* and *lpr* mice indicated that both Fas and FasL (CD95/CD95L) are expressed on lung epithelial cells, but not on immune hematopoietic cells *(117,118)*. Many types of bacteria are able to induce apoptosis of the host cells in vitro, but participation of Fas/FasL in this process is well documented only for *S. aureus (121)*.

The FasL-Fas interaction was shown to play a role in the pathogenesis of *Helicobacter pylori* infection *(119)*: *gld* mice were unable to induce apoptosis of infected gastric epithelial cells and failed to produce sufficient amounts of IFN-γ. This subsequently led to more severe disease, atrophy of gastric epithelium, and premalignant phenotype. Fas signaling is important in *Listeria monocytogenes* infection for killing infected liver and spleen cells. In this mechanism of resistance, Fas collaborates with other molecules, such as perforin, since mice with a double deficiency in perforin and Fas had a more severe phenotype than any of the single knockouts *(120)*.

4.1.5. Ox40/Ox40L

Knockout studies implicated the role of Ox40L expressed on APCs, as well as Ox40 expressed on T-cells, as important contributors to costimulation *(59)*.

There is only limited information on the role for Ox40/Ox40 L in host defense. Akiba et al. *(60)* have reported that administration of monoclonal antibody (MAb) to Ox40L abrogated disease progression in a subcutaneous *Leishmania major* model. During the course of *Leishmania* infection in wild-type mice, Ox40 is expressed by CD4 T-cells, whereas Ox40L is expressed by DCs, promoting the detrimental shift to Th2 response. Blocking of Ox40L leads to the suppression of Th2 response and, as a result, to the healing of disease. Mice with deletion of the Ox40 system may be more susceptible to Th2-inducing types of infectious agents such as worms and protozoa. Owing to lack of costimulation, Ox40 knockout mice are resistant to experimental autoimmune encephalomyelitis *(141a)*.

4.1.6. CD40/CD40L

CD40L and its receptor CD40 define an important costimulatory pathway for interacting T- and B-cells, as well as for interaction of lymphocytes with DCs. Accordingly, formation of protective immunity against *Leishmania amazonensis* is dependent on CD40/CD40L interaction. The features of the CD40L-CD40 knockout phenotype are higher bacterial burden, prolonged time of clearance, lack of IFN-γ, and diminished nitric oxide production *(110)*. Another infectious model in which CD40-deficient mice have a phenotype is malaria *(113)*. After challenge with *P. berghei*, which induces the brain stage of murine malaria in wild-type mice, CD40-deficient mice are resistant to infection, apparently because of decreased lymphocyte activation and recruitment. CD40L/CD40 interactions are also implicated in resistance against various viruses *(114–116)*. The recent finding that BAFF and APRIL can partially compensate for the absence of CD40 costimulation by DCs *(142)* suggests that the susceptibility of double knockout mice (CD40/BAFF, CD40/APRIL) may be more pronounced than that of mice with inactivation of CD40 alone.

4.2. Contrasting Roles of TNF and TNFR Family Members in Cancer

Because of their multiple effects on cell differentiation, proliferation, activation, migration, costimulation, and cell death, TNF and TNFR family members affect many physiologic processes, including reversible tissue remodeling, homeostasis, and certain aspects of host defense. It is not inconceivable that these gene products may affect carcinogenesis, tumor progression, and metastasis, while, on the other hand, they may also play a limited role in natural resistance to tumors.

4.2.1. Tumor Necrosis Factor

TNF was discovered because of its association with spectacular effects of experimental tumor therapy in an animal model *(1)*. Nevertheless, TNF-null mice and do not show an enhanced growth of spontaneous tumors. It should be noted that pro- or antitumorigenic potential of TNF ablation on the cancer-prone background, such as $p53^{-/-}$ or $p53^{+/-}$ mice, has not yet been reported.

TNF and LT (*see* below), through effects on chemokines and lymphoid tissue organization, have a profound effect on natural killer (NK) cell recruitment. As a result, TNF-null mice have a significantly decreased ability to reject transplantable tumors in the peritoneal cavity through an NK-dependent mechanism *(143)*.

On the negative side of the equation are the effects of TNF on tumor initiation and promotion in the skin carcinogenesis model. TNF-null mice are significantly more resistant to several experimental protocols of carcinogenesis *(37,38)*. The underlying mechanism is associated with the autocrine effects of TNF on keratinocyte proliferation and on inflammation. The tumor-promoting effects of TNF in vivo are proposed to result from chronic inflammation and are mediated by AP-1 and protein kinase C-α (PKC-α) *(144)*. No direct effects of TNF ablation on malignant progression have been observed *(37)*. Similarly, both TNFRI- and TNFRII-null mice were reported to show significant reduction of skin tumorigenesis induced by ultraviolet radiation, as revealed in the hairless SKH-1 model *(145)*. Additionally, TNFRI-null mice, but not TNFRII-null mice, are relatively resistant to liver carcinogenesis, implying a role for TNF in proliferation of hepatic stem cells at an early pre-neoplastic stage *(146)*. Overall, in spite of its name, TNF appears to contribute to carcinogenesis.

4.2.2. FAS (Apo-1)

lpr and *gld* mice develop splenomegaly and lymphadenopathy and die prematurely *(147)*. *lpr* is actually a leaky mutation, and therefore the engineered Fas knockout mouse has a more severe phenotype *(55)*. Old *gld* mice on several genetic backgrounds develop B-cell malignancies, suggesting the role of a Fas-FasL interaction in control of the B-cell population *(58)*. Intact Fas signaling is required for successful cancer treatment both in humans and in mice, including experimental therapy by IL-12/pulse IL-2, in which case Fas promotes destruction of both tumor and neovascular endothelial cells *(148)*.

Studies with melanoma cell lines transplanted to *lpr* or *gld* mice provide considerable evidence for the role of Fas-mediated killing of immune effector cells in tumor-bearing mice *(149)*. As a result, tumors grew faster in wild-type and *gld* mice than in *lpr* mice. This and other findings have been generalized to a concept of *tumor counterattack*, suggesting that tumor cells can kill the effector immune cells (see ref. *150* for review), although the relevance of these findings for human cancer has been questioned *(151)*. On the other hand, recent data indicate that FasL expression on tumor cells promotes tumor rejection and provides protection from subsequent tumor challenge. DCs expressing Fas play a critical role in this phenomenon, and they are resistant to Fas-mediated cytotoxicity *(152)*.

4.2.3. LT-LT-βR System

In an experimental metastasis model, LT-α contributes to protection from tumor growth through an NK cell-dependent mechanism resulting in control of leukocyte trafficking and recruitment *(153,154)*. These effects may be secondary to LT-α's influence on the microenvironment of lymphoid tissues discussed earlier, although LT-α also contributes to production of NK cells from bone marrow *(153,155)*.

Triggering of LT-βR results in activation of NF-κB and apoptosis of several tumor cell lines, in spite of the fact that LT-βR lacks the death domain. Several groups considered recombinant ligands and reagents that could trigger this receptor as a potential anticancer treatment *(156–159)*. However, in the experiments utilizing LT-βR and LT-α/LT-β double knockout mice, it was shown recently that solid tumors expressing LT-βR may receive stimulating signals from not-yet-identified host cells expressing surface LT to produce proangiogenic factors enhancing tumor growth *(160)*. These data may indicate that blocking, rather than triggering, the LT-βR signaling pathway may be beneficial for treatment of some types of tumors. In this regard it is interesting that combined TNF/LT-deficient mice when bred on a cancer-prone background show delalyed tumorigenesis (our unpublished observation).

4.2.4. TRAIL (Apo-2L)-DR System

TNF-related apoptosis-inducing ligand (TRAIL; Apo-2L) is a nonsecreted homolog of TNF that acts through death receptors, such as DR4 and DR5. Like TNF, TRAIL can transmit both activating/proliferating and apoptotic signal *(83)*. In humans, engineered soluble TRAIL showed significantly lower systemic toxicity, compared with TNF, and is considered to be a "better TNF"; it is currently undergoing clinical trials. This lower toxicity is presumably owing to the pattern of expression of the receptor molecules DR4 and DR5, but also probably to the presence of decoy receptors DcR1 and DcR2, which bind TRAIL but do not provide a cytotoxic signal. In the murine system, ortholog was firmly identified as a signaling receptor. Although TRAIL-null mice are grossly normal and were not reported to develop spontaneous tumors, the contributions of TRAIL dysfunction on a genetically cancer-prone background as well as the role of TRAIL-mediated cytotoxicity in vivo have yet to be assessed.

Most interestingly, TRAIL was implicated recently in immune surveillance against tumors in experiments using both blocking reagents *(161)* and TRAIL knockout mice *(82)*. Specifically, TRAIL (Apo-2L) is expressed on the cell membrane of NK cells, and its expression is enhanced by IL-2, IL-15 *(162)*, and type I interferons *(163)*. TRAIL knockout mice showed enhanced growth of NK-sensitive transplantable tumors, enhanced metastasis, and poor response to experimental therapy. Additionally, these mice showed a higher frequency of spontaneous fibrosarcomas in response to the chemical carcinogen methylcholanthrene *(82)*. T cells also require TRAIL for graft-vs-tumor activity *(163a)*. Overall, experiments with mouse models indicate that TRAIL may play an important protective role against cancer.

4.2.5. APRIL, BAFF/BAFF-R, BCMA, and TACI

APRIL was the first cytokine from the TNF family to be described as a tumor-promoting agent *(164)*. APRIL was shown to interact with two receptors, BCMA and TACI, but not with BAFF-R. "Biochemical knockout" produced by injection of soluble BCMA reagent inhibits experimental tumor growth in nude mice *(165)*. APRIL knockout mice are grossly normal (Varfolomeev, Kischkel, and Ashkenazi, personal communication). The relevance of these pathways for cancer awaits further studies on APRIL, BCMA, and TACI null mice *(70,75)*.

4.2.6. Other Pathways

Since several knockout mice with dysfunction of members of the TNF and TNFR families [LT-α, LT-β, LT-βR, receptor activator of NF-κB (RANKL), RANK ligand (RANKL)] show defects in the development of peripheral lymphoid tissues, such as lymph nodes, it is conceivable that the spread of tumor cells may be significantly altered in these mice, although this issue has not yet been systematically addressed. Recent reports on RANKL expression by myeloma cells suggested an important role of RANKL-mediated bone destruction in myeloma progression *(166)*.

5. Conclusions

Members of the TNF and TNFR families play diverse roles in homeostasis of the immune system and in host defense, as well as in morphogenesis. A remarkable expansion and diversification of these families in evolution argues for their important role in mammalian organism. We believe that many additional functions that remain masked in currently available mutant mice owing to the redundancy of signaling pathways will be discovered in mice engineered to be multiply deficient for these cytokines or receptors.

Acknowledgments

We are very grateful to Drs. J.J. Oppenheim and N. Rice for critically reading and improving the manuscript. This work has been funded in part with U.S. Federal funds from the National Cancer Institute, National Institutes of Health, under contract no. NO1-CO-12400. The contents of this publication do not necessarily reflect the view or policies of the Department of Health and Human Services, nor does mention of trade names, commercial products, or organizations imply endorsement by the U.S. Government. S. A. N. is an International Research Scholar of the Howard Hughes Medical Institute. S. I. G. is a recipient of INTAS fellowship YSF 2002-0235. D. V. K. acknowledges support from the Russian Foundation for Basic Research (grant 02-04-49105a).

References

1. Carswell, E. A., Old, L. J., Kassel, R. L., Green, S., Fiore, N., and Williamson, B. (1975) An endotoxin-induced serum factor that causes necrosis of tumors. *Proc. Natl. Acad. Sci. USA* **72,** 3666–3670.
2. Lejeune, F. J., Ruegg, C., and Lienard, D. (1998) Clinical applications of TNF-alpha in cancer. *Curr. Opin. Immunol.* **10,** 573–580.
3. Gray, P. W., Aggarwal, B. B., Benton, C. V., et al. (1984) Cloning and expression of cDNA for human lymphotoxin, a lymphokine with tumour necrosis activity. *Nature* **312,** 721–724.
4. Granger, G. A. and Kolb, W. P. (1968) Lymphocyte in vitro cytotoxicity: mechanisms of immune and non-immune small lymphocyte mediated target L cell destruction. *J. Immunol.* **101,** 111–120.
5. Ruddle, N. H. and Waksman, B. H. (1968) Cytotoxicity mediated by soluble antigen and lymphocytes in delayed hypersensitivity. I. Characterization of the phenomenon. *J. Exp. Med.* **128,** 1237–1254.
6. Fu, Y. X. and Chaplin, D. D. (1999) Development and maturation of secondary lymphoid tissues. *Annu. Rev. Immunol.* **17,** 399–433.
7. Locksley, R. M., Killeen, N., and Lenardo, M. J. (2001) The TNF and TNF receptor superfamilies: integrating mammalian biology. *Cell* **104,** 487–501.
8. Pfeffer, K., Matsuyama, T., Kundig, T. M., et al. (1993) Mice deficient for the 55 kd tumor necrosis factor receptor are resistant to endotoxic shock, yet succumb to *L. monocytogenes* infection. *Cell* **73,** 457–467.
9. Rothe, J., Lesslauer, W., Lotscher, H., et al. (1993) Mice lacking the tumour necrosis factor receptor 1 are resistant to TNF-mediated toxicity but highly susceptible to infection by *Listeria monocytogenes. Nature* **364,** 798–802.
10. De Togni, P., Goellner, J., Ruddle, N. H., et al. (1994) Abnormal development of peripheral lymphoid organs in mice deficient in lymphotoxin. *Science* **264,** 703–707.

11. Banks, T. A., Rouse, B. T., Kerley, M. K., et al. (1995) Lymphotoxin-alpha-deficient mice. Effects on secondary lymphoid organ development and humoral immune responsiveness. *J. Immunol.* **155,** 1685–1693.
12. Pasparakis, M., Alexopoulou, L., Episkopou, V., and Kollias, G. (1996) Immune and inflammatory responses in TNF alpha-deficient mice: a critical requirement for TNF alpha in the formation of primary B cell follicles, follicular dendritic cell networks and germinal centers, and in the maturation of the humoral immune response. *J. Exp. Med.* **184,** 1397–1411.
13. Marino, M. W., Dunn, A., Grail, D., et al. (1997) Characterization of tumor necrosis factor-deficient mice. *Proc. Natl. Acad. Sci. USA* **94,** 8093–8098.
14. Korner, H., Cook, M., Riminton, D. S., et al. (1997) Distinct roles for lymphotoxin-alpha and tumor necrosis factor in organogenesis and spatial organization of lymphoid tissue. *Eur. J. Immunol.* **27,** 2600–2609.
15. Chen, G. and Goeddel, D. V. (2002) TNF-R1 signaling: a beautiful pathway. *Science* **296,** 1634–1635.
16. Wajant, H. (2002) The Fas signaling pathway: more than a paradigm. *Science* **296,** 1635–1636.
17. Roschke, V., Sosnovtseva, S., Ward, C. D., et al. (2002) BLyS and APRIL form biologically active heterotrimers that are expressed in patients with systemic immune-based rheumatic diseases. *J. Immunol.* **169,** 4314–4321.
18. Yin, L., Wu, L., Wesche, H., et al. (2001) Defective lymphotoxin-beta receptor-induced NF-kappaB transcriptional activity in NIK-deficient mice. *Science* **291,** 2162–2165.
19. Shinkura, R., Kitada, K., Matsuda, F., et al. (1999) Alymphoplasia is caused by a point mutation in the mouse gene encoding NF-kappa B-inducing kinase. *Nat. Genet.* **22,** 74–77.
20. Karin, M. and Lin, A. (2002) NF-kappaB at the crossroads of life and death. *Nat. Immunol.* **3,** 221–227.
21. Senftleben, U., Cao, Y., Xiao, G., et al. (2001) Activation by IKKalpha of a second, evolutionary conserved, NF-kappa B signaling pathway. *Science* **293,** 1495–1499.
22. Dejardin, E., Droin, N. M., Delhase, M., et al. (2002) The Lymphotoxin-beta receptor induces different patterns of gene expression via two NF-kappaB pathways. *Immunity* **17,** 525–535.
23. Coope, H. J., Atkinson, P. G., Huhse, B., et al. (2002) CD40 regulates the processing of NF-kappaB2 p100 to p52. *EMBO J.* **21,** 5375–5385.
24. Kayagaki, N., Yan, M., Seshasayee, D., et al. (2002) BAFF/BLyS Receptor 3 binds the B cell survival factor BAFF ligand through a discrete surface loop and promotes processing of NF-kappaB2. *Immunity* **17,** 515–524.
25. Janeway, C. A. Jr. and Medzhitov, R. (2002) Innate immune recognition. *Annu. Rev. Immunol.* **20,** 197–216.
26. Moreno, E., Yan, M., and Basler, K. (2002) Evolution of TNF signaling mechanisms. JNK-dependent apoptosis triggered by Eiger, the *Drosophila* homolog of the TNF superfamily. *Curr. Biol.* **12,** 1263–1268.
27. Koni, P. A. and Flavell, R. A. (1998) A role for tumor necrosis factor receptor type 1 in gut-associated lymphoid tissue development: genetic evidence of synergism with lymphotoxin beta. *J. Exp. Med.* **187,** 1977–1983.
28. Kuprash, D. V., Alimzhanov, M. B., Tumanov, A., Anderson, A. O., Pfeffer, K., and Nedospasov, S. A. (1999) TNF and lymphotoxin beta cooperate in the maintenance of secondary lymphoid tissue microarchitecture but not in the development of lymph nodes. *J. Immunol.* **163,** 6575–6580.
29. Scheu, S., Alferink, J., Potzel, T., Barchet, W., Kalinke, U., and Pfeffer, K. (2002) Targeted disruption of LIGHT causes defects in costimulatory T cell activation and reveals cooperation with lymphotoxin beta in mesenteric lymph node genesis. *J. Exp. Med.* **195,** 1613–1624.
30. Kuprash, D. V., Alimzhanov, M. B., Tumanov, A. V., et al. (2002) Redundancy in TNF and LT signaling in vivo: mice with inactivation of the entire TNF/LT locus versus single knockout mice. *Mol. Cell. Biol.* **22,** 8626–8634.
31. Korner, H., Cretney, E., Wilhelm, P., et al. (2000) Tumor necrosis factor sustains the generalized lymphoproliferative disorder (gld) phenotype. *J. Exp. Med.* **191,** 89–96.
32. Yan, M., Wang, L. C., Hymowitz, S. G., et al. (2000) Two-amino acid molecular switch in an epithelial morphogen that regulates binding to two distinct receptors. *Science* **290,** 523–527.

33. Sean Riminton, D., Korner, H., Strickland, D. H., Lemckert, F. A., Pollard, J. D., and Sedgwick, J. D. (1998) Challenging cytokine redundancy: inflammatory cell movement and clinical course of experimental autoimmune encephalomyelitis are normal in lymphotoxin-deficient, but not tumor necrosis factor-deficient, mice. *J. Exp. Med.* **187,** 1517–1528.
34. Neumann, B., Luz, A., Pfeffer, K., and Holzmann, B. (1996) Defective Peyer's patch organogenesis in mice lacking the 55-kD receptor for tumor necrosis factor. *J. Exp. Med.* **184,** 259–264.
35. Le Hir, M., Bluethmann, H., Kosco-Vilbois, M. H., et al. (1996) Differentiation of follicular dendritic cells and full antibody responses require tumor necrosis factor receptor-1 signaling. *J. Exp. Med.* **183,** 2367–2372.
36. Kontoyiannis, D., Pasparakis, M., Pizarro, T. T., Cominelli, F., and Kollias, G. (1999) Impaired on/off regulation of TNF biosynthesis in mice lacking TNF AU- rich elements: implications for joint and gut-associated immunopathologies. *Immunity* **10,** 387–398.
37. Moore, R. J., Owens, D. M., Stamp, G., et al. (1999) Mice deficient in tumor necrosis factor-alpha are resistant to skin carcinogenesis. *Nat. Med.* **5,** 828–831.
38. Suganuma, M., Okabe, S., Marino, M. W., Sakai, A., Sueoka, E., and Fujiki, H. (1999) Essential role of tumor necrosis factor alpha (TNF-alpha) in tumor promotion as revealed by TNF-alpha-deficient mice. *Cancer Res.* **59,** 4516–4518.
39. Erickson, S. L., de Sauvage, F. J., Kikly, K., et al. (1994) Decreased sensitivity to tumour-necrosis factor but normal T- cell development in TNF receptor-2-deficient mice. *Nature* **372,** 560–563.
40. Wang, B., Fujisawa, H., Zhuang, L., et al. (1997) Depressed Langerhans cell migration and reduced contact hypersensitivity response in mice lacking TNF receptor p75. *J. Immunol.* **159,** 6148–6155.
41. Lucas, R., Juillard, P., Decoster, E., et al. (1997) Crucial role of tumor necrosis factor (TNF) receptor 2 and membrane-bound TNF in experimental cerebral malaria. *Eur. J. Immunol.* **27,** 1719–1725.
42. Sam, H., Su, Z., and Stevenson, M. M. (1999) Deficiency in tumor necrosis factor alpha activity does not impair early protective Th1 responses against blood-stage malaria. *Infect. Immun.* **67,** 2660–2664.
43. Ruuls, S. R., Hoek, R. M., Ngo, V. N., et al. (2001) Membrane-bound TNF supports secondary lymphoid organ structure but is subservient to secreted TNF in driving autoimmune inflammation. *Immunity* **15,** 533–543.
44. Koni, P. A., Sacca, R., Lawton, P., Browning, J. L., Ruddle, N. H., and Flavell, R. A. (1997) Distinct roles in lymphoid organogenesis for lymphotoxins alpha and beta revealed in lymphotoxin beta-deficient mice. *Immunity* **6,** 491–500.
45. Alimzhanov, M. B., Kuprash, D. V., Kosco-Vilbois, M. H., et al. (1997) Abnormal development of secondary lymphoid tissues in lymphotoxin beta-deficient mice. *Proc. Natl. Acad. Sci. USA* **94,** 9302–9307.
46. Futterer, A., Mink, K., Luz, A., Kosco-Vilbois, M. H., and Pfeffer, K. (1998) The lymphotoxin beta receptor controls organogenesis and affinity maturation in peripheral lymphoid tissues. *Immunity* **9,** 59–70.
47. Tumanov, A. V., Kuprash, D. V., Lagarkova, M. A., et al. (2002) Distinct role of surface lymphotoxin expressed by B cells in the organization of secondary lymphoid tissues. *Immunity* **17,** 239–250.
48. Wu, Q., Wang, Y., Wang, J., Hedgeman, E. O., Browning, J. L., and Fu, Y. X. (1999) The requirement of membrane lymphotoxin for the presence of dendritic cells in lymphoid tissues. *J. Exp. Med.* **190,** 629–638.
49. Kawabe, T., Naka, T., Yoshida, K., et al. (1994) The immune responses in CD40-deficient mice: impaired immunoglobulin class switching and germinal center formation. *Immunity* **1,** 167–178.
50. Xu, J., Foy, T. M., Laman, J. D., et al. (1994) Mice deficient for the CD40 ligand. *Immunity* **1,** 423–431.
51. Renshaw, B. R., Fanslow, W. C. 3rd., Armitage, R. J., et al. (1994) Humoral immune responses in CD40 ligand-deficient mice. *J. Exp. Med.* **180,** 1889–1900.
52. Grewal, I. S. and Flavell, R. A. (1998) CD40 and CD154 in cell-mediated immunity. *Annu. Rev. Immunol.* **16,** 111–135.
53. Watanabe-Fukunaga, R., Brannan, C. I., Copeland, N. G., Jenkins, N. A., and Nagata, S. (1992) Lymphoproliferation disorder in mice explained by defects in Fas antigen that mediates apoptosis. *Nature* **356,** 314–317.

54. Takahashi, T., Tanaka, M., Brannan, C. I., et al. (1994) Generalized lymphoproliferative disease in mice, caused by a point mutation in the Fas ligand. *Cell* **76,** 969–976.
55. Adachi, M., Suematsu, S., Kondo, T., et al. (1995) Targeted mutation in the Fas gene causes hyperplasia in peripheral lymphoid organs and liver. *Nat. Genet.* **11,** 294–300.
56. Adachi, M., Suematsu, S., Suda, T., et al. (1996) Enhanced and accelerated lymphoproliferation in Fas-null mice. *Proc. Natl. Acad. Sci. USA* **93,** 2131–2136.
57. Chervonsky, A. V., Wang, Y., Wong, F. S., et al. (1997) The role of Fas in autoimmune diabetes. *Cell* **89,** 17–24.
58. Davidson, W. F., Giese, T., and Fredrickson, T. N. (1998) Spontaneous development of plasmacytoid tumors in mice with defective Fas-Fas ligand interactions. *J. Exp. Med.* **187,** 1825–1838.
59. Chen, A. I., McAdam, A. J., Buhlmann, J. E., et al. (1999) Ox40-ligand has a critical costimulatory role in dendritic cell: T cell interactions. *Immunity* **11,** 689–698.
60. Akiba, H., Miyahira, Y., Atsuta, M., et al. (2000) Critical contribution of OX40 ligand to T helper cell type 2 differentiation in experimental leishmaniasis. *J. Exp. Med.* **191,** 375–380.
61. Jember, A. G., Zuberi, R., Liu, F. T., and Croft, M. (2001) Development of allergic inflammation in a murine model of asthma is dependent on the costimulatory receptor OX40. *J. Exp. Med.* **193,** 387–392.
62. Kopf, M., Ruedl, C., Schmitz, N., et al. (1999) OX40-deficient mice are defective in Th cell proliferation but are competent in generating B cell and CTL responses after virus infection. *Immunity* **11,** 699–708.
63. Amakawa, R., Hakem, A., Kundig, T. M., et al. (1996) Impaired negative selection of T cells in Hodgkin's disease antigen CD30-deficient mice. *Cell* **84,** 551–562.
64. DeYoung, A. L., Duramad, O., and Winoto, A. (2000) The TNF receptor family member CD30 is not essential for negative selection. *J. Immunol.* **165,** 6170–6173.
65. Kurts, C., Carbone, F. R., Krummel, M. F., Koch, K. M., Miller, J. F., and Heath, W. R. (1999) Signalling through CD30 protects against autoimmune diabetes mediated by CD8 T cells. *Nature* **398,** 341–344.
66. Hendriks, J., Gravestein, L. A., Tesselaar, K., van Lier, R. A., Schumacher, T. N., and Borst, J. (2000) CD27 is required for generation and long-term maintenance of T cell immunity. *Nat. Immunol.* **1,** 433–440.
67. Thompson, J. S., Bixler, S. A., Qian, F., et al. (2001) BAFF-R, a newly identified TNF receptor that specifically interacts with BAFF. *Science* **293,** 2108–2111.
68. Schiemann, B., Gommerman, J. L., Vora, K., et al. (2001) An essential role for BAFF in the normal development of B cells through a BCMA-independent pathway. *Science* **293,** 2111–2114.
69. Yan, M., Brady, J. R., Chan, B., et al. (2001) Identification of a novel receptor for B lymphocyte stimulator that is mutated in a mouse strain with severe B cell deficiency. *Curr. Biol.* **11,** 1547–1552.
70. Xu, S. and Lam, K. P. (2001) B-cell maturation protein, which binds the tumor necrosis factor family members BAFF and APRIL, is dispensable for humoral immune responses. *Mol. Cell. Biol.* **21,** 4067–4074.
71. Mackay, F. and Browning, J. L. (2002) BAFF: a fundamental survival factor for B cells. *Nat. Rev. Immunol.* **2,** 465–475.
72. Yan, M., Marsters, S. A., Grewal, I. S., Wang, H., Ashkenazi, A., and Dixit, V. M. (2000) Identification of a receptor for BLyS demonstrates a crucial role in humoral immunity. *Nat. Immunol.* **1,** 37–41.
73. Yan, M., Wang, H., Chan, B., et al. (2001) Activation and accumulation of B cells in TACI-deficient mice. *Nat. Immunol.* **2,** 638–643.
74. Schneider, P., Takatsuka, H., Wilson, A., et al. (2001) Maturation of marginal zone and follicular B cells requires B cell activating factor of the tumor necrosis factor family and is independent of B cell maturation antigen. *J. Exp. Med.* **194,** 1691–1697.
75. von Bulow, G. U., van Deursen, J. M., and Bram, R. J. (2001) Regulation of the T-independent humoral response by TACI. *Immunity* **14,** 573–582.
76. DeBenedette, M. A., Wen, T., Bachmann, M. F., et al. (1999) Analysis of 4-1BB ligand (4-1BBL)-deficient mice and of mice lacking both 4-1BBL and CD28 reveals a role for 4-1BBL in skin allograft rejection and in the cytotoxic T cell response to influenza virus. *J. Immunol.* **163,** 4833–4841.

77. Kwon, B. S., Hurtado, J. C., Lee, Z. H., et al. (2002) Immune responses in 4-1BB (CD137)-deficient mice. *J. Immunol.* **168,** 5483–5490.
78. Tamada, K., Ni, J., Zhu, G., et al. (2002) Cutting edge: selective impairment of CD8+ T cell function in mice lacking the TNF superfamily member LIGHT. *J. Immunol.* **168,** 4832–4835.
79. Dougall, W. C., Glaccum, M., Charrier, K., et al. (1999) RANK is essential for osteoclast and lymph node development. *Genes Dev.* **13,** 2412–2424.
80. Kong, Y. Y., Yoshida, H., Sarosi, I., et al. (1999) OPGL is a key regulator of osteoclastogenesis, lymphocyte development and lymph-node organogenesis. *Nature* **397,** 315–323.
81. Fata, J. E., Kong, Y. Y., Li, J., et al. (2000) The osteoclast differentiation factor osteoprotegerin-ligand is essential for mammary gland development. *Cell* **103,** 41–50.
82. Cretney, E., Takeda, K., Yagita, H., Glaccum, M., Peschon, J. J., and Smyth, M. J. (2002) Increased susceptibility to tumor initiation and metastasis in TNF-related apoptosis-inducing ligand-deficient mice. *J. Immunol.* **168,** 1356–1361.
83. Ashkenazi, A. and Dixit, V. M. (1999) Apoptosis control by death and decoy receptors. *Curr. Opin. Cell Biol.* **11,** 255–260.
84. Sedger, L. M., Glaccum, M. B., Schuh, J. C., et al. (2002) Characterization of the in vivo function of TNF-alpha-related apoptosis-inducing ligand, TRAIL/Apo2L, using TRAIL/Apo2L gene-deficient mice. *Eur. J. Immunol.* **32,** 2246–2254.
84a. Lamhamedi-Cherradi, S. E., Zheng, S. J., Maguschak, K. A., Peschon, J., and Chen, Y. H. (2003) Defective thymocyte apoptosis and accelerated autoimmune diseases in TRAIL(–/–) mice. *Nat. Immunol.* **4,** 255–260.
85. Ronchetti, S., Nocentini, G., Riccardi, C., and Pandolfi, P. P. (2002) Role of GITR in activation response of T lymphocytes. *Blood* **100,** 350–352.
86. Srivastava, A. K., Pispa, J., Hartung, A. J., et al. (1997) The Tabby phenotype is caused by mutation in a mouse homologue of the EDA gene that reveals novel mouse and human exons and encodes a protein (ectodysplasin-A) with collagenous domains. *Proc. Natl. Acad. Sci. USA* **94,** 13069–13074.
87. Tucker, A. S., Headon, D. J., Schneider, P., et al. (2000) Edar/Eda interactions regulate enamel knot formation in tooth morphogenesis. *Development* **127,** 4691–4700.
88. Koppinen, P., Pispa, J., Laurikkala, J., Thesleff, I., and Mikkola, M. L. (2001) Signaling and subcellular localization of the TNF receptor Edar. *Exp. Cell. Res.* **269,** 180–192.
89. Yan, M., Zhang, Z., Brady, J. R., Schilbach, S., Fairbrother, W. J., and Dixit, V. M. (2002) Identification of a novel death domain-containing adaptor molecule for ectodysplasin-A receptor that is mutated in crinkled mice. *Curr. Biol.* **12,** 409–413.
90. Naumann, T., Casademunt, E., Hollerbach, E., et al. (2002) Complete deletion of the neurotrophin receptor p75NTR leads to long-lasting increases in the number of basal forebrain cholinergic neurons. *J. Neurosci.* **22,** 2409–2418.
91. Kindler, V., Sappino, A. P., Grau, G. E., Piguet, P. F., and Vassalli, P. (1989) The inducing role of tumor necrosis factor in the development of bactericidal granulomas during BCG infection. *Cell* **56,** 731–740.
92. Flynn, J. L. and Chan, J. (2001) Immunology of tuberculosis. *Annu. Rev. Immunol.* **19,** 93–129.
93. Flynn, J. L., Goldstein, M. M., Chan, J., et al. (1995) Tumor necrosis factor-alpha is required in the protective immune response against *Mycobacterium tuberculosis* in mice. *Immunity* **2,** 561–572.
94. Tsenova, L., Bergtold, A., Freedman, V. H., Young, R. A., and Kaplan, G. (1999) Tumor necrosis factor alpha is a determinant of pathogenesis and disease progression in mycobacterial infection in the central nervous system. *Proc. Natl. Acad. Sci. USA* **96,** 5657–5662.
95. Wilhelm, P., Ritter, U., Labbow, S., et al. (2001) Rapidly fatal leishmaniasis in resistant C57BL/6 mice lacking TNF. *J. Immunol.* **166,** 4012–4019.
96. Ehlers, S., Benini, J., Kutsch, S., Endres, R., Rietschel, E. T., and Pfeffer, K. (1999) Fatal granuloma necrosis without exacerbated mycobacterial growth in tumor necrosis factor receptor p55 gene-deficient mice intravenously infected with *Mycobacterium avium*. *Infect. Immun.* **67,** 3571–3579.
97. Hultgren, O., Eugster, H. P., Sedgwick, J. D., Korner, H., and Tarkowski, A. (1998) TNF/lymphotoxin-alpha double-mutant mice resist septic arthritis but display increased mortality in response to *Staphylococcus aureus*. *J. Immunol.* **161,** 5937–5942.

98. Grau, G. E., Fajardo, L. F., Piguet, P. F., Allet, B., Lambert, P. H., and Vassalli, P. (1987) Tumor necrosis factor (cachectin) as an essential mediator in murine cerebral malaria. *Science* **237,** 1210–1212.
99. Rudin, W., Eugster, H. P., Bordmann, G., et al. (1997) Resistance to cerebral malaria in tumor necrosis factor- alpha/beta-deficient mice is associated with a reduction of intercellular adhesion molecule-1 up-regulation and T helper type 1 response. *Am. J. Pathol.* **150,** 257–266.
100. Li, C. and Langhorne, J. (2000) Tumor necrosis factor alpha p55 receptor is important for development of memory responses to blood-stage malaria infection. *Infect. Immun.* **68,** 5724–5730.
101. Senaldi, G., Yin, S., Shaklee, C. L., Piguet, P. F., Mak, T. W., and Ulich, T. R. (1996) *Corynebacterium parvum-* and *Mycobacterium bovis* bacillus Calmette-Guérin-induced granuloma formation is inhibited in TNF receptor I (TNF-RI) knockout mice and by treatment with soluble TNF-RI. *J. Immunol.* **157,** 5022–5026.
102. Kusters, S., Tiegs, G., Alexopoulou, L., et al. (1997) In vivo evidence for a functional role of both tumor necrosis factor (TNF) receptors and transmembrane TNF in experimental hepatitis. *Eur. J. Immunol.* **27,** 2870–2875.
103. Olleros, M. L., Guler, R., Corazza, N., et al. (2002) Transmembrane TNF induces an efficient cell-mediated immunity and resistance to *Mycobacterium bovis* bacillus Calmette-Guérin infection in the absence of secreted TNF and lymphotoxin-alpha. *J. Immunol.* **168,** 3394–3401.
104. Roach, D. R., Briscoe, H., Saunders, B., France, M. P., Riminton, S., and Britton, W. J. (2001) Secreted lymphotoxin-alpha is essential for the control of an intracellular bacterial infection. *J. Exp. Med.* **193,** 239–246.
105. Engwerda, C. R., Mynott, T. L., Sawhney, S., de Souza, J. B., Bickle, Q. D., and Kaye, P. (2002) Locally up-regulated lymphotoxin-alpha, not systemic tumor necrosis factor-alpha, is the principle mediator of murine cerebral malaria. *J. Exp. Med.* **195,** 1371–1377.
106. Suresh, M., Lanier, G., Large, M. K., et al. (2002) Role of lymphotoxin alpha in T-cell responses during an acute viral infection. *J. Virol.* **76,** 3943–3951.
107. Benedict, C. A., Banks, T. A., Senderowicz, L., et al. (2001) Lymphotoxins and cytomegalovirus cooperatively induce interferon-beta, establishing host-virus detente. *Immunity* **15,** 617–626.
108. Trueb, R., Brown, G., van Huffel, C., Poltorak, A., Valdez-Silva, M., and Beutler, B. (1995) Expression of an adenovirally encoded lymphotoxin-beta inhibitor prevents clearance of *Listeria monocytogenes* in mice. *J. Inflamm.* **45,** 239–247.
109. Berger, D. P., Naniche, D., Crowley, M. T., Koni, P. A., Flavell, R. A., and Oldstone, M. B. (1999) Lymphotoxin-beta-deficient mice show defective antiviral immunity. *Virology* **260,** 136–147.
110. Soong, L., Xu, J. C., Grewal, I. S., et al. (1996) Disruption of CD40-CD40 ligand interactions results in an enhanced susceptibility to *Leishmania amazonensis* infection. *Immunity* **4,** 263–273.
111. Campbell, K. A., Ovendale, P. J., Kennedy, M. K., Fanslow, W. C., Reed, S. G., and Maliszewski, C. R. (1996) CD40 ligand is required for protective cell-mediated immunity to *Leishmania major.* *Immunity* **4,** 283–289.
112. Kamanaka, M., Yu, P., Yasui, T., et al. (1996) Protective role of CD40 in *Leishmania major* infection at two distinct phases of cell-mediated immunity. *Immunity* **4,** 275–281.
113. Piguet, P. F., Kan, C. D., Vesin, C., Rochat, A., Donati, Y., and Barazzone, C. (2001) Role of CD40-CVD40L in mouse severe malaria. *Am. J. Pathol.* **159,** 733–742.
114. Andreasen, S. O., Christensen, J. E., Marker, O., and Thomsen, A. R. (2000) Role of CD40 ligand and CD28 in induction and maintenance of antiviral CD8+ effector T cell responses. *J. Immunol.* **164,** 3689–3697.
115. Whitmire, J. K., Flavell, R. A., Grewal, I. S., Larsen, C. P., Pearson, T. C., and Ahmed, R. (1999) CD40-CD40 ligand costimulation is required for generating antiviral CD4 T cell responses but is dispensable for CD8 T cell responses. *J. Immunol.* **163,** 3194–3201.
116. Thomsen, A. R., Nansen, A., Christensen, J. P., Andreasen, S. O., and Marker, O. (1998) CD40 ligand is pivotal to efficient control of virus replication in mice infected with lymphocytic choriomeningitis virus. *J. Immunol.* **161,** 4583–4590.
117. Hotchkiss, R. S., Dunne, W. M., Swanson, P. E., et al. (2001) Role of apoptosis in *Pseudomonas aeruginosa* pneumonia. *Science* **294,** 1783–1783a.
118. Grassme, H., Kirschnek, S., Riethmueller, J., et al. (2000) CD95/CD95 ligand interactions on epithelial cells in host defense to *Pseudomonas aeruginosa*. *Science* **290,** 527–530.

119. Jones, N. L., Day, A. S., Jennings, H., Shannon, P. T., Galindo-Mata, E., and Sherman, P. M. (2002) Enhanced disease severity in *Helicobacter pylori*-infected mice deficient in Fas signaling. *Infect. Immun.* **70,** 2591–2597.
120. Jensen, E. R., Glass, A. A., Clark, W. R., Wing, E. J., Miller, J. F., and Gregory, S. H. (1998) Fas (CD95)-dependent cell-mediated immunity to *Listeria monocytogenes. Infect. Immun.* **66,** 4143–4150.
121. Baran, J., Weglarczyk, K., Mysiak, M., et al. (2001) Fas (CD95)-Fas ligand interactions are responsible for monocyte apoptosis occurring as a result of phagocytosis and killing of *Staphylococcus aureus. Infect. Immun.* **69,** 1287–1297.
122. Garcia, I., Miyazaki, Y., Araki, K., et al. (1995) Transgenic mice expressing high levels of soluble TNF-R1 fusion protein are protected from lethal septic shock and cerebral malaria, and are highly sensitive to *Listeria monocytogenes* and *Leishmania major* infections. *Eur. J. Immunol.* **25,** 2401–2407.
123. Garcia, I., Miyazaki, Y., Marchal, G., Lesslauer, W., and Vassalli, P. (1997) High sensitivity of transgenic mice expressing soluble TNFR1 fusion protein to mycobacterial infections: synergistic action of TNF and IFN-gamma in the differentiation of protective granulomas. *Eur. J. Immunol.* **27,** 3182–3190.
124. Adams, L. B., Mason, C. M., Kolls, J. K., Scollard, D., Krahenbuhl, J. L., and Nelson, S. (1995) Exacerbation of acute and chronic murine tuberculosis by administration of a tumor necrosis factor receptor-expressing adenovirus. *J. Infect. Dis.* **171,** 400–405.
125. Jacobs, M., Brown, N., Allie, N., and Ryffel, B. (2000) Fatal *Mycobacterium bovis* BCG infection in TNF-LT-alpha-deficient mice. *Clin. Immunol.* **94,** 192–199.
126. Bean, A. G., Roach, D. R., Briscoe, H., et al. (1999) Structural deficiencies in granuloma formation in TNF gene-targeted mice underlie the heightened susceptibility to aerosol *Mycobacterium tuberculosis* infection, which is not compensated for by lymphotoxin. *J. Immunol.* **162,** 3504–3511.
127. Bopst, M., Garcia, I., Guler, R., et al. (2001) Differential effects of TNF and LTalpha in the host defense against M. bovis BCG. *Eur. J. Immunol.* **31,** 1935–1943.
128. Neumann, B., Machleidt, T., Lifka, A., et al. (1996) Crucial role of 55-kilodalton TNF receptor in TNF-induced adhesion molecule expression and leukocyte organ infiltration. *J. Immunol.* **156,** 1587–1593.
129. Murray, H. W., Jungbluth, A., Ritter, E., Montelibano, C., and Marino, M. W. (2000) Visceral leishmaniasis in mice devoid of tumor necrosis factor and response to treatment. *Infect. Immun.* **68,** 6289–6293.
130. Nashleanas, M., Kanaly, S., and Scott, P. (1998) Control of *Leishmania major* infection in mice lacking TNF receptors. *J. Immunol.* **160,** 5506–5513.
131. You, L. R., Chen, C. M., and Lee, Y. H. W. (1999) Hepatitis C virus core protein enhances NF-kappaB signal pathway triggering by lymphotoxin-beta receptor ligand and tumor necrosis factor alpha. *J. Virol.* **73,** 1672–1681.
132. Magez, S., Radwanska, M., Beschin, A., Sekikawa, K., and de Baetselier, P. (1999) Tumor necrosis factor alpha is a key mediator in the regulation of experimental *Trypanosoma brucei* infections. *Infect. Immun.* **67,** 3128–3132.
133. Hodge-Dufour, J., Marino, M. W., Horton, M. R., et al. (1998) Inhibition of interferon gamma induced interleukin 12 production: a potential mechanism for the anti-inflammatory activities of tumor necrosis factor. *Proc. Natl. Acad. Sci. USA* **95,** 13806–13811.
134. Haas, E., Grell, M., Wajant, H., and Scheurich, P. (1999) Continuous autotropic signaling by membrane-expressed tumor necrosis factor. *J. Biol. Chem.* **274,** 18107–18112.
135. Kratz, A., Campos-Neto, A., Hanson, M. S., and Ruddle, N. H. (1996) Chronic inflammation caused by lymphotoxin is lymphoid neogenesis. *J. Exp. Med.* **183,** 1461–1472.
136. Sacca, R., Cuff, C. A., Lesslauer, W., and Ruddle, N. H. (1998) Differential activities of secreted lymphotoxin-alpha3 and membrane lymphotoxin-alpha1beta2 in lymphotoxin-induced inflammation: critical role of TNF receptor 1 signaling. *J. Immunol.* **160,** 485–491.
137. Cuff, C. A., Schwartz, J., Bergman, C. M., Russell, K. S., Bender, J. R., and Ruddle, N. H. (1998) Lymphotoxin alpha3 induces chemokines and adhesion molecules: insight into the role of LT alpha in inflammation and lymphoid organ development. *J. Immunol.* **161,** 6853–6860.

138. Netea, M. G., van Tits, L. J., Curfs, J. H., et al. (1999) Increased susceptibility of TNF-alpha lymphotoxin-alpha double knockout mice to systemic candidiasis through impaired recruitment of neutrophils and phagocytosis of *Candida albicans*. *J. Immunol.* **163,** 1498–1505.
139. Lucas, R., Tacchini-Cottier, F., Guler, R., et al. (1999) A role for lymphotoxin beta receptor in host defense against *Mycobacterium bovis* BCG infection. *Eur. J. Immunol.* **29,** 4002–4010.
140. Montrasio, F., Frigg, R., Glatzel, M., et al. (2000) Impaired prion replication in spleens of mice lacking functional follicular dendritic cells. *Science* **288,** 1257–1259.
141. Prinz, M., Montrasio, F., Klein, M. A., et al. (2002) Lymph nodal prion replication and neuroinvasion in mice devoid of follicular dendritic cells. *Proc. Natl. Acad. Sci. USA* **99,** 919–924.
141a. Ndhlovu, L. C., Ishii, N., Murata, K., Sato, T., and Sugamura, K. (2001) Critical involvement of OX40 ligand signals in the T cell priming events during experimental autoimmune encephalomyelitis. *J. Immunol.* **167,** 2991–2999.
142. Litinskiy, M. B., Nardelli, B., Hilbert, D. M., et al. (2002) DCs induce CD40-independent immunoglobulin class switching through BLyS and APRIL. *Nat. Immunol.* **3,** 822–829.
143. Smyth, M. J., Kelly, J. M., Baxter, A. G., Korner, H., and Sedgwick, J. D. (1998) An essential role for tumor necrosis factor in natural killer cell-mediated tumor rejection in the peritoneum. *J. Exp. Med.* **188,** 1611–1619.
144. Arnott, C. H., Scott, K. A., Moore, R. J., et al. (2002) Tumour necrosis factor-alpha mediates tumour promotion via a PKC alpha- and AP-1-dependent pathway. *Oncogene* **21,** 4728–4738.
145. Starcher, B. (2000) Role for tumour necrosis factor-alpha receptors in ultraviolet-induced skin tumours. *Br. J. Dermatol.* **142,** 1140–1147.
146. Knight, B., Yeoh, G. C., Husk, K. L., et al. (2000) Impaired preneoplastic changes and liver tumor formation in tumor necrosis factor receptor type 1 knockout mice. *J. Exp. Med.* **192,** 1809–1818.
147. Cohen, P. L. and Eisenberg, R. A. (1991) Lpr and gld: single gene models of systemic autoimmunity and lymphoproliferative disease. *Annu. Rev. Immunol.* **9,** 243–269.
148. Wigginton, J. M., Gruys, E., Geiselhart, L., et al. (2001) IFN-gamma and Fas/FasL are required for the antitumor and antiangiogenic effects of IL-12/pulse IL-2 therapy. *J. Clin. Invest.* **108,** 51–62.
149. Hahne, M., Rimoldi, D., Schroter, M., et al. (1996) Melanoma cell expression of Fas(Apo-1/CD95) ligand: implications for tumor immune escape. *Science* **274,** 1363–1366.
150. Igney, F. H. and Krammer, P. H. (2002) Immune escape of tumors: apoptosis resistance and tumor counterattack. *J. Leukoc. Biol.* **71,** 907–920.
151. Chappell, D. B., Zaks, T. Z., Rosenberg, S. A., and Restifo, N. P. (1999) Human melanoma cells do not express Fas (Apo-1/CD95) ligand. *Cancer Res.* **59,** 59–62.
152. Tada, Y., Wang, J., Takiguchi, Y., et al. (2002) Cutting edge: a novel role for Fas ligand in facilitating antigen acquisition by dendritic cells. *J. Immunol.* **169,** 2241–2245.
153. Ito, D., Back, T. C., Shakhov, A. N., Wiltrout, R. H., and Nedospasov, S. A. (1999) Mice with a targeted mutation in lymphotoxin-alpha exhibit enhanced tumor growth and metastasis: impaired NK cell development and recruitment. *J. Immunol.* **163,** 2809–2815.
154. Smyth, M. J., Johnstone, R. W., Cretney, E., et al. (1999) Multiple deficiencies underlie NK cell inactivity in lymphotoxin-alpha gene-targeted mice. *J. Immunol.* **163,** 1350–1353.
155. Iizuka, K., Chaplin, D. D., Wang, Y., et al. (1999) Requirement for membrane lymphotoxin in natural killer cell development. *Proc. Natl. Acad. Sci. USA* **96,** 6336–6340.
156. Browning, J. L., Miatkowski, K., Sizing, I., et al. (1996) Signaling through the lymphotoxin beta receptor induces the death of some adenocarcinoma tumor lines. *J. Exp. Med.* **183,** 867–878.
157. Degli-Esposti, M. A., Davis-Smith, T., Din, W. S., Smolak, P. J., Goodwin, R. G., and Smith, C. A. (1997) Activation of the lymphotoxin beta receptor by cross-linking induces chemokine production and growth arrest in A375 melanoma cells. *J. Immunol.* **158,** 1756–1762.
158. Wu, M. Y., Wang, P. Y., Han, S. H., and Hsieh, S. L. (1999) The cytoplasmic domain of the lymphotoxin-beta receptor mediates cell death in HeLa cells. *J. Biol. Chem.* **274,** 11868–11873.
159. Rooney, I. A., Butrovich, K. D., Glass, A. A., et al. (2000) The lymphotoxin-beta receptor is necessary and sufficient for LIGHT-mediated apoptosis of tumor cells. *J. Biol. Chem.* **275,** 14307–14315.
160. Hehlgans, T., Stoelcker, B., Stopfer, P., et al. (2002) Lymphotoxin-beta receptor immune interaction promotes tumor growth by inducing angiogenesis. *Cancer Res.* **62,** 4034–4040.

161. Takeda, K., Hayakawa, Y., Smyth, M. J., et al. (2001) Involvement of tumor necrosis factor-related apoptosis-inducing ligand in surveillance of tumor metastasis by liver natural killer cells. *Nat. Med.* **7,** 94–100.
162. Kayagaki, N., Yamaguchi, N., Nakayama, M., et al. (1999) Expression and function of TNF-related apoptosis-inducing ligand on murine activated NK cells. *J. Immunol.* **163,** 1906–1913.
163. Sato, K., Hida, S., Takayanagi, H., et al. (2001) Antiviral response by natural killer cells through TRAIL gene induction by IFN-alpha/beta. *Eur. J. Immunol.* **31,** 3138–3146.
163a. Schmaltz, C., Alpdogan, O., Kappel, B. J., et al. (2002) T cells require TRAIL for optimal graft-versus-tumor activity. *Nat. Med.* **8,** 1433–1437.
164. Hahne, M., Kataoka, T., Schroter, M., et al. (1998) APRIL, a new ligand of the tumor necrosis factor family, stimulates tumor cell growth. *J. Exp. Med.* **188,** 1185–1190.
165. Rennert, P., Schneider, P., Cachero, T. G., et al. (2000) A soluble form of B cell maturation antigen, a receptor for the tumor necrosis factor family member APRIL, inhibits tumor cell growth. *J. Exp. Med.* **192,** 1677–1684.
166. Pearse, R. N., Sordillo, E. M., Yaccoby, S., et al. (2001) Multiple myeloma disrupts the TRANCE/osteoprotegerin cytokine axis to trigger bone destruction and promote tumor progression. *Proc. Natl. Acad. Sci. USA* **98,** 11581–11586.

Index

H

I

N

O

GPSR Compliance
The European Union's (EU) General Product Safety Regulation (GPSR) is a set of rules that requires consumer products to be safe and our obligations to ensure this.

If you have any concerns about our products, you can contact us on

ProductSafety@springernature.com

In case Publisher is established outside the EU, the EU authorized representative is:

Springer Nature Customer Service Center GmbH
Europaplatz 3
69115 Heidelberg, Germany

www.ingramcontent.com/pod-product-compliance
Ingram Content Group UK Ltd.
Pitfield, Milton Keynes, MK11 3LW, UK
UKHW051131260726